Grappling With Death

The Union Second Corps Hospital at Gettysburg

Grappling With Death

The Union Second Corps Hospital at Gettysburg

Roland R. Maust

Morningside
2001

ISBN: 0-89029-337-6

Morningside House, Inc.
260 Oak Street
Dayton, Ohio 45410
(800) 648-9710
Fax: (937) 461-4260
http://www.morningsidebooks.com
E-mail: msbooks@erinet.com

To Karen
My Beloved and My Friend

Table of Contents

Maps

"If we die in this battle, we will have died for the right.
There's just one thing.
I hope I die quick. I hope I don't have to die
In the hospital.
There is one thought that to me is worse than death."
This, they say over and over.
"It is the thought of being buried as they bury us here
After a battle. Sometimes they barely cover us."

Stephen Vincent Benet
John Brown's Body

"I have often thought it would be profitable for some if a competent observer would recount the scenes at the rear of a fighting army removing from the field after a great battle."

Joshua Lawrence Chamberlain

The Passing of the Armies

FOREWORD

"I remember we went through a small piece of open timber, where our doctors were posted, and as we went by we shook hands with them, and exchanged little pleasantries," wrote Lt. Charles Fuller of the movement of his regiment up to the battleline on July 2, 1863, in an obscure little Pennsylvania town named Gettysburg. "I remember saying to them, 'We'll see you again later.' I tried to say this with a jaunty air, but down in my shoes I did not feel a bit jaunty. I think we all felt that this should be a death grapple. . . ."

Indeed it was going to be a death grapple, one that would continue for days, months, years, even decades for those wounded on that field. It was a grapple to stop the bleeding in time, lying on the field with hot lead trimming the heads off the wheat stalks by your head, or seeing those coming to your aid shot dead in their tracks, a struggle to get someone, anyone, to carry you off the field before the enemy reached your position, or shouting out for assistance after the cover of darkness had fallen, unable to walk and surrounded by only the dead and dying, with the sound of half-wild hogs rooting among the bodies. It was a grapple with death to survive the clumsy efforts at rescue by well-meaning soldiers, as wounds reopened under their ham-handed ministrations. It was a bone-jarring, teeth-gritting grapple with death just to hang on to consciousness and life during the ride in an ambulance nicknamed "avalanche."

At the field hospital, a new grapple began, as thousands of injured soldiers clamored for the medical care of mere dozens of surgeons. For many, that care included amputation of the wounded extremity, and the life and death wrestling match with shock, infection, and inclement weather began in earnest. For those too weak or too injured to live, there were last-minute struggles to get one last word or letter to that mother, that wife or sweetheart before it was forever too late; often working with dying breath to make sure that their body would be identified. The many thousands of relatives trying to reach Gettysburg had to strive to overcome destroyed railroads, stolen wagons, and critical shortage of lodging, only to begin the all too frequent, ultimately lonely, search for that one, silent grave.

For the hardy (and sometimes lucky) survivors, the grapple to hang on to life often hinged on getting transportation to a general hospital for further treatment.Another white-knuckle ride in an ambulance or splintery farm wagon ended at the rickety, single-line railroad heading east out of town. Drafty boxcars that reeked of manure and swayed dangerously, transmitting each jarring crash of the couplings to the broken men inside, carried thousands of soldiers from the battlefield to the big city general hospitals. There, the grapple for life and sanity started all over again.

This is the story of the hospitals of the Union Second Corps. In a time period that we look back on with aghast and dismay, where "laudable pus" and hospital fevers were the norm, when antisepsis and microbes were totally unknown, this hospital had an incredible 86.6 percent survival rate following the battle of Gettysburg. In spite of enormous, almost overwhelming, difficulties, the Second Corps hospitals succeeded because of the tough, compassionate dedication of its surgeons, and the selfless sacrifices of a small group of volunteers, men and women, who cared enough to come to a town that could be smelled from miles away as dead men and animals began to decompose in the sweltering summer heat.

To understand these hospitals, one must know something of the lives of the soldiers, surgeons, and civilians that met there, and of the battle that brought them together (which, for many, was the defining point of their lives). For some, where, and even how, they were wounded served as the deciding factor between life and death.

This is a timeless story of ordinary men and women, caught in events that swirl far beyond their control, who triumphed over seemingly impossible odds. It is a story of medicine in the midst of overwhelming catastrophe, where people swirl kaleidiscopically into the limelight for an hour, or for several days, and then vanish into the background of history.

Here is the story of the Union Second Corps hospitals, as they grappled with death before, during, and after the bloody battle of Gettysburg.

Part 1
The March

An Army on the move is a weary sight,
Fifteen miles of wagons, guns and dirty men
Along the roads, starting and stopping,
Stretching an ear, when officers gather
In conference near. Trotting to prod
Some laggards on, or sitting
To watch their marathon.

Requiem
W. J. Tancig

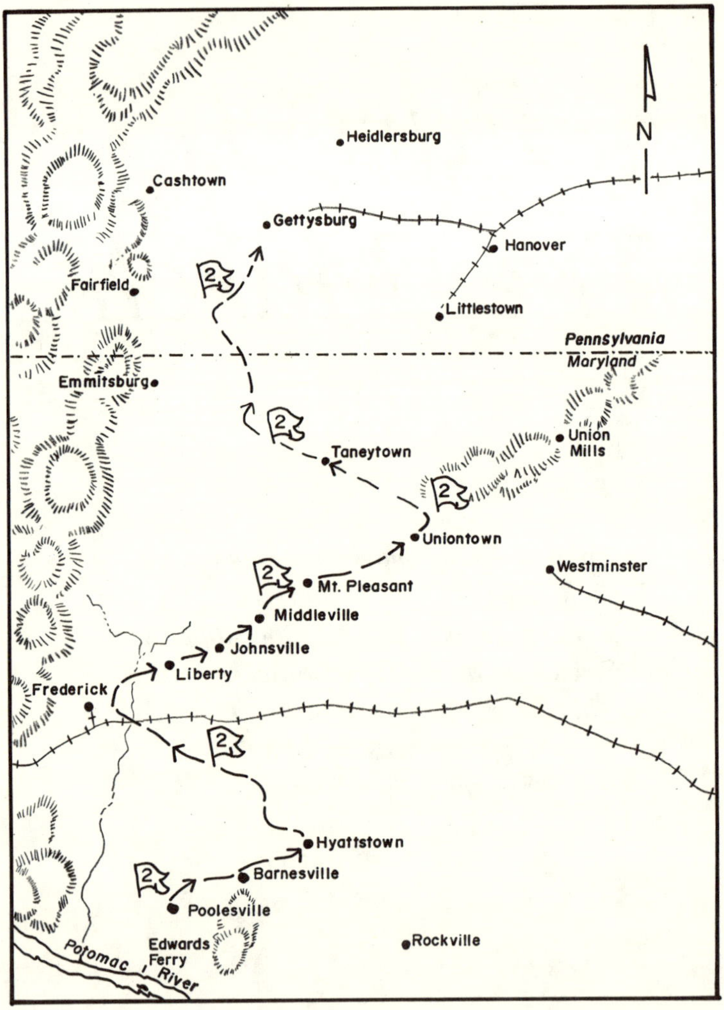

Map by John Heiser

Route of the Second Corps from the Potomac River to Gettysburg.

PRELUDE

MONDAY, JUNE 29: MORNING — TUESDAY, JUNE 30: LATE AFTERNOON

"Marching for . . . a position"

Captain Thomas Livermore

"Field after field and wood after wood were reached and passed, and at last we realized the fact that it was not a good camping-ground we were marching for, but a position, and those of us who stuck called all our determination and hurried on through the shadows. But there was little heard in the ranks but the tread of feet, the clanking of arms and equipment, and an occasional oath or grumble from some tired mortal."[1]

For the men of the Union Second Corps, June 29, 1863, was rapidly degenerating into a grueling test of physical endurance. "Our pace was rapid and the most rigid orders to keep the ranks closed up were enforced," wrote Capt. Thomas Livermore of the 5th New Hampshire Volunteers; "we even were obliged to keep the regulation twenty-eight inches only between the men and their file leaders in fording streams, and no one of us was permitted to stop long enough to remove our shoes or stockings, and as we forded several early in the day and drenched our feet and their apparel, we became footsore very easily on the hard roads. But the country was green and cheerful, and from the elevated land on which our road lay we got the most beautiful views of the valleys and the blue mountains on the north of us; the crops were smiling; the grass was green; the lands seemed to be improved and

1. Thomas Livermore, *Days and Events, 1860-1866* (Boston: H. Mifflin Company, 1920), p. 235.

cultivated in the highest style of art when compared with the forbidding soil of Virginia on which we had spent many months. . . ."[2]

"The country is very hilly and the roads in many places in bad order," recorded an Ohio soldier. "The general run of the ridges is east and west, so that as we are marching almost due north we are continually going up and down hill."[3]

As lovely vistas of hills and swales unfolded around them, Captain Livermore, a native of Illinois, was having his hands full just keeping his small command in line. "My men came to me one after another to say that they were tired out and could go no further. For I had made the rule that I would forgive no man who left the ranks on the march without first reporting to me his inability to go farther, thereby insuring a knowledge of the cause of absence and at the same time making the confession a hinderance to a too easy giving up. . . ."[4]

But young Livermore had other, more personal, things on his mind this muggy June day than just the comportment of his company. Several days previously, while waiting at Thoroughfare Gap, he had been approached by Col. R. N. Batchelder, chief quartermaster of the Second Corps, and former quartermaster of Livermore's own 5th New Hampshire regiment. Batchelder asked the captain if he might be interested in joining the corps staff—the chief of ambulances post was open, and the quartermaster felt he could secure the position for his regimental comrade. "The position of chief of ambulances, I was informed, gave me quarters and recognition as belonging to the staff of corps headquarters, gave me horses without expense, gave me an independent command of considerable magnitude, plenty of transportation, and comfortable quarters."[5]

Of course, there was always the life to which Livermore was now accustomed: "That very day I had perspired in a hot and dusty march; that night I should lie on the ground with little if any shelter; my coffee would be drunk if at all from a tin cup; my meal would be rounded out with a slice of salt pork, salt beef, or fresh-killed meat boiled in an iron pot, and hardtack; if it rained while we were marching I should be soaked and my feet would be clogged with mud. . . ."[6]

---

2. *Ibid.*, p. 234.
3. Thomas Francis Galwey, *The Valiant Hours: Narrative of "Captain Brevet," an Irish-American in the Army of the Potomac*, ed. W. S. Nye (Harrisburg, Pennsylvania: Stackpole Books, 1961), p. 96.
4. Livermore, *Days and Events*, p. 235.
5. *Ibid.*
6. *Ibid.*

Although knowing full well the unwillingness of Col. Edward E. Cross, the acting brigade commander and former head of the 5th New Hampshire regiment, to release any men on detached service, Captain Livermore was also aware that there was presently a surplus of officers in the regiment. Livermore compromised by asking his immediate superior to be allowed to take the offer. "I at once walked over to [Lieutenant] Colonel [Charles E.] Hapgood, who was then commanding our regiment, and told him of the offer, and that if he consented I would accept. He without the slightest hesitation said: 'Yes, Captain, take it. It's a good chance for you and we have plenty of officers and can spare you without injury to the regiment,' or words to the same effect." Livermore at once told Quartermaster Batchelder, who rode away telling the captain that he would personally see to his detachment. No sooner had Batchelder left than Hapgood walked over to talk to Cross. After conversing for a few moments, Hapgood sent for Livermore and promptly withdrew his permission. The New Hampshire captain reluctantly agreed to stay on with the regiment, but there was no way to reach the quartermaster colonel with news of the rescinded approval.[7]

To further add to his uncertainty, Livermore had stopped by Second Corps headquarters a few days later [June 28th] to check on his new posting, having heard that someone else had been appointed chief of ambulances. Colonel Batchelder received him graciously, introduced him to Dr. Alexander N. Dougherty, the corps medical director, only to find that the order had indeed just been cut detailing another officer to fill the vacancy. Batchelder, in no uncertain terms, made it clear that Livermore was the man he wanted, and sent the captain on his way with personal assurances that the opening would be his.[8]

Now the young New Hampshire captain trudged north on a seemingly endless road, granting permission to an ongoing stream of his men to fall out of the ranks, and wondering in exactly what position he would find himself serving by week's end.

It was a lean, stripped-down Second Corps marching north that day. The continuing heat throughout the trek from Falmouth, Virginia, had

7. *Ibid.*, pp. 227-29.
8. *Ibid.*, p. 233.

prompted the men to discard all but the most necessary baggage, forcing them to reevaluate just how much equipment they were willing to lug the long, dusty miles each day. "Every morning our place of bivouac were marked by long rows of piles of burning clothing and blankets, but notwithstanding these reliefs many a knapsack was cut off on the road when the panting wearer could no longer keep up with his command and carry his burden. While in Virginia this property was religiously burned to keep it from falling into the hands of the enemy; but in Maryland we were more careless. I saw four horse express wagons following our columns and gathering up fragments, but who the gatherers were we never knew."[9]

Those that held on to their full issue of equipment were carrying musket, ammunition, knapsack, cartridge box, shelter tent, woolen blanket, rubber blanket, overcoat, extra shirt, drawers, socks, canteen, and rations: a total of fifty-seven to sixty pounds of gear to carry while dressed in an itchy wool uniform in the seventy-plus degree weather.[10]

In addition to the standard issue of military hardware, Capt. Jeremiah Z. Brown and Pvt. David Polliard of Company K, 148th Pennsylvania Volunteers, struggled along with an additional burden: a rucksack full of potatoes. "The evening before, I had bought a peck of potatoes from the officers' wagon, hoping to enjoy a good breakfast, but the bugle sounded the march before the potatoes were cooked. Comrade Polliard proposed to carry them, so that we might have them for dinner. He put them in his knapsack, and we started."[11]

---

9. Benjamin W. Thompson, *Personal Narrative of Experiences in the Civil War, 1861-1865* (manuscript owned by John A. Thompson, copy of original typescript in the 111th New York Vertical File, Gettysburg National Military Park), pp. 29-30. "The loss in the whole army must have reached a million dollars," continued Thompson, "for which these poor fellows never received a cent, the survivors of the battle having to [reequip] themselves at their own expense, consuming an average of over a [full] pay."
10. J. H. Douglas, *Report on the Operations of the Sanitary Commission During and After the Battles at Gettysburg, July 1st, 2d, and 3d, 1863. Sanitary Commission No. 71.* (Washington, D.C.: Privately Printed, 1863), p. 8, copy in the U.S. Sanitary Commission Vertical File, Gettysburg National Military Park.
11. Joseph W. Muffly, *The Story of Our Regiment: a History of the 148th Volunteers* (Des Moines, Iowa: Kenyon Print and Manufacturing Co., 1904), p. 798.

Dr. Justin Dwinelle, regimental surgeon of the 106th Pennsylvania Volunteer Infantry, commented on the rigorous marches when he sat down to write his brother on June 20: "I take up my hospital near Potomac Creek Station the evening of the 14th, and after a hot dusty and night and day march I arrived here just before dark last night. . . . The first thirty hours of one march we did not stop to rest."[12]

During the rapid movements, the wagons were kept consistently to the rear of the corps, instead of traveling with the brigades or divisions. Officers were forced to do without their personal luggage; forge, repair, forage, and supply wagons, even ambulances and medical trains, were bringing up the dusty rear of the line. Perhaps most important was the fact that the commissary wagons were separated from the very troops they were to supply. The men were issued rations in a sporadic manner, and in multiple-day portions. It was an unfortunate soldier who ate his allotment too quickly, and found himself a few mornings later marching on an empty stomach under a blistering sun. "Before crossing the Potomac we received six days rations, and again at Taneytown a small ration of hardtack was issued," wrote one veteran of that grueling march.[13]

Muggy, humid heat meant dry roads, and the passage of the many thousand men, wagons, and artillery stirred up vast amounts of dust. "At times we could scarcely see the men immediately in front of us. Great clouds of dust rose around us—I thought one might write in them, they were so thick." Even the movements of the enemy, carefully screened behind guarded mountain passes, were betrayed by the dry weather. "Great clouds of dust were seen in the West, where Lee's army was marching."[14]

As the dreadful march continued, sunstroke and heat exhaustion became widespread, particularly among the grimy footsoldiers. "The ambulances were crowded everyday and numbers asked for

---

12. Dr. Justin Dwinelle, letter to brother, June 20, 1863, courtesy of Scott Michael Dwinelle. Justin Dwinelle's name appears as both "Dwinell" and "Dwinelle" on various documents. His mother had added the final "e" to the family name, and even Dwinelle's aides were not consistent in their spelling of his name on the documents they prepared.

13. Galwey, *The Valiant Hours*, p. 112.

14. J. H. W. Stuckenberg, *I'm Surrounded by Methodists: The Civil War Diary of a Lutheran Chaplain*, ed. David T. Hedrick and Gordon Barry Davis (Gettysburg, Pennsylvania: Thomas Publications, 1994), pp. 121-22; J. H. W. Stuckenberg, lecture delivered in Warren, Pennsylvania, on January 6, 1864, The Stuckenberg Collection, Gettysburg College [hereafter referred to as the "Warren Lecture"].

admittance who were refused. Those that gave out were afraid to stop and rest because they were in great danger of being taken by the rebels. So they dragged their sick bodies and weary, sore limbs along until they fell by the road side, panting for breath, some [conscious], others on the point of death, and all suffering terribly. . . . Water was often scarce, and generally very poor." "Numbers of wells by the roadside were observed filled with stones; the water was always muddy and bad, and could be had only at long distance from the road."[15]

Occasionally, as if to vary the breathless aridness, an intermittent downpour would transform the dusty roadway into a winding muddy morass. "We had rather rough times marching here," wrote Ohio hospital steward Charles H. Merrick on June 27; "the first of the march was hot and dusty—now it is very muddy and the roads almost impassable." The sultry June weather, however, soon dried the mud and returned the gritty taste of dust to everyone's mouth as they trudged along the narrow dirt roads.[16]

The soldiers sought every opportunity to relieve the monotony of the long, tedious marches, and, at the same time, make their own situation easier. "Numbers of cavalry horses had been abandoned by their riders, who only required a few days' rest to recruit, and again they were ready for duty. They were to be seen all along our route, undisturbed by the passing column, except when caught by some of the foot soldiers. It was amusing to observe the ingenious arrangements meant to answer for the horses' trappings: a piece of old tent-canvas was soon converted into an admirable bridle; another piece of the same shelter kept the saddle (a blanket) in its place; thus mounted, he would be delighted; and day by day added the number of this escort."[17]

That peck of potatoes seemed to gain weight with every passing mile as the march dragged on over the rolling Maryland landscape.

15. Stuckenberg, Warren Lecture; Anna Holstein, *Three Years in Field Hospitals of the Army of the Potomac* (Philadelphia: J. B. Lippincott & Co., 1867), as quoted in E. F. Conklin, *Women at Gettysburg 1863* (Gettysburg, Pennsylvania: Thomas Publications, 1993), pp. 256-57.

16. Charles H. Merrick, letter to his sister Min Merrick, June 27, 1863, William P. Palmer Collection, Container 1, Folder 3, MSS 3088, Western Reserve Historical Society, Cleveland, Ohio.

17. Conklin, *Women at Gettysburg*, p. 257.

Captain Brown eyed Private Polliard as he let out a grunt and shifted the knapsack to a more comfortable position. "It was a very warm day, the march was rapid, and about noon Polliard said, 'I wish they would stop. These potatoes are getting heavy.'"[18]

As afternoon gradually faded into evening, some of the more compassionate officers began dismounting so that their men could use their horses as a form of mobile support. Much of the afternoon, Chaplain William Henry Stevens of the 148th Pennsylvania, an imposing man at six-foot-one, with jet black hair and steel gray eyes, had put his own horse "at the disposal of the foot-sore." It was not uncommon, his men had learned, to spot the chaplain, "trudging along, leading his horse, which was covered from head to tail, with twenty-five or more knapsacks."[19]

However, not even animals were immune to the debilitating nature of the June marches. "Horses and mules fell dead in the road. Our Col's dog gave out and was left; but the men with their loads had to march on."[20]

Now the Second Corps continued pushing northward, uncharacteristically confining it's movement to just one narrow country road. Infantry, artillery, and trains marched doggedly onward in a long, single-file parade of misery and exhaustion, curling like a long dry snake over the undulating countryside.[21]

It had been evident by early morning that June 29 would be another stifling day. "The roads were in very good condition, neither muddy nor dusty, still it was sultry and drizzled rain most of the day." Wool uniforms clung to the marching men like damp, suffocating blankets in the muggy weather.[22]

Capt. Benjamin W. Thompson, Company F, 111th New York, had come up with his own way to help keep his men in line. "Men would fall

18. Muffly, *The Story of our Regiment*, p. 798.
19. *Ibid.*, pp. 191, 196-97.
20. Stuckenberg, Warren Lecture.
21. John H. Rhodes, *The History of Battery B, First Regiment Rhode Island Light Artillery, in the War to Preserve the Union, 1861 - 1865* (Providence, R. I.: Snow & Farnham, Printers, 1894), p. 197. Usually, the army would move each division along different roads to converge at some predetermined place.
22. Muffly, *The Story of Our Regiment*, p. 171.

out every few rods, declaring they could not go another step, but by coaxing and carrying their muskets for them, and more by keeping up a constant stream of funny stories, and songs, we were able to hold them on for miles. Much of the day I carried one or two musket beside my own heavy belt, and furnished more than my share of the hilarity for the regiment."[23]

Thompson was particularly angry about the men not being allowed to throw up hasty bridges, or remove their shoes, before fording streams. "The old Second Corps marched from Monocacy Junction to Uniontown, Maryland, thirty three miles, and waded every stream, on the way. . . . We had marched a mile or two when we came to a ford of the Monocacy River which we had to cross. There were good fences and flattened logs upon which our men could have crossed almost or quite dry shod. But we were brought down to quick time, arms on the right shoulder, and marched directly through the stream, hip deep to the tallest of us. Fearing our Colonels would neglect his brutal order, he left an aide at the ford to enforce it, while he rode forward to keep the column in motion."[24]

"He" was Second Corps commander Maj. Gen. Winfield Scott Hancock. But in all fairness, and in marked contrast to Captain Thompson's harsh view of General Hancock, the entire situation was the result of simple clerical error. "The Second Corps was to have moved at 4 A.M., but through a blunder on the part of a bearer of dispatches the orders were not received till 6 A.M., and it was 8 o'clock before the Corps was in motion." Hancock, not known for his patience, was highly perturbed, as was Meade—the Second Corps commander reported to Meade that the hapless headquarter's clerk "has already been brought to punishment. I took every precaution. . . . I shall try to make up the most of it by short cuts and rapid marching."[25]

Consequently, in an attempt to compensate for the four-hour setback, Hancock pushed his command thirty-two miles to Uniontown,

---

23. Thompson, *Personal Narrative*, p. 31.

24. *Ibid.*, p. 30. This was probably Linganore Creek, or another stream near Frederick, although it may have been one of the branches of the Monocacy River.

25. Almira Hancock, *Reminiscences of Winfield Scott Hancock by his Wife* (New York: Charles L. Webster & Co., 1887), p. 184; United States War Department, *The War of the Rebellion: A Compilation of the Official Records of the Union and Confederate Armies*, 70 vols. in 128 parts (Washington, D.C.: Government Printing Office, 1880-1901), series 1, vol. 27, pt. 3, pp. 395-96. (Hereafter cited as *OR*. All citations are from Series

just two miles short of the assigned destination of Frizzelburg, where darkness and grinding fatigue finally precluded going any further. To make matters even worse, the delay in the Second Corps' departure had in turn held up the Fifth Corps, which could not leave until the Second had cleared the way, consequently making it only as far as Liberty on the 29th.[26]

Now, the "short cuts and rapid marching" had led to cutting corners in the proper care of the troops. After marching straight through the ford, the dust and road grime on the men's clothing quickly took on the pasty consistency of glue. "This caused the dust and fine gravel to adhere to their trousers, which soon found its way into the worn shoes, causing many of them to become footsore." Devastation to the feet of marching men in wool stockings and often ill-sized shoes was quick to follow. "It is an invariable rule after troops have forded a stream, unless under the enemy's fire, to halt them long enough to take off their shoes, wring out their stockings and wipe their feet. But Hancock marched us several miles at a rapid pace before he allowed us a breath. By that time the feet of nearly every man and officer were blistered and many could just hobble."[27]

Captain Thompson was an officer who cared deeply for his men, and had planned ahead for the needs and exigencies of his command. "My men were completely exhausted and I spent the whole halt in doctoring their feet and administering whiskey, of which I had procured two canteens of the surgeon that morning."[28] But the arduous march of June 29 was far from over.

The march had certainly started innocuously enough. The column had moved out of its bivouac around 8:00 a.m., wrote Lt. Col. Richards

---

I.); David L. Ladd and Audrey J. Ladd, eds., *The Bachelder Papers: Gettysburg in Their Own Words*, 3 vols. (Dayton, Ohio: Morningside, 1994-95), p. 1348; Edwin B. Coddington, *The Gettysburg Campaign: A Study in Command* (New York: Charles Scribner's Sons, 1968; reprint, Dayton, Ohio: Morningside Bookshop, 1979), pp. 227-28.

26. Hancock, *Reminiscences of Winfield Scott Hancock*, p. 184; *OR.*, pt. 3, 395-96; Ladd, *The Bachelder Papers*, p. 1348; Coddington, *The Gettysburg Campaign*, pp. 227-28.

27. Charles D. Page, *History of the Fourteenth Regiment Connecticut Volunteer Infantry* (Meriden, Connecticut: The Horton Printing Company, 1906), p. 133; Thompson, *Personal Narrative*, p. 16.

28. Thompson, *Personal Narrative*, p. 16.

McMichael of the 53rd Pennsylvania, "passed over the Monocacy Creek on the bridge at the railroad station, and marched on the Frederick pike until within a few miles of the city, when the column headed to the right, repassed the Monocacy, and continued marching northward. . . ."[29]

The recrossing of that particular waterway became a focal point of festering discontent throughout the entire Second Corps. The trouble started when the troops were ordered to "bulge" the stream, as marching through a ford without first removing shoes was called. The outrage was compounded by the fact that two large foot logs were in place at the ford, hewn flat on top and floored with planking. The men could easily cross without even getting wet.[30]

Each unit, in its turn, had its own story to tell of that ford. When Captain Livermore's commander, Colonel Cross, reached the stream, he sat mounted along one side of the road with a staff officer on the other side, supervising the wading of his men. Some of the men made some snide remarks, and Colonel Cross, thinking he knew who said it, lashed out with the flat of his sword. Twenty-one-year-old Cpl. George J. Duffy, Company G of the 148th Pennsylvania, took the blow directly on the neck. One of the men muttered: "I'll bet if Colonel [James A.] Beaver were here he would not dare do that."[31]

Upon reaching the stream with the 148th Pennsylvania Volunteers, seventeen-year-old Pvt. Lemuel Osman of Company C tried to beat the odds of getting blistered feet. "I pulled my shoes off, so that I would not get sand in them, and tied them together. The current was strong, every man was pressing forward for himself and, in the confusion, my shoe strings came open and away went my shoes. I was in a bad way but was compelled to march on without any covering for my feet."[32]

Brig. Gen. Alexander S. Webb's Second Brigade of Gibbon's Second Division encountered a totally different welcome to the now dreaded ford. When the lead elements of his brigade, the 106th

29. *OR*, vol. 27, pt. 1, p. 411.

30. Glenn Tucker, *Hancock the Superb* (Indianapolis: The Bobbs-Merrill Company, 1960), p. 128.

31. Muffly, *The Story of Our Regiment*, p. 716. Colonel Beaver was severely wounded in the side at Chancellorsville, and had not yet returned to the regiment.

32. *Ibid.*, p. 602. On the morning of July 2, Osman met a man coming from the hospital, carrying an extra pair of shoes. "I told him what had happened to mine and he gave me a pair. I thanked him very much. They didn't fit very well, for they were No. 10's and I wore No. 7's. They answered the purpose, however."

Pennsylvania, halted to remove their shoes, Webb ordered them forward. In an effort to show his willingness to suffer with his troops, the newly-minted twenty-eight-year-old brigadier general rode out into the middle of the stream, vaulted from his horse, and stood silent and watchful in midstream as his entire brigade, shoes and all, sloshed across. An Irishman of the 69th Pennsylvania was singularly unimpressed. As he waded past his commander, he muttered: "Sure it's no wonder ye can stand there when ye are leather up to your waist." The water and comment obviously did nothing to sweeten Webb's temper, for he spotted one of his men walking across the stream on a nearby log and had the captain summarily arrested. It took an official medical certification from a regimental surgeon of the man's chronic rheumatism to persuade the fuming general to release him.[33]

When Brig. Gen. William Harrow's First Brigade of Gibbon's command reached the water, it found Col. Charles H. Morgan sitting on horseback and carefully noting what was happening. Morgan was Hancock's inspector general and chief of staff, and was notorious for his harshness with the troops. As lead elements of the 1st Minnesota approached, Morgan told their commander, Col. William Colvill, to close up ranks and march straight through. Despite their colonel's orders, some men broke ranks to cross the planked-over logs to the other side, highly perturbing Inspector General Morgan.

The 15th Massachusetts, next in line, saw what was coming, and balked at crossing. Colonel Morgan gave them the same order. When the men were finally allowed to stop and wring out their socks, Morgan rode by the two intermixed regiments. The Massachusetts men greeted him with a hearty groan, and an irate Colonel Morgan blew up. Thinking these men were all attached to the Minnesota regiment, Hancock's officer personally arrested Colonel Colvill and stripped him of his command. Morgan then rode to General Harrow, who was in temporary command of the division, making sure that he confirmed Colvill's arrest.[34]

---

33. Joseph R. C. Ward, *History of the One Hundred and Sixth Regiment, Pennsylvania Volunteers* (Philadelphia: Grant, Faires & Rodgers, 1883), pp. 149-50.

34. Return I. Holcombe, *History of the First Regiment, Minnesota Volunteer Infantry* (Stillwater, Minnesota: Easton & Masterson, 1916), pp. 348-50; John Quinn Imholte, *The First Volunteers: History of the First Minnesota Volunteer Regiment* (Minneapolis: Ross and Haines, 1963), pp. 114-15; Tucker, *Hancock the Superb*, pp. 128-29.

Finally, the last of Hancock's men sloshed their way across the now-infamous ford, leaving the way clear for the wagons and trains to cross. It was, however, a far more gloomy and footsore corps that continued to tramp their way toward the Keystone State.

"On, on we marched, the sun beating down with almost tropical power, the roads now a stifling cloud of dust and anon filled with cobble stones over which the footsore men were constantly stumbling." "We passed through several small, but pleasant and picturesque villages," wrote one artilleryman of the tedious march. One was even named Mt. Pleasant, "a very nice little village, but the Inhabitants were not to be seen. . . ."[35]

Nine miles after starting out, the column was marching through Liberty, and reached Johnsville six miles later. Johnsville proved to be "the collective title of a dozen cheerful looking residences, situated along the road at an average distance of one-fourth mile apart." After eighteen long, grueling miles, the weary men were allowed to fall out for a brief rest in Middleville. It was readily apparent to the winded infantrymen that they were in for some "big marching."[36]

"The very names of the towns we passed through were reviving, such as Liberty, Uniontown, etc., and they seemed almost like New England in their neatness. I recollect a negro, who had come from Virginia with us, as he trudged along beside the ranks, and who hearing some one inquire how far it was to Liberty, said, with a broad grin, 'It's a long way to liberty, sah!'"[37]

---

35. Thompson, *Personal Narrative*, pp. 30-31; Rhodes, *The History of Battery B*, p. 197; Robert L. Bee, "Fredericksburg on the Other Leg: Sergeant Ben Hirst's Narrative of Important Events, Gettysburg, July 3, 1863," in *The Third Day at Gettysburg & Beyond*, ed. Gary Gallagher (Chapel Hill: University of North Carolina Press, 1994), p. 138.
36. Letter of Levi J. Fritz, *Montgomery Ledger*, August 4, 1863; Pennsylvania Gettysburg Battlefield Commission, *Pennsylvania at Gettysburg: Ceremonies at the Dedication of the Monuments Erected by the Commonwealth of Pennsylvania to Mark the Positions of the Pennsylvania Commands Engaged in the Battle*, ed. John P. Nicholson, 2 vols. (Harrisburg Pennsylvania: William Stanley Ray, State Printer, 1904), vol. 1, p. 305.
37. Livermore, *Days and Events*, p. 235. The corps ultimately passed through Frederick City, Mt. Pleasant, Liberty, Jamestown, Union Bridge, ending up in Uniontown, Maryland. William Kepler, *History of the Three Months' and Three Years' Service from April 16th, 1861, to June 22d, 1864, of the Fourth*

However, "many pleasant incidents occurred during the day to lighten the toil and severity of that long march. At every farm house, and in every village, along our route, the people, old and young, stood in front of their homes with buckets of water, baskets of bread, cakes and other eatables, which they distributed among the boys as they passed, until their provisions were all gone, meantime speaking words of welcome, sympathy and encouragement. Such demonstrations we had not been accustomed to farther south in Dixie."[38]

Another soldier jotted in his diary: "We were greeted all day with smiles, kind words and refreshed with water and cakes and other things grateful to the taste of a soldier. May this page live a thousand years to record the goodness of the loyal hearts of Maryland."[39]

For the most part, the country lanes through which the corps now moved were in better repair than the much-traveled thoroughfares of Virginia, and "cherries are plenty on the road." "While on the march we found the trees loaded with cherries and other fruits. Everything was pleasing to the eye and palate, but we could not tarry long enough to enjoy the fruit or flowers." The weary soldiers ate what little they could pluck from the heavily-laden trees as they marched by.[40]

The thought of actually being back on Northern soil once more kept many weary soldiers moving. "The fact of getting into Pennsylvania during the day seemed to have a wonderful effect on the spirits of all the men of the regiment," wrote the commander of the 116th Pennsylvania Volunteers, "and frequent inquiries were made during the day for the State line from the farmers who lined the fences by the way and gazed in wonder at the passing column. 'Where does this road run to,' asked one of the men. 'Oh,' replied the intelligent citizen, 'it runs straight on!'"[41]

Regiment Ohio Volunteer Infantry in the War for the Union (Cleveland, Ohio: Leader Printing Company, 1886; reprint, Huntington, West Virginia, Blue Acorn Press, 1992), p. 123.

38. Muffly, *The Story of our Regiment*, pp. 533-34.

39. *Ibid.*, p. 703.

40. Theodore Reichardt, *Diary of Battery A, First Regiment Rhode Island Light Artillery* (Providence, Rhode Island: N. Bangs Williams, Publisher, 1865), p. 94; Jacob H. Cole, *Under Five Commanders, or A Boy's Experience with the Army of the Potomac* (Paterson, New Jersey: News Printing Company, 1906), p. 191.

41. St. Clair A. Mulholland, *The Story of the 116th Regiment Pennsylvania Volunteers in the War of the Rebellion. The Record of a Gallant Command.* (Philadelphia, Pennsylvania: F. McManus Jr. and Company, Printers, 1903), p. 118. In actuality, the Second Corps did not reach Pennsylvania until the morning of July 1.

The men seemed determined to make the very best impression as they trudged steadily northward through town after borough after hamlet. "On nearing villages, colors were unfurled and bands played lively airs. Instantly new life would pervade the exhausted troops. Guns . . . were brought to position, limping steps became firm . . . the line straightened itself and the men were soldiers all over." When out of sight of cheering shopkeepers and waving ladies, the effects of blistered feet and raw fatigue reasserted themselves once again.[42]

Not even the prospect of crossing the Mason-Dixon line could counteract the debilitating effects of the day's exertions, since many had already reached or exceeded their limits of physical endurance. The First Brigade band of the Third Division had been hit particularly hard by the march—all of the musicians, save one, had collapsed by the wayside. Only grocer-turned-drummer George Washington Lambert of the 14th Indiana continued to stagger along, carrying his drum, and supported by a comrade who helped hold drum and drummer alike in a mostly vertical position as they tottered along.[43]

For their part, the men were quick to give voice to their frustration and misery as the road continued to unfold before them. "From early morning through afternoon to evening, and then till midnight, the press was forward," remembered Capt. Gilbert Frederick of the 57th New York. "The men then declared that Hancock would not stop until he got to Harrisburg. [Lieutenant] Colonel [Alford B.] Chapman was very patient, and said it was a soldier's privilege to grumble."[44]

There were moments of pleasant companionship along the way, but these seemed to be mostly confined to those favored few who were mounted on horseback. Capt. Josiah M. Favill, staff aide to Brig. Gen. Samuel K. Zook of the Third Brigade, First Division, was at the head of

42. Arabella M. Willson, *Disaster, Struggle, Triumph. The Adventures of 1000 "Boys in Blue," August, 1862, to June, 1865* (Albany, New York: The Argus Company, Printers, 1870), p. 54.

43. Journal of George Washington Lambert, entry for June 29, 1863, Indiana Historical Society.

44. Rev. Gilbert Frederick, Captain, 57th New York Volunteers, "Dedication of Monument, 57th Regiment Infantry, Historical Notes," October 6, 1889, New York Monuments Commission for the Battlefields of Gettysburg and Chattanooga, *Final Report on the Battlefield of Gettysburg*, comp. and ed. William F. Fox, 3 vols. (New York: J. B. Lyon Company, 1900), p. 419. [Hereafter cited as *New York at Gettysburg*.]

the column, riding with his commander. "The day was beautiful, but the sun much too hot for comfort," wrote the New Yorker. Inspired by Chaucer's Canterbury pilgrims, the general himself suggested to his staff that each do something to help entertain the others as the column wound its tedious way northward. "I unexpectedly made quite a hit by relating a lot of Ovid's metamorphoses, which some of them had never heard before and thought very wonderful." Obviously quite pleased with himself, the youthful aide failed to note what others of his group contributed.[45]

Being on a general's staff did have its perks—Favill could stop from time to time to socialize and get some refreshment. "Occasionally we dismounted and walked, and at times rode out of the column to neighboring houses to chat with the natives, get a cool drink of water, and perhaps chat with the girls of the establishment." Contrary to the murmured gripes and complaints of the footsore infantry, Favill felt that "nothing can be more delightful and interesting than campaigning in a civilized country at this season of the year."[46] But then Favill had not waded hip-deep through a river either.

"In passing through these towns, we usually resume the regular step, and with bands playing, colors flying make a stunning appearance. The Fifty-second [New York], as in days gone by, although with fewer voices, sing their memorable songs, which creates more enthusiasm than do the bands."[47] With more an air of parade than forced march, Favill and entourage rode north as the sinking sun cast lengthening shadows over the rolling landscape.

"I never have made so long a march as that before or since, and I perhaps have never been so tired, but it was a principle with me never to give out on a march," wrote Captain Livermore, "and I reached the camp, with perhaps half my company, at two o'clock in the morning, near Uniontown, after marching thirty-two miles. That may not be a great walk for an unencumbered pedestrian, and armies have doubtless gone further in one march, but I thought that, considering our wet feet, our loads, and the worry of walking in a column in a June (almost July)

45. Josiah M. Favill, *The Diary of a Young Officer* (Chicago: R. R. Donnelly & Sons, Company, 1909), p. 241.

46. *Ibid.* It is hard to believe that Captains Favill and Thompson were actually involved in the same march, so different were their experiences.

47. *Ibid.*

day in Maryland, it was a wonderful march, and so did the commander of the army, who congratulated us in orders the next day."[48]

That treasured peck of potatoes now felt as though it had been magically transformed into a full bushel. Private Polliard was staggering under the dead weight, and he let Captain Brown know his displeasure in no uncertain terms. "As the march continued, he said, 'If we don't stop soon, I will have to throw them away,' but I took his gun and carried it for him for several hours. . . ."[49]

Carrying all those muskets for his men was starting to take a heavy toll on Captain Thompson. "As night drew on my own powers began to flag. My men could not be kept in line and one by one they dropped by the wayside to rest and sleep. I commanded the color company and the colors could not halt, so I nerved myself and a few of my most resolute men to 'see the colors through to camp.' We were every moment expecting orders to go into camp, but none came and on we staggered. About eight o'clock I found myself unable to go further unaided and pressed forward to the adjutant, who was mounted, and supported myself for some distance by holding on to his horse's mane. At length I fell in the road unconscious and was carried to a house not far away, where I rested until morning."[50]

The heavy drum was finally the undoing of bandsman Lambert and his faithful friend. The instrument began to literally come apart at the seams, so the exhausted pair gathered together the bits and pieces, detoured to a roadside barn, and, after reassembling the drum, collapsed in the fragrant hay.[51]

The unfortunate men of the 4th Ohio found themselves as the rearguard of the wagon train. One soldier described the duty of guarding the trains as "an extremely disagreeable task. A well-drilled

48. Livermore, *Days and Events*, p. 235.

49. Muffly, *The Story of Our Regiment*, p. 798.

50. Thompson, *Personal Narrative*, p. 31.

51. Lambert journal, June 29, 1863. Barns were proving to be overwhelming enticements to the weary men. "We climbed a fence and made our way to a large barn on the side of a hill, which we could just discern through the night and the rain," wrote Thomas Galwey of the 8th Ohio. "We had expected to find the barn empty of everything but cattle and feed; but on getting there we were welcomed to a hay bed by forty or fifty used-up stragglers." Galwey, *The Valiant Hours*, p. 97.

body of soldiers can march for hours without either losing or gaining enough distance to make the march irregular, but it is very difficult to train mules to do the same. What is more, they have to pull loads over very bad roads. The head of a wagon train comes to a slough, then goes through it slowly, each wagon halting or checking its pace as it arrives, to prevent collision with the one in front. But having passed the obstacle it is necessary to take up the trot to catch up with the wagons in front, already over. And so it goes. . . . Imagine, then, the feelings of the infantry who have been detailed to guard the wagon train. Two men go with each wagon. Of course they walk, creep, run or halt, just as the wagon which they accompany walks, creeps, runs, or halts, and in twelve or fifteen hours this becomes not only monotonous but maddening."[52]

While the corps moved out at 8:00 a.m., the 4th did not even budge until 1:30 p.m., and then only to eat the dust of the entire corps and eight miles of toiling wagons. By nightfall, the rains began, dry roads quickly turned into muddy quagmires, and the Ohioans feet were soon squishing in soggy shoes. Friendly families along the way proffered warm food and hearty encouragement, but the round-the-clock march would not end for the sleepy, drenched Ohioans until nearly daybreak on the 30th.[53]

"Slowly but steadily the long dark-blue heaving mass for miles dragged its slow length along," wrote one veteran of that arduous trek. "The sun slowly sank to rest in the far west, but there was no rest for us; in the beautiful twilight we kept marching on. By 8 o'clock, P.M., we had marched twenty-eight miles. Many of the troops were exhausted and lay by the roadside. Everybody was very tired. We even believed that some of our soldiers would have given utterance to more or less profane words, but they were too much exhausted to speak."[54]

Trailing the Second Corps by nightfall was a dazed conglomeration of filthy and bedraggled men. "The day began with route-march, and ended with go-as-you-please. The different regiments became mingled with the stragglers, and when the last regimental staff had passed,

52. Galwey, *The Valiant Hours*, p. 95.

53. Kepler, *Fourth Ohio Volunteers*, p. 123.

54. Letter of Levi J. Fritz, *Montgomery Ledger*, August 4, 1863.

there followed an army of the lame, the halt, the sick, and, last of all, the born tired. The ambulances were full of both officers and men."[55]

By now, even dedicated, committed marchers who never straggled were feeling the overwhelming weariness taking its toll. "My feet were very sore," wrote one Ohio soldier. "Generally, I am one of the best marchers in our company which, by the way, is considered one of the best marching companies in the brigade. Seldom is a Hibernian seen amongst the stragglers. About dark, not knowing how soon I might give out, I got a pass from our Surgeon. But I kept up with my company for another couple of hours. Finally I could not put one foot before another. I was utterly done out, so sticking my pass in my hat band, and telling my sergeant of my intentions, I stepped out from the ranks and lay down on a spot of grass in the angle of a fence. In a minute or two I dropped asleep."[56]

Not even the surgeons themselves were immune to straggling and falling out. Surgeon William Warren Potter of the 57th New York, which had been guarding a bridge over the Monocacy River the previous night, was hurrying with his command to overtake the fast-moving Second Corps. "Sometime during the night, being tired and hungry, I reined into a lot, and sat down on a cock of hay with Capt Rose, our commissary of subsistence. Discovering a cow in the field near by, for it was moonlight, we got one of the soldiers to milk her and, after refreshing ourselves with hardtack and milk, we soon fell asleep."[57]

Scuttlebutt had been circulating along the line that Uniontown (or Union Bridge, as it was also known) was to be the ultimate destination for the day. For those stalwart and faithful few that wearily dragged into the Maryland village in late hours of July 29th, or the wee hours of June 30th, there was the reward of water, cookies, fresh bread, cherries, milk, even entire meals, some at nominal prices, most free of charge.[58]

"By some hocus pocus the town gradually neared us," remembered one dazed marcher. "We moved our wearied limbs so slowly that we

---

55. Frederick, "Dedication of Monument," p. 419.
56. Galwey, *The Valiant Hours*, p. 97. Hibernian is the Latin name for a native of Ireland.
57. William Warren Potter, *Three Years with the Army of the Potomac: A Personal Military History* (Buffalo: n. p., 1888), p. 57.
58. Coddington, *The Gettysburg Campaign*, p. 228.

almost stood still." "Liquid refreshments were freely offered at the gates and porches," recalled another, "while kind words lightened the hearts of the weary soldiers, crowding onward to battle for the Union."[59]

But still the column kept plodding onward, with no visible signs of stopping, or even pausing. Sgt. Ben Hirst of the 14th Connecticut vividly recounted his arrival (and departure) from the town in a letter to his wife. "When about sunset we arrived at Union Bridge we began to think we had done for one day, but no; Close up is still the word, and we passed through the Village as if the devil was after us. . . ."[60]

By this point in the marathon march, the very infrastructure of the Second Corps was coming unraveled. "Now we have marched 27 miles since sunrise, and still no sign of Camping and now they we begin to Growl and to fall out first one gives up, then another, then they begin to fall out in twos and threes, but still I move along as best I can. By and by whole Companies seem to drop out, officers and men together, but still no one can answer that often asked: how much further. . . ."[61]

With Uniontown steadily receding into the night, Sergeant Hirst finally reached his limit, emotionally as well as physically. "~~Ilebe~~ Ilebe [*sic*] Damd [*sic*] if I can go any further, and away goes my Gun over the . . . fence and for a few minutes I give way to bitter thoughts as I rest my head upon my hands. Who is to blame for this marching us Past all endurance, oh it is our new Corps Commander (General Hancock) who wants to show that we can outmarch as well as outfight anything in the army. But no that cannot be it. It is the cursed Rebels, who not daring to attackt [*sic*] us where we could chastise them have stole a march upon us and now threaten to carry the War to our own Homes. Yes that is it and with the thought I get my Gun again and trudge along for a few more weary miles and I got rewarded for my perseverance for I soon saw the advance was encamped for the rest of the night, and me and John [his brother] were soon asleep by the road side, having marched with 3 days rations and 60 rounds of ammunition over 34 miles. . . ."[62]

Rest was uppermost in benumbed minds of everyone in the tottering column. "We halted, as I have said, near Uniontown (it was a

---

59. Letter of Levi J. Fritz, *Montgomery Ledger*, August 4, 1863; Page, *History of the Fourteenth Connecticut*, p. 133; Rhodes, *The History of Battery B*, p. 197.
60. Bee, "Fredericksburg on the Other Leg," p. 138.
61. *Ibid.*
62. *Ibid.*

little beyond that place in a piece of woods on the side of a hill), and lay down there to rest our aching members." Some, like Lt.Charles Fuller of the 61st New York, were so exhausted that they dropped right where they stopped: "As soon as arms were stacked I stretched out without unrolling my blankets, and I knew nothing till the next morning, when I was awakened by the sun shining into my eyes."[63]

The thirty-two mile Potato Marathon was finally over for the stalwart Capt. Jeremiah Z. Brown and Pvt. David Polliard of the 148th Pennsylvania. "When we halted, about ten o'clock at night, with but four men of the company to stack arms, we dropped down on the ground, forgetting all about the potatoes, and went sound asleep."[64]

Some, however, were reminded that they were still part of a military organization in a state of war, dead tired or not. William Lochren of the 1st Minnesota remembered being so "weary that we dropped down for sleep without care for supper, [Lt. Chris] Heffelfinger and I, as usual, doubling and sharing our blankets. We had just lain down when I heard my name called by the adjutant to go with the picket detail. It seemed impossible to move again, but there was no help for it; and I thought I could detect in Heffelfinger's profuse and sincere condolences an undertone of satisfaction that the lot had fallen on me rather than on him. I could not blame the feeling, and gathered the grumbling detail . . . we went about three miles farther and posted pickets. Morning was long in coming."[65]

Throughout the remaining hours of darkness, men dribbled into camp by ones and twos, staggering, limping, and filthy with road grime. "The stragglers came up during the night. Utterly worn out by the toilsome march, their clothes wet from perspiration, numbers of the boys simply dropped down on the bare ground, as they reached the place of bivouac, pulled a rubber blanket or a piece of shelter tent over

63. Livermore, *Days and Events*, p. 236; Charles A. Fuller, *Personal Recollections of the War of 1861 as Private, Sergeant and Lieutenant in the 61st Regiment, New York Volunteer Infantry* (Sherburne, New York: News Job Printing House, 1906), p. 91.

64. Muffly, *The Story of Our Regiment*, p. 798.

65. William Lochren, "The First Minnesota at Gettysburg," *Glimpses of the Nation's Struggle* (St. Paul, Minnesota: D. D. Merrill Company, 1893), vol. 3, p. 46.

them, and fell asleep in a moment, without making coffee or partaking of a mouthful of food."[66]

"The night having been quite cool, many of the boys caught a severe cold; and they would have been in poor condition to resume the march the following morning, but fortunately for them, the Corps remained in camp all day."[67]

"On the morning of the 30th, reveille was not sounded until six o'clock, affording the men extra time to rest from their march of the previous day." As it was, dawn of the last day of June came far too early for the fatigued men of the Second Corps. "We rose from the ground on the next morning rested, but stiff and sore," noted Thomas Livermore. Lieutenant Fuller, after sleeping without blankets on the bare ground all night, found himself "so stiff it took some time to get on my legs, but, after moving about for a while, I was all right."[68]

Captain Thompson regained consciousness in the house to which he had been carried the previous night. "With the dawn of day I was up and begged a substantial breakfast of the good Samaritan who lodged me, and then pressed on to overtake my regiment. I found them encamped about half a mile beyond where I fell out and learned that of all our regiment the mounted officers, the colors and some twenty men were all who had been able to endure to the end."[69]

Drummer Lambert and his companion, bits and pieces of hay sticking out of their hair and clothing, hurried to catch up to the First Brigade in the first light of morning. They were shocked by the fragmentary remnant of the once proud brigade they found. "We would not have known whether it was the brigade or a squad of stragglers had not the flag been waving in the breeze." Thomas Galwey of the Third Brigade found that more than two-thirds of his 8th Ohio regiment had fallen out along the roadside.[70]

Even parts of the Irish Brigade had fared poorly in the grueling march. "The Major of one battalion of our brigade turned round to give orders to his men and found he had but one man to command," related Color Sgt. Peter Welsh of the 28th Massachusetts Volunteer Infantry in a letter to his wife. Welsh had doggedly endured the march, but was

---

66. Muffly, *The Story of Our Regiment*, p. 534.
67. *Ibid.*
68. Rhodes, *The History of Battery B*, p. 197; Livermore, *Days and Events*, p. 236; Fuller, *Personal Recollections*, p. 92.
69. Thompson, *Personal Narrative*, p. 31.
70. Lambert journal, June 29, 1863; Galwey, *The Valiant Hours*, pp. 97-98.

"the only man of my company that was able to cook coffe [*sic*] after we halted[.] i [*sic*] went over half a mile for water and had my supper before i [*sic*] lay down[.]"[71]

"When I awoke it was daylight," recalled Surgeon Potter in later years, "my horse had straggled off a little way, and was grazing in a clover field. I was alone, Capt Rose had gone, and I could see no troops anywhere; so I mounted my horse and rode on. I soon came across the regt, and then stopped at a farm house where I got breakfast, and fed my horse some grain purchased of a farmer. At this house I wrote a letter home at 5 o'clock A. M. which I mailed at Union Bridge, Md., a small village near by which was, however, called Uniontown in our orders."[72]

And what of the persistent Capt. Jeremiah Z. Brown and Pvt. David Polliard of the 148th Pennsylvania? The well-traveled potatoes proved to be quite delicious. "We had them for breakfast . . . the next morning."[73]

It was fortunate indeed that battle was not pending for Hancock's weary corps; the command was literally scattered along the entire length of the march route. "We lay at Uniontown all day—the 30th of June, awaiting the arrival of our stragglers. They came first a few at a time, then in squads, and towards noon it became almost a continuous stream. I do not remember ever having seen such a lame, stiff, footsore crowd as we gathered that day." "All day long the stragglers were coming up, and one by one rejoined their regiments. A motley, dirty crowd they were; for having fallen in their tracks and slept, an early start was made to find their camps, mostly without washing or cleaning."[74]

"Weather very hot; remained all day in bivouac, awaiting orders. During the day the lame ducks came up and rejoined their colors,"

71. Peter Welsh, *Irish Green and Union Blue: The Civil War Letters of Peter Welsh, Color Sergeant, 28th Regiment Massachusetts Volunteers*, eds. Lawrence Frederick Kohl and Margaret Cosse Richard (New York: Fordham University Press, 1986), p. 109.
72. Potter, *Three Years with the Army of the Potomac*, p. 57.
73. Muffly, *The Story of Our Regiment*, p. 798.
74. Thompson, *Personal Narrative*, p. 31; Frederick, "Dedication of Monument," p. 419; Potter, *Three Years with the Army of the Potomac*, p. 57.

added Captain Favill caustically, not the least bit footsore since he had ridden with General Zook the entire length of the previous day's march.[75]

As the men gathered for morning roll call, the following congratulatory message was publicly read:

HEADQUARTERS, SECOND ARMY CORPS,
June 29, 1863.

Circular

The major-general commanding the corps thanks the troops under his command for the great exertion they have made this day in achieving a march of a full thirty-three miles.

This severe labor would have only been exacted of them from urgent necessity.

It was required by the Major-General commanding the Army, who has expressed his appreciation of the manner in which the duty has been performed.

(Signed,) Major-General HANCOCK
By order of
W. G. Mitchell,
ADC, AAAG

There is no record that the weary troops received the reading of this missive with any great enthusiasm.[76]

The business of the army had to continue, fatigue or no. "We took advantage of this time to make the regular monthly muster. I wrote my four rolls sitting by a stone fence," remembered Captain Thompson, "and resting my paper on a flat rock." Captain Livermore had slightly better office facilities for his paperwork: "We sat down on the ground and wrote upon cracker boxes, and I believe that I completed a rather dirty and perhaps incomplete roll, as it seems to me that our baggage was not up with us, so that we could not get at our books, though it may have been otherwise." The Second Corps happily mustered for pay in the afternoon while resting in their camps, an event that helped the men focus on something other than their aching feet and stiff muscles.[77]

---

75. Favill, *Diary of a Young Officer*, p. 242.
76. Rhodes, *The History of Battery B*, pp. 197-98. Mitchell served as Hancock's aide de camp and acting assistant adjutant general.
77. Thompson, *Personal Narrative*, p. 31; Livermore, *Days and Events*, p. 236; Kepler, *Fourth Ohio Volunteers*, p. 123.

Some of the men availed themselves of the lull in marching, and a pocketful of crisp army scrip, to visit the hamlet of Uniontown. William J. Burns of the Philadelphia Brigade jotted his impressions down in his diary that night: "Visited the town—plenty of fresh bread, cakes, pies—plenty of cherries along the route." The largess of the citizens seemed to know no bounds, and bottles of alcohol, no doubt intended for medicinal purposes only, were shortly making their way through some regiments. "Whiskey is very abundant round here," noted one soldier, in a masterpiece of understatement.[78]

In retrospect, many of the men were mystified by the harshness of the June 29 march. "I cannot see any use of it, as when the Brigade arrived[,] it was composed almost solely of those who rode," wrote 8th Ohio hospital steward Charles H. Merrick to his sister. "In our Regiment there was only nineteen men by actual count. Some companies [were] not represented at all. But the Generals[,] I suppose[,] will see that the papers make a great blow about the wonderful march. . . ."[79]

Except for the final move to Gettysburg on July 1, the marathon march of June 29 was the culmination of a series of large scale movements of the Second Corps since the departure from Falmouth. One artillerist, keeping a running total of the distance covered by the corps, noted down in his June 30 entry: "We have marched one hundred and thirty-nine miles since the fourteenth of June."[80]

The cumulative effect of these grueling marches would have a far reaching impact on the abilities of the men to hold up under the rigors of the coming battle. "It is said that 1,000 men in the Second Corps were physically disabled for weeks thereafter," said Rev. Gilbert Frederick, D.D. (a captain of the 57th New York Volunteers in 1863) to a regimental reunion twenty-six years later. "Even many who went into the battle of Gettysburg, and did good service under its stimulus, after it was over

78. William J. Burns diary, June 30, 1863, Philadelphia Brigade Vertical File, Gettysburg National Military Park; Reichardt, *Diary of Battery A*, p. 94.

79. Charles H. Merrick, letter to his sister Min Merrick, July 1, 1863, William P. Palmer Collection, Container 1, Folder 3, MSS 3088, Western Reserve Historical Society, Cleveland, Ohio.

80. Reichardt, *Diary of Battery A*, p. 94.

were sent to the hospitals at Washington and Baltimore for general repairs."[81]

"Details of the approach to Gettysburg are given to throw light upon the worn out condition of our men from long marches, loss of sleep, lack of rations, which were largely consumed from issue made before starting; absence of supply trains far to the rear; no commissary to fall back upon except the haversack," chronicled one regimental historian. "[These] will give the civilian an idea how far spent the physical man was when we went into the fight and kept it up three days."[82]

"The previous March of the corps from Falmouth was unusually severe," wrote Surgeon Justin Dwinelle, who would serve as chief surgeon of the Second Corps Hospital in the days ahead, "and it suffered greatly from dust, heat, and protracted marches. The endurance of the men was remarkable considering it was their first march of any account after the winter's encampment. We can but conclude that after the battle the men were much exhausted and but illy prepared to bear up under the shock of wounds, and the subsequent exhaustion of the System."[83] Only the coming days would prove just how perceptively accurate Dr. Dwinelle's assessment was.

---

81. Frederick, "Dedication of Monument," p. 419.
82. Muffly, *The Story of Our Regiment*, p. 171.
83. Dr. Justin Dwinelle, Manuscript report of the Second Corps Hospital operations during the Battle of Gettysburg, MSC 129, National Library of Medicine, Bethesda, Maryland [hereafter cited as *Medical Report*].

CHAPTER 1

TUESDAY, JUNE 30: EVENING — WEDNESDAY, JULY 1: MIDNIGHT

"I'll die first" . . . "so will I"

Men of the 4th Ohio

With still no word from Quartermaster Batchelder about his tentative appointment as the chief of the Second Corps Ambulance Corps, nineteen-year-old Captain Livermore immersed himself in the daily routine of army life. "In the evening of June 30 I was sent on picket. My picket line was in a wheatfield about half a mile from our bivouac, and that part which came under my command was perhaps a quarter of a mile long. The wheat was tall and ripe and afforded luxurious resting-places for those who were permitted to lie down. My own post was at a farmer's house with a few men held in reserve. The farmer, notwithstanding his wheat was sadly being injured by our tramping, was very friendly and insisted upon my coming into his house to sleep, which would have been a luxury, but I did not deem it compatible with discipline or duty when my command were outdoors and in front of the enemy, so I lay on his barn floor with hay or straw for a couch with the rest, which itself was far better than what I had been accustomed to for some time."[1]

The circumstances of life, however, were about to drastically change for the young New Hampshire officer. "In the middle of the night, Lieutenant Dan Cross, who was serving on the staff (at division headquarters, I think), came around to my post and informed me that I was appointed as chief of ambulances of the corps. The news,

1. Livermore, *Days and Events*, p. 237.

although not surprising, was grateful. In the morning, before or about daylight, the farmer invited me to breakfast with him, which I did, and his table was spread with all the preserves and sauces his house could muster, I should think, in honor of the occasion. As soon as I had finished, I bade the good soul good-bye, and collecting my command marched to camp."[2]

A distinctly frosty welcome was awaiting him at regimental headquarters. "When I got there an aide of Colonel Cross's staff came over and informed me that the colonel sent word that I was detailed as chief of ambulances of the corps, and I would report at the headquarters of the corps; that he had recommended another officer for the position, but as his recommendation had probably not reached corps headquarters yet, the detail had not been made, but as soon as it did I would doubtless be relieved, the propriety of which I would undoubtedly see. . . . I thought the latter part of his message needlessly and purposely calculated to remind me of my supposed powerlessness to oppose his wishes, and for the first and last time I was perhaps disrespectful to him, when I sent word to him, in answer to his suggestion that I doubtless would see the propriety of my being sent back on his recommendation, that I didn't see it [at all]."[3]

The choice of the conscientious Livermore over another officer would prove to be a most fortunate one for the many Second Corps wounded in the horrific days of July that lay just ahead. Unfortunately, his raw inexperience would also directly lead to the death of a number of men through a bizarre chain of events.

Captain Thompson found that "the morning of July first was one of those periods of uncertainty as to the whereabouts of the enemy which generally precedes a great battle. The signal corps had been flashing orders from the hill tops all night and we were under arms by dawn. Yet we were not moved until near nine A.M., and then our brigade, which had led the Corps from Monocacy was ordered to guard the Corps wagon train in the rear," taking over for the frazzled 4th Ohio and their companions in the Gibraltar Brigade. "We had taken this position and had marched some distance when, by the rapid dashing about of aides from the General Staff, and the rapid change of direction of the wagon

2. *Ibid.*
3. *Ibid.*

train, which was started on the run to the rear, we knew something was up. . . ."[4]

Something was indeed up. The Second Corps had been ordered to march the remaining seven miles to Taneytown on July 1st, where army headquarters were located, or to press on to Gettysburg or Emmitsburg, as the situation demanded. "At eleven o'clock, A.M. on that day, the 2nd Corps was halted at Taneytown, which is thirteen miles from Gettysburg, South; and there awaiting orders, the men were allowed to make coffee and rest." As the corps reached Taneytown, "it stacked arms and prepared to bivouac on the supposition that its days work was done."[5]

Initial reports of an unplanned clash just up the road at Gettysburg were already beginning to filter in to army headquarters. When General Hancock reported to his commanding officer as the Second Corps settled in at its new camp, General Meade took the opportunity to extensively brief him concerning his overall strategy of the campaign. After detailing his plans to mass the army behind Pipe Creek, just south of Taneytown, Meade dismissed the Second Corps commander.[6]

Events were about to take a very dramatic turn, however. Back at the Second Corps bivouac, "the men were busy preparing their coffee when a mounted officer came through the camp at a furious pace. His horse was reeking with perspiration, and both horse and rider gave unmistakable evidence that they were the bearers of portentous news. All eyes were turned on the ominous messenger as he dashed up to corps headquarters, flung himself from his saddle, and delivered a message to the corps commander."[7]

---

4. Thompson, *Personal Narrative*, p. 32.
5. Frank L. Byrne and Andrew T. Weaver, eds., *Haskell of Gettysburg: His Life and Civil War Papers* (Kent, Ohio: The Kent State University Press, 1989), pp. 98-99; reprint, New York: Bantam Books, 1992), p. 149; Azor H. Nickerson, "Personal Recollections of Two Visits to Gettysburg," *Scribner's Magazine*, vol. 14, no. 1 (1893): 19; Tucker, *Hancock the Superb*, pp. 130-31; Isaac R. Pennypacker, *General Meade* (New York: D. Appleton and Company, 1901), p. 150; Hancock, *Reminiscences of Winfield Scott Hancock*, p. 188.
6. *Report of the Joint Committee on the Conduct of the War, 2nd Session, 38th Congress*, 2 vols. (Washington, D.C.: Government Printing Office, 1863, 1865; reprint New York: Kraus Reprint Company, 1977), Gen. Winfield Scott Hancock, March 22, 1864, vol. 1, pp. 403-4; Gen. George Gordon Meade, March 5, 1864, vol. 1, p. 330. [Hereafter cited as *Conduct of the War*.]
7. Nickerson, "Personal Recollections of Two Visits to Gettysburg," p. 19.

The messenger was Capt. Stephen M. Weld, staff aide to Maj. Gen. John Reynolds of the First Corps, who had been detailed by his commander to ride posthaste to army headquarters with the news of heavy Confederate forces at Gettysburg. "The enemy are advancing in strong force, and I fear they will get to the heights beyond town before I can," relayed the First Corps commander. Reynolds' parting words to his courier emphasized the extreme urgency of the situation: "Don't spare the horse—never mind if you kill him."[8]

As Captain Weld now stood before General Meade, the enormous threat posed by the presence of the entire Confederate army at a major crossroads directly between the Union Army of the Potomac and Washington, D.C. was clearly evident. "Good God!," exclaimed Meade; "if the enemy gets Gettysburg, we are lost." Only minutes later, a dispatch arrived from Brig. Gen. John Buford, a Union cavalry commander heavily engaged with the enemy forces: "I am positive that the whole of [Lt. Gen.] A. P. Hill's force is advancing." While General Meade was busy pondering these messages, Maj. William Riddle, General Reynolds' aide-de-camp, arrived at headquarters with the sobering news of the death of the First Corps commander. This news shook Meade to his very core—not only was Reynolds' a trusted army commander, but a close personal friend as well.[9]

It was time to act, and act decisively. With Army chief-of-staff Maj. Gen. Dan Butterfield in tow, Meade paid a surprise visit to Hancock's headquarters. It was clear that the fighting was rapidly escalating into a major battle outside of Gettysburg; Meade immediately dispatched Hancock to the crossroads village at 1:10 p.m. to "assume command of the corps there assembled, viz., the Eleventh, First [both at Gettysburg], and Third, at Emmitsburg . . . in consequence of the death of Major-General Reynolds." The commanding general chose to remain behind for the time being, apparently still hoping that the main action would take place along the easily defensible terrain of Pipe Creek.[10]

---

8. George Gordon Meade, *The Life and Letters of George Gordon Meade, Major General United States Army*, ed. George Gordon Meade, 2 vols. (New York: Charles Scribner's Sons, 1913), vol. 2, p. 35.
9. *Ibid.*; Stephen Minot Weld, *War Diary and Letters*, (Boston: Privately Published, 1912), pp. 231-32; Freeman Cleaves, *Meade of Gettysburg* (Norman: University of Oklahoma Press, 1960; reprint, Dayton, Ohio: Morningside Press, 1980), p. 135; *OR*, vol. 27, pt. 1, p. 702; James C. Biddle to General Alexander S. Webb, November 31, 1886, Alexander S. Webb Collection, Yale University.
10. Coddington, *The Gettysburg Campaign*, pp. 284-85; Byrne and Weaver, *Haskell of Gettysburg*, p. 99; *Report of the Joint Committee on the Conduct*

"Hancock always was the most energetic and impetuous of generals," remembered one of his soldiers. "In the execution of an order he imparted his vigorous personality to everything and everybody about him, from the chief of staff to the orderly who brought him his horse. . . . It did not seem to us that a minute had elapsed from the time the messenger arrived before we received the order to 'fall in;' and even while our ranks were being formed, the general with his whole staff, dashed out upon the road toward Gettysburg."[11]

After transferring command of the corps to Brig. Gen. John Gibbon of the Second Division, Hancock clattered away in an ambulance with a "poor little map" of the Gettysburg area spread out before him, studying the terrain he would soon be called upon to defend, and mulling over Meade's proposed battle plans. His personal staff—Second Corps chief-of-staff Lt. Col. Charles H. Morgan, Maj. William G. Mitchell, a few personal aides, and a small group of signal officers—mounted up to ride escort as the ambulance disappeared up the road to Gettysburg.[12]

The medical vehicle proved slow transport for the impatient Hancock, and he soon folded up the map, and called for his horse. He quickened the pace towards the crossroads town, sharply scanning the topography for any tactical advantages. Four miles south of Gettysburg, the group encountered traffic coming the opposite direction—it was an ambulance bearing the body of First Corps commander John Reynolds, accompanied by one solitary outrider. Reminded anew of the serious job ahead, the general and his staff rode on in total silence until they reached the battlefield.[13]

Back in Taneytown, while the 4th Ohio was halted, "an order [was] read notifying us of the resignation of [Maj.] General [Joseph] Hooker and the appointment of General Meade as Commander in Chief of the

---

of the War, Gen. Winfield Scott Hancock, March 22, 1864, vol. 1, pp. 403-5; Meade, *Life and Letters*, vol. 1, p. 330.

11. Nickerson, "Personal Recollections of Two Visits to Gettysburg," p. 19.
12. *Report of the Joint Committee on the Conduct of the War*, Gen. Winfield Scott Hancock, March 22, 1864, vol. 1, pp. 403-5; *OR*, vol. 27, pt. 1, pp. 367-68; Hancock, *Reminiscences of Winfield Scott Hancock*, p. 188.
13. Francis A. Walker, *History of the Second Army Corps in the Army of the Potomac* (New York: Charles Scribner's Sons, 1886), pp. 265-66; Hancock, *Reminiscences of Winfield Scott Hancock*, p. 188.

Army of the Potomac, also urging the duty of defending our homes and driving back the invaders. . . . The men seemed to think the order too tame, and we ought to *destroy* the invader instead of driving him back. There was an apparent distrust on the part of the men, who had always seemed more anxious for 'real business' than their general officers." With that formality out of the way, the men moved out on the road to Gettysburg.[14]

Being assigned to the ambulance corps, and actually finding the ambulance corps in the hodgepodge of wagon trains on the road, would prove to be two entirely different things. "I hurriedly donned my dress coat, packed my valise, and hastened to corps headquarters," wrote Captain Livermore of that exciting day. "When I got there I found the camp struck and the general and his staff gone, as the corps was already on the march, but luckily Colonel Batchelder was there, and seeing me, he at once in the kindest manner furnished me one of his horses and directed me where to find my command, which was on the route with the corps. I mounted and rode ahead at a rapid rate past troops and trains to find my train."[15]

Livermore was still marveling at his good fortune. "My feelings were certainly as buoyant and cheerful, with this change in my circumstances, as they ever were afterwards at any promotion. My legs were still sore from tramping in the column; I had just arisen from a barn floor which was far more comfortable than my usual bed; I had for a writing-desk but the day before the end of a cracker box; the mess I had left was neither inviting nor bountiful, and I was lucky to see my valise with spare clothing once in two or three days; my command was thirty men, and my wishes were bounded in their effects by my company limits. But now, speeding away on a spirited and strong-limbed horse, I looked at marches with indifference. I knew that my quarters would be in comparatively spacious tents at headquarters of the corps; that my baggage would be with me every night; my bed would be comfortable; my mess far better than I had known; my command two or three hundred men, a dozen officers, and a large train; and my position in all respects far more comfortable than that I had held."[16]

---

14. Kepler, *Fourth Ohio Volunteers*, pp. 123-24.
15. Livermore, Days and Events, p. 238.
16. *Ibid.*

"The duties of chief of ambulances I had only been informed about in a general way. I knew that he had a general direction of all the trains; that he was to see that every one in his command were busied in gathering the wounded; and that he was to superintend discipline in general. I had also shared in a feeling prevalent among the infantry that the men and officers of the ambulance train habitually kept away from danger and only came up to get the wounded when they could in safety; and certainly as far as my own regiment was concerned, I think we never had seen the ambulance men near us in a fight, and our wounded had shifted for themselves until well out of range unless our own musicians or men had carried them away. From what I subsequently learned I am satisfied that at Chancellorsville, at least, Lieutenant Anderson and his command had behaved in the bravest manner, but at the time I took command I had fully made up my mind to make the ambulance corps learn what fighting was from actual experience."[17]

The captain was making excellent time along the crowded road, and soon drew up on the headquarter trains. "The column was on the road to Taneytown, and at a point several miles southeast of that place I reached my train and, passing to the head of it, found the officer in command, Lieutenant Sullivan, and took command. He was pleasant and imparted information to me as I inquired about details of conducting the affairs of the corps." So, moving toward battle, Livermore set out to learn all he possibly could about his new command in the shortest amount of time.[18]

Strict orders had been issued in the Second Corps forbidding foraging in the friendly countryside. One notable exception to this order was the case of Jacob H. Cole of the 57th New York Volunteers. "As we were nearing Gettysburg a flock of geese came near the road and, as is usual with geese, they commenced to hiss. As they all looked plump and fat, I could not resist the temptation to run my bayonet through one. As I did so General Zook [commander of Cole's brigade, and boyhood friend of General Hancock] happened to ride up, and seeing me with the goose on my bayonet, he drew his sabre and spurred toward me, pretending to strike me. I did not wait, but with the

17. *Ibid.*
18. *Ibid.*

goose still on the bayonet started on the double quick to my company. After getting among the boys I took the goose off the bayonet and carried it in my hands until I reached camp."[19]

Drummer George Washington Lambert of the 14th Indiana, reunited now with the First Brigade band, and triumphantly playing his repaired drum, was making his way through the tiny hamlet of Harney. A festive spirit pervaded the town; townsfolk flocked to their front yards to witness this incredible event, and to pass comments back and forth.

"Ah me!," marveled one; "I can't begin to see the end of 'em." "La me," replied his neighbor; "I guess we will get to see something now." The citizenry gaped at the specter of an ambulance rolling by against the current of marching men, one lone outrider providing a somber escort. The band moved to the side to let the vehicle pass, soberly looked in at the body of General Reynolds, then mutely marched on.[20]

As the ambulance passed through the 148th Pennsylvania Volunteers, Pvt. George W. McIlhattan of Company G was heard to mutter, as much to himself as to his fellow soldiers: "Boys, if the rebels are killing Generals they will not have much respect for us little fellows."[21]

Galvanizing news was filtering back from the front of the column of the clash at Gettysburg. "Everyone turned to his neighbor to know what had occurred or was occurring. The answer sped through the ranks with the speed and shock of an electric current: 'The battle is on at Gettysburg; General Reynolds has been killed; General Meade has ordered Hancock to go at once to the front to assume command, representing him'—the corps to follow as fast as its many legs could carry it."[22]

---

19. Jacob H. Cole, *Under Five Commanders*, p. 190.
20. Lambert journal, July 1, 1863, Indiana Historical Society.
21. Muffly, *The Story of Our Regiment*, p. 716.
22. Nickerson, "Personal Recollections of Two Visists to Gettysburg," p. 19. It seems highly unlikely that all of these facts were known to the troops at the time—Nickerson, writing years later, apparently lumped them all together in his memory.

"A new spirit animated our stiff and footsore corps and we started with all speed for the front. We made a forced march that afternoon, the length of which I never knew," wrote Captain Thompson in retrospect; "but we were marched under General Meade's especial orders and fared well compared with our previous experience. We marched three miles and rested five minutes alternately. Two of my men were barefooted—their feet swollen so badly they could not get their shoes on, but those men came into camp that night, one to meet his death the next day and the other to be disabled by a sword on the third instant. I was suffering considerable from varicose veins and swollen limbs, but was greatly helped by the adjutant, who several times dismounted and gave me a rest on his horse's back."[23]

Others in the column were using their horses to aid the footsore marchers. William Henry Stevens, the Methodist Episcopal chaplain of the 148th Pennsylvania, had once again made his mount available to the weary men of his regiment, and ended up walking much of the thirty-five miles to Gettysburg with the soldiers of his regiment. "The heat was intense and the dust several inches deep, rising and settling everywhere and filling the eyes, ears and throat." The thoughtful chaplain also carried the muskets and gear of the men to spell them as they slogged doggedly onward toward the distant sound of firing.[24]

"The column moved rapidly forward; there was no straggling, no need of commands, no urging to 'close-up;' the ripening cherries and apples, and the abundance of forage, enticed but few from their places; every man was ready to do his duty, now that he knew it as never before, no difference who was in command. Soon the booming cannon could be heard and the smoke seen rising to the right of the two spurs toward which we were hastening. Little was said; every one was thinking. . . ."[25]

The ambulance with the remains of General Reynolds, still accompanied by its solitary mounted attendant, continued its spectral journey back along the Second Corps route of march, a ghostly forerunner of horrors soon to come. "About the middle of the afternoon we met the body of General Reynolds," wrote another

23. Thompson, *Personal Narrative*, p. 32.
24. Muffly, *The Story of Our Regiment*, p. 197.
25. Kepler, *Fourth Ohio Volunteers*, p. 124.

witness to this grisly vehicle from Gettysburg; "none were disposed to ask questions; but little could be learned, save that he was killed early in the action, and that nearly the entire of Lee's force was at Gettysburg. There was profounder silence than ever; no more jokes, and as usual before a battle, hundreds of playing cards were strewn along the road."[26]

Captain Livermore had been making good use of the march toward Gettysburg, pumping every bit of information on the Second Corps ambulance corps out of the officer from whom he had assumed command. Livermore had to work fast, for taking over so crucial a command in the face of battle carried with it the responsibility for thousands of lives. And there was a great deal to learn.

"The ambulance corps consisted of three trains, one for each division of the army corps. Each train consisted of forty two-horse ambulances (in the proportion of three ambulances to each regiment, I think), with a few for the artillery, several wagons with four horses to carry forage and rations in, and a forge wagon for repairs and horseshoeing, with several old-style four-horse ambulances. The men were selected proportionately from the regiments, and consisted of a driver for each ambulance and wagon, two stretcher-carriers for each wagon, and several blacksmiths and supernumeraries. The train of each division was commanded by a first lieutenant, and under him were a second lieutenant from each brigade in the division (three in all usually, never over four), and a sergeant from each brigade, the lieutenants and sergeants all being mounted. The total force of the ambulance corps was, in round numbers, 13 officers, 350 to 400 men, and 300 or more horses, with a little over 100 ambulances and 10 or 12 forage and forge wagons; and these were my command."[27]

---

26. *Ibid.* The practice of card playing and gambling were seriously deprecated by the morality of the 1860s. When soldiers faced the prospect of upcoming combat and the possibility of being killed in battle, they often cleaned out their knapsacks of anything incriminating that might be sent home to grieving relatives. Having survived the clash, it was easy enough to secure a new set of playing cards.
27. Livermore, *Days and Events*, pp. 239-40. More specifically, the staff complement of an ambulance corps was one captain, three first lieutenants, nine second lieutenants, thirty-six sergeants, and three hundred and sixty privates. At Gettysburg, privates were armed with Colt Army model 1860

But despite the imposing number of personnel, horses and wagons, Livermore's command centered around the ambulance vehicle itself.[28] "Each two-horse ambulance was a stout spring wagon very much like an ordinary express or grocer's wagon, with sides a little higher than theirs along each side. Inside this wagon were two seats the whole length, like those of an omnibus, stuffed and covered with leather. Hinged to the inner edges of each of these seats was another leather-covered seat, which could be raised and supported horizontally on a level with the first seats, and, as they filled all the space between the first seats, thus made a couch on which three men could lie lengthwise of the ambulance. In the rear end of the ambulance under each seat was a water keg with the end out and containing a faucet, which contained fresh water for the wounded. In front, under the driver's seat, was a supply of beef stock, and I believe bandages and other hospital stores. On each side of the ambulance there was hung a canvas-covered stretcher to carry the wounded on, and the whole ambulance was neatly covered with white canvas on bows."[29]

.44 caliber revolvers. All officers and non-commissioned officers were mounted. [General Order No. 147, *OR*, vol. 11, pt. 1, pp. 217-29.]

28. The ambulance concept was an innovative step forward, having never been used in the United States prior to this war. Two years before the outbreak of hostilities, the United States Medical Board uncharacteristically fell in with the latest European concept of providing wagons set aside specifically for the transport of the sick and wounded. After field tests of a four-wheeled model received favorable reviews, the government mistakenly concluded that the two-wheeled model would provide better transport for the wounded, and immediately set about issuing four times as many two-wheeled ambulances as four-wheelers. It proved to be a wonderful pleasure carriage for officers on holiday, a splendid portable headquarters for general staff, but, unfortunately, a terrible conveyance for those in pain. Its design caused it to sway with a rocking motion absolutely excruciating to the battered men inside, and had a spring "suspension" that provoked soldiers to nickname them "avalanche" due to the jolting ride it provided. One soldier wrote that ambulances "shake what there is left of a fellow to jelly." Horace H. Cunningham, *Field Medical Services at the Battles of Manassas (Bull Run)*, University of Georgia Monographs, no. 16 (University of Georgia Press, 1968), p. 3; Hannah Ropes, *Civil War Nurse, The Diary and Letters of Hannah Ropes*, ed. John R. Brumgardt (Knoxville: The University of Tennessee Press, 1980), p. 42.

29. Livermore, *Days and Events*, p. 240. Each regiment was allotted three ambulances (one four-horse and two two-horse) and a transport wagon. Only one two-horse ambulance was assigned to each artillery battery. Two two-horse vehicles were attached to corps headquarters. A sergeant oversaw ten privates (four drivers and six stretcher bearers) in each regimental detachment. [General Order No. 147, *OR*, vol. 11, pt. 1, pp. 217-19.]

The command that Livermore assumed was in excellent running order. "The horses were all good ones and well kept; the men were stout, and the officers were intelligent. Each division train was complete in itself and could, independently of the other, follow its own division, equipped to supply its own forage and rations, make its own repairs, and, in short, act alone. Each one had a separate organization and made a separate report. The lieutenant commanding each division train was responsible for the horses, wagons, and all its property, and made returns of them and the men to the chief of ambulances. The officers of each train camped, marched, and lived with it. . . . The ambulance trains of each division had been, by orders from army headquarters, put under the command of a captain who was to be attached to corps headquarters, and they were to be entirely free from the control of the division commanders, and it was to this position I had been appointed."[30]

It had been a crash course for Captain Livermore in ambulance protocol, and the accompanying responsibility that its commander now faced as he rode to Taneytown. "I learned that my duties were to direct the ambulance corps in all things, but that I was to be one of the staff of the general commanding the corps, and in matters relating to the care of property, discipline, marches, reports, etc., I was to receive orders from the general through the adjutant-general's chief quartermaster, and in matters pertaining to the collection, care, and transportation of the wounded I was to receive directions from the medical director. In practice I found that I was not only at liberty, when my duties about the ambulance corps permitted, to act as aide to the general on the march, in camp, and in battle, but my services as such were acceptable. My horses and horse equipment were to be furnished from my trains. . . . I did not learn all this at once upon joining the train as I have related, but found out enough to start with."[31]

Halting the ambulance corps in the outskirts of Taneytown, and drawing it up in park for the night, Livermore took the opportunity to ride into town. He found what he saw of the community to be "uninteresting," but was intrigued by the scurrying of multiple mounted officers around army headquarters. Livermore finally took conscious note of the faint background noise he had been hearing—"the sound of rapid artillery firing some miles ahead of us toward Gettysburg. . . ."[32]

30. *Ibid.*, pp. 240-41.
31. *Ibid.*, pp. 241-42.
32. *Ibid.*, p. 242.

As the head of the marching columns drew on toward Gettysburg, the going became increasingly difficult for the weary men of the Second Corps. "Early in the afternoon, we could see way off in the air, beyond the Round Top, bursting shells and clouds of smoke[,] and soon found the road blocked up with baggage wagons driven to the rear by panic-stricken drivers who with the greatest difficulty could be induced to give up the road to our artillery and ambulances."[33]

General Gibbon, left in command of the corps by Hancock, quickly resorted to more direct methods when reason and logic failed to resolve the problem. "We had finally to tear down the fences and force the drivers, with drawn pistols, to park the wagons in the fields. Clearing the road in this way, vehicles and artillery traveled the road, whilst the infantry marched, when it could, in the open field alongside."[34]

This roadblock cleared, the corps continued to press on toward the ominous sounds of battle.

The sound of the firing was not lost on the men of the 4th Ohio. "We were passing over a rise of ground, whence the guns could be heard more distinctly and the smoke seen more clearly, when one of the boys, in a sad tone, remarked: 'What if they whip us this time?' Instantly a strong, manly voice replied, 'They won't; I'll die first.' 'Here, I,' added another; 'So will I,' said a third; immediately those in hearing closed up, four abreast, and thus it was through a considerable part of the regiment, keeping perfect step, seeming to shake the very earth with their determined tread. The 'Old Fourth' was ready to go into the jaws of death and compel a victory."[35]

Some men did indeed feel that this would be their final battle, and were busy making appropriate plans. Officers sold favorite horses, while men of all ranks made arrangements with friends to dispose of watches, keepsakes, valuables, or to send that dreaded letter to wife, sweetheart, or mother. One young Pennsylvanian had written a short note, and carried it with him as he marched toward his home state:

---

33. John Gibbon, *Personal Recollections of the Civil War* (New York: n.p., 1903; reprint, Dayton, Ohio: Morningside, 1978), p. 132.
34. *Ibid.*
35. Kepler, *Fourth Ohio Volunteers*, p. 124.

To all whom it may concern:

Should I, in the providence of God, be killed or seriously wounded, or in any way hurt while on this movement, please write a note to my dear father, Jacob Beidelman, Bloomburg, Pa., informing him of the fact; and may the Lord reward you for the same.

Yours truly,
George Washington Beidelman
Co C 1st Cala Regt[36]

"Die they did," grimly noted one regimental historian with the sharp clarity of hindsight, "some of our noblest."[37]

Ambulance commander Captain Livermore, upon hearing the faraway cannonade, quickly returned to his ambulances. "After a short halt our camp, which we had supposed was for the night, was broken, and the whole corps again took to the route. We marched through Taneytown and toward the quarter in which we heard the firing."[38]

Their resumed march soon took them on into Pennsylvania. Some Keystone units gave three cheers and rousing huzzahs for their home State when they spied the stone marker at the state line. Others felt that distinct differences, whether real or imagined, was immediately noticeable. "The face of the country in Pennsylvania was not as pleasing as in Maryland, and the people were not nearly as friendly toward us in their conduct, and it was said that some of our men paid them for water from their wells."[39]

The 4th Ohio, now the lead regiment, had the best view of what was ahead. As the day drew toward its close, "firing ceased, and no more smoke was seen to rise; our brigade was in advance of the corps; just at dark we met our Corps Commander, General Hancock, in whose generalship and judgment all had unbounded confidence; the column was halted a few moments after dark."[40]

---

36. Catherine H. Vanderslice, *The Civil War Letters of George Washington Beidelman* (New York: Vantage Press, 1978), p. 178. Early in the war, the 1st California Regiment was redesignated the 71st Pennsylvania. Many of the men, however, still proudly continued to refer to it by it's earlier name.
37. Kepler, *Fourth Ohio Volunteers*, p. 124.
38. Livermore, *Days and Events*, p. 242.
39. *Ibid.*
40. Kepler, *Fourth Ohio Volunteers*, p. 124.

Hancock quickly brought Colonel Carroll up to date on the present situation, concluding with the fact that "we could stack arms, rest for the night and take position early in the morning. Just as the General was riding away Carroll asked: 'General, have we a good position?' and received the instant reply, in a firm tone, 'If Lee does not attack before all our forces are up, we can hold the position against the whole Confederacy.'"[41]

After passing along orders to General Gibbon concerning the bivouac and deployment of the Second Corps, Hancock spurred southward to personally report on the July 1 action to General Meade.[42]

"We immediately marched into a meadow to the right of the road and a patch of woods near the foot of the two mountain spurs, and stacked arms. The evening was balmy and beautiful, though somewhat hazy, but with sufficient moonlight to enable one to discern any object." For the Buckeye troops, the long march to Gettysburg was over.[43]

Captain Thompson and his men found their camping ground nearby, but not nearly as idyllic. "As the sun was setting, we filed off the Taneytown road near Round Top into a piece of very broken ground covered with rocks, underbrush and a few trees. Without fire or lights we munched a few crackers and stretched our exhausted bodies on the ground for the night." Some regiments were not allowed fires, others were permitted to build only small ones due to the proximity of the enemy.[44]

Jacob H. Cole, still carrying his purloined goose, had just reached the place where the 57th New York was to bivouac when an order came to immediately report in person to General Zook, commander of the Third Brigade, First Division, Second Corps. "I went and he asked me about the goose, saying at the same time that he was surprised to think that one of his men would disobey orders, and again asked me why I had done so. I said, 'General, as we passed that flock of geese they

41. *Ibid.*, pp. 124-25.
42. Gibbon, *Personal Recollections*, pp. 132-33.
43. *Ibid.*, p. 125.
44. Thompson, *Personal Narrative*, p. 33; William J. Burns diary, July 1, 1863, Philadelphia Brigade Vertical File, Gettysburg National Military Park.

began to hiss at us and I knew at once they were rebels, and thought it my duty to capture a rebel at any time. I did so and have brought him to your headquarters, and now await your decision.'"

After a moment, no doubt trying to keep from laughing at Cole's quick improvisation, Zook announced his decision. "He said, 'You may leave your prisoner here and go to your tent.'" No doubt the general and his staff closely "interrogated" the "prisoner" in short order.

Heading back to camp without his choice prize, Cole set about the routine evening duties of the company. "As soon as we had halted for the night, the usual detail of men was made—some to get water, others to make fires, and others to do the cooking. I was one to get water, but lost my supper, as I was so tired I fell asleep while I was waiting for the supper to be cooked and did not wake up until called in the morning to get ready to take our position on the battlefield."[45]

"Everything was comparatively quiet; not a shot did we hear. Yet there was the lumbering roll of the artillery moving up to available positions for the morning and the loud shouts of men losing one another in the dark, in their search for water for their everlasting coffee. What would an American soldier do without his coffee?" mused Thomas Galwey of the 8th Ohio. These unfortunate troops had just settled for the night in bivouac when they were rousted up again and moved still further north to the area near Powers Hill.[46]

Being with the trains to the rear, Captain Livermore and his ambulances did not arrive until much later. "We continued our march until somewhere near midnight. When we halted I was directed to bring up ambulances for the general and staff to sleep in at the headquarters, which was near a house at the roadside."[47]

So the wearied men of the Second Corps, fatigued by yet another march, settled down for a brief, and for some their last, night of sleep in the fields and among the rocks of the Pennsylvania countryside.

45. Cole, *Under Five Commanders*, pp. 190-91.
46. Galwey, *The Valiant Hours*, p. 100.
47. Livermore, *Days and Events*, p. 242.

Part 2
The Battle

These were Hancock's men, the men of the Second Corps,
Eleven States were mixed there, where Minnesota stood
In battle-order with Maine, and Rhode Island beside New York.
The metals of all the North, cooled into an axe of war.

John Brown's Body
Stephen Vincent Benet

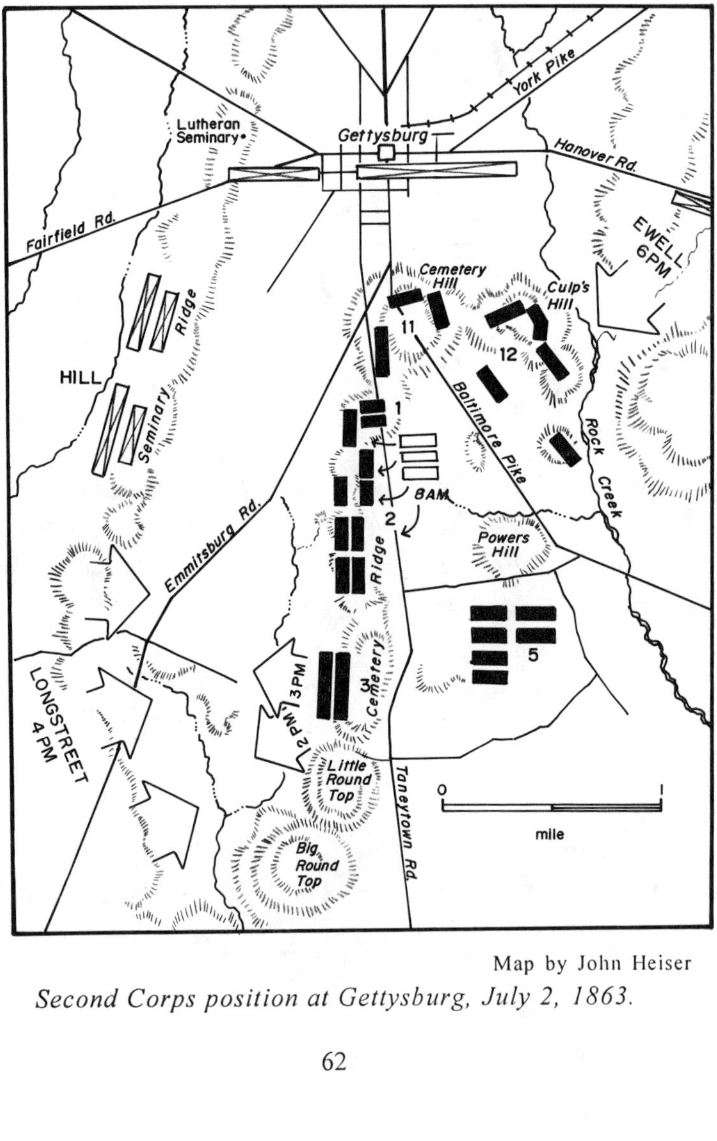

Map by John Heiser

Second Corps position at Gettysburg, July 2, 1863.

CHAPTER 2

WEDNESDAY, JULY 1: MIDNIGHT—THURSDAY, JULY 2: 8:30A.M.

"Ready for the reception of his wounded"

Dr. Richard Swanton Vickery

Not all of Hancock's corps found release and forgetfulness in sleep. Lt. Frank Aretas Haskell, staff aide to General Gibbon of the Second Division, had been busy directing troops into bivouac since nine o'clock on the evening of July 1. "The night before a great pitched battle, would not ordinarily, I suppose, be a time for much sleep to Generals and their staff officers. We needed it enough,—but there was work to be done.—This war makes strange confusion of night and day! I did not sleep at all that night. . . . At midnight Genl. Meade and Staff rode by Gnl. Gibbon's Head Quarters, on their way to the field; and in conversation with Gnl. Gibbon, Gnl. Meade announced that he had decided to assemble the whole army before Gettysburg, and offer the enemy battle there. The 2nd Corps would move at the earliest day light, to take up its position."[1]

For the exhausted soldiers, reveille came uncomfortably early on July 2. "We were roused from our slumbers at about 3 o'clock, ordered to get breakfast and to be ready to go to the front at quarter past four." "[We] made small fires of twigs to cook our coffee and bacon; [however,] we discovered that we were out of rations. I had lost my

1. Byrne and Weaver, *Haskell of Gettysburg*, pp. 102-3.

haversack in the hustle of the day before," lamented Captain Thompson, "and my breakfast, like that of many of my men, consisted of crackers and coffee—and it was the last until the afternoon of the Third."[2]

"We were all astir early in the morning and would have been on the road by daylight but for some detention caused by delay in the leading division," remembered General Gibbon, still in command of Hancock's Second Corps. "We got off, however, soon after, and to facilitate the march and shorten the column, the road was left, as before, to the artillery and ambulances, the infantry marching through the grain and grass fields on each side. In this way the corps reached the field about 6 o'clock."[3]

As usual, hurry up and wait were the order of the day. "We started soon after the hour designated, halted shortly after daylight—to the rear and left of Cemetery Hill—for more than an hour, awaiting orders; in the meantime there was a disposition to get a glimpse across the hill, 'to see how the land lay' and the position of the enemy; not much could be seen that might indicate the presence of an enemy save an occasional shot fired from a wheatfield, half a mile to the front and left of our positions." The Second Corps was "halted temporarily by the side of the Taneytown Road upon which it had marched, while some movements of other troops were being made, to enable it to take position in the order of battle."[4]

"The morning was thick, and sultry, the sky overcast with low, vapory clouds. As we approached all was astir upon the crests near the Cemetery, and the work of preparation was speedily going on. Men looked like giants there in the mist, and the guns of the frowning Batteries so big, that it was a relief to know that they were our friends."[5]

"I remember we went through a small piece of open timber, where our doctors were posted, and as we went by we shook hands with them, and exchanged little pleasantries," wrote Lt. Charles Fuller of the movement of his regiment up to the battleline. "I remember saying to them, 'We'll see you again later.' I tried to say this with a jaunty air, but down in my shoes I did not feel a bit jaunty. I think we all felt that this should be a death grapple. . . ."[6]

---

2. Kepler, *Fourth Ohio Volunteers*, p. 126; Thompson, *Personal Narrative*, pp. 33-34.
3. Gibbon, *Personal Recollections*, p. 133.
4. Kepler, *Fourth Ohio Volunteers*, p. 126; Byrne and Weaver, *Haskell of Gettysburg*, p. 103.
5. Byrne and Weaver, *Haskell of Gettysburg*, p. 103.
6. Fuller, *Personal Recollections*, p. 92.

After pausing briefly, the corps "moved up and took position, its right resting upon the Taneytown Road at the left of the Eleventh Corps and extending in a line thence (nearly a half a mile) almost due south toward the Round Top, with its divisions in the following order, from right to left: the 3d, Gnl. Alex. Hays;—the 2nd (Gibbon's) Gnl. [William] Harrow, (temporarily) [since Gibbon was given command of the corps when General Hancock rode forward to Gettysburg];—the 1st, Gnl. [John C.] Caldwell. The formation was, in line by brigade in column, the brigades being in colum [*sic*] by regiment, with forty paces interval between regimental lines. . . . The intervals between them, some of which were left wide, [were] for the posting of the batteries. . . . Five Batteries, in all twenty-eight guns, were posted. . . . I have been thus specific in in [*sic*] the description of the posting and formation of the 2nd Corps," wrote staff aide Haskell with some satisfaction, "because they were works that I assisted to perform; and also that the other Corps were similarly posted with reference to the strength of the lines, and the intermixing of Infantry and Artillery."[7]

"At sunrise we [111th New York] were marched to our place in line, just in rear of the brow of Cemetery Hill and to the left of the Eleventh Corps. We inspected and cleaned our arms, had every man supplied with cartridges and waited for the fight to begin." "About 8 o'clock the brigade [First Brigade of the Third Division] was formed in line of regiments, right in front, with the Fourth Ohio in advance; marched forward into position. . . . Men soon busied themselves getting their arms in the best possible order, blankets and cartridge-boxes into comfortable position."[8]

"These dispositions were all made early, I think before eight o'clock, in the morning," wrote Lieutenant Haskell; "skirmishers were posted well out all around the line, and put in readiness for battle." Some of those skirmishers were men of the 4th Ohio. Their flankers, along "with two other companies, were sent across and down the hill, under the direction of Colonel Carroll, and took position near the Emmitsburg Road, where they remained until relieved by [companies] G and I and the Eighth Ohio."[9]

---

7. Byrne and Weaver, *Haskell of Gettysburg*, pp. 106-7.
8. Thompson, *Personal Narrative*, p. 34; Kepler, *Fourth Ohio Volunteers*, p. 126.
9. Byrne and Weaver, *Haskell of Gettysburg*, p. 108; Kepler, *Fourth Ohio Volunteers*, p. 126.

"Orders were issued that no man or officer should show himself on the hill. In the main it was observed, but knots of officers would get up where they could see and as surely find themselves a target for a shell from the enemy." Time had begun to drag, and the men sought anything to occupy their attention. "A sharpshooter had made his burrow behind a stump in front of our regimental line," wrote Captain Thompson, "and a few of us who had ventured over there began to question him about his—to me—novel arm. Said he—'Put your field glasses to your eyes—Yes—do you see that single horseman just coming out of the woods which covers the enemy? Well, keep your eyes on him.' He discharged his piece and in a moment that horseman, so far away that we could hardly distinguish him with the naked eye, dropped from his steed with a Yankee bullet in his body. Our group, and perhaps, that shot, brought a shell which fell in the regiment. Fortunately it did not explode, but it created quite a sensation . . . it had only gone through our bass drum and knocked a knapsack into a bundle of rags."[10]

So the men of the Second Corps occupied themselves as best they were able, waiting to see what the day would bring.

Captain Livermore was up early, intent on getting his command fully prepared for the coming conflict. "We were roused before light, and in march of a mile or so we reached the open country in the rear of the cemetery of Gettysburg and there our corps went into line of battle. As I rode up on this ground I saw many troops moving around, cooking coffee and getting breakfast near their stacked arms."[11]

Of primary importance was getting the Second Corps Ambulance Corps into position and ready to deal with any situation as it developed. "I placed the main portion of my train at a house on the right-hand side of the Taneytown road, around a house near which was an orchard. As this house was a little to the left of the left rear of the 1st Division, I think it was Mr. [Michael] Frye's [*sic*] or Jacob Swisher's or Sarah Patterson's. At any rate, it was a house of considerable dimensions and its vicinity afforded clear ground for the park. As soon as the train was established, I sent up to the rear of each

10. Thompson, *Personal Narrative*, p. 34.
11. Livermore, *Days and Events*, p. 243.

division a detachment of ambulances, perhaps a dozen in number, and officers to direct them, and they sent stretcher-carriers to each brigade, having instructed the officers to have all the wounded brought to the house where the park was."[12]

To guarantee that the ambulances were ready, and, no doubt, to assure his own mind, Livermore personally toured the knots of parked ambulances scattered along the backside of Cemetery Ridge, checking that the kegs of water were topped off, the supply of beef stock was on board, bandages and the few other basic medical supplies were under the front seat, and that each had its two stretchers properly hung on the side. He also paused along the way to chat with the attendants, three privates for each ambulance, making sure that they knew their duties once the battle began. Satisfied by what he found, Livermore restlessly rode up to the ridge to check out the battlelines.[13]

The Second Corps Medical Department was also off to an early start on this July morning, checking out likely sites to set up medical facilities. But they were already laboring under a severe disability, even before the outbreak of day's hostilities. While the hospital wagons containing panniers of dressings, some medicines, surgical appliances, and medical equipment had already arrived, the supply wagons bearing all the cooking supplies, personal and hospital tents, basins, cots, blankets, and miscellaneous accoutrement did not come up to the field with the hospital. And they weren't simply delayed along the road, either.

On June 19, the number of medical wagons had been slashed, over Medical Director Jonathan Letterman's adamant protests, to just six per division by the then-commanding General Hooker. Letterman tried to maneuver around Hooker's order by creating a twenty-five wagon reserve supply train, under the command of Medical Purveyor Jeremiah B. Brinton. But when the newly-minted commanding general George Meade took charge, he ordered all trains except ambulances and ammunition, to the rear. There they camped between Union Mills and Westminster, Maryland, the division medical wagons as well as Brinton's reserve train. So much for getting around orders.

12. *Ibid.*
13. *Ibid.*, pp. 243-44.

On the second day of fighting, Meade ordered them even further back. As a military man, his primary concern was to win the battle while protecting all vulnerable equipment and supplies. He needed the roads open and available for the rapid movement of men and materiel to the front, or to the rear in case of battlefield disaster.

It was only "after much persuasion" that Meade allowed Letterman to bring up half the medical supply wagons to the battlefield. Letterman seethed: "Without proper means, the Medical Department can no more take care of the wounded than the army can fight a battle without ammunition. The Medical Department had these means, but military necessity deprived it of a portion of them, and would not permit the remainder to come to the field." Brinton and the reserve train drove hard, but they would not roll into Gettysburg until late on July 4; the rest of the Second Corps wagons would not appear until July 7—much too late for those who had died for lack of those very supplies. Letterman pointed out bitterly: "Lost supplies can be replenished, but lives lost are gone forever."[14]

With the hospital tents, cots, blankets, and baggage far to the rear around Westminster, Maryland, and the Taneytown Road running roughly parallel with the backside of Cemetery Ridge, the homes and farmsteads along the thoroughfare became prime hospital locations for appropriation by the Second Corps doctors.

One experienced assistant surgeon detailed the multitude of things that had to be considered when choosing a location for a field depot:[15]

---

14. Jonathan Letterman, M.D., *Medical Recollections of the Army of the Potomac.* (New York: D. Appleton and Co., 1866), p. 156.

15. Richard Swanton Vickery, although not serving with the Second Corps at Gettysburg, already had plenty of battlefield experience under his belt by the time he penned these words. Born in Ireland in 1831, Vickery studied medicine in Dublin before immigrating to the United States in 1851. In 1860, he enrolled in the University of Michigan's School of Medicine, but the coming of war interrupted his studies. Enlisting as a private in the 2nd Michigan, he worked with the hospital corps before becoming an assistant surgeon on August 8, 1862. His regiment served in the Peninsula Campaign, battled at Second Bull Run and Fredericksburg, helped capture Jackson, Mississippi, and defend Knoxville, Tennessee.

In the winter of 1863-1864, Vickery used the lull in fighting to complete his medical coursework at the University of Michigan. He detailed the nuts and bolts of contemporary field hospital work in his thesis "On the Duties of the Surgeon in Action," which appears here in part.

1) "It should be as near the Regiment as possible, so that the wounded may be promptly attended to."

2) "It should be as secure as possible from shot and shell. In these days of rifled small arms and artillery, it cannot be out of the range but by taking advantage of inequalities of the ground, getting behind some hill or knoll, comparative safety may be obtained and shelter from the heaviest fire: and there are few positions a Regiment can be in[,] in which a practiced eye will not discern some slight cover, close enough to be serviceable for that purpose. The advantages of this are that his attendants are cool and attentive to their duties, not watching the coming shot or shell with one eye and the patient with the other—that the wounded just in from the hot strife have a grateful feeling of safety, and are not agitated by seeing men fall around them—and last [but] not least, that the Surgeon himself, however brave, will be able to discharge his duty more clearly, steadily and quietly than if under direct fire. . . ."

3) "If he can establish himself where the Ambulances can drive up, it will save his stretcher bearers much work, and ensure that the wounded will be moved speedily to the Division Depot [hospital]."

4) "Other advantages which it would be well to look to in the selection of a site, though they are not indispensable, are water and shelter—such as trees or a building, if a storm or a hot southern sun should beat down on the field."

5) "If there is time it would be well also to have something laid on the ground to place the wounded on—such as straw, hay, corn stalks, or even pine tops or brush of any kind."[16]

After graduating in March of 1864, Vickery returned to his regiment in Virginia, participating in the battle of the Wilderness and the siege of Petersburg (where he was severely wounded on July 30 at the Crater). On September 1, he was promoted to surgeon of his regiment, but received a medical discharge on March 11, 1865. But he was back in the army by 1867 as an assistant surgeon, and there he would stay until his retirement in 1895 as a surgeon with the rank of major.

Even after departing the military, he continued to his medical career, serving as chief physician of the Soldiers Home in Hampton, Virginia, until shortly before his death in 1906 at Riverton, New Jersey. Bentley Historical Library, Michigan Historical Collections, University of Michigan at Ann Arbor, Michigan; reprinted as Richard Swanton Vickery, "On the Duties of the Surgeon in Action," ed. Albert Castel, *Civil War Times Illustrated*, vol. 17, no. 3 (June 1978), pp. 13-14.

16. Vickery, "On the Duties of the Surgeon in Action," pp. 18-19.

With these guidelines in mind, the Second Corps Medical Department headed up the Taneytown Road. Corps and divisional staff were intent on finding spacious sites with easy access, somewhat removed from the battle, for their division (and ultimately corps) hospitals. Assistant surgeons, each armed with his pocket case or "surgeon's field companion" of instruments, and accompanied by an orderly carrying hospital knapsacks filled with up to twenty pounds of aid station supplies, kept their eyes peeled for anything close-up to the rear of the battlelines that could be pressed into service as a temporary aid station.[17]

The first farm they encountered was that of Jacob Weikert, situated behind the Big and Little Round Tops on the west side of the road. This 102-acre farm, with its large bank barn, carriage house, and eight room stone house, had already been grabbed by the Fifth Corps surgeon-in-charge as a hospital site, so the Second Corps medical men kept on moving northward.[18]

Farther up the Taneytown Road, on the same side of the road just south of Blacksmith Shop Road, was the farmstead of Leonard Bricker and his family. Fifth Corps surgeons had also staked out this property, so the frustrated aid station men from the Second Corps continued to push on.[19]

They finally got lucky at the farm of Sarah Patterson, laying south of the Granite School House Road on the east side of the Taneytown Road. None of the other corps had moved into the buildings sitting well back from the road, so it was decided to locate the Second Division Hospital at the capacious stone barn and surrounding orchard. There was also enough room left over to set up a temporary aid station on the grounds.[20]

---

17. George Worthington Adams, *Doctors in Blue* (New York: Henry Schuman, Inc., 1952; reprint, Dayton, Ohio: Morningside, 1985), p. 66.
18. Edward L. Munson, M.D., Major, Medical Department, United States Army, "The Army Surgeon and His Work," *The Photographic History of the Civil War*, ed. Francis T. Miller, 10 vols. (New York: Review of Reviews co., 1911; reprint New York: Castle Books, n.d.), vol. 7, pp. 230, 236; Dr. Clinton Wagner, letter to George Torney, August 7, 1911, Gettysburg National Military Park. The Weikert farm would also be used by the Second and Third Corps as a hospital site, especially after the Fifth Corps moved back farther from the battle lines at about 9:00 a.m. on July 3. [See Chapter 7]
19. Gregory Coco, *A Vast Sea of Misery: A History and Guide to the Union and Confederate Field Hospitals at Gettysburg, July 1-November 20, 1863* (Gettysburg, Pennsylvania: Thomas Publications, 1988), p. 68.
20. Coco, *A Vast Sea of Misery*, p. 67.

Just to the north, in a curve of the Taneytown Road, lay the farm of the Jacob Swisher family. Appropriated by the doctors for an aid station, this was most probably one of the hospitals of General Alexander Hays' division. The Twelfth Corps had been eyeing the building the previous day, but had not located a dressing station there, so the Second Corps quickly snatched it up.[21]

Further to the north, also on the east side of the road, lay the small farm of Michael and Sarah Frey, tucked into the corner formed by the Granite School House Road and the Taneytown Road. The Third Corps had already claimed the property for one of their aid stations, so the surgeons had to look further up the road for medical sites. Captain Livermore, however, saw the potential of the smooth approaches and open land of the Frey, Swisher, and Sarah Patterson farms, and located his ambulance park in one of these three farmyards.[22]

Forty-year-old William Patterson and his forty-one-year-old wife Lydia fled their house on the east side of the Taneytown Road, about eight hundred yards north of the Granite School House Road, when it became obvious that they were within range of the Confederate artillery. The seventy-five acre farm, with its spacious barn, was a fine addition to the growing number of aid stations of the Second Corps.[23]

The Jacob Hummelbaugh home, across the road and just north of the Patterson homestead, was a modest frame-covered log house about 1100 yards up the road from the Granite School House Road and Taneytown Road junction. Hummelbaugh, a local shoemaker and farmer, and his family had hastily evacuated the house, leaving behind a partially consumed meal on the table in their hasty departure. It was here that Dr. Alfred T. Hamilton, 148th Pennsylvania, laid out his regimental aid station.[24]

The fieldstone home of the Peter Frey family, due north of the Hummelbaugh's, and under the shadow of Cemetery Ridge, was quickly seized by the 108th New York Infantry as a regimental primary station. Dr. Francis Wafer and several other surgeons laid out their medical supplies there, and prepared to receive the wounded.[25]

---

21. *Ibid.* These temporary field hospitals were known interchangeably as aid stations, dressing stations, primary stations, and advance depots. There were sixteen identified Union burials at the Swisher farm, many from Hay's division.
22. *Ibid.*, p. 66; Livermore, *Days and Events*, p. 243.
23. Coco, *A Vast Sea of Misery*, p. 65.
24. *Ibid.*, pp. 64-65; Muffly, *The Story of Our Regiment*, p. 172; Jacob Hummelbaugh Farm Vertical File, Gettysburg National Military Park.
25. Coco, *A Vast Sea of Misery*, p. 63.

The Frey's next-door neighbor was the widow Lydia Leister. The Union surgeons probably cast longing glances at the white clapboard house and outbuildings on the west side of the road, within eight hundred feet of the troops, yet comparatively sheltered by the ridge behind it. Unfortunately, the army's new commander, General Meade, had already set up his headquarters at the tiny farmhouse late on July 1, so the property was known to be off limits.[26]

The two-story log house of Widow Catherine Guinn was the closest Second Corps aid station to town, just south of the junction of the Emmitsburg and Taneytown Roads. Elderly "Katie" Guinn had little choice in the commandeering of her home since the battle lines were a scarce hundred yards to the west. Built in 1776, the house was taken over by Hays' division as a temporary aid station, with Dr. Harry M. McAbee overseeing the site.[27]

For those regiments without the shelter of a house, barn, or shed of their own, or even shared with another regiment, aid stations were set up in orchards, in groves of trees, and under the protecting cover of a scattering of rocks. All were intent on getting ready, before the shooting started in earnest, to receive the wounded men that surely would soon come staggering over the nearby ridge.[28]

After securing a location for the primary station, the assistant surgeon charged with supervising the facility set about preparing for the arrival of casualties. There were numerous details which the assistant surgeon needed to personally attend to when setting up his aid station: "He wants to have the wounded as they fall, picked up as rapidly as possible and brought to the Depot which he shall select, there to be cared for and dressed, and forwarded quickly to the Division Hospital in the rear."[29]

First priority was to check the status of his stretchers. "For a Regiment of five or six hundred men he should have at least four stretchers—those generally issued now with light canvas bottoms, and with transverse iron bars at the head and foot, the side poles being

26. *Ibid.*, pp. 62-63.
27. *Ibid.*, pp. 61-62.
28. William Warren Potter, "Reminiscences of Field-Hospital Service with the Army of the Potomac," *Buffalo Medical and Surgical Journal* (October/November 1889), pp. 15-16.
29. Vickery, "On the Duties of the Surgeon in Action," p. 16.

stout enough to be firm, are the best. They have not so much of that springing motion to every step of the bearers which is so disagreeable and sometimes torturing to the wounded man.... If it happens that there are no stretchers, blankets or shelter tents stretched between two poles will make a good substitute. Failing even these a man can be carried, though not so comfortably or so easily, on a blanket held by four men at the corners, or seated on the crossed arms of two stout men."[30]

The stretcher men were under the supervision of their officers on the battlefield side of their journey, and under the direction of the assistant surgeon at the aid station end of the trip. Their job was to care for the removal of the non-walking wounded from the field, giving no excuse for able-bodied soldiers to leave the field in order to help wounded comrades to the rear. Stretchermen were to move as rapidly and smoothly as possible, so that the wounded man was removed from the field promptly, and with a minimum of painful jostling. The litter teams also helped direct the walking wounded to the regimental aid station. "The stretcher bearers must be looked to, of whom there should be four to each stretcher. After reserving one or two of his Hospital attendants for other duties, he [the assistant surgeon] will have three or four of them act in this capacity. The Drum corps and the Regimental Band, if there is one, are always on the eve of a battle ordered to report to the Surgeon for duty, but the less he calculates on aid from them the better. With few exceptions, they are generally worthless as stretcher bearers, many of them being young lads incapable of such fatiguing duty. These may be sufficient while the wounded are but few and come in slowly, but more help will soon be required when the combat thickens and some dashing charge or close firing brings them to the rear by dozens. In that case the Surgeon will find the Pioneers [construction and engineering troops] the best and most reliable aid. Generally numbering about ten under charge of an experienced sergeant, all able-bodied men accustomed to standing fire, they form a really effective corps of stretcher bearers, and can generally be procured for that purpose if required on application to the Commanding Officer of the Regiment."[31]

---

30. *Ibid.*
31. *Ibid.*, pp. 16-17. Stretcher bearers, while ideally intended to provide quick removal of the wounded to medical facilities, were viewed with mixed feelings by the troops, who sarcastically called them "angels of mercy." Every regiment was required to provide anywhere from twenty-five to thirty men for stretcher duty. No intelligent regimental commander was about to give up that many top-notch soldiers; consequently, only those considered

With these basics under control, the aid station surgeon should next "see to the condition of his Hospital Knapsack with its dressings, ligatures [surgical thread], sponges, stimulants &c. . . ." The orderly would have begun unpacking the meager collection of supplies and equipment as soon as a site for the station was chosen. Pails, basins, and sponges were laid out for cleansing the wounds; lint, bandages, splints, and tourniquets were put to one side to bind up the injured; chloroform, opium, morphine, and a modest supply of whiskey were on hand to numb the pain.[32]

Finally, a last minute check of "his Instruments—a good pocket-case with perhaps a bullet forceps, being nearly all the instruments he is likely to need."[33]

"These things being all considered he [the aid station surgeon] is ready for the reception of his wounded. . . ."[34] Now all the men of the aid station could do was wait for the shooting to start.

Further to the south and barely to the rear of the aid stations, the division hospitals were getting ready to receive the wounded that would soon be forwarded from the assistant surgeons at the aid stations. The division field hospitals of the Second Corps were initially set up in an opening in the woods spreading back from the junction of the Taneytown and Granite School House Roads, with fluttering red or yellow flags marking them as medical facilities. All three of the divisional facilities were jointly headquartered at the Granite School

---

unusable in a fight were assigned. He would usually delegate loafers, rogues, cowards, musicians, or any other non-combatants, and it was not uncommon to see them heading to the rear immediately upon the sound of gunfire.

32. *Ibid.*, p. 19; Stewart Brooks, *Civil War Medicine* (Springfield, Illinois: Charles C. Thomas, 1966), p. 34. See Gordon Dammann, *Pictorial Encyclopedia of Civil War Medical Instruments and Equipment, Volume I* (Missoula, Montana: Pictorial Histories Publishing Company, 1983), p. 32.

33. Vickery, "On the Duties of the Surgeon," p. 19. A pocket or folding surgical kit was a roll up or fold up leather or cloth wallet. It contained sewn-in slots for scalpels and a very few of the most basic medical tools to administer emergency first aid on the field. See Dammann, *Pictorial Encyclopedia of Civil War Medical Instruments and Equipment*, pp. 25-28, and *Pictorial Encyclopedia of Civil War Medical Instruments and Equipment, Volume II* (Missoula, Montana: Pictorial Histories Publishing Company, 1988), pp. 58-59 for examples of pocket surgical kits.

34. Vickery, "On the Duties of the Surgeon in Action," p. 19.

House on Granite School House Road. Each division was encamped separately, radiating out to the south and west of the schoolhouse. "The Hospital of the Second Division was located before the battle commenced at the stone barn and orchard of Miss Sally [Sarah] Patterson on the Taneytown Road immediately in the rear of the Second Corps which occupied the left centre of the line of battle," reported Dr. Justin Dwinelle of the 106th Pennsylvania Infantry, surgeon-in-charge of the Second Division Hospital. "The Third Division Hospital was at a barn on the same road some forty rods to the right [of the Sarah Patterson farm], and the First Division Hospital was located at first to the right and rear of the Third in the edge of the woods near the stone School house."[35]

The division hospitals were alive by now with intense activity as the two enemy forces prepared for combat. The Army of the Potomac had been forced to learn by mid-1863 the value of pooling its resources and the knowledge of its surgeons in hospitals by brigade, or even division, rather than merely by regiment. The regimental compliment of medical staff varied, but most often was made up of one surgeon and one or two assistant surgeons.[36] The regimental hospital had been the standard in field care in the early part of the war, but grossly unsanitary conditions, uneven knowledge and skill of the few regimental medical men, lack of even rudimentary supplies in time of crisis, and refusal to treat wounded not from that particular regiment had led to the vastly improved care provided in the combined hospitals at Gettysburg.

The advent of Surgeon Jonathan Letterman as medical director of the Army of the Potomac had speeded along this change as he reorganized the commissary system to supply entire divisions rather than only individual regiments. Under the divisional hospital concept, one assistant surgeon from each regiment operated a dressing station immediately behind that regiment's front lines, while the remaining medical staff gathered at the division hospital. There the duties were divided up between the medical men.

While under the regimental hospital system any surgeon who felt like trying his hand at surgery was allowed. Now only one out of about fifteen doctors, and those only the most medically proficient, were on the actual surgical team in the divisional setup. This led to some hard feelings at first, but ultimately provided consistent, standardized care

35. Dwinelle, *Medical Report.*

36. A requirement of one regimental surgeon and two assistant surgeons would officially be mandated by an act of Congress later in the year.

within each hospital. (The regimental hospital did continue throughout the war, however, as the standard care facility for the sick and slightly wounded in Union armies).[37]

A surgeon-in-charge headed up each division hospital, and administered the division's medical care and all associated supervisory paperwork. He "will exercise general supervision, under the Medical Director of the Corps, over the medical affairs in his division. He will see that the officers are faithful in the performance of their duties in the hospital and upon the field, and that, by the ambulance corps, which has heretofore been so efficient, the wounded are removed from the field carefully and with dispatch. Whenever his duties permit, he will give his professional services at the hospital—will order to the hospital as soon as located all the hospital wagons of the brigades, the hospital tents and furniture, and all the hospital stewards and nurses. He will notify the Captain commanding the ambulance corps, or, if this be impracticable, the First Lieutenant commanding the Division ambulances, of the location of the hospital."[38]

To help carry the heavy bureaucratic load, two administrative aides, both assistant surgeons, were detailed to each divisional surgeon-in-charge. These staff members would actually oversee the hands-on, day-to-day functionings of the facility.

One assistant dealt primarily with the physical workings of the hospital—he oversaw the dispensary, hospital instruments, medicines, and stores; monitored the pitching of the tents (when available); and made sure that straw, fuel, water, blankets and other necessities were provided. After seeing that adequate shelter was provided, he then turned his attention to the hospital kitchen. To get it up and functioning, he had full access to all hospital mess chests and the emergency rations carried in the ambulances. "The supplies of beef stock and bread in the ambulances, and of arrowroot, tea, etc., in the hospital wagon, will enable him to prepare quickly a sufficient quantity of palatable and nourishing food. All the cooks, and such of the Hospital Stewards and Nurses as may be necessary, will be placed under his orders for these purposes."[39]

The other handled the mountains of forms, records, and reports generated by a field hospital and demanded by the bureaucracy of war, as well as maintaining the hospital record. It was his responsibility "to

37. Adams, *Doctors in Blue*, pp. 63-65, 88; Vickery, "On the Duties of the Surgeon in Action," p. 15.
38. *OR*, vol. 19, pt. 1, pp. 115-16.
39. *Ibid.*, p. 115.

keep a complete record of every case brought to the hospital, giving the name, rank, company, and regiment; the seat and character of injury; the treatment; the operation, if any be performed; and the result; which will be transmitted to the Medical Director of the Corps, and by him sent to this office. This officer will also see to the proper interment of those who die, and that the grave is marked with a head-board, with the name, rank, company, and regiment legibly inscribed upon it. He will make out two tabular statements of wounded, which the surgeon-in-chief of division will transmit within thirty-six hours after the battle, one to this office [Medical Director, Army of the Potomac] (by a special messenger, if necessary) and the other to the medical director of the corps to which the hospital belongs."[40]

Three of the most able regimental doctors in the division chosen for their "surgical skill, sound judgement, and conscientious regard for the highest interests of the wounded," and with no regard of rank or seniority, were detailed by the surgeon-in-charge to perform or supervise all major operations. "In all doubtful cases, they will consult together, and a majority of them shall decide upon the expediency and character of the operation." Three other medical officers were detailed to the surgical team, "to act as assistants to each one of these officers, who will report to him and act entirely under his direction. It is suggested that one of these assistants be selected to administer the anaesthetic." The senior man, known as the chief operator, headed up this six-man surgical team.[41]

Those doctors not actively involved in surgery would be setting up to serve as wound dressers and general assistants. Surgical instruments for both major and minor operations were being laid out. Operating tables were unloaded from the hospital wagon and set up under the shelter of trees, or in the shade of tarpaulins or shelter tents tied to branches or upright poles, to ward off the fierce rays of the July sun.

Meanwhile, the hospital stewards not assigned to aid stations would have the hospital medical chests open, laying out vials of stimulants, bottles of medicinal whiskey or brandy, and supplies for surgery. Water would be boiling over campfires for tea, coffee, and soup, and the hospital sponges would be put in to soak.[42]

---

40. *Ibid.*
41. *Ibid.*
42. Adams, *Doctors in Blue*, pp. 48, 66; Brooks, *Civil War Medicine*, p. 32. With 18 regiments in the First Division, and 13 regiments in each of the Second and Third Divisions, the Second Corps should ideally have had approximately 132 trained medical personnel to deal with the massive

The snafu with the medical wagon train, marooned far to the rear, began to be felt almost immediately, even as the division hospitals were being set up. "Our cooking department was early extemporized, We having to rely almost entirely for cooking utensils on the Farmers in the immediate vicinity. It was impossible to obtain rations from the commissary Dept, But by taking possession of the contents of a number of unclaimed haversacks and an Ox in an ajoining [*sic*] field with some Beef stock furnished from the ambulances, and small lots of provisions from several other sources, We were able to provide Tea & Coffee and Beef soup for all the wounded as fast as they arrived."[43]

Every conceivable contingency was taken into consideration, even the ever-present specter of ignominious defeat and rout. "Previous to an engagement, a detail will be made by Medical Directors of Corps of a proper number of Medical Officers, who will, should a retreat be found necessary, remain and take care of the wounded. This detail Medical Directors will request the Corps Commanders to announce in orders."[44]

Dr. Alexander N. Dougherty was the medical director of the Second Corps, and administratively oversaw all medical and surgical aspects of the three divisional hospitals. Captain Livermore of the ambulance corps had a real fondness for his new messmate and fellow member of the general staff, as is evident in his written portrait of the physician. "The doctor was a very fat man, and the picture of good-nature. His uniform, which was never, or very seldom, renewed, did not serve to lengthen his short and broad figure, and he rode a very fat and sturdy black horse as phlegmatic and good-natured as he. . . . Dr. Dougherty was . . . learned in medicine and literature, and an inveterate punster. His wife was his great admiration, and he showed us her picture, which proved her a very good-looking lady, and used to read us choice

---

inflow of wounded. Unfortunately, resignations, sickness, and long leaves of absence were pandemic among the surgical staff of the Army of the Potomac. In January of 1863, one divisional medical director in the Army of the Potomac reported that more than half of his divisional staff were absent from their posts, and some had been away for more than a year. The Second Corps was indeed fortunate if there were a hundred surgeons and assistant surgeons present for duty at Gettysburg. Adams, *Doctors in Blue*, pp. 45-46.

43. Dwinelle, *Medical Report*.

44. *OR*, vol. 19, pt. 1, p. 116.

passages from her letters, which he lauded as the production of an extraordinary woman. He . . . smoked a meerschaum pipe, which he filled often. His face was fair and much covered with a full light-brown beard, and his blue eyes would twinkle with humor. . . . The doctor . . . was not one of those members of the medical profession who so rigidly sheltered their bodies by the privilege of being non-combatants as never to visit the field in time of battle, but was noted for his frequent presence under fire, where he encountered danger rather with the equanimity of a philosopher than the martial spirit of the professed fighting man."[45]

Each of the three division hospitals had its own divisional medical director as well, all answerable directly to Doctor Dougherty. The medical director of the First Division, which had set up shop in the edge of the woods near the school house, was Surgeon R. C. Stiles, of the United States Volunteers. While it remained in this outdoor setting, the surgeon-in-charge was Dr. William W. Potter of the 57th New York Infantry, a highly-opinionated surgeon who had grown up in a family of physicians in rural New York. Dr. Charles Squire Wood, former New York City physician and now surgeon of the 66th New York Volunteers, served as the chief operator.[46]

Dr. J. Franklin Dyer, regimental surgeon of the 19th Massachusetts Volunteers, filled the post of Second Division medical director. Divisional Surgeon-in-Charge Dr. Justin Dwinelle, 106th Pennsylvania Volunteers, supervised the facility at Sarah Patterson's capacious barn and orchard, while Dr. Nathan Hayward, the photogenic surgeon of the 20th Massachusetts Volunteers, oversaw the actual medical treatment of patients as chief operator.[47]

---

45. Livermore, *Days and Events*, pp. 259-60, 309.
46. Dwinelle, *Medical Report*; Louis C. Duncan, *The Medical Department of the United States Army in the Civil War* (Washington, D.C.: U.S. Government Printing Office, 1910; reprint, Gaithersburg, Maryland: Olde Soldier Books, Inc., 1987), p. 271; Coco, *A Vast Sea of Misery*, pp. 181, 183. The position of surgeon-in-charge for the First Division would be taken over after leaving the Taneytown Road area by Assistant Surgeon Charles T. Kelsey of the 64th New York.
47. Dwinelle, *Medical Report*; Duncan, *The Medical Department of the United States Army*, p. 271. Second Division medical director Franklin J. Dyer of the 19th Massachusetts would assume Dwinelle's surgeon-in-charge duties when Dwinelle was appointed surgeon-in-charge of the combined Second Corps Hospitals. Dr. Nathan Hayward seems to hold the record of all Second Corps surgeons for the number of photographs he posed for—singlely, with his medical staff, with the 20th Massachusetts officers, etc., etc.

The Third Division contained the only Second Corps brigade made up entirely of Western troops. Parkersburg native Isaac Scott, surgeon of the 7th Regiment from the brand new state of West Virginia, was the Third Division's medical director, and he carefully monitored the work of Surgeon-in-Charge Ebenezer Day of the 39th New York Infantry "Garabaldi Guards," and Chief Operator (and Methodist Episcopal minister) Harry McKindree McAbee, 4th Ohio Volunteer Infantry, at a barn adjacent to the other two divisions.[48]

With everything as ready as possible at the three divisional hospitals, all the staff could do now was listen to the distant spattering of gunfire and wonder how bad it would be this time.

All the preparations taking place along the Taneytown Road were clearly visible to the troops looking down over the rearward crest of Cemetery Ridge. The aid stations could be clearly seen setting up opposite each regiment, displaying their distinctive small scarlet flag. "Surgeons were busy riding about selecting eligible places for Hospitals, and hunting streams, and springs, and wells. Ambulances and the Ambulance men were brought up near the lines, and stretchers gotten ready for use.—Who of us could tell but that he would be the first to need them?" noted Lieutenant Haskell somberly.[49]

All other departments and commands were also making final dispositions for battle. "The Provost Guards were busy driving up all stragglers, and causing them to join their regiments. Ammunition wagons were driven to suitable places, and pack mules bearing boxes of cartriges [*sic*]; and the commands were informed where they might be found. Officers were sent to see that the men had each his hundred rounds of ammunition. Generals and their Staffs were riding here and

48. Dwinelle, *Medical Report*; Duncan, *The Medical Department of the United States Army*, p. 271; Coco, *A Vast Sea of Misery*, p. 179. In fact, Surgeon Isaac Scott did such a fine job overseeing medical care in the Third Divison that he received special commendation in the after-action report of his divisional commander, General Hays: "I cannot omit the high recommendation of credit which is due Dr. Isaac Scott, medical director of the division, and all his assistants. No case of neglect or evasion of their duties has come to my notice." *OR*, vol. 27, pt. 1, p. 454.

49. John Day Smith, *The History of the Nineteenth Regiment of Maine Volunteer Infantry, 1862-1865* (Minneapolis: The Great Western Printing Company, 1909), pp. 97-98; Byrne and Weaver, *Haskell of Gettysburg*, p. 111.

there among their commands to see that all was right.—A staff officer, or an orderly might be seen galloping furiously in the transmission of some order or message."[50]

As for the troops themselves, they filled the downtime as best suited each man's mood. At Ziegler's Grove, the northern extremity of the Second Corps line, Lt. Thomas Galwey used the time of enforced waiting to record what was going on in his own unit. Born in 1846 in London to a family with ancient Irish roots, Galwey had immigrated to Cleveland, Ohio, in 1851, settling on a farm along present-day Euclid Avenue. A slight youth at five feet, four inches, with just a hint of downy beard and a thick, dark mop of hair, Galwey had apparently inflated his age when enlisted in the Hibernian Guard Company of the 8th Ohio. Meticulous in personal habits, Galwey made daily entries, often illustrated with his own drawings and maps, in leather-bound notebooks which he carried with him in his knapsack. "Some of us are writing letters to our loved ones, which might be found in our haversacks if we lose our lives in this coming battle. I am making little pencil sketches and jotting down notes of my feelings."[51]

Looking south along the crest of Cemetery Ridge, "the men stacked their arms—in long bristling rows they stood along the crests—and were at ease. Some men of the 2nd and 3rd Corps pulled down the rail fences near and piled them up for breast-works in their front. Some loitered,—some went to sleep upon the ground,—some, a single man carrying twenty canteens slung over his shoulder, went for water,—some made them a fire and boiled a dipper of coffee,—some with knees cocked up enjoyed the soldier's peculiar solace, a pipe of tobacco,—some were mirthful and chatty, and some were serious and silent."[52]

"All, all was ready. And yet the sound of no gun had disturbed the air or ear today."[53] That, however, was about to change.

---

50. Byrne and Weaver, *Haskell of Gettysburg*, p. 111.
51. Galwey, *The Valiant Hours*, foreword, p. 102.
52. Byrne and Weaver, *Haskell of Gettysburg*, pp. 111-12.
53. *Ibid.*, p. 111. Haskell was speaking figuratively, for occasional potshots were being exchanged by skirmishers since early morning. See Kepler, *Fourth Ohio Volunteers*, p. 126.

Chapter 3

THURSDAY, JULY 2: 8:30 A.M.—THURSDAY, JULY 2: NIGHTFALL

"Men fell at every step"

Capt. Benjamin W. Thompson
111th New York Volunteers

Washington, D.C.

Even with communication at a minimum from Gettysburg, word was out on the streets of Washington that combat was already taking place somewhere in the vicinity of the Pennsylvania-Maryland state line. "A battle is in progress," wrote Ellen Orbison Harris; "I fear the results are unsatisfactory. An evident reluctance to forward hospital stores to Hanover or Gettysburg, where the conflict is supposed to rage, betokens a want of confidence in the position or the strength of our forces."[1]

As secretary of the Philadelphia Ladies Aid Society, Mrs. Harris had taken it upon herself to serve as "their worker among the soldiers." After serving in the field hospitals at Chancellorsville, she had accompanied the evacuation of the wounded to Falmouth, Virginia. There she had received a personal request from Pennsylvania governor Andrew J. Curtin for her services in anticipation of a Confederate invasion of the North.

Following a short visit to Harrisburg, this "pale, quiet, delicate woman, often an invalid for months, and almost always a sufferer. . . ."

1. *Fifth Semi-Annual Report of the Ladies Aid Society of Philadelphia with Letters and Extracts from Letters from the Secretary of the Society Written from Various Places While Attending to the Sick and Wounded of the Union Army* (Philadelphia: C. Sherman & Son, 1863), p. 12. [Hereafter cited as *Report of the Ladies Aid Society*.]

packed her bags, and headed for the nation's capital. From there she could move quickly to wherever her services were most needed. For now, however, there was nothing to do but await further news from the battlefield.[2]

Baltimore, Maryland

Andrew Cross and other members of the Christian Commission had also been carefully monitoring the news from the battlelines. The Commission had worked closely with the Army of the Potomac over the past months, laboring to meet the shortfalls of the army commissary department, while ministering also to the spiritual needs of the soldiers.[3] A forward supply base had been set up at Frederick, Maryland; as the army continued to advance toward Pennsylvania, the base leap-frogged to keep up with the fast-moving troops.

On July 2, plans were made to advance the supply operation to Westminster, Maryland. "That day the announcement was made that there had been an engagement near Gettysburg, and General Reynolds killed; that appearances were unfavorable for our army. Everything looked gloomy, but there was no time for delay. We immediately got our stores in readiness to start."[4]

Going into a battle zone was always dangerous work, and agents of the Commission went at once to seek passes, transportation, and whatever other assistance could be secured from the army. "On calling on Colonel [James L.] Donaldson, the Quartermaster in Baltimore, he readily and promptly gave us what facility he could, as well as advice. He

---

2. Conklin, *Women at Gettysburg*, pp. 186, 189; L. P. Brockett and Mary C. Vaughn, *Women's Work in the Civil War: A Record of Heroism, Patriotism and Patience* (Boston: R. H. Curran, 1867), p. 149.
3. Founded by the Young Men's Christian Association (Y.M.C.A.) in 1861, the Christian Commission was a privately operated organization, roughly equivalent to the Salvation Army. With their stated purpose of supplying the "spiritual and temporal welfare" of the troops, they worked with the army to supplement shortcomings in the military supply system, while distributing testaments, tracts, and encouraging and evangelizing the troops on a personal level. Many of their workers were volunteer clergymen. Frederick Law Olmsted, *The Papers of Frederick Law Olmsted; Volume IV: Defending the Union: The Civil War and the U.S. Sanitary Commission 1861-1863*, ed. Jane Turner Censer (Baltimore: The Johns Hopkins University Press, 1986), p. 651.
4. Andrew Cross, *The War and the Christian Commission* (Baltimore: Privately Printed, 1865), p. 11.

would have furnished a wagon and ambulances to take our goods to the battle-field, but from the depredations of guerrillas and [Confederate Maj. Gen. J. E. B.] Stuart's cavalry, advised us not to take that way, but the military road, which was the railroad to Westminster. He gave us an order on the railroad President and Superintendent."[5]

With the necessary papers in hands, the Commission representatives hurried back to their depot to gather their supplies for the long trip to Gettysburg.

Westminster and Frederick, Maryland

Another volunteer group, the Sanitary Commission, was already several steps ahead of the Christian Commission in transporting supplies to the Army of the Potomac. With a goal of providing physical and medical necessities, the Sanitary Commission, under the steerage of a number of prominent Northern personalities, had secured high-level permission to attach their supply wagons directly to the army's wagon train.

The Commission was a model of efficient organization—nearly five hundred agents were constantly in the field, moving when the army moved, assisting at base hospitals, and manning supply stations within easy reach of the army. A Sanitary Commission representative accompanied each corps of the northern army, closely monitoring any shortfalls in the military commissary system. Needed supplies, running the gamut from medicines to forage for the animals, were requisitioned from the accompanying Sanitary wagons, and promptly delivered to the individual corps.[6]

With inside information on the movements of the army, the far-flung resources of the Sanitary Commission were alerted to the probability of impending battle. "Sanitary stores" were warehoused in New York,

5. *Ibid.*
6. J. H. Douglas, *Report on the Operations of the Sanitary Commission During and After the Battles at Gettysburg, July 1st, 2d, and 3d, 1863. Sanitary Commission No. 71.* (Washington, D.C.: Privately Printed, 1863), pp. 1-2, copy in the U. S. Sanitary Commission Vertical File, Gettysburg National Military Park. The Sanitary Commission was much like the modern-day Red Cross. However, unlike the grassroots Christian Commission, which drew its support largely through local churches, the Sanitary Commission was a high-profile national organization. Its leadership was composed of numerous influential businessmen and politicians, and their voice was heard in the highest circles of national government.

Philadelphia, Baltimore, Harrisburg, Washington, and Frederick, Maryland; two highly-trained men, one in Philadelphia, the other in Baltimore, were standing by, awaiting only the notification by telegraph of where the battle was taking place in order to rush the stockpiled goods to the scene. Like the Christian Commission, local supply dumps called "flying depots" shadowed and anticipated the movements of the vast military machine, setting up shop along the eastern flank of the army, then packing up and dashing ahead to pitch camp once again.[7]

Westminster and Frederick, Maryland, with their immediate access to railroad lines and the outside world, both saw sprawling Sanitary Commission supply bases spring up almost overnight. Knowing that enemy troops were operating in the area, the Commission sent forward some initial supply convoys to the advancing army, but left the bulk of their supplies in the relative safety of Maryland. Elaborate precautions were put into place to insure that the stores would reach the army; wagons were sent over different routes, and dispatched at various times to avoid any roving patrols of enemy cavalry.

But even with these painstaking safeguards in place, two shipments were intercepted by Confederates. The first, a wagon loaded with supplies for Harpers Ferry, was captured, and the Sanitary representative shipped directly off to Libby prison. The second shipment represented a far more serious loss—Dr. Alexander McDonald, senior man in charge of all the operations at Gettysburg, was captured with his personal staff in the vicinity of Emmitsburg, and also promptly sent off to Richmond. Valuable time was lost while a new command team was brought in.[8]

Now, as the sun was rising on another hot July morning, two heavily-laden Sanitary Commission wagons were on the road from Frederick to the small rural community of Gettysburg. Their cargo of lint, chloroform, sponges, bandages, beef soup and brandy was going to be badly needed by the time the sun began to approach the other horizon.[9]

---

7. *Ibid.*, p. 8; Katherine Prescott Wormeley, *The United States Sanitary Commission. A Sketch of Its Purposes and Its Work. Compiled from Documents and Private Papers* (Boston: Little, Brown, and Company, 1863), p. 122; *The Sanitary Commission of the United States Army: A Succinct Narrative of Its Works and Purposes* (New York: Published for the Benefit of the United States Sanitary Commission, 1864), pp. 148-49.
8. Douglas, *Report on the Opperation of the Sanitary Commission*, pp. 8-9; *The Sanitary Commission of the United States Army*, p. 149.
9. *The Sanitary Commission of the United States Army*, p. 151.

With a roar, the peacefulness of the early morning was shattered by Confederate forces off to the Union right, out of sight of the men of the Second Corps. "Before nine A.M. the right of our army's line, resting on Culps Hill, north and east of the Cemetery, was savagely attacked by [Lt. Gen. Richard S.] Ewell's Corps. The hill hid the forces from our sight, but the roar of small arms and cannon was continuous and betokened a severe battle. We could see our men and guns at intervals, being moved in to assist and our interest was intense. By noon the firing almost completely ceased and we learned that Ewell's Corps had been repulsed and he had withdrawn his force to his former position."[10]

So a quiet morning of spectating drew to a close for the men of Company F, 111th New York Volunteer Infantry. "The day wore on, the weather still sultry, and the sky overcast, with a mizzling effort at rain." "There was a lull for a time and by diligent search of our pockets and haversacks we got coffee enough to give a swallow or two apiece to our regiment—but no food. We gave our belts a hitch and all who smoked indulged vigorously while we awaited events."[11]

After getting his ambulance operations in order, Captain Livermore restlessly headed north toward Gettysburg along the Second Corps lines, working diligently to learn the lay of the land. He rode all the way to the cemetery grounds, then back again in last minute checking and double checking of his preparations. "Toward noon I was down in front of Colonel [Samuel S.] Carroll's brigade of the 3rd Division, and saw some lively skirmishing between our skirmishers and the rebels in the vicinity of the Emmitsburg road and had occasion to direct the stretcher-carriers in carrying away some wounded. . . . My men behaved very well and took the wounded away where the enemy's bullets flew savagely."[12]

---

10. Thompson, *Personal Narrative*, p. 34. Although this seemed to be a resumption of "severe battle" from the perspective of the men along the Second Corps line, this affair was actually a rather minor affair over on the Union right.
11. Byrne and Weaver, *Haskell of Gettysburg*, p. 111; Thompson, *Personal Narrative*, p. 35.
12. Livermore, *Days and Events*, pp. 244-45.

While nothing much was happening for the men of the Second Corps on the hilltop, things were anything but boring out on the skirmish line. "During all the morning—and the night, too—the skirmishers of the enemy had been confronting those of the 11th, 1st, and 12th corps. . . . About nine o'clock in the morning, I should think, . . . some rifled guns in the Cemetery at the left of the 11th Corps, opened fire,—almost the first shots of any kind this morning,—and when it was found they were firing at a Rebel line of skirmishers merely, that were advancing upon the left of that, and the right of the 2nd Corps, the officer in charge of the guns was ordered to cease firing, and was rebuked for having fired at all. These skirmishers soon engaged those of the right of the 2nd Corps, who stood their ground and were reinforced to make the line entirely secure. The Rebel skirmish line kept extending further and further to their right,—toward our left,—they would dash up close upon ours, and sometimes drive them back a short distance, in turn to be repulsed themselves,—and so they continued to do until their right was opposite the extreme left of the 3rd Corps. By these means they had ascertained the position and extent of our line,—but their own masses were still out of view."[13]

The skirmishing was especially sharp in front of Brig. Gen. Alexander Hays' Third Division, and the men of Col. George L. Willard's Third Brigade were in the thick of it. The terrain between the opposing forces, while composed of mildly rolling ridges, offered no significant cover for the men except for the William Bliss Farm. Complete with bulletproof brick barn, it lured both Union and Rebel skirmishers, and elements of the 39th New York "Garabaldi Guards" and 126th New York had been dispatched to this area.[14]

Both units advanced, but it was the 39th, skirmishing on the north side of the Bliss farmstead, that succeeded in drawing conspicuous attention to themselves. For some reason, the Garabaldis carried their flag out to the picket line with them, then uncharacteristically stood in full view of the enemy while skirmishing. Colonel Willard promptly sent out to have the flag brought back to the main lines, but the damage had already been done. The Confederates had little trouble drawing a bead on the exposed New Yorkers during their four hour stint on the line.

---

13. Byrne and Weaver, *Haskell of Gettysburg*, p. 113.

14. *OR*, vol. 27, pt. 1, p. 369; Harry W. Pfanz, *Gettysburg: The Second Day* (Chapel Hill: University of North Carolina Press, 1987), p. 65.

While the 39th lost fifteen killed and eighty wounded in the fighting of July 2 and 3, twenty-nine percent of that loss was sustained in the skirmishing on July 2.[15]

Farther up the line, Colonel Carroll's First Brigade pickets were strung out in front of Ziegler's Grove. There, "the skirmishing became quite brisk, Companies G and I of our [4th Ohio] regiment, in command of Captain [Peter] Grubb, were advanced to the front and somewhat to the left," wrote the historian of the 4th Ohio Volunteers of that morning's work. "They soon drove the enemy before them, and took position to the left of an old frame house, shielding themselves behind fence rails and ridges. The entire force of the Eighth Ohio was soon sent to their right, when the enemy was again driven a short distance and a new position occupied."[16]

The firing continued sporadic all along the line. "Sometimes stray shots, then again volleys, now rattling fire all along the front, and smoke would be seen here and there in the distant foliage" was the way Col. St. Clair Mulholland of the 116th Pennsylvania described the action. So the morning passed in the deadly give-and-take pastime of skirmishing, and the July 2 bloodletting began in earnest.[17]

The first trickle of casualties started making their way to the rear: some by stretcher, some walking or assisted by comrades from the skirmish lines. At this point, the number was so slight that the surgeons had little problem providing prompt care for the wounded as they arrived at the regimental aid facilities.

Dealing with hemorrhage proved to be a surprisingly small problem. "[The aid station surgeon] finds in his knapsacks a formidable array of tourniquets and compresses, yet it is very rarely that he will be obliged to use them. Men will be brought in who have bled a great deal—enough perhaps to saturate their clothing and the stretcher or blanket on which they lie—yet by the time they get to the Surgeon it [the bleeding] is generally stopped, or so nearly as to require nothing more than a light wet compress and a bandage not too tightly applied. . . .

15. Ezra D. Simon, *A Regimental History, the One Hundred and Twenty-fifth New York State Volunteers* (New York: Ezra D. Simons, 1888), p. 10; Pfanz, *Gettysburg: The Second Day*, pp. 65-67; *OR*, vol. 27, pt. 1, pp. 177, 472.

16. Kepler, *Fourth Ohio Volunteers*, p. 127.

17. St. Clair A. Mulholland, *The Story of the 116th Regiment Pennsylvania Infantry* (Philadelphia: F. McManus Jr. & Company Printers, 1899), p. 135.

The exception to this are mostly in the case of wounds in the head or face. . . . Then a compress can nearly always be applied so as to check the bleeding until the patient gets to the Division Hospital."[18]

Regimental aid stations had developed a general rule of thumb for bleeding wounds: "Where a large artery is wounded the man generally dies before he can be moved—smaller arteries speedily become blocked up from the amount of bruising and disorganization of tissue caused by a rifle ball."[19]

The spirits of the wounded men carried to the regimental aid facilities continued high, even in the face of serious wounds. "The ardor and fury of the fight stimulating every nerve and fibre of the body, and making every drop of blood flow quicker has not yet quite died away, and it is many hours before its effects altogether pass off. Wounds of the intestines or any of the abdominal viscera are generally the most depressing—those of the thorax and head next—fractures of the limbs in proportion to their nearness to the trunk, and injuries of the joints in proportion to their size." To restore flagging spirits, it was the common practice of the day to give most men "medicinal spirits" to drink—frequently, it "will be eagerly sought after by the wounded."[20]

Surprisingly, apart from the sound of battle, the aid stations were relatively quiet places. "[The surgeon] hears as a general rule only low moans escaping involuntarily, and an occasional expression of an impatient wish that the Doctor would get round quickly to dress the wound—the poor fellow expecting relief from him that he often cannot give. When a large nerve or plexus of nerves has been bruised, or partially divided, we sometimes hear expressions of acute pain, [but] not often otherwise."[21]

After the wounded were stabilized, they were removed to their respective division hospital as rapidly as possible by stretcher or ambulance. "The wounded began to arrive at the [division] Hospital about eleven O'clock A.M. They were composed mostly of portions of Regiments which had been sent out early in the day as skirmishers. A considerable number of them were from the Third Corps. The operating staff of the second Division were able to keep up with their operations for several hours."[22]

---

18. Vickery, "On the Duties of the Surgeon in Action," p. 20.
19. *Ibid.*
20. *Ibid.*, p. 21. Giving alcohol to badly injured men is a practice that makes modern medical men cringe.
21. *Ibid.*
22. Dwinelle, *Medical Report.*

Things had been quiet for so long at the First Division Hospital that Surgeon-in-Charge William Warren Potter had lain down for a nap after breakfast, sleeping until about noon. After a midday meal, "taking advantage of the dullness and quietude," Potter rode over to Meade's headquarters and spent half an hour visiting with the officers there. He then wandered up to the crest of the ridge, entertaining himself with a borrowed set of field glasses, scanning the distant enemy lines and watching the limited activity of the northern troops. As the wounded began arriving by ones and twos, the leading medical man of the First Division was no where to be found.[23]

On the crest of Cemetery Hill, the afternoon was quickly shaping up to be just as monotonous as the morning had been. "Some were sleeping near the stacked guns, others writing, some wandered away a few rods to get a better view of what was impending. The middle of the afternoon had passed; the pickets had become remarkably quiet; camp followers, clerks, orderlies, aides, colonels and generals, were becoming quite bold—taking observations, watching the smoke of the firing on the picket line and of the occasional booming of a gun on the extreme left, and closely scanning objects a mile or so west of them moving in the deepening shade of the trees. . . ."[24]

The men of the 1st Minnesota were in the uncomfortable position of having occasional enemy shells land in their ranks from several separate enemy batteries. The regiment was "just behind the crest of the ridge, to the left of the cemetery; a few rods to the left, and in front of a small white building near the Baltimore Pike, having the appearance of a summer house, and which I understood was occupied a part of the day by General Meade," wrote Col. William Colvill. "The artillery of the enemy commanded this position from the direction of Gettysburg, and from behind [Culp's Hill] and also from the low ground in front of Round Top, so that the shells crossed each other over us, and we lost several men during the day from such as happened to drop in the ranks." Sgt. John W. Plummer noted wryly that "the way the ambulances, hospital men, stragglers and darkies did skedaddle for the rear,

23. Potter, *Three Years with the Army of the Potomac*, pp. 58-59.

24. Kepler, *Fourth Ohio Volunteers*, p. 127. While used extensively during the Civil War as a unit of measurement, the "rod" is almost obsolete in our day. It is equal to 5.5 yards, or 16.5 feet.

was amusing to those old fellows who had got used, somewhat, to such things as shells. . . ."[25]

"Somewhat after one o'clock, P.M.—the skirmish firing had nearly ceased now,—a movement of the 3rd Corps occurred. . . ." A great deal of curiosity was in evidence over this activity of Maj. Gen. Daniel E. Sickles' corps, the erstwhile neighbor of the Second. "The Third Corps had moved in on our left, but, instead of prolonging our line, General Sickles had moved out to Peach Orchard knoll nearly half a mile in front to our left." "It was magnificent to see those ten or twelve thousand men,—they were good men—with their Batteries, and some squadrons of Cavalry upon the left flank, all in battle order, in several lines, with flags streaming, sweep steadily down the slope, across the valley, and up the next ascent, toward their destined position!" "As far to the left as the eye could see, batteries of artillery, ambulance trains and stretcher carriers moved in parallel lines in rear of the troops, while staff officers and orderlies flew back and forth directing the movements or bearing orders." "[General Sickles] and General Meade sat on their horses, probably discussing this move, which was evidently contrary to General Meade's plan, when the Corps was struck by an assault of Lee's forces outnumbering them three or four to one. We were able to see a battle in which we were not participants."[26]

Fidgety Ambulance Chief Livermore continued to nervously prowl the lines as the day wore on, bringing him again in contact with his antagonistic brigade commander. "Toward sundown (possibly not later than three o'clock) I happened to ride to my regiment, which was sta-

25. William Colvill, letter to John R. Bachelder, June 9, 1886, John B. Bachelder Papers, New Hampshire Historical Society, Concord, New Hampshire; John W. Plummer, letter to his brother, n.d., *Minneapolis Atlas*, August 26, 1863, Newspaper Clippings, Gettysburg National Military Park. The "small white building near the Baltimore Pike" was most likely the Widow Pfeffer House, where Meade set up headquarters on July 4 after being shelled out of Widow Leister's House during the July 3 Confederate cannonade. A photograph of this house was part of the set of views taken by Frederick Gutekunst when he visited Gettysburg [see Chapter 12]. [William A. Frassanito, *Early Photography at Gettysburg* (Gettysburg, Pennsylvania: Thomas Publications, 1995), pp. 225-29.]

26. Byrne and Weaver, *Haskell of Gettysburg*, pp. 116, 117; Thompson, *Personal Narrative*, p. 35; Robert L. Stewart, *History of the One Hundred and Fortieth Regiment, Pennsylvania Volunteers* (Philadelphia: Regimental Association, 1912), p. 99.

tioned near the left of the Second Corps, and passed a few words with Colonel Cross, who was then commanding the 1st Brigade, in which the regiment was. He spoke pleasantly, and after surveying the field in front of us, in which there did not seem to be anything transpiring in the way of fighting, he laughingly said to me, alluding to my ambulances, 'We shan't want any of your dead carts here to-day!' I was glad to be joked by him, because I did not wish to have him cherish ill-feelings toward me on account of my receiving and accepting the staff appointment, and I concluded from this that he had not conceived much if any animosity toward me."[27]

Satisfied with what he found of the preparations of his regiment, Captain Livermore moved on. "I rode away, and I do not think it was ten minutes before the sounds of rapid artillery firing and musketry drew my eyes toward the Peach Orchard, where I saw our artillery, as I think, advancing and firing, and evidently from the quick reports and flashes it was hotly engaged."[28]

Shortly before 5:00 p.m., orderlies came dashing along the Second Corps line, at least one a staff aide of General Meade in search of Hancock. The Second Corps commander was ordered to dispatch a division to Maj. Gen. George Sykes, commander of the Fifth Corps, to help stem the imminent breakthrough of Confederate forces through Sickles' weakening lines. Hancock quietly told Brig. Gen. John C. Caldwell of the First Division to prepare his men.[29]

Father William Corby, chaplain of the 88th New York, requested permission of his commander to address the men. As the troops stood to "order arms," Corby explained that he was about to deliver general absolution to the men, and urged them to do their fullest duty this day. At Corby's request, caps were removed and held in the left hand, while the men held their weapons in their right hand and knelt on their right knee. Standing on a large rock in order to be seen and heard by the men, the chaplain raised his right hand and pronounced the ancient Latin words: "*Eqo Te Absolvo.*" General Hancock and others observing the solemn ceremony removed their hats as well, and the quiet dignity of the absolution proceeded as the sounds of battle roared in the back-

27. Livermore, *Days and Events*, p. 247.
28. *Ibid.*
29. Stewart, *History of the One Hundred and Fortieth*, p. 101.

ground. Colonel Mulholland of the 116th Pennsylvania wrote that the "scene was more than impressive, it was awe-inspiring."[30]

Another onlooker was greatly inspired by Father Corby's service, so much so that he sought to have a similar service in his own regiment. "Seeing the Irish Brigade bowed in prayer and feeling deeply impressed with the idea that many might enter the battle never to return, I asked permission of Col [Hiram Loomis] Brown to hold worship before entering the battle," wrote Lutheran chaplain J. H. W. Stuckenberg of the 145th Pennsylvania. "He willingly acquiesced. 'Attention' was called. After a few remarks we joined in prayer. The occasion was a very solemn one—it was the last prayer in which some of our regt joined."[31]

When it became evident that part of the Second Corps would be sent to the aid of Sickles' men, Captain Livermore rode over to personally supervise that portion of the ambulance corps. "Soon after [the firing broke out] I learned that the 1st Division of our corps had been ordered to hasten to the scene of this fight, and I at once proceeded to ascertain if the ambulances and stretcher-carriers had gone with them. I pursued the track of the division to the left and through some oak woods, and was evidently close upon them.[32] I found that the ambulances and stretcher-carriers had left the posts at which they were stationed and followed the division, but while pursuing the division through these woods I found some of the stretcher-carriers lagging behind, evidently afraid to go after the division, I accordingly made them go along with me until I had got them up to the division or close to it and well under the artillery fire, which was uncomfortably savage."[33]

Livermore had no way of knowing whether the entire corps would be fully engaged within a few minutes, or not. So, after shepherding his men into their proper positions, the Second Corps ambulance commander rode back to monitor the ambulance and stretcher work in the other two divisions, leaving the frontline conduct to Lieutenant Anderson, 53rd Pennsylvania, head of the First Division ambulance train.[34]

30. Nicholson, *Pennsylvania at Gettysburg*, p. 623; Mulholland statement to Bachelder, John B. Bachelder Papers; Stewart, *History of the One Hundred and Fortieth*, p. 101.
31. Stuckenberg, *I'm Surrounded by Methodists*, p. 136.
32. Captain Livermore was probably near the Jacob Weikert Farm, just to the north of the Valley of Death and the Wheatfield area.
33. Livermore, *Days and Events*, p. 247.
34. *Ibid.*, pp. 241, 247-48.

Once he had ascertained that the other divisional ambulance trains and stretcher-bearers were ready to move at a moment's notice, Livermore paused to watch the action unfolding below. Caldwell's First Division of the Second Corps was moving in to fill the hole left by the fleeing Third Corps. "The line stood up in perfect array and fired rapidly. The smoke of their rifles encircled them, the flashes lighted up the field upon which the shadows of evening were advancing, and the scene resembled one of those battles which are seen in pictures, where the lines of battle are formed with mathematical exactness, but which were rarely witnessed in our war, in which thick woods, hills, valleys, and rivers were so frequently in the fields of battle."[35]

Division by division, the Second Corps was being inexorably sucked into the battle — first General Caldwell and his First Division went charging into the Wheatfield, then fragmented bits and pieces of General Gibbon's Second Division were sent out to plug holes in the dissolving battleline; soon the Third Brigade of General Hays' Third Division was called on to go in against the oncoming Confederate attack.

"Before 6 o'clock the firing on the left was more rapid, accompanied by the whirr of musketry, while troops could be seen hurrying forward over the plain from our side; in a few minutes more[,] there was unusual activity among the strange spectres in the shadows of the trees on our front, then a puff of smoke, a shot went over our heads, then came another, and a third scattered a stack of guns of the rear regiment, the Seventh [West] Virginia, plunging a bayonet into a comrade's side and another cut a comrade of the Fourth [Ohio] in twain; now there was hurrying to and fro, men for their companies and their guns, disinterested eye-witnesses, generals and staff for shelter over the brow of the hill. . . . There was meager chance for shelter; General Hays and staff had just dismounted back of us, but across the brow of the hill, when a solid shot plowed through an orderly's horse. The batteries in front of us were now replying vigorously; the enemy's skirmishers were making it hot for our pickets; whizzing shot and whirring shell, plunging and ricocheting among and over us. . . ."[36]

35. *Ibid.* pp. 251-52.

36. Kepler, *Fourth Ohio Volunteers*, p. 128.

General Hancock rode up to Col. Clinton D. MacDougall's regiment, personally ordering the 111th New York to advance to Sickles' aid. "As we looked, suddenly the order came to 'Fall in'—and we were marched behind our line to the left until we came to the low place between Cemetery Hill and Little Round Top. The Third Corps were pouring through the gap to the rear, closely pursued by a line of rebel infantry who were firing rapidly. It was difficult to keep a line in the face of these squads of flying men who were not moved by Hancock's shouted orders or his blistering curses. I opened my company and let four men carry General Sickles, minus a leg, to the rear. Our brigade commander, Colonel [George L.] Willard of the 125th, N. Y. Inf, who had been a Regular, was equal to the occasion. He placed markers and lined us up as if we were on parade instead of under a perfect storm of missiles from minie balls to bursting shells. Our position was just in rear of [a] line of cannon which were holding back the enemy by a very vigorous fire of shell and canister."[37]

"Before he had given us any command to move a rebel shell took off Col Willard's head right in front of our line and his Adjutant General's horse was killed by another.[38] The command devolved upon Col [Eliakim] Sherrill of the 126th N.Y., he immediately ordered us forward and forward we charged to the Plum Run thicket, where we were ordered to lie down, a rebel line of battle being on the other side of the alders, not over a rod away."[39]

The men of the 111th New York found themselves in the uncomfortable and lethal position of laying face to face across Plum Run from the enemy, firing at each other at point blank range. "The constant rain of missiles at this point was terrific. A large number of cannon at close range were pouring shell and shrapnel and canister upon us without intermission, and in our whole front was a line of riflemen giving us minie balls with such rapidity that it seemed as if nothing could live an instant exposed to their fire. One of our Lieutenants held his sword in the air for a minute and the blade was cut off just above the hilt."[40]

The deadly stalemate was finally broken by the command for the New Yorkers to move forward. "Into this hell of destruction we were ordered to charge. Our men sprang to their feet, pushed through the Plum Run Thicket of alders and ran over a line of rebels lying just the

---

37. Thompson, *Personal Narrative*, pp. 35-36.
38. Colonel Willard was actually decapitated after, not before, the counterattack through the Plum Run swale.
39. Thompson, *Personal Narrative*, p. 36.
40. *Ibid.*

other side of the run, then swung out into the open, a ready mark for the enemy and pushed for the Peach Orchard in our front, alive with Confederates. Men fell at every step."[41]

Chaplain Stuckenberg, after leading his men from the 145th Pennsylvania in worship, had gone in search of his horse and provisions which had been sent to the rear. "After hunting for more than an hour in the hot sun I found our [First] Division Hospital in the woods and my horse near it. I was very tired and after dinner lay down to rest. But immediately the heavy thunder of cannon was heard on the front. This was about 3 P.M. I jumped up, took my canteen and some bandages and hastened to go to the regiment. But coming to the top of the hill the shells fell between the regt and myself, and I thought it folly to expose myself. I remained on this hill for a while, attending to some of the wounded men, watching the prisoners who came in and the fight generally as much as possible. But soon my position became too much exposed. The shells came nearer and nearer, some exploding just in front of me, others passing over my head and pieces falling far and near around me. One struck the ground a short distance before me and threw its pieces and earth and rocks high in the air."[42]

The chaplain continued working on Cemetery Ridge, ministering to the wounded as they came reeling up the slope, dressing their wounds as best he could with his small stock of medical supplies. The shells passing over his position were causing quite a commotion in the rear. "Some shells fell near the place where my horse was. A kind of panic seized the 'bummers' and others all of whom were hurried further back."[43]

41. *Ibid.*
42. Stuckenberg, *I'm Surrounded by Methodists*, pp. 77-78.
43. *Ibid.*, p. 78. By "bummers," Stuckenberg means skulkers, seeking safety in the rear. "Hospital bummers" were a highly specialized breed of soldiers, skilled at distancing themselves from any fighting by being "sick." "The favorite disease was 'diarrhoea,' which became chronic in a week. . . . The regular prescriptions were numbered six, nine, and eleven, which were blue pill, quinine, and vinium. We soon learned 'vinium' meant either wine or brandy." So practiced were these "diarrhoea cases" that they could step into the sick call line just where "vinium" would be dispensed, since the surgeons gave out prescriptions of numbers six, nine, and eleven in a regular rotating order. Abner Small, *The Road to Richmond - The Civil War Memoirs of Major Abner Small of the 16th Maine Volunteers; With His Diary as a Prisoner of War*, ed. Harold Adams Small (Berkeley: University of California Press, 1939), pp. 187-88.

The overshot shells were also making it impossible for the surgeons in the First Division Hospital to do their work. "The first position of our hospital had become untenable, by reason of being in range of the enemy's fire," wrote First Division Surgeon-in-Charge William Warren Potter. Instead of staying at his post, Potter had been up on Cemetery Ridge sightseeing when the hospital came under fire. He belatedly remembered his duties and headed back to the medical facility only when he saw Sickles' corps under severe attack.[44]

"Arriving at the place where I had left the hospital not a person was to be found, and no traces of it could be discovered. I began searching for it, and soon found its new location near a stream, protected by a ridge from great danger of shells, though we were somewhat nearer the lines than before. It seems that, during my absence, the hospital was literally shelled out of its first position, and this new place was sought out as a necessity." The many wounded from the First Division were being rushed to the hospital, the "quietude" of the morning now only a vague memory.[45]

"The hospital was moved hastily," continued Stuckenberg. "I moved my horse, took him farther back to the side of a hill under cover of some high rocks. Leaving my horse there in charge of some of our regiment, I went to assist the wounded."[46]

The ambulance corpsmen and stretcher men now had their hands full evacuating the wounded. One injured infantryman related that "those of the wounded who could do so limped to the shelter of some great rocks, and here their worse injured fellows were soon gathered. Whence the stretcher bearers came we could not have told. . . . The ambulances come presently and the wounded are placed in them."[47]

Sometimes, however, the evacuation process was just as hazardous as the front line fighting. Ambulances made nice large targets for cannoneers, especially when traveling in trains of multiple vehicles. "Hardly are they under way when a Confederate gunner sees them and a shell,

44. Potter, "Reminiscences of Field-Hospital Service with the Army of the Potomac," p. 15.
45. Potter, *Three Years with the Army of the Potomac*, p. 59.
46. Stuckenberg, *I'm Surrounded by Methodists*, p. 78.
47. James L. Bowen, "On the Gettysburg Field," *The Philadelphia Times*, June 28, 1—, Newspaper Clippings, Volume 6, Hospitalization after Gettysburg: Personal Accounts Vertical File, Gettysburg National Military Park.

followed quickly by others, renews our peril. The drivers bend low and lash their horses. A wheel is struck; another piece of iron goes through the top of an ambulance, making an ugly rent. Away goes the train, driven like mad, across the fields, trying to get out of range. The vehicles plunge into a gully with a lurch, and are jerked out only to bound over a hillock, pitching from side to side, barely maintaining an upright position, but going forward at a gallop till at length a valley is reached where the Confederate artillery cannot make afraid."[48]

Rough rides of this kind were absolutely devastating to the bleeding passengers inside. "One side of my companion's face has been torn away by a piece of shell and both of my legs are damaged. As a consequence, the promiscuous rolling and tossing about in our narrow quarters has been extremely unpleasant, and we are relieved to find ourselves safe in the shelter of the division hospital."[49]

As wounded and demoralized troops streamed to the rear from Sickles' crumbling position, fresh reinforcements from the First Division of the Second Corps hastily rushed in to shore up the sagging Union line. Second Lt. Charles A. Fuller of Company C, 61st New York Volunteer Infantry, was hurrying with his brigade, commanded by Col. Edward Cross, into an innocuous-looking wheatfield owned by a local farmer.

"In the early part of the day I remarked to a number of the men near by that when some one of them was knocked down I was going to take his musket and get into the firing line. We were in this wheatfield and the grain stood almost breast high. The Rebs had their slight protection, but we were in the open, without a thing better than a wheat straw to catch a Minnie bullet that weighed an ounce. Of course, our men began to tumble. They lay where they fell, or, if able, started for the rear."[50]

"Near to me I saw a man named Daily go down, shot through the neck. I made a movement to get his gun, but at that moment I was struck in the shoulder. It did not hurt and the blow simply caused me to step back. I found that I could not work the arm, but supposed that hurt was a flesh wound that had temporarily paralyzed it, and that it was not serious enough to justify my leaving the fighting line. So, I remained and did what I could in directing the firing."[51]

---

48. *Ibid.*
49. *Ibid.*
50. Fuller, *Personal Recollections*, pp. 94-95.
51. *Ibid.*, p. 95.

The brigade was standing on a slight rise in the ripening grain, trading shots with the approaching Confederates. Colonel Cross, after issuing orders to be ready to advance, dropped with a bullet in the abdomen. Lieutenant Fuller, standing behind his company directing the fire, also made a splendid target. "Sometime after this, I felt a blow on the left leg, and it gave way, so that I knew the bone was broken. This stroke did not hurt, and I did not fall, but turned around and made a number of hops to the rear, when my foot caught in the tangled grain and I went down full length. . . ."[52]

Lying prostrate in the trampled grain, with balls cutting the heads from wheat stalks still standing around him, Fuller spotted two men from the regiment, making for the rear. "I yelled out to them, 'Drag me back.' They heeded the order, or entreaty, and one man grabbed one arm, and the other man the other arm, and they started back with me between them, not on any funeral gait, but almost on a run. My right arm was sound, but the left one was broken at the shoulder joint, and on that side it was pulling on the cords and meat. I wobbled much as a cut of wood drawn by two cords would have. These men pulled me back in this fashion for a number of rods, and until I thought they had pulled me over a rise of ground like a cradle knoll, when I shouted, 'Drop me,' and they dropped, and went on without note or comment."[53]

Satisfied that he was out of the line of fire, at least for the moment, the twenty-one-year-old lieutenant looked to his wounds. "I had a tourniquet in my haversack, and with my one serviceable arm, I worked away till I got it out, and did the best I could to get it around my leg; for anything I knew I was bleeding to death, and, if possible, I wanted to check the flow of blood. I think my effort did not amount to much."[54]

Having done all he could to attend his own injuries, Fuller lay back to await developments in the fighting.

The 148th Pennsylvania, another regiment of the First Division rushing forward with Lieutenant Fuller's 61st New York, was also taking

52. Charles A. Hale, "With Colonel Cross at the Wheatfield," John Rutter Brooke Papers, Historical Society of Pennsylvania, Philadelphia, Pennsylvania; reprinted in *Civil War Times Illustrated*, vol. 13, no. 5 (August 1974), p. 36; Fuller, *Personal Recollections*, p. 95.

53. Fuller, *Personal Recollections*, p. 95.

54. *Ibid.*, pp. 95-96.

heavy casualties. "About the middle of our battle in the wheat field I caught a piece of Confederate shell on the large tendon above the knee with force enough to give me quite a whirl, and with shock enough to make me feel down to find if the leg were on or off," wrote Adjutant J. W. Muffly years later, the incident still distinct in his memory. "I limped back to the rear of a huge rock that afforded good shelter for our wounded, where I found quite a number of the boys with a variety of wounds. Just after me came a sergeant badly hurt in the shoulder, who begged me to remove his knapsack. Next came another with blood spurting from a shot through the wrist."[55]

Adjutant Muffly discovered that he had been unspeakably lucky in the Wheatfield that day, and was even able to look back with humor and grace upon the dangerous situation. "After fixing them both up as best I could, I examined my own case and found it to be only a bad bruise of the tendon, sore enough but not serious. I limped back to the Regiment and 'fought it out on that line.' I was obliged to mount my horse for a week on the right side, which is, of course, the wrong side, the left side being the right side—cavalry paradox. . . . A comrade seeing my difficulty in marching handed me his canteen and said, 'Take a drink of this, Adjutant, it will do you good.' I took two big swallows of commissary whiskey—my first and last taste of liquor during the service, and I must admit that it did me good."[56]

Off to the right, the 57th New York, part of General Zook's Third Brigade, was pushing into the other end of the ruined wheatfield. A Confederate brigade (probably Brig. Gen. J. B. Kershaw's South Carolinians at this point) was rushing toward a widening hole in the line, and Zook's brigade hustled to head them off. "When about four o'clock, the order came to move, the Fifty-Seventh fell in, filed left, went into the woods and was soon under fire. As we pushed forward a bullet struck my right arm and passed through, . . ." wrote Jacob H. Cole of that deadly afternoon. "When I was shot in the arm, the feeling was the same as though I had been struck on the elbow—a feeling of numbness came into the arm—and I turned to the comrade by my side and asked him why he had hit me. He said: 'I did not hit you, but you have

55. Muffly, *The Story of Our Regiment*, p. 245.
56. *Ibid.*, pp. 245-46.

been shot and you had better go to the rear.' I laughed at him and said I was not hurt bad enough to do so."[57]

Cole's humor was to be short-lived, however. "As we charged into the wheatfield a shell exploded and shattered my right leg and killed two of my comrades. . . . After my leg was shattered I fell down, laying for a few minutes unconscious, and when I came to my senses, I found I was surrounded by the enemy and a rebel officer was standing over me with one foot on my wounded leg. I pleaded with him to step off my wounded leg. He said in answer to my pleadings, drawing his sword, 'You d— Yankee, I will cut your heart out,' and as he raised his sword a ball came from the direction of Little Round Top and cut him through the throat, and he fell beside me dead." With the death of their officer, the other Confederates moved on, leaving the young Union soldier alone on the field with the still-twitching body of his tormentor, and surrounded by only the dead and dying.[58]

The battle was still raging over on the other side of the wheatfield. Laying incapacitated with wounds to the arm and leg, Lieutenant Fuller of the 61st New York "heard a line of battle approaching from the rear. As the men came in sight I sang out, 'Don't step on me, boys!' Those in range of me stepped over and on they went, to take their medicine. I understand they rushed forward and fought the enemy in advance of the line we occupied. It was not many minutes after these troops passed me that the rattle of musketry was again heard from that wheat field. It was kept up for a good while, and then it died down. No body of our men went back past me."[59]

Like Jacob Cole lying prostrate further up the field, this young Northern officer was also about to have an close encounter with the enemy. "After a while I was aware that a skirmish line was coming from the front, and soon discovered that the skirmishers were not clothed in blue. The officer in command was mounted and rode by within a few feet of me." Fighting broke out behind Fuller's position, "and a short time after these gentlemen in gray moved back in the same manner they

57. Cole, *Under Five Commanders*, p. 202.
58. *Ibid.*, pp. 202-3.
59. Fuller, *Personal Recollections*, p. 96. The men who "stepped over" Lieutenant Fuller were part of Col. John R. Brooke's Fourth Brigade, First Division, Second Corps.

had advanced, greatly to my relief. I did not fancy remaining their guest for any length of time."[60]

"As the Rebs went back, a nice looking young fellow, small of stature, with bright black eyes, whose face was smutted up with powder and smoke, came along where I lay. My sword was on the ground beside me. He picked it up, and said, 'Give me that scabbard!' I said, 'Johnny, you will have to excuse me, as my arm is broken and I can't unbuckle my belt.' He made no comment, but went off with my sword. Then matters quieted down, and there was no sound to be heard in that vicinity, except groanings of the wounded."[61]

With men dropping at an alarming rate out in the Wheatfield and the surrounding areas, the seriously wounded desperately needed to be evacuated to primary aid stations before they bled to death. Whenever there were insufficient hands available for carrying stretchers or dressing wounds, regimental musicians were on call, waiting to fill the gap. "The musicians of our Division were formed into a squad or command under a Sergeant and Lieutenant, for the purpose of caring for the wounded, and assisting the surgeons in their work," remembered Drummer John B. Holloway of Company D, 148th Pennsylvania Volunteers.[62]

"On the 2d day of July, 1863, at 4:00 P.M., the battle opened, and Colonel McKeen told us to go to a certain rock that afforded some shelter, to assist Dr. [Alfred T.] Hamiliton in dressing the wounds of those who were wounded on the field," wrote Drummer Nathaniel Beerly of Company B, 148th Pennsylvania Volunteers. "While there the ambulance corps came along with some twenty stretchers, one more than they had men for, so Lawrence Bathhurst called on me to go along, and we followed our Division into the wheat field close to Little Round Top, and on the right of me about five or six feet, an orderly Sergeant was shot through the thigh. We took him about one mile to the field hospital, returned and helped others until the sun set on that terrible day."[63]

60. *Ibid.*
61. *Ibid.*
62. Muffly, *The Story of Our Regiment*, p. 331.
63. *Ibid.*, p. 325.

The Confederate attack continued to roll its way northward, sucking ever more of the Second Corps into the fight. The First Division had gone to the rescue of the now-shattered Third Corps, and the men of the Second Division to the immediate right of the First were watching the fighting moving steadily toward their position. "We saw them [Third Corps] falling back and the enemy advancing," wrote Capt. John "Jack" G. B. Adams of the 19th Massachusetts. "Lieut Sherman Robinson and I were lying side by side watching the battle. 'Some one must go and help them, Jack,' said Robinson. At that moment a staff officer rode up to Colonel [Arthur F.] Devereaux, and then we heard the familiar command, 'Attention, 19th!' 'We are in for it,' said Robinson. . . ."[64]

"With the 42nd New York, we double-quicked to a point where the line had broken and the rebels were advancing on our flank. I was in command of the color company, had just removed the covering from the colors when a regiment to our left broke; with other officers I rushed to rally them, and was returning to my place in line when I went down. I heard an officer say, 'Jack is down,' before I really knew that I was shot."[65]

No stretchermen were available, the regiment was falling back, and the enemy line was relentlessly bearing down on where the wounded officer lay bleeding. There was no time to be lost if Captain Adams was to be gotten to a field hospital. "I could not rise, and Sergeant Smith and Private Collopee came to me. 'Put him on my back, Smith,' said the latter, and under a terrible fire he carried me from the field. Our lines fell back as fast as we could go. . . . Everything indicated that we were again defeated, but when our men arrived at the stone wall, by unanimous consent they turned about, and with that wild hurrah that only Yankee soldiers can give, drove the rebels beyond our former lines."[66]

Since the 19th had moved so far to the left to aid Sickles' men, its position was now in front of the Third Corps field hospitals, and the faithful private headed straight for the nearest one. "I expected that Collopee would be obliged to drop me, and I should fall into the hands of the rebels, but he kept on and landed me in the field hospital of the 3rd corps."[67]

"I found myself surrounded by men wounded and dying. An assistant surgeon was in charge and I asked him to look at my wound. He

---

64. J. G. B. Adams, *Reminiscences of the Nineteenth Massachusetts Regiment* (Boston: Wright & Potter Printing Company, 1899), p. 66.
65. *Ibid.*
66. *Ibid.*, pp. 66-67.
67. *Ibid.*, p. 66.

did, and said that I could not live twenty-four hours. I suggested that he stop the blood, as he might be mistaken, but he had no time to waste on me and went along. Upon examination I found that I was wounded in three places, and all were bleeding badly, but I could not tell where the bullets had entered or come out."[68]

"The battle was yet raging; men were coming in thick and fast, the last arrivals being mostly rebels. Collopee had waited until the surgeon said I should die, when he rushed back to the regiment with the information. In a short time Lieut Mose Shackley appeared before me with one of his company named Younger. 'Jack, old boy, they say you are going to die, and I thought you would like a canteen of coffee before you passed up your check,' said Mose."[69]

Lieutenant Shackley, for one, still nourished a healthy antagonism toward the rebels, even fallen ones. "'What are you lying on?' he asked, as it was quite dark. I replied, 'Only the ground:' and going to a rebel who was slightly wounded but was comfortable, having a rubber blanket under and a woolen blanket over him, he said, 'There is a darned sight better man than you are, with no blanket under or over him,' and captured one for me. Making me as comfortable as possible, urging me to keep a stiff upper lip, he said he would like to remain with me, but there was lots of fun at the front, and he must return."[70]

So Capt. Jack Adams pulled the confiscated blanket around him, listened to the expressions of pain and suffering in this strange corps hospital, and idly mused in the dark about just how long it would be before he bled to death.

Into this mass confusion of bleeding men and laboring doctors rolled the welcome sight of two Sanitary Commission wagons. These wagons, heavy with medicines, surgical supplies, and foodstuffs, "arrived from Frederick at the moment of the assault of Longstreet upon the left wing of the loyal army, and were driven under fire to reach the collections of wounded in the rear. As one of them came to a point where several hundred sufferers had been taken from the ambulances and laid upon the ground behind a barn and in an orchard, less than a thousand yards in the rear of our line of battle, on the left wing, then

68. *Ibid.*, p. 67.
69. *Ibid.*
70. *Ibid.*

fiercely engaged, a surgeon was seen to throw up his arms, exclaiming, 'Here is the Sanitary Commission, now we shall be able to do something.' He had nearly exhausted all his supplies; and the brandy, beef soup, sponges, chloroform, lint and bandages, which were at once furnished him, were undoubtedly the means of saving many lives."[71]

The wagons were under the supervision of Sanford Hoag, an experienced agent of the Commission, and were loaded to capacity with a virtual cornucopia of supplies. "As soon as the surgeons had decided upon the different areas where the Corps Hospitals were to be formed, Mr. Hoag moved the wagons to them at once," remembered Maj. J. C. Bush, another Sanitary Commission agent riding along with Hoag, "and commenced to issue our stores, which consisted chiefly of concentrated beef soup, stimulants, crackers, condensed milk, concentrated coffee, corn starch, farina, shirts, drawers, stockings, towels, blankets, quilts, bandages and lint. We hastened from one hospital to another, as rapidly as possible, issuing to each a portion of our stores, until the supply was nearly exhausted. . . ."[72]

Seeing that their two wagons would barely begin to meet the pressing needs of the hospitals, Major Bush left the wagons in charge of Hoag, and set off in search of the nearest telegraph. It was imperative that the outside world be informed immediately of the desperate needs at Gettysburg.

Still the Confederate juggernaut kept coming. As General Hancock rode north of the Wheatfield toward the "copse of trees" on Cemetery Ridge, he could see a disaster in the making. Shattered remnants of the Third Corps continued fleeing to the rear, pursued by some 1600 men of Cadmus Wilcox's brigade. There simply were not enough Union troops on hand to stop the hemorrhage. Hancock immediately sent a dispatch to General Gibbon, acting commander of the Second Corps, urgently requesting reinforcements.

As they rode behind the lines, Hancock, accompanied by staff aide Capt. W. D. W. Miller, drew the attention of the oncoming enemy's infantry, and a hail of bullets went their way. Hancock escaped unharmed, but two of the bullets struck Captain Miller. Hancock promptly

71. *The Sanitary Commission of the United States Army*, p. 151.
72. Douglas, *Report of the Operations of the Sanitary Commission*, p. 11.

sent his aide off to seek medical care while Hancock attempted to slow the enemy attack.[73]

The only infantry at hand were the 262 men of the 1st Minnesota. Frustrated, Hancock exclaimed: "My God! Are these all the men we have here?" Turning to their commander, Colonel Colvill, Hancock unflinchingly sent the undersized regiment head-on against the onrushing brigade.[74] Even though they knew that most of them would never survive the encounter, the Badgers, nevertheless, fixed bayonets, closed ranks, and charged headlong into the enemy.[75]

The scrap was fierce and determined. Unflinchingly, the Minnesotans traded shots and blows with grit and determination in the face of certain destruction. Seconds were dearly bought, minutes measured in lifetimes, but the Confederate attack finally began to stall and lose its momentum. The determined resistance of the 1st Minnesota Volunteers gave the Union commanders valuable minutes to hurry fresh troops forward, but at a terrible price to the westerners. "What Hancock had given us to do was done thoroughly," recorded one fortunate survivor of that bloody encounter. "The regiment had stopped the enemy. . . . But at what sacrifice! . . . Of the two hundred and sixty-two men who made the charge, two hundred fifteen lay upon the field . . . forty seven were still in line, and not a man was missing."[76]

---

73. A. M. Gambone, *Hancock at Gettysburg . . . and beyond.* (Baltimore: Butternut and Blue, 1997), p. 97.
74. The three officers and twenty-eight men of Company L were serving as skirmishers, and fifty-six men from Company C were detached for divisional duties. [See Appendix 1.]
75. "Minnesota at Gettysburg," Winfield Scott Hancock Papers, Scrapbook of his death and obituaries, United States Army Military History Institute, Carlisle Barracks, Pennsylvania; Letter of Winfield Scott Hancock to Francis A. Walker, November 5, 1885; Letter of Winfield Scott Hancock to ?, November 16, 1885, Civil War Library and Museum, Philadelphia.
76. William Lochren, "Narrative of the First Regiment," *Minnesota in the Civil and Indian Wars, 1861-1865* (St. Paul, Minnesota: Pioneer Press Company, 1891), vol. 1, p. 36. Fortunately, Hancock would later personally commend the men involved in the July 2 charge; unfortunately, he would mistakenly identify the 1st Minnesota as the 111th New York Volunteer Infantry. In his defense, he had ordered the 111th New York to charge a little earlier in the afternoon, and they too did a tremendous job in the face of overwhelming odds; he simply confused the two regiments.

With the onset of night, ever increasing fatigue, and a lack of reinforcements, the Southern assault gradually shuddered to a halt, then reluctantly receded toward the distant rebel lines. Behind them lay a terrible swath of death and destruction cut deeply into the Union lines. The three corps involved in plugging the hole at the Peach Orchard salient had lost nearly 9,000 men in the late afternoon struggle. Casualties in the three divisions of the Second Corps totaled about 2,800, with 1,275 of them from Brig. Gen. John C. Caldwell's First Division alone. The two divisions of Sickles' Third Corps had lost 593 officers and men killed, 3,029 wounded, and 589 missing. Virtually all of the 2,187 casualties sustained by the Fifth Corps in the entire three day battle were taken in attempting to close the breached lines on July 2.[77]

Although the 111th New York had taken tremendous losses in its toe-to-toe slugfest with the rebels on July 2, similar scenes were witnessed along much of the Second Corps line, with similar casualties. The corps had been severely mauled by the attacking Confederates, its command structure largely devastated.

The First Division lost three of its four brigade commanders: Col. Edward E. Cross of the First Brigade, the victim of a sharpshooter, went down with a mortal abdomen wound; Brig. Gen. Samuel K. Zook of the Third Brigade fell with a similar wound; Fourth Brigade Col. John R. Brooke was fortunate to escape with only a debilitating ankle wound. Col. Orlando H. Morris, 69th New York, was also sidelined with a nonlethal wound, while Col. Richard P. Roberts, 140th Pennsylvania, fell dead after reminding his men to never forget that they were Pennsylvanians and to fire low. Lt. Col. Henry C. Merwin, commanding two companies of the 27th Connecticut, and Col. Hiram L. Brown, 145th Pennsylvania, fell at almost the exact same moment.

The Second Division lost Col. John H. Ward of the 15th Massachusetts, overseeing the action while supported by his wooden leg and cane, and Lt. Col. James Huston, heading the 82nd New York, both mortally wounded. Col. Paul J. Revere, grandson of the Revolutionary War patriot, was killed at the head of the 20th Massachusetts. Lt. Col. Max "Jack of Diamonds" Thoman, 59th New York commander, also

---

77. Pfanz, Gettysburg: The Second Day, pp. 429-30, 553-54. Casualty figures for the July 2 fight are difficult to determine with accuracy since some Union reports make no distinction between the losses of July 2 and July 3. The 2,800 figure is Caldwell's losses reported for July 2, plus half those of Hays' and Gibbon's divisions and the corps artillery reported for the two day period.

received a mortal wound. The 1st Minnesota lost Col. William Colvill (shot through the shoulder and foot), Lt. Col. Charles P. Adams (shot through the chest and leg), Maj. Mark N. Downie, all of its field officers, and 215 of 262 men. Col. William De Witt Baxter fell while leading the 72nd Pennsylvania "Fire Zouaves" near the soon-to-be-famous copse of trees.

The Third Division lost significantly less commissioned officers. Most notable was Col. George L. Willard, commander of the Third Brigade, Third Division, who was killed instantly by a shell as he led his men.

Adjt. J. W. Muffly of the 148th Pennsylvania probably summed up the condition of much of the Second Corps troops as the surging Confederate attack finally ground to a halt: "The men showed the effects of the relaxation from the terrible strain and excitement of battle in an unusual degree. We were panting, pale, except where powder-marked, and in a state of general collapse."[78]

After pausing to watch the Second Corps advancing on the enemy, Livermore was off again, this time to personally conduct the retrieval of the wounded from the front lines. "Having performed such duties as I found necessary I left this part of the field, and, going to my [ambulance] park, prepared to go to the scene of the battle of the 1st Division in the woods. It was now past twilight, and at this moment I was grieved and surprised to see coming across the Taneytown road hundreds and perhaps thousands of the 1st Division of our corps in hasty retreat and great disorder. There was no organization among them, and they bore the appearance of having been broken by the enemy. . . . I started with a party of my men for the woods where the 1st Division had fought, to collect all the wounded who had not been brought out."[79]

"It was now dark and the firing had ceased . . . but under the guidance of some of the men who had helped to bring out the wounded, we reached the wheatfield, where we came to a little house to which many of the wounded and dead had been brought. . . .[80] I was here informed

78. Muffly, *The Story of Our Regiment*, p. 246.

79. Livermore, *Days and Events*, p. 253.

80. This was most probably the Jacob Weikert Farmhouse. Located just north of the Valley of Death, at the southern end of the Weikert Woods, this was the same area where Captain Livermore had needed to drive up the laggardly stretcher-bearers of the First Division earlier in the afternoon.

that our skirmish line was posted in the wheatfield a few yards in front of us, and... I concluded that it was not prudent to go farther toward the enemy than into and half across the wheatfield... I accordingly made sure that there were no wounded left inside the skirmish line...."[81]

The wounded now streamed to the rear in search of the regimental aid stations, which were not always easy to find in the heat, noise, smoke, and confusion of the battle, and now lay concealed by the deepening darkness. The ambulance drivers, as well as the walking wounded, were fortunate if there were posted markers they could follow, directing them to the medical facilities. One eyewitness recorded: "We noticed as we were going through the woods a red flag alongside a board on which we read: '1700 wounded down this way.'"[82]

The influx of men needing medical attention now far exceeded the abilities of the few regimental aid station personnel, and an increasing backlog began to develop. In a situation like this, "[t]he Surgeon . . . should appoint his Hospital Steward, or, if he is not there, one of the most experienced of his attendants to receive them as they come in, get them placed as comfortably as possible, and cut away the bloody clothing and sponge the wounds—all in readiness for [the surgeon's] examination. Another of the attendants might accompany him with dressings, adhesive plaster, &c. and still another will be well employed in administering water to the wounded, and stimulants to the cases designated by the Surgeon—taking care not to pour them in too liberally. A sponging of the wound with cold water—especially in warm weather—removing any clotted blood or shreds of clothing, will be most grateful to the patient, and should generally be the first thing attended to."[83]

81. *Ibid.* Livermore later regretted the implicit trust he placed in the word of others that night. "I did not explore our skirmish line to the left or right, and this is now a source of regret to me. I relied upon the statement of some of my men that the division had fought in the wheatfield, and my own regiment had fought entirely in the woods on the left. Had I known this I should have made an effort to reach the positions occupied by the division in the fight by riding along the skirmish line to the right and left, but I think it is highly probable that at this hour our skirmish lines were not as far advanced as these positions and my efforts would have been useless."
82. Coco, *A Vast Sea of Misery*, p. 188.
83. Vickery, "On the Duties of the Surgeon in Action," p. 21. Unfortunately, the sponging greatly increased the chance of infection since the same sponge was used on patient after patient.

The division hospitals further to the rear were also quickly swamped by the sheer volume of wounded. "About four o'clock the wounded arrived in such large numbers [that] we soon had an accumulation of cases requiring amputation. The operators were keeped [*sic*] at work untill [*sic*] late in the evening and untill they were compelled to desist from their labors from exhaustion. The other Surgeons of the Division who had been detailed to the Hospital were busily engaged during the day performing the various duties which had been assigned them."[84]

Now, as the sun faded to a faint red glow over the ghastly fields of Gettysburg, the wounded continued trudging to the rear.

The evening air was "laden with mist and pervaded by the strange musty smell peculiar to battlefields immediately after battle." Out toward the Emmitsburg Road "on every side lay the cold stiffened bodies of our dead soldiers, sometimes two or three forming ghastly groups together—in most unnatural attitudes together—Sometimes lying naturally and as if asleep—occasionally a wounded man [not] able to move would draw our attention by plaintive moans or a request for water. These we comforted with the assurance that the ambulances would find them in a few minutes."[85]

"The fight done, the sudden revulsion of sense and feeling follow. . . . How strange the stillness seems! The whole air roared with the conflict but a moment since,—now all is silent, not a gunshot is heard — and the silence comes distinctly, almost painfully to the senses. . . . And how look those fields? . . . They were beautiful this morning. They are desolate now,—trampled by countless feet of the combattants [*sic*],—plowed and scarred by shot and shell, the orchards splintered, the fences prostrate, the harvests trodden in the mud."[86]

"And more dreadful than the sight of all this, thickly strewn over all their length and breadth, are the habiliments of the soldier,—the knapsacks, cast aside in the stress of the fight, or after the fatal lead had struck;—haversacks, yawning with the rations, the owner will never call for; canteens of cedar of the Rebel men of Jackson and cloth-covered tin of the men of the Union;—blankets and trowsers, and

84. Dwinelle, *Medical Report*.
85. Adolphus F. Cavada diary, entry for July 2, 1863, The Historical Society of Pennsylvania, Philadelphia, Pennsylvania.
86. Byrne and Weaver, *Haskell of Gettysburg*, pp. 127-28.

coats, and caps; and some are blue and some are gray;—muskets, and ramrods, and bayonets, and swords, and scabbards, and belts, some bent and cut by the shot, or shell;—broken wheels, exploded caissons, and limber-boxes, and dismantled guns;—and all these are sprinkled with blood;—horses, some dead, a mangled heap of carnage, some alive, with a leg shot clear off, or other frightful wound, appealing to you with almost more than brute gaze as you pass;—and last, but not least numerous, many thousands of men,—and there was no rebellion here now,—the men of South Carolina were quiet by the side of those of Massachusetts,—some composed with upturned faces, sleeping the last sleep, some mutilated and frightful, some wretched, fallen, bathed in blood, survivors still and unwilling witnesses of the rage of Gettysburg."[87]

A large number of gravely wounded men still lay on the field where they had fallen, many unreachable in the deadly no-mans-land between the two warring armies. Jacob H. Cole of the 57th New York, unable to walk because of his injuries, looked out past the dead Confederate officer by his side at the trampled field of wheat in which he lay. "As darkness crept in to cover the scene of blood and death, the musketry fire ceases, the artillery fire languishes, and the pall of smoke drifts away on the rising night breeze. The second day's battle is over here. [I am] Wearied by the long march and heavy fighting and suffering from my wounded leg and arm, and the moans of others suffering from wounds came across the battlefield and could not be shut out even by covering my head. . . . But weariness at last asserted itself and I fell asleep until morning."[88]

Second Lieutenant Fuller of the 61st New York was also trapped on the ruined field, trying to come to grips with the broken condition of his body. "As long as I lay perfectly quiet, I was not in much pain, but if I attempted to stir the pain was severe. I had heard that wounded men always suffered from thirst, but I was not specially thirsty, and I wondered at it. I did not have any desire to groan, and take on, as many about me were doing. So I wondered if I were really badly hurt, and if I could groan, if I wanted to. I determined to try it, and drew in a good breath, and let out a full grown-man groan. I was satisfied with the

87. *Ibid.*, p. 128.
88. Cole, *Under Five Commanders*, pp. 203-4.

result and then kept quiet. This action on my part will read like the performance of a simpleton, and I would not record it, but for the fact that it was the freak and experience of one man, helpless on the battlefield. . . ."[89]

Fuller, however, was not content to spend the night on the field, and set about trying to figure out some way to get carried to a hospital. "After a time I was satisfied our people were establishing a picket line some way to my rear. I succeeded in securing the attention of a sergeant. He told me the number of his regiment, which was a new Pennsylvania regiment. I told him I wanted to get back out of this debatable belt of land between the skirmish lines. He said he would go and see his officer." This done, the New York lieutenant lay back and waited.[90]

"In a little while he came back with a Lieutenant. He was a good hearted man, and commiserated with my condition, and inquired what he could do for me. I told him my present anxiety was to get to the rear of our skirmish line—that where I then lay was like to be fought over again, and any little thing would, at least, set the pickets firing at one another. I told him I thought if he and the sergeant would make a chair of their hands, as children often do, they could carry me between them. With difficulty they got me up, and their hands under me, and started, but the broken leg hung down, and caught in the trampled wheat, and I told them I couldn't go it." The two men gently laid Lieutenant Fuller back down on the ground.[91]

The would-be Good Samaritans were not about to give up, though. "Then the Lieutenant said he would carry me on his back. I noticed he had braced up with commissary, and his legs were not wholly reliable, but I thought he could manage me as a pack. So he squatted, and the sergeant helped me get on his back with my arm around his neck. Then he attempted to raise me up, but my weight and the tanglefoot were too much, and we all went down in a heap together, I under."[92]

Enough was enough; Lieutenant Fuller could take no more of the agony his "rescuers" were inflicting on him. "As soon as I could express myself in words, I told the men, if they would straighten me out

---

89. Fuller, *Personal Recollections*, pp. 96-97.
90. *Ibid.*, p. 97
91. *Ibid.*
92. *Ibid.* When someone (especially officers) had been drinking, it was said that "he had braced up with commissary." The chief source of alcohol in the army was the commissary department, and drinking to give a false sense of courage was a prevalent problem with some officers in the army.

and cover me up with my blanket, I would excuse them with thanks for their kind intentions. This they did, and left me with no one in sight."[93]

"It now grew dark rapidly and soon there was as little light as at any time that night. I was wide awake, and my thoughts went on excursions the wide world around." The young officer, broken arm and shattered leg arranged as comfortably as possible, settled in for a very long, dark night.[94]

"The night roll call was a sad one," remembered Capt. Benjamin W. Thompson of that horrible evening. "More than a third of our regiment present for duty fell in this charge [one hundred eighty five out of three hundred ninety]. In the entire battle our losses amounted to seventy three per cent of our force present—a loss only exceeded in modern times by the First Minnesota, which in this battle lost eighty two per cent of its force present for duty."[95]

Captain Thompson and the battle-blackened survivors of the 111th New York were finally marched to the rear, only to be ordered peremptorily back again to the front by the ever-present General Hancock himself. "This countermarch was more for spleen than for sense as, in a short time, orders came through the proper channels, and we dragged our weary bodies back to our former place in line. Without meat, bread or coffee, we cast ourselves down on the ground as thoroughly worn out and exhausted in mind, body, brain and stomach as men could well be."[96]

"Nor was there much in the situation to stir our enthusiasm. One of our best corps was badly broken up and demoralized, and the day had only been saved from total defeat by these terribly desperate counter charges which we have been describing, and we had developed a force of the enemy that clearly outnumbered us. We had saved the left, and night closed on a drawn battle, but God only knew who would be victors tomorrow."[97]

---

93. *Ibid.*
94. *Ibid.*
95. Thompson, *Personal Narrative*, p. 37.
96. *Ibid.*, p. 39.
97. *Ibid.*

CHAPTER 4

THURSDAY, JULY 2: NIGHTFALL—FRIDAY, JULY 3: ABOUT 1:00 P.M.

"Acres of ground covered with wounded"

Sgt. Thomas P. Meyer,
148th Pennsylvania Pioneer Corps

As the exhausted men of the Second Corps attempted to get some badly needed sleep, a strange lullaby floated up from the rear of Cemetery Ridge. "All the bands in the army were ordered up and placed between the troops and the hospitals. They played by detachments all night to drown the cries of the wounded and those who were being operated upon. They played 'When this cruel War is over' for hours together, and while we sympathized with the sentiment we execrated the doleful and monotonous music."[1]

The repetitious music also helped cover the rustle and muted clinking of stealthy movement. "All night long were heard the tramp of moving troops, the low rumble of the wheels of ambulances, the ammunition and supply trains, and the artillery over the stony roads. The sharp command of the officers, the curses of the teamsters heard above the murmur of many voices, the groans of the wounded and dying made a medley of weird and discordant sounds."[2]

From far out to the front, however, came an entirely different serenade—the eerie ululation of voices that sent cold chills up the spines of those within earshot: "The most doleful sounds that broke the night stillness were the cries for water and help that came from the

1. Thompson, *Personal Narrative*, p. 39.
2. Muffly, *The Story of Our Regiment*, pp. 538-39.

poor sufferers on the field who were in an agony lest they should be missed in the search and left to perish unaided."[3]

It was shaping up to be a very long night.

Out on the skirmish line, with only a ditch to serve as shelter, the men of the 8th Ohio were settling in for an uncomfortable and tedious night. "Night soon came on and put a stop to any more serious fighting. But the crack of the rifle, along with the singing of the bullets and the roar of the shells passing over one's head like a train of carts crossing a bridge, continued throughout the night. As we lay on our backs courting sleep, we could at any time, if we opened our eyes, see the skies crossed with a network of the fiery traces of shells going and coming, like shooting stars, between the artillery of both sides."[4]

The night again reverberated as Ewell's Confederate troops stormed Culp's Hill. For the Ohioans, on solitary duty far to the front, the nighttime action enigmatically took place to their rear, prompting Lt. Thomas Galwey to write that "this was, to say the least, very interesting to us who were firing an occasional shot at the skirmishers in our front and were now and then startled by a shell coming from the enemy behind us."[5]

This was getting to be very familiar ground to these men. "I had been on the line with my company until about nine o'clock, when I was relieved by another company, but at midnight we were again sent out to that fatal fence." Midnight, however, saw the return of quiet to the field. Except for a solitary Rebel courier who unwittingly bumbled into the Union skirmishers, the wee hours of Friday passed quietly enough for Galwey and his men. "At four in the morning (Friday, July 3) I was relieved, and took my company back to the ditch of the road, where we stretched out and slept. How we slept!"[6]

J. H. W. Stuckenberg of the 145th Pennsylvania was determined to do his part in helping comfort and care for the ongoing flood of casualties. The twenty-eight-year-old chaplain set out through the

3. Thompson, *Personal Narrative*, p. 40.
4. Galwey, *The Valiant Hours*, pp. 103-4.
5. *Ibid.*, p. 104.
6. *Ibid.*, pp. 106-8.

hospitals and aid stations to minister to the men of his regiment, starting with the First Division Hospital immediately to the rear. "Our hospital was at the foot of the hill. Going toward it, the first one of the first wounded men I saw was Col [Hiram L.] Brown, wounded in the right arm above the elbow. I led his horse to the hospital, where his wound was examined and the cheerful announcement was made that his arm need not be amputated. As Dr. [George L.] Potter put his fingers in the wound to discover the extent of the injury, Col B was writhing in pain—his suffering evidently being intense. About the same time Col [*sic*] [Samuel K.] Zook was carried to the hospital on a stretcher, mortally wounded." (Brigadier General Zook had been brought from the field by ambulance, accompanied by his aides. Knowing that the wound was fatal, and that nothing could be done except make the patient as comfortable as possible, the First Division surgeons sent him by stretcher to a small house on the Baltimore Pike).[7]

"Col Brown requested me to hunt the Adjutant who was very badly wounded. I at once started towards the field of battle." The chaplain accordingly headed off in the darkness toward the Union right. "At the 11th Corps hospital I found Adj [John D.] Black wounded through the breast, mortally Dr. [J. S.] Whillden [*sic*] thought.[8] He looked very feeble, said little and that in a voice scarcely audible. He thought himself that he could scarcely live till morning, said he suffered greatly, was willing and ready to die and longing for death to relieve him. I asked him whether he had any words for his parents? 'Tell them,' he replied, 'that I fell in a noble cause.' 'I have been a bad boy,' he said, 'but God is merciful.' He was calm and seemed perfectly resigned to his fate. Some effects about his person and his sword he requested me to send home to his parents."[9]

---

7. Stuckenberg, *I'm Surrounded by Methodists*, p. 78; *The Philadelphia Times*, January 6, 1864; Potter, "Reminiscences of Field-Hospital Service," p. 15; Potter, *Three Years with the Army of the Potomac*, pp. 59-60; Douglas D. Zook, "A Biographical Sketch of Samuel K. Zook," *The Bulletin of the Historical Society of Montgomery County* [Pennsylvania], vol. 23, no. 2 (Spring 1982): 121; Josiah M. Favill, *The Diary of a Young Officer Serving with the Armies of the United States During the War of the Rebellion* (Chicago: R. R. Donnelley & Sons Co., 1909), pp. 246-48. Zook carried the rank of brigadier general, not colonel, at Gettysburg.
8. Adjutant Black was most probably in the Eleventh Corps field hospital at the George Spangler Farm. [Gregory A Coco, *A Vast Sea of Misery*, pp. 105-7.] However, somewhere along the line, the assistant surgeon from his regiment, J. S. Whildin, was able to examine his wounds.
9. Stuckenberg, *I'm Surrounded by Methodists*, p. 78.

"I also saw Capt [John W.] Reynolds at this hospital, wounded on the left side of the head. He was much excited—elated because our regt had done so well and had driven the rebels before them. I found many more here of the wounded of our regt. As many as could easily be moved I directed to be taken to our [Second] corps hospital, others were made as comfortable as possible."[10]

The aid stations and division hospitals were working at full speed now, struggling to keep pace with the incoming wave of casualties from Thursday's fight. "I stopped at a dozen or more of the great Pennsylvania barns, looking more like large factory buildings than our New England barns," wrote Vermont Lt. George Grenville Bennett, staff aide to Vermont Brig. Gen. George J. Stannard, who stumbled onto the hospitals while on a frustrating nighttime search for the ammunition train. "Each of them was a field hospital; its floor covered with mutilated soldiers, and surgeons busy at the lantern-lighted operating tables."[11]

As the wounded continued to stream in, all buildings were soon full, and the overflow crowded around the shadowed doorways. "By the door of one of them was a ghastly pile of amputated arms and legs, and around each of them lay multitudes of wounded men, covering the ground by the acre, wrapped in their blankets and awaiting their turns under the knife. I was stopped hundreds of times by wounded men, sometimes accompanied by a comrade but often wandering alone, to be asked in faint tones the way to the hospital of their division, till the accumulated sense of the bloodshed and suffering of the day became absolutely appalling. It seemed to me as if every square yard of the ground, for many square miles, must have its blood stain."[12]

Even in the difficult circumstances under which they were laboring, the hospitals were striving to sort out the tangle of wounded from

---

10. *Ibid.*
11. George G. Benedict, *Army Life in Virginia—Letters from the Twelfth Vermont Regiment and Personal Experiences of Volunteer Service in the War for the Union* (Burlington, Vermont: Free Press Association, 1895), p. 171.
12. *Ibid.*, pp. 171-72.

other corps, transporting them, whenever possible, back to their own medical facilities. For Capt. Jack Adams of the 19th Massachusetts, in a Third Corps field hospital, word of his evacuation came "late at night, when a surgeon came with an ambulance, and said I must be moved to the 2d corps hospital, as this was too near the line of battle. Having no stretchers they placed me on a board, and loaded me in."[13]

Captain Adams' trip proved to be short and potentially fatal. "This movement started my wounds bleeding again, and I thought that the words of the assistant surgeon would prove true, but they drove me a mile I should judge, and dumped me by the road side with other wounded. I remained here until the next noon." Now stranded between hospitals at an ambulance collection point, again bleeding from his three separate wounds, and too badly injured to walk the remaining distance to the Second Corps Hospitals, Adams could only stretch out on the hard ground, wrapped in his Confederate blanket, and wait.[14]

After personally overseeing the collection of the wounded in the wheatfield area, Captain Livermore returned in the pitchy darkness to the Union positions on Cemetery Ridge to supervise the efforts of his other ambulance teams. "Riding back to the other divisions I found a great deal to do in superintending the collection and dispatch of the wounded to the hospital. While engaged in this work I received word that Colonel Cross had been mortally wounded and that he desired to see me. Nothing but the most imperative duty could have detained me from him, but the removal of the many wounded who might perish, if not cared for, was of that character, and I found myself unable to go to him until midnight, when I rode to the spot where he lay. It was a little dell, possibly one through which a little stream ran, between the Taneytown road and the Baltimore road, and from a quarter to half a mile from my [ambulance] park going toward Gettysburg. Here under the shelter of some boulders lay a large number of our wounded and dead who had been brought from the field. They lay upon the ground covered with their blankets, and the living were nearly all silent, having fallen asleep from fatigue. I picked my way among their prostrate forms to the spot where the colonel lay, and inquiring of an officer of my

13. Adams, *Reminiscences of the Nineteenth Massachusetts*, pp. 67-68.
14. *Ibid.*, p. 68.

regiment, whom I saw, which was the colonel, he pointed him out to me, indicating that he was dead."[15]

"I went to him and turned the blanket back from his face, and saw that it was true that he was dead. The moonlight or starlight enabled me to see his features distinctly. They were placid and exceedingly lifelike, and it was hard to persuade myself that the flush of life had gone from them. His lofty forehead was smooth, his long, silky beard lay upon his breast undisheveled, and he looked more as he would if he slept than seemed possible. . . . He sent for various members of the regiment, myself included, and also my little boy Charlie, to bid us farewell. . . . I was oppressed with great regret that I had failed to see Colonel Cross before he died, but I took his sending for me as proof that my course had not given such offense to him as to forfeit his friendship."[16]

"Sitting beside the colonel listening to what the officer told me about him at midnight, surrounded by many wounded, was a sad experience and one which can never forsake my memory; among the other circumstances which I recall is this, that lying close by us was a lieutenant of the 2nd New Hampshire Volunteers mortally wounded (I think his name was Patch), and it was a mournful thing to think of his dying there, not only away from home, but away from those of his own regiment who might have cared for him."[17] The same fate was in store for many of the men strewn over the battlefield on that sad night.

Beside the ambulancemen, chaplains, and doctors, another group of men were getting precious little sleep on this miserable July night. These were the pioneer troops, combat engineers who were assigned the grisly duty of locating, identifying, and burying the dead from the regiments in their brigade. Sgt. Thomas P. Meyer of the 148th Pennsylvania, First Brigade, First Division of the Second Corps, saw more than his share of dead men before the night was over.

---

15. Livermore, *Days and Events*, p. 254.
16. *Ibid.*, pp. 254-55. "The boy, Charlie Fullerton, . . . had come to serve my lieutenant and myself at Falmouth, and had remained with us until I left the regiment, chose to go with me to the staff, so that I was provided with a very good servant." [p. 274.]
17. *Ibid.*, p. 255. Lt. Charles W. Patch, thirty-one-year-old native of Portsmouth, New Hampshire, was mortally wounded in the abdomen and died July 10.

"According to orders received at eleven o'clock at night, I took the pioneers of the Regiment, with picks, shovels and sperm candles, back to an open air field hospital, behind a rocky bluff on Rock Creek, a mile to our right rear where several thousand wounded had been carried during the day while the battle was in progress, to sort the dead from the living and to bury them.[18] We reached the hospital designated and *found acres of ground* covered with wounded, and among them, many who had died after being brought here from the field. The pioneers of the 148th were the only men on duty at this point during the night."[19]

"We lit our candles and examined the situation. This was an awful place. The most able writer could not give the slightest shadow of an idea of this dreadful charnel scene; the awful sights in the wheat field and death valley thickly strewn over with weapons, cannon, broken gun carriages, thousands of dead men and horse, mutilated in all manner of form and degree, when we left in the early evening were incomparable behind this scene of suffering and death. Here the dead and wounded lay promiscuously side by side, and close together, in long rows, on the bare wet ground, the feet of one row nearly touching the heads of the next row, the Union and Confederate in separate rows."[20]

"All was darkness; not a torch or candle burning. For some unknown reason, there were no surgeons in attendance on the wounded at this place during this night, at least not from midnight to 3:00 A.M., during which time we were at work there; yet about half of them had their wounds dressed, lying on the bare ground, unsheltered, uncovered, many of them nearly naked. Here the men in hundreds of cases dressed each other's wounds, making bandages out of drawers taken from their bodies for the purpose. Many a soldier gave drawers and shirt from his body to bandage the wounds of his comrades. Men wounded in the legs had pant legs cut off, some close to the body, leaving the legs entirely naked and uncovered. There were no blankets or tents, absolutely nothing. Many lay entirely helpless in the scorching sun and rain till the skin was scalded and burned into

---

18. This was the Second Corps Hospital, already in the process of evacuating its facilities by the Taneytown Road. The final movement would take place during the heavy shelling preceding the Pickett-Pettigrew-Trimble charge on July 3.
19. Muffly, *The Story of Our Regiment*, p. 460. Italics are Meyer's.
20. *Ibid.*

pealing blisters in the faces, and worse in the parts of the body, tender and unaccustomed to exposure to the sun."[21]

While deeply touched by the needs of the men they encountered, the 148th Pioneers were particularly in search of men from their own unit. "We found, by the dim light of our sperm candles, many of the 148th boys. Some had their wounds dressed and were sleeping soundly, among them Amos Erhart, of Company A, like the rest, few clothes, no cover, with a nasty hole through the thigh just grazing the femoral artery; the pant leg cut off at the body, shoe and stocking gone, the naked leg as cold as ice, his head much lower than his body, the wound nicely dressed and not bleeding. He was sleeping quietly, and as soundly as anyone could in the best bed. I put a flat stone under his head to put him in a more comfortable position and stop the rattle in his throat. Manassas Gilbert, also of Company A, was found here sitting on the ground with his back against a tree, with a bullet in his shoulder, but wide awake. Deep moans of agony in continuous chorus, were heard, but in all this vast number of desperately wounded men there was not a tear or a single noisy outcry."[22]

Everyone attending Cross' body had either wandered away or nodded off when Sergeant Meyers' pioneer corps made their sweep through the facility collecting the dead for burial. "Some of my men carried out the dead and laid them in rows, heads all one way, and the one against the other," wrote Meyers. "About the third man carried out was the tyrant commander of our Brigade, Colonel Cross, of the 5th New Hampshire Regiment, killed in the woods near the wheat field. We did not bury him."[23]

While one detail collected and laid out the dead, another started the gruesome task of interring their friends and neighbors from back home. "Some of the men buried the dead thus laid in rows; a shallow grave about a foot deep, against the first man in a row, and he was then laid

---

21. *Ibid.*, p. 461.
22. *Ibid.*
23. *Ibid.*, pp. 461-62. Cross' body was embalmed and sent home to Lancaster, New Hampshire, where his casket, draped with the U.S. flag, on which rested his cap and sword, lay in state on the wide covered porch at his family's home. The colonel was buried July 9 with full military and Masonic honors at the local cemetery, attended by a vast crowd of friends, relatives, lodge members, and the village band. [William Child, *A History of the Fifth Regiment New Hampshire Volunteers in the American Civil War, 1861-1865*, (Bristol, New Hampshire: R. W. Musgrove, Printer, 1893), pp. 212-13.]

down into it; a similar grave was dug where he had lain. The ground thus dug up served to cover the first man, and the second was laid in a trench, and so on, so the ground was only handled once. This was the regular form of burial in our battlefields; it is the most rapid, and is known as trench burial, and is employed where time for work is limited."[24]

And so the Pioneer Corps of the 148th Pennsylvania labored on, performing a tender last service for their dead, on into the early morning hours of July 3.

For Frank Haskell, staff aide to Second Division commander John Gibbon (now once again in charge of the entire Second Corps with Hancock's temporary appointment to command the wounded Sickles' Third Corps), it was shaping up to be another long night.[25] "Near eleven o'clock, the enemy wearied with his disastrous work, desisted; and thereafter until morning not a shot was heard in all the armies. . . . After evening came on, and from reports received, all was known to be going satisfactorily upon the right, Gnl Meade summoned his Corps Commanders to his Head Quarters for consultation."[26]

Haskell accompanied Gibbon to the command summit at the Widow Leister House. "The mean little room where they met,—its only furniture consisted of a large, wide bed in one corner; a small pine table in the center, upon which was a wooden pail of water, with a tin cup for drinking, and a candle, stuck to the table by putting the end in tallow melted down from the wick; and five or six straight-backed, rush-bottom chairs. The Generals came in,—some sat, some kept walking or standing, two lounged upon the bed,—some were constantly smoking cigars."[27]

24. *Ibid.*, p. 462.
25. *Conduct of the War*, General Winfield Scott Hancock, March 1, 1864, vol. 1, p. 407 and March 22, 1864, p. 502; *OR*, vol. 27, pt. 1, p. 370; Hancock, *Reminiscences of Winfield Scott Hancock*, p. 196. Sickles had appointed Maj. Gen. David B. Birney, commander of the First Division of the Third Corps, as Sickles' replacement when his leg was almost totally ripped off by a cannonball. However, when Meade learned of the appointment, he overrode Sickles and detailed Hancock instead to shore up the deteriorating situation in the Third Corps.
26. Byrne and Weaver, *Haskell of Gettysburg*, p. 131.
27. *Ibid.*, p. 134.

After some two hours, and a unanimous decision to stay on the heights and fight it out at Gettysburg, the council dissolved, and the officers went their several ways. "Night, sultry and starless, droned on; and it was almost midnight that I found myself peering my way from the line of the 2nd Corps, back down to the General's Head Quarters, which were in an Ambulance in the rear, in a little peach orchard. All was silent now, but the sound of the Ambulances, as they were bringing off the wounded; and you could hear them rattle here and there about the field and see their lanterns. I am weary and sleepy almost to such an extent as not to be able to sit my horse."[28]

At last, after almost two days of continuous activity, Haskell reached Second Corps headquarters, and, with the help of his servant, settled in for the night. "Generals Hancock and Gibbon, [as well as Maj. Gen. John Newton, temporary commander of the First Corps,] were asleep in the Ambulance. . . . 'George, make my bed here upon the ground, by the side of this Ambulance.—Pull off my sabre and my boots,—that will do!' Was ever princly [*sic*] couch, or softest down so soft as those rough blankets, there upon the unroofed sod? At midnight they received me for four hours delicious, dreamless oblivion of weariness and of battle. So to me ended the 2nd of July."[29]

Lt. Charles A. Fuller, incapacitated by a broken arm and shattered leg, was still laying awake out between the hostile skirmish lines, listening to the night sounds and wondering how soon morning would arrive. "I think it must have been midnight—for hours I had heard no sound but the groanings of the men lying on the field about me. All at once I heard a voice. It came from the mouth of Phil Comfort, a private of Co A. Phil had always been one of the incorrigibles. He would get drunk, and brawl, and fight on the slightest provocation, but he also had the credit of doing much for the wounded of the regiment. I do not know what Phil's business was, out there between the picket lines at

28. *Ibid.*, p. 135.

29. *Ibid.*, pp. 135, 136; Gibbon, *Personal Recollections*, p. 145. C. H. Morgan, of Hancock's staff, disagrees with Haskell as to where General Hancock spent the night. "The council having adjourned, General Hancock laid down on the porch at army headquarters to snatch a little sleep." [Hancock, *Reminiscences of Winfield Scott Hancock*, p. 206.] "George" was George Hamlin, Haskell's personal servant, who had traveled with Haskell since 1861. [Byrne and Weaver, *Haskell of Gettysburg*, p. 136, note.]

midnight of that day. I suspect he may have been there for the purpose of accommodating any corpse that was desirous of being relieved of any valuables he was possessed of, fearing they might be buried in an unmarked grave with his dead body. I never asked Phil about the orders, or from whom they came, that sent him into hailing distance of my place of repose, but I made haste to call Phil up to me."[30]

"He responded to my call, and in a moment was staring down at me in the starlight. He said, 'Why, Lieutenant, that's you, ain't it!' I admitted the allegation, and said I wanted to get out of here. He replied that he would go for a man and stretcher, and return as soon as possible, and off hc went. Before long he was back with man and stretcher, and after much working they got me loaded and started for a point at which ambulances were assembling. I was set down in the dooryard of a house built of hewed logs, whitewashed. . . ." After finally managing to leave the ghostly solitude of the battlefield, Lieutenant Fuller was waiting again, this time for an ambulance to take him to the nearest aid station.[31]

Having witnessed friends, classmates, relatives, and bosom buddies blown away, seemingly at random, other Second Corps troops set out on late night forays across the battlefield. They carried dark

30. Fuller, *Personal Recollections*, p. 98.

31. *Ibid.* The area over which the men had fought was usually so littered with the strewn bodies of dead and wounded, or choked with boulders, brush, or uneven ground as to make driving a vehicle virtually impossible. The wounded were carried to the nearest level spot inside Union lines and deposited there for pick up by the ambulance corps. [Theodore B. Gates, *The "Ulster Guard" [20th N. Y. State Militia] and the War of the Rebellion. Embracing a History of the Early Organization of the Regiment; Its Three Months' Service; Its Reorganization and Subsequent Service; A Chronological Record of Every March, Place of Encampment or Bivouac, with Distances Marched; Account of Proceedings of Detachment on Veteran Furlough; Flag Presentations, &c.; Complete Roster During Entire Service; Officers and Companies on Special Duty; Lists of Killed and Wounded; &c.; &c. Together with a Brief Treatise Upon the Origin and Growth of Secession; The Militia System, and the Dependence of the Federal Government Upon it in the Beginning of the War; With a Critical History of the First Battle of Bull Run; Campaign of Gen. Pope; McClellan's Maryland Campaign; Battle of Fredericksburg; Hooker's Chancellorsville Campaign; Gettysburg Campaign; and a Glance at the Campaign from the Rapidan to Appomattox Court House* (New York: Benjamin H. Tyrrel, Printer, 1879), p. 460.]

lanterns, or candles carefully shielded from enemy eyes, and searched for familiar faces, or a recognizable ring or hat or coat when faces were blurred or removed by flying projectiles. Some secured permission first; others simply melted quietly into the darkness. "All night, some of the officers and men were, by special permission, employed assisting the Surgeons in hunting for the dead and wounded," recalled J. Smith Brown, adjutant of the 126th New York.[32]

Searching for downed family, friends, or fellow soldiers over unfamiliar terrain, where shattered trees loomed and shell-plowed fields and discarded military hardware tripped the unwary, was not a task for the faint of heart. "Nothing could be more dismal and appalling than searching over a battle-field in a dark night for a friend or comrade. To turn up one dead cold face after another to the glimmering light of a lantern, and see it marred with wounds and disfigured with blood and soil, the features, perhaps, convulsed by the death-agony, the eyes vacant and staring,—surely that friendship must be, indeed, stronger than death which would prompt to such an office, yet it was often undertaken, and even by women! Dismal, too, the sight of the dark battleground, with lanterns twinkling here and there, 'like the wisp on the morass!'"[33]

Chaplain Stuckenberg knew that a number of men from his regiment were still out in the field where the regiment had fought earlier in the day. Determined to see what he could do to physically relieve them and spiritually minister to them, he set out from the Eleventh Corps Hospital, "and with Dr. [Assistant Surgeon D. W.] Richards [of the 145th Pennsylvania] started for the battle field where our regt had fought, hoping to find some of our wounded. We met a number of regts leaving the field and saw two guns drawn off by hand. It was dark and the road was not very good."[34]

"We soon came to a house full of wounded men," noted Chaplain Stuckenberg in his diary, "with only one or two well ones to wait on them. We went on farther, over fields and rocks and stone walls and through woods not knowing whither our course would lead us. We met

32. Arabella M. Willson, *Disaster, Struggle, Triumph: The Adventures of 1000 "Boys in Blue," From August, 1862, to June, 1865* (Albany, New York: Argus co., printers, 1870), p. 178.

33. *Ibid.*

34. Stuckenberg, *I'm Surrounded by Methodists*, p. 78.

few soldiers, heard but little noise. The very stillness was fearful and oppressive. A dread came upon [me] as I neared the ground where the desperate fighting had taken place in the afternoon. At any moment I might stumble on some corpse or fall over some wounded man. We frequently stopped to listen for groans, but heard none till we came to another house."[35]

If the conditions in the aid stations were frightful, the situation in the individual houses and sheds where the wounded had crawled or been carried for shelter were absolutely horrifying. "I asked for the wounded of our regt and found one man answering my call. I passed through between the wounded men outside the house, entered the house, with difficulty passed in the dark through a room in which were some wounded men, and entered another room. On a bed suffering terribly lay [Pvt. Frank M.] Forbes of Company G, wounded through the breast. He begged us to dress his wounds, but as there was no candle to be had, this was out of the question. I gave him some whiskey to stimulate him and then left him promising if possible to have him removed to our Hospital, where I had the pleasure of seeing him the next morning."[36]

There was still the possibility of men lying on the field, so badly wounded that they were unable to reach the crowded shelter of this small building, so Stuckenberg and Richards pressed on. "I left the many wounded at their house (no physicians to attend them, no candle even, though they were taken away as fast as the ambulances could carry them) and went further to the front. Back of the house we saw the first corpse. Scarcely had we passed it when a bullet from the rebels whistled past us and warned us to proceed no further, for our picket line was but a short distance in front of us. In again passing the house we had just left we heard subdued, but constant groaning near the barn. I found a rebel there, seriously wounded, who gave no answer to the question, whether I could do anything for him? he being perhaps unconscious and near his end."[37]

---

35. *Ibid.*
36. *Ibid.*, p. 79. Stuckenberg mistakenly identified Pvt. Frank M. Forbes, wounded through the right lung actually belonged to Company I. [*Erie Weekly Gazette*, July 16, 1863; Carded Medical Records, National Archives and Records Administration] This may be the same "little house to which many of the wounded and dead had been brought" that Livermore visited in his trip to the wheatfield, most likely the home of the Jacob Weikert family. [Livermore, *Days and Events*, p. 253.]
37. *Ibid.*

"In passing from the field we learned that a wounded man was lying all alone in the woods. We carried him to a place easily to be found, and sent a stretcher for him. We went back to the [First Division] hospital, where I found quite a number of our wounded." The chaplain continued to minister to the men until exhaustion finally overtook him. "I then went to bed. Seldom had I been so tired. Nature had endured all it could and now coveted the balmy restorer—sleep."[38]

So, surrounded by the murmur of many voices, and the groans and cries of the wounded, with the tread of the stretchermen and clatter of the incoming ambulances as a backdrop, and the monotonous strains of "When this Cruel War is Over" to lull his rest, Chaplain J. H. W. Stuckenberg drifted off to sleep.

Lieutenant Fuller lay at the ambulance collection point, bleeding from his two serious wounds, watching the wounded continue to arrive and the loaded ambulances clatter away into the darkness. "After an hour's waiting, I was loaded into an ambulance without taking me from my stretcher. This was fortunate for me, as I kept it until it was swaped [*sic*] for a new one two weeks later. The stretcher kept me from the ground, and was an important factor in my recovery. A man was placed beside me shot through the body. He was in an agony of pain, and it was impossible for him to restrain his groans."[39]

"When the ambulance started, it went anywhere but in a good road, and as it bumped over logs and boulders, my broken leg would thresh about like the mauler of a flail. I found it necessary to keep it in place by putting the other one over it. At last we stopped and were unloaded." The young lieutenant was pulled out, stretcher and all, and laid among the growing number of wounded around the First Division Hospital in the edge of a woods, near the old schoolhouse on Granite School House Road. Once again, Fuller was forced to wait, this time to have his wounds examined. The New Yorker checked the tourniquet on his leg by groping in the dark, then lay back to rest as best as possible until it was his turn with the doctors.[40]

38. *Ibid.*
39. Fuller, *Personal Recollections*, p. 98.
40. *Ibid.*

"The Ambulances commenced their work as soon as the battle opened," commented staff aide Frank Haskell, "the twinkling lanterns through the night and the sun of to-morrow saw them still with the same work unfinished."[41]

Any weary infantryman or cannoneer, roused from sleep by the harsh clatter of passing ambulances and their groaning passengers throughout the long night hours, would have looked down upon a strange scene of grisly horror and sprectral beauty. "Hundreds of ambulances" and "surgeons, hospital stewards, and stretcher-bearers without number" methodically covered the scarred landscape where battle had just taken place. From the far side of the field "came the Confederate surgeons and their assistants," and they "soon filled the mile-square space between the two armies with wandering jets of light." Like hovering fireflies, "these wandering lights were seen all through the night, and when morning came the work of relief was still unfinished."[42]

"Long after midnight the ambulance corps were busy picking up the wounded and hauling their groaning loads to the rear," remembered Captain Thompson of that horrible night. "Every house and barn for a mile or more in our rear were taken for hospitals and long rows of poor fellows lay on the ground awaiting their turn to undergo probing, dressing and perhaps amputation."[43]

(Only one corps ambulance officer's report of the night's activities was ever published. Capt. James A. Bates, Fifth Corps ambulance commander, reported that eighty-one of his crews worked throughout the night. By 4:00 a.m., they had recovered all of the wounded behind the picket line, and transported 1,300 casualties to the Fifth Corps divisional hospitals beyond the Taneytown Road. With approximately 2,800 casualties in the Second Corps as compared with the nearly 2,100 in the Fifth Corps, Livermore's crews were probably wrapping up their night's work of gathering and transporting the wounded a little after sunrise, as Haskell recorded).[44]

Captain Livermore continued to personally direct the work of removing the wounded from the field until the very early hours of July 3.

---

41. Byrne and Weaver, *Haskell of Gettysburg*, pp. 128-29.
42. George A. Bruce, *The Twentieth Regiment of Massachusetts Volunteer Infantry 1861-1865* (Boston: Houghton, Mifflin and Company, The Riverside Press, Cambridge, 1906), pp. 283-84.
43. Thompson, *Personal Narrative*, p. 39.
44. *OR*, vol. 27, pt. 1, p. 597.

He dryly commented: "I believe that I found enough to do to prevent my sleeping more than an hour or two on this night."[45]

Very few vehicles were rolling that night other than the ambulances. The bivouac of Lt. Tully McCrea and the men of Lt. George A. Woodruff's 1st United States Artillery, Battery I, had finally quieted for the night, men and horses stolidly enduring what promised to be a dark, hungry night. "All the wagons of the army, except ammunition wagons, had been sent back to Westminster, seventeen miles to the rear, so as to leave the roads clear in case the Army of the Potomac had to retreat," recalled Tully years later, "and orders were given that none should be allowed to go to the front. Our wagons had the rations for the men and forage for the horses, and we carried with the battery only three days' supply. This supply was exhausted on the evening of July 2nd, and the officers were wondering where they were to get food for the men and horses the next day."[46]

The hush of early morning lay over the artillery camp after the "terrible fight on the 2nd. . . . About two o'clock that night while we were lying on the ground getting what sleep we could, a wagon drove into camp. Sergeant Stewart, the Quartermaster Sergeant, who was in charge of the wagons, waiting for the small hours of the morning, had managed to slip past the guards with his wagon and was there with three days' rations and forage for his battery. He had disobeyed orders, but he had supplied his battery with the necessary food. Before daylight he was back in the wagon camp and no one was the wiser."[47]

There was little sleep to be had for the staff at the 148th Pennsylvania Volunteers aid station that night. Set up at the Hummelbaugh homestead under the guidance of Assistant Surgeon Alfred T. Hamilton, the bustling medical facility was even running its own commissary, with twenty-one-year-old hospital attendant Pvt. Davy

45. Livermore, *Days and Events*, p. 258.

46. Tully McCrea, *Dear Belle: Letters from a Cadet & Officer to his Sweetheart, 1858-1865*, ed. Catherine S. Crary (Middletown, Connecticut: Wesleyan University Press, 1965), p. 207.

47. *Ibid.*

McIlhattan of Company G making “slapjacks” for staff and patients from a half barrel of flour discovered in the attic. The frame building was soon redolent with the warm fragrance of fresh pancakes, giving the severely wounded patients (mostly from the decimated Third Corps) some welcome distraction from the magnitude of their injuries.[48]

The overflow of casualties quickly spilled beyond the small house, into the outbuildings, and then even out over the surrounding boulder-strewn pastures. In response to the backlog of patients at the division hospitals, Hamiliton had greatly expanded the medical care provided here beyond its assigned duty of quickly stabilizing the wounded for removal to the hospitals in the rear. Adjt. J. W. Muffly of the 148th, hobbling badly after being struck in the left calf by a spent piece of a Confederate shell, discovered that fact in a most unpleasant way: “During the night of the 2d as I approached the little house—now the field hospital—I stepped on something that felt so peculiar that I stopped and picked it up. It proved to be an arm. Happening to look at the west window I saw an outline of a pyramid of some sort, which on examination I found was a pile of hands, arms, feet and legs which the surgeons had thrown out in their work and which now reached the window sill.”[49]

“During the fight I saw Colonel Cross of the 5th New Hampshire, a little in the rear of the line of works at the time of his wound,” recorded Doctor Hamilton of the previous afternoon, “—the twelfth battle wound—a white bandage tied around his top-head. I thought of the occasion when he struck [Cpl. George J.] Duffy, of Company G, with his sword while on the march to Uniontown [at the fording of the creek on June 29].”[50]

Now, with the coming of night, Doctor Hamilton had one very famous, and equally cantankerous, patient under his care. Stretcher-bearers had come upon Confederate Brig. Gen. William Barksdale on the field and carried him to the nearest aid station—the Hummelbaugh Farm. The general had fallen at the head of his Mississippi troops in the assault on Colonel Willard’s brigade, and now lay surrounded by the very men his troops had attacked.

The house was full when the stretcher team arrived, so someone made up a pallet of a few blankets on which to position the general until

48. Muffly, *The Story of Our Regiment*, p. 172.

49. *Ibid.*, p. 245.

50. *Ibid.*, p. 173. See the account of the encounter between Colonel Cross and Corporal Duffy in the prelude.

he could be seen by the surgeon. Principal Musician Robert A. Cassidy was busy assisting Hamilton in receiving the incoming casualties, examining their varied wounds by candlelight. Cassidy tried to give his Confederate patient some water from a canteen, but Barksdale could not sit up. Handing the candle to a bystander, Cassidy gave the general water with a spoon. The Southerner identified himself to the young musician, and Cassidy at once called over Doctor Hamilton.[51]

"I attended General Barksdale of Mississippi," reported the surgeon, noting his diagnosis of the patient's injuries; "he was shot through the left breast from behind, and the left leg was broken by two missiles. He was brought by some staff orderly to my temporary hospital. I gave him what I had to relieve him. He asked several times whether I considered his wound necessarily mortal. I told him I did. . . . He was large, corpulent, refined in appearance, bald, and his general physical and mental make up indicated firmness, endurance, vigor, quick perception and ability to succeed whether as politician, civilian, or warrior. He told me he was a member of Congress under [Presidents Franklin] Pierce and [James] Buchanan."[52]

Barksdale looked every bit the haughty politician and general that he was. "He was dressed in jeans of their choice. His short roundabout was trimmed on the sleeves with gold braid. The Mississippi button, with a star in the center, closed it. The collar had three stars on each side next the chin. Next his body was a fine linen or cotton shirt which was closed by three studs bearing Masonic emblems. His pants has two stripes of gold braid, half an inch broad, down each leg."[53]

Surgeon Hamilton prescribed morphine to help ease Barksdale's suffering, and Cassidy administered it. "Thus conditioned the politician and warrior was laid on the sacred soil of Pennsylvania to breathe his last."[54]

"In front of the house lay General Barksdale mortally wounded," remembered Adjutant Muffly of his late night visit to the hospital, "his breast torn and one leg shattered by grape shot. . . . 'Bring me water, cold water,' he would say. 'When I am well I am a great lover of water,

---

51. Robert A. Cassidy to Mrs. Barksdale, n. d., *Mississippi Index*, June 13, 1866, Ethelbert Barksdale Papers, Mississippi Department of Archives and History; Harry W. Pfanz, *Gettysburg: The Second Day*, pp. 434-35.
52. Muffly, *The Story of Our Regiment*, p. 173.
53. *Ibid.*
54. Robert A. Cassidy to Mrs. Barksdale; Muffly, *The Story of Our Regiment*, pp. 173-74.

and now when I am shot all to pieces and burning with fever, I must have cold water.' Then he would break out, 'Yes, you think you have whipped us, but wait till morning and you will hear Ewell thundering in your rear.' . . . Alternately begging for water, which a drummer boy was giving him with a spoon, and cursing the Yankees, it was a most pathetic sight."[55]

After a time, Barksdale lost consciousness, and Cassidy moved on to care for the wounded still streaming in to the aid station. Chaplain William Henry Stevens of the 148th Pennsylvania stopped by the general's pallet frequently during his rounds that night, ministering to the dying soldier/statesman.[56]

By morning, the fiery Southerner was dead. "I saw his body soon after the life had left it, . . ." wrote Lt. George G. Benedict of the 12th Vermont; "his vest thrown open disclosed a ball hole through the breast, and his legs were bandaged and bloody from gunshots through both of them. He had fought without the wig which Speaker Grow once knocked off in the Hall of Representatives, and his bald head and broad face, with open unblinking eyes, lay uncovered in the sunshine. There he lay alone, without a comrade to brush the flies from his corpse."[57]

Scroungers had already taken all of value about the general's person, whether for souvenirs of the noteworthy Confederate, or simply as barter to trade with some other scavenger. Musician Cassidy was able to find one remaining coat button and the general's sword strap, a few precious mementoes which he was able to present to Barksdale's widow in 1866.[58]

Some time later, the general was buried in a temporary grave under a little peach tree between the Hummelbaugh and Leister houses, "near General Meade's headquarters." At the head of his grave was the following inscription, written unceremoniously in pencil on the top of a cardboard box tacked to a stake: "Brigadier General Barksdale of Mississippi McLaw's division, Longstreet's Corps Died on the morning of 3rd July, 1863 Eight years a representative in United States Congress. Shot through the left breast, and left leg broken below the knee." Chaplain Stevens attended the general at the burial,

---

55. Muffly, *The Story of Our Regiment*, p. 245.
56. Robert A. Cassidy to Mrs. Barksdale; Muffly, *The Story of Our Regiment*, p. 197.
57. Benedict, *Army Life in Virginia*, pp. 169-70.
58. Robert A. Cassidy to Mrs. Barksdale.

commending his Southern soul to God while his remains were unceremoniously interred in Northern soil.[59]

Assistant Surgeon Albert Vander Veer was also struggling to keep up with the wounded flowing into his aid station, just up the Taneytown Road from Doctor Hamilton's facility. "The wounded were brought back and our temporary hospital was located in a farm house that had been built for many years, of stone. We worked through the night with the aid of candles and oil lamps."[60]

"During the day I had taken care of many of the wounded behind a stone wall. Beside being assistant surgeon of the 66th New York Volunteers, I was placed in charge of the sick and wounded of the 22nd Connecticut and almost the first one I had to treat was Colonel Chaplin who was brought back wounded through the chest but sunk rapidly from internal hemorrhage and died without our being able to more than relieve him more or less from pain."[61]

Dr. Harry McKindree McAbee had his own unique problems as he struggled to keep up with the ongoing tide of wounded at the aid station on the property of the Widow Guinn, still further up the Taneytown Road toward town. The wounded, falling back from the fighting around the cemetery, were naturally attracted to the two-story log home of the widow. But the seventy-two-year-old lady, who adamantly refused to move out of the home that her husband had lovingly built, was not making it any easier on the frazzled Canton,

59. *Ibid.*; Benedict, *Army Life in Virginia*, pp. 169-70; Muffly, *The Story of Our Regiment*, p. 197. Barksdale was one of two Confederates buried at the Hummelbaugh aid station after the battle. [Gregory Coco, *Wasted Valor: The Confederate Dead at Gettysburg* (Gettysburg, Pennsylvania: Thomas Publications, 1990), p. 85.]

60. Albert Vander Veer, Vander Veer Papers, DB 560, Albany Institute of History and Art, Albany, New York, transcribed copy in the 66th New York Infantry Vertical File, Gettysburg National Military Park. This was almost certainly the Peter Frey House, where Surgeon Francis Wafer was also working.

61. *Ibid.* There was no 22nd Connecticut or Colonel Chaplin in the Second Corps. It is possible that Vander Veer was referring to the 27th Connecticut, whose leader, Lt. Col. Henry C. Merwin, was killed on July 2.

Ohio, surgeon. She physically threatened any soldiers she found lurking near her house, even "beating up" one hapless fellow she cornered in her basement after he soiled her clean laundry. By July 4, her home would be perforated thirteen times by shot and shell, one just barely missing the feisty, elderly resident.[62]

Hundreds of wounded were already laid out on the grounds and in the outbuildings by early afternoon on July 2. Sgt. Frank B. Nickerson of the 8th Ohio related what it was like at the aid station later that night: "Surgeon McAbee was constantly at work, and it was midnight before he reached me: having asked a few questions and promised to specially care for me at daybreak, he turned to a mere boy on my left—a Confederate—not more than seventeen years old; death's pallor was on his brow and the blood flowing from his mouth; he was moaning pitifully, in striking contrast to the silent way so many were suffering and dying all around."[63]

The quiet Ohio surgeon was also a Methodist Episcopal minister back home, and he showed complete impartiality in his concern for and treatment of friend and foe alike. "Dr. McAbee seemed touched with his youthful appearance and disquietude of mind, and said to him, 'My poor fellow, you cannot be helped; you can live but a little time.' The boy broke out in a despairing cry, 'My poor mother, what will she do? I cannot die, I cannot die. She will never know what became of me. I was shot on the skirmish line and no one knows it.' The Surgeon wrote in his notebook his name as a member of a Georgia regiment, and his mother's address, and promised, if possible, to write to his mother, and then knelt down by his side, holding the lantern in his blood-stained hand; with the other he took a pocket Bible from his pocket and read the first fourteen verses of the Fourteenth of St. John, and then offered up a prayer for the soul that was passing away, in such a simple, earnest language that helped the faith of all."[64]

So the pastor turned surgeon labored throughout the night, ministering physically where he could aid the wounded with his medical skills, and spiritually where he could not.

The wounded that were stable enough to be moved from the aid stations were being transported by stretcher, ambulance, and even on

62. Coco, *A Vast Sea of Misery*, pp. 61-62.
63. Kepler, *Fourth Ohio Volunteers*, p. 193.
64. *Ibid.*, pp. 193-94.

foot to the division hospitals clustered in the vicinity of the Granite School House. "I think at Midnight there were none who had not been provided with good nourishing food," reported Dr. Justin Dwinelle of the Second Division Hospital's work that night. "We were successful in finding sufficient hay for bedding for all of them."[65]

Surgeon Dwinelle, unlike some Civil War doctors, was deeply concerned with the care and needs of the men entrusted to his care, and saw to it that all were made as comfortable as conditions allowed. "At night the wounded occupied the large barn and the ground under the trees in the orchard. . . . The day had been moderately warm and most of the time the sun was obsured [*sic*] by clouds. The night was not cool enough to cause any great degree of Suffering to the men on that account. Those that lay out doors were as well & perhaps better than those in the barn, they being less crowded and having a purer atmosphere. Nearly all were covered with blankets, Rubber cloths, and shelter tents."[66]

For now, the Second Division Hospital was running smoothly, even with the absence of supply wagons. This facility, like many of the division hospitals, treated a diverse group of wounded as the battle progressed: "As near as I can judge, we had five hundred wounded men that night, most of whom belonged to the Second Division. The remainder was composed of men from the other Divisions of our corps, the Third Corps, & Confederates."[67]

Just down the road from Justin Dwinelle's location, the Third Division Hospital had its share of wounded in and around the barn it was occupying. "I worked in the hospital until three in the morning," remembered Assistant Surgeon Pierre D. Peltier of the 126th New York, "slept an hour on the ground and was awakened by firing near at hand."[68]

At the neighboring First Division Hospital, surgeon-in-charge William Warren Potter had returned from attending to the dying General Zook. "After working till the small hours of the morning of the 3d, I laid down and obtained a little sleep, but was up and at it again by day-light. After assisting at many operations, as well as making a

---

65. Justin Dwinelle, *Medical Report.*
66. *Ibid.*
67. *Ibid.*
68. Louis C. Duncan, *The Medical Department of the United States Army*, p. 241.

number myself to spell the chief operator, I once more repaired to General Zook's side, finding him still alive, but sinking rapidly."[69]

After working burial detail for almost four hours, Sgt. Thomas P. Meyer of the 148th Pennsylvania Pioneer Corps called it quits for the night at the new Second Corps Hospital site along Rock Creek. "At about three o'clock in the morning, our candles were all burned up and we returned to a similar field hospital, just to the rear of our division battle lines, with about twelve hundred wounded. Here we lay down for a short rest; we had had little chance for rest or sleep day or night for two weeks, and we were very much fatigued."[70]

Trying to get any rest while camped beside a fully-functional divisional field hospital was a dicey proposition at best. "Here the wounded seemed to be in greater distress. The endless and louder moans were indicative of intense suffering. The voice of a boy was heard in prolonged wails and screams, high above the rest. His voice became hoarse and husky, but as morning came he was more quiet, and a little later entirely still. I imagined he had fallen asleep."

"As soon as it was light enough I went over and asked the wounded lying near, 'Where is the boy that was in such agony during the night?'"

"A wounded soldier raised himself on his elbow, pointing over a few others and said, 'That is him; he is now dead.'"

"I went over to him. He was a boy about sixteen, smooth faced as a woman and handsome. He was dead; one of his feet was torn into an unrecognizable mass of flesh, bone and sinew. Gangrene was evidently the immediate cause of death. Early amputation would have saved the boy's life. Here many had died of their unattended wounds during the night."

"Many of the badly wounded were chloroformed to have their wounds dressed. When the operations were finished they were carried away, and laid out on the ground. There was no time to assist them in

69. Potter, *Three Years with the Army of the Potomac*, p. 60. For more on General Zook, see Chapter 16: "The Union Wounded of the Second Corps Hospital."

70. Muffly, *The Story of Our Regiment*, p. 462.

resuscitation, and many never woke again. Many strangled to death for the want of a little assistance at the proper time."[71]

James Moore, Company G of the 108th New York Volunteers, was awake early at the hospital, aroused by the throbbing in his wounded ankle. The 108th had had the dubious distinction of supporting Battery I of the 1st U.S. Artillery the previous day, posted so close to Lt. George A. Woodruff's guns that they were actually between the cannon and their limbers. No amount of remonstrance or complaint of either artillerymen or infantrymen seemed to do any good. The Union battery immediately drew Confederate counterfire, and although the 108th took no active part in firing on the enemy, the luckless regiment suffered almost fifty percent casualties from incoming artillery fire. James Moore was one of the luckier ones.[72]

Since he couldn't sleep, the New Yorker pulled out some paper and started a letter:

> July 3rd/63
> Pennsylvania
>
> My Dear Friend,
>
> I am sorry to have to inform you that I got wounded again. This time in the ankle. The bone is not broke, thank God, and perhaps I may soon be able to be about again. But it pains. It is very painful but we must put up with it and I am very thankful to God to have escaped so easy. It is heart rending to listen to the cries of the poor fellows during the night that is past and this morning possibly some dozens of

---

71. *Ibid.* This is the only reference that this author has discovered to any widespread anesthesia-related deaths following surgery in the Second Corps Hospitals at Gettysburg. Whether Sergeant Meyer saw this himself, or whether he was merely relating rumors, is unclear. Overall Civil War surgical statistics reflect an extremely low anesthesia-related death rate, apparently due in large part to the administration of chloroform and/or ether in areas such as open-air tent hospitals and well-ventilated general hospital surgeries. Even if Meyer's report is true, the overwhelming influx of shattered men from the battlefield simply made it impossible to provide much personalized attention during surgical recovery.

72. *New York at Gettysburg*, vol. 2, p. 780; *OR*, vol. 27, pt. 1, p. 465; William L. Haskin, *The History of the First Regiment of Artillery* (Portland, Maine: B. Thurston and Company, 1879), p. 170.

them has been laid in their final resting places. At about 5 o'c AM this morning the cannonading commenced and I trust God will give us the victory. At present we just hold our own, no more.[73]

The faint light of dawn found Lieutenant Fuller of the 61st New York still waiting to have his wound examined at the First Division Hospital by the edge of the woods. "In due time light broke in the East, and a little later I could roll my head and take in some of the surroundings. Most of the wounded of the regiment had been gathered at this place, and we made by far the largest part of it. Many of the men were so hurt that they could move about, and they all came and made me an early morning call."[74]

With the improving light, many of the surgeons were making their rounds through the hospital, searching out men from their own commands. "After a time two of our regimental doctors appeared. They cut open my trouser leg, found where the bullet went in, and, I think, put a strip of adhesive plaster over the wound, and they did the same with the shoulder. It was clear to my mind that the leg, at least, must come off. I expressed my opinion and said, I thought it would be better to do it at once, than to wait till inflammation set in. At my request they promised me that they would see to it that I should be among the first operated on."[75]

Friends from the regiments were coming back over the ridge to the hospitals along the Taneytown Road—some sent on orders, many coming on their own—seeking news of their wounded comrades. "While in this place my life long friend and companion, Lieut Isaac Plumb, came to me. We had been side by side since the organization of the regiment, and, until now, neither of us had been badly hurt. He told me that he saw me as I went down, and sang out, 'Uncle Fuller, that's good for sixty days.' He said I made up quite a face, as if it hurt." Plumb

---

73. James Moore letter, July 3, 1863, copy in the 108th New York Vertical File, Gettysburg National Military Park, copied by permission of the United States Army Military History Institute (USAMHI), Carlisle, Pennsylvania, original at the University of Rochester. All underlinings are those of James Moore; such underlinings were frequently used to communicate additional information between members of secret societies.

74. Fuller, *Personal Recollections*, p. 99.

75. *Ibid.*

had been more fortunate—the bullet that knocked him down had harmlessly imbedded itself in a ring of keys in a vest pocket, leaving only a nasty throbbing bruise.[76]

Cheered by his friend and other wounded companions from his regiment, the early morning hours passed pleasantly as Fuller waited again, this time to have his leg amputated.

Chaplain Stuckenberg had also risen early, and now he too was busy working his way through the crowded First Division Hospital, seeking out the wounded of his regiment. "In visiting the hospital on the morning of the third, I found the doctors and [male] nurses busily engaged with the wounded, scattered around in all directions, some lying on blankets, some on straw, a few on stretchers, others on the bare ground. [Pvt.] E Allen of Co G, shot through [the] abdomen suffered terribly.[77] Some of the intestines protruded through the wound and some of their contents would occasionally flow out, producing a horrible stench. Adj [John D.] Black was much easier and looked much better. The Col was walking about, doing well; he started for Baltimore this day. It was very evident that our regiment had again suffered severely, though the extent of our loss was not yet known—many of our men wounded being still missing."[78]

After doing all he could at the hospital, the chaplain headed up the ridge to check on the remnants of the 145th Pennsylvania, still in line of battle. "It was very small—66 men and officers, commanded by Capt [Moses W.] Oliver. Though saddened by their heavy loss, they were in good spirits because they had driven the rebels and taken 75 or 100 prisoners. It evident that another engagement would take place that day."[79]

The previous night's activities had taken a severe toll on Stuckenberg's health. "I was not well, had not been for some days. I withdrew to the neighborhood of our Hospital and tried to sleep. But

76. *Ibid.* Wounds of a minor nature could be good for up to a sixty day leave of absence.

77. Pvt. Erastus Allen died of his wounds the next day, and is buried in the Gettysburg National Cemetery. Chaplain Stuckenberg personally buried the young private.

78. Stuckenberg, *I'm Surrounded by Methodists*, p. 78.

79. *Ibid.*

soon our right, immediately in front of me, was heavily engaged by Ewell's corps, formerly Jackson's." Unable to sleep, and having nothing that immediately needed his attention, the chaplain climbed the slopes to one of the batteries that was engaging the enemy, and spent the rest of the morning watching Maj. Gen. Henry W. Slocum personally direct the artillery fire.[80]

"Despite all these night horrors most of us slept like logs until day dawn[ed]," remembered Benjamin W. Thompson forty-seven years later. Even the early morning firefight by the men on Culp's Hill to regain positions lost to the Confederates at nightfall, and sharp skirmishing in front of the Second Corps right, seems not to have disturbed the exhausted slumbers of most of the Second Corps.[81]

The sun was coming up brazen in the east, quickly obscured by a cover of stratocumulus clouds that promised another breathless and sultry day; at 7:00 a.m., the temperature was already seventy-three degrees, and rising steadily. "We were waked to receive, not food or coffee, but sixty rounds each of ball cartridge, a suggestive hint for the day's work before us. Oh, how fiercely hungry we were that Friday morning, July Third, 1863. We took our belts up several inches and smoked our pipes continuously. Without the sedative effect of tobacco, it seemed as if we could not have endured the fast. Some of the boys prowled into other corps and brought back a little coffee, but most of us had nothing but cold water for breakfast, a species of total abstinence which was not popular at that time and place."[82]

"The men were roused early, in order that their morning meal might be out of the way in time for whatever should occur," wrote Lieutenant Haskell of that Friday morning's activities. "Then ensued the hum of an army, not in ranks, chatting in low tones, and running about and jostling among each other, rolling and packing their blankets and tents. They looked like an army of rag-gatherers, while shaking these very useful articles of the soldier's outfit,—for you must know that rain and mud in conjunction have not had the effect to make them very clean;

80. *Ibid.*

81. Thompson, *Personal Narrative*, p. 40; Byrne and Weaver, *Haskell of Gettysburg*, pp. 136-37.

82. Michael Jacobs, weather records, Gettysburg National Military Park; Thompson, *Personal Narrative*, p. 40.

and the wear and tear of service have not left them entirely whole. . . . They packed their knapsacks, boiled their coffee, and munched their hard bread, just as usual,—just like old soldiers, who know what campaigning is; and their talk is far more concerning their present employment,—some joke or drollery,—than concerning what they saw or did yesterday."[83]

Washington, D.C.

Ellen Orbison Harris of the Philadelphia Ladies Aid Society had risen before the sun, hoping to catch any new developments from the front. "Waked this morning to learn that the peaceful village of Gettysburg was the scene of a terrible battle. I went early to the War department to beg permission to carry forward a car-load of stores; besought with tears the privilege. Experiences of the saddest kind have taught me that everything is needed to meet the wants of the battle-field immediately after an engagement."[84]

In spite of her on-site experience and excellent credentials, her request was denied. This was still a man's war, and the recommendations of even the most skilled volunteer female nurses did not carry very much weight. "My entreaties were in vain; so I left Washington with a sad heart and harrowing forebodings. . . ." In spite of physical limitations, Harris was a very determined woman; if the War Department would not help her, she would simply have to go on her own.

Within hours, she was on the train to Baltimore. Instead of the desired "car-load of stores," she was only able to gather together one box of chloroform and a single box of stimulants for her trip.[85]

Baltimore, Maryland

The representatives of the Christian Commission were still trying to get out of Baltimore with their medical supplies. It had all started so well, at least at first. "We had our goods sent to Calvert Station, then re-shipped at the Relay, and that evening [July 2] placed in a car with General Meade's mail for Westminster or the army."[86]

---

83. Byrne and Weaver, *Haskell of Gettysburg*, p. 139.
84. *Report of the Ladies Aid Society*, p. 12.
85. *Ibid.* Brockett and Vaughn, *Woman's Work in the Civil War*, p. 158. For more on Mrs. Harris' precarious health, see Appendix 3.
86. Cross, *The War and the Christian Commission*, p. 11.

Then the delays began. Dealing with the military was always a case of hurry up and wait, and now the waiting began in earnest for the impatient Christian Commission representatives. "After we secured them [the supplies] in the cars at the Relay at 10 o'clock at night, we had to wait for a train, walking the platform or sitting about the cars until 7 o'clock the next morning [July 3]. We were so fortunate before the train started as to get some breakfast, through the kindness of Mrs. Samuel Barnes."[87]

The military railroad finally produced a locomotive and tender for the stranded carriages. However, being a government freight train, and not a passenger train, presented a challenge in seating for the small group. "We first entered a burden car, but soon found it would be more comfortable, though a little more dangerous, on the top. Tired of walking all night, and anxious to get on in any way, the top of the car became quite comfortable."[88]

Then there were more holdups as various trains assembled by the tracks leading out of town. The shaky single-line track of the Western Maryland Railroad, built from scrap-iron rails on poor supports, ran from Baltimore to Union Bridge, Maryland, through Westminster without a single adequate siding to pull over on as trains passed from the other direction. Lack of telegraph lines for communication and coordinating schedules along this stretch of track proved to be a further hindrance.

To move the maximum amount of supplies to the embattled Army of the Potomac, Brig. Gen. Herman Haupt, in charge of the military's rail support system, devised an innovative system of multiple train convoys. Borrowing all the rolling stock he could lay his hands on from neighboring railways, and throwing out the normal schedules, Haupt started running three convoys of five to six trains, moving one right after the other and under heavy guard, to and from Westminster daily. As soon as each group of trains cleared the junction at Baltimore on their return trip, the next convoy rolled out for Westminster.[89]

---

87. *Ibid.*

88. *Ibid.*

89. Thomas Weber, *The Northern Railroads in the Civil War, 1861-1865* (Columbia University, New York: King's Crown Press, 1952), pp. 163-64. It would be a very long trip for Cross and his men; due to a delay at the Baltimore end, the trip to Westminster took thirty hours to complete. [J. H. Douglas, *Operations of the Sanitary Commission*, p. 9.] General Haupt estimated that, by using this multiple train convoy system employing approximately five ten-car trains in each trip, he was able to move 1,500

As the various locomotives and their loads trundled into position along the tracks leading out of town, no one paid any particular attention to freight car #816, coupled into one of the trains. When word confirming a battle at Gettysburg had reached the highly-organized Sanitary Commission at Washington, representatives there were poised for action. Quickly loading a boxcar with medicines, foodstuffs, and sanitary supplies, the car rolled out of Washington within hours, while fighting still raged along Cemetery Ridge. Making the connection in Baltimore, the boxcar was now in this same early morning convoy, awaiting clearance from the yard master to move out for Westminster.[90]

Finally, the wait was over. The lead locomotive shuddered into motion, the couplings of its train snapping tight in rapid-fire succession. As the first train cleared the junction, the next in line eased open the throttle and steamed forward. Each train, in its turn, ponderously moved out of the yard, in close order and heavily-guarded formation. Gradually picking up as much speed as the rickety rail line would allow, the trains rattled, clattered and swayed their way towards Westminster. The men of the Christian Commission tenaciously hung on to the roof of their boxcar, feeling the rising sun of July 3 hot on their backs as gritty soot and cinders from the locomotive smokestack rained down on them.

Gettysburg, Pennsylvania

The 111th New York gathered together its shrunken ranks, and again faced another day on the skirmish line. "No one could divine what the enemy was about or where he would strike next. His skirmish lines were particularly active and the sharpshooters began to make it unpleasant to be seen long in one place on Cemetery Hill. One division

---

tons of military supplies to Westminster each day, while evacuating 2,000 to 4,000 wounded on the return trip. [Herman Haupt, *Reminiscences of General Herman Haupt* (Milwaukee: Wright and Joys Co., Engravers, Printers, 1901), pp. 213-16, 236.]

90. Douglas, *Operations of the Sanitary Commission*, p. 9. A representative of the Sanitary Commission, William A. Hovey, was on the first passenger train out of Washington after news of the battle was received in the capital, charged with overseeing the safety of boxcar #816. Due to the delays of the military convoy, he was able to arrive in Baltimore just in time to catch the departing supply trains, and so reached Westminster with the men of the Christian Commission.

[company] after another of my regiment had served its tour on the skirmish line when last of all the color division, which ordinarily does not skirmish, was ordered out."[91]

Now the bloody business left off as night fell yesterday began again in earnest; if possible, even more deadly and vindictive than before. "Line fighting is barbarous, but skirmishing is savage—nay, devilish," wrote one veteran of the hazardous duty. "To juke and hide and skulk for men and deliberately aim at and murder them one by one is far too bloodthirsty business for Christian men. Yet, so much of the wild animal is there in the best of us that if you ask twenty old soldiers which they prefer, at least nineteen of them will say: 'Give me the skirmish line by all odds.'"[92]

Despite being the color company of the regiment, Thompson's men gave a good account of themselves on the picket line that morning. "My men were fine marksmen, having a good deal of target practice during their months of picket duty, and they made such an impression upon the rebels opposite them that their line was speedily reinforced, and some prisoners which we took told us that they all thought we belonged to a regiment of sharpshooters. The enlisted men on both sides were all lying on the ground and had bits of fence or pits to cover them. They fired by aiming at the puffs of smoke which were made by discharging the pieces."[93]

For officers, however, the luxury of cover was not provided, and Captain Thompson was finding out just how dangerous that could be on the skirmish line. "The officers, standing or walking along the line, were conspicuous targets and I soon found that a group of sharpshooters were getting my range too near for safety or comfort. So I tried strategy. I would drop on my back in the tall timothy and lie still for a minute; then roll to right or left a rod or two and then get up and look after my men until some close shot warned me to drop again. I had the timothy heads cut off by bullets over my head a number of times."[94]

In time, Thompson grew tired of the subterfuge and took matters into his own hands. "Finally, I borrowed a rifle from one of my men and took a shot at the sharpshooters who were devoting themselves especially to me. It was the only shot fired by myself in battle during the war, and it appeared to be effective, for there were three men in the

---

91. Thompson, *Personal Narrative*, p. 40.
92. *Ibid.*
93. *Ibid.*, pp. 40-41.
94. *Ibid.*, p. 41.

party and I very soon saw two of them carrying the other man to the rear, and after that I had no trouble with the sharpshooter's bullets."[95]

The 126th New York, sister regiment of Thompson's 111th New York, also took a fearful beating on the skirmish line. Capts. Charles M. Wheeler, Orin J. Herendeen and Isaac Shimer were all shot dead, a lieutenant severely wounded, and "many of the rank and file were killed and wounded." So devastating was the musketry fire that when Captain Herendeen's body was finally recovered, "his head looked," wrote one messmate, "as if he had been beaten by some ruffian with a club until he was dead."[96]

The nasty front-line sniping slowly fizzled out and died around 11:00 a.m. Lt. George Yost summed up the feelings of many of the exhausted men as they rotated out of the picket line: "I would do anything rather than skirmish with those fellows. I never want to do it again. I will charge and repel charges but don't put me in that place again."[97]

Even as a new day was breaking, the hospitals were already running full bore, struggling to treat the casualties of yesterday's clash, as well as fresh casualties produced by skirmish fire in the early half light. "During the morning of the third we succeeded in getting a sufficient supply of coffee, sugar, crackers, salt, and salt-pork from several Regimental Commissaries," noted Second Division Surgeon Justin Dwinelle. "From early in the morning until noon the Operating Surgeons were at work constantly at four different tables. The slighter wounds were dressed as fast as possible by the Surgical and other help we had on hand in expectation of an attack on our immediate front to take place in the latter part of the day."[98]

Musicians from the various regiments were also hard at work. Organized into squads at the divisional level, their job, when not providing colorful instrumental renditions, "was to put up and take down the hospital tents and arrange the tables for operations; provide a plentiful supply of water, clean up the operating instruments, hold

95. *Ibid.*

96. Willson, *Disaster, Struggle, Triumph*, p. 180; George Yost, letter to his father, July 4, 1863, copy in the 126th Vertical File, Gettysburg National Military Park.

97. George Yost to his father, July 4, 1863.

98. Dwinelle, *Medical Report*.

the limbs while being amputated and bury these amputated limbs. We usually dug a hole a few rods away from where the operations were performed, and in these holes we put limb after limb until sufficiently full, then covered them up and made an additional limb grave. . . . It frequently fell to our lot to go out on the battle lines, during an engagement, with stretchers and gather up the wounded."[99]

On this early July morning, the musicians had been detailed as temporary medical aides and requisition officers for the Medical Department. Drummer Nathaniel Beerly of Company B, 148th Pennsylvania Volunteers, recalled: "The next day our time was employed at the amputating table and in getting hay or straw to lay the wounded on, and a squad of men were detailed to procure the same and the Doctor told me to estimate the cost or damage and report the amount and the owner's name, but the farmer refused to let us have any, so we forcibly opened the barn and took the same and I reported the amount taken, with the owner's name to the Doctor."[100]

Over at the First Division Hospital, there were so many wounded that the surgical facilities had to be expanded. Lieutenant Fuller, anxious to have his injured leg dealt with, watched the proceedings with great interest. "After a time the division operating table was set up in the edge of a piece of timber not very far away. I was on thc watch, expecting every minute to be taken out, but waited and waited and no one came for me. I became quite impatient at this delay. I saw one after another brought on, carried up, and taken away, and I was not called for. This aroused my stock of impatience, of which, I naturally always had quiet [*sic*] enough."[101]

The young officer was determined to have his wounded leg amputated as soon as possible, and nothing was going to deter him. Fuller finally decided to take matters into his own hands. "At last I asked my friend Porter R. Whitney and another man to take me down to the table. I made up my mind, if the mountain did not go to Mahomet, the next best thing was for the prophet to go to the mountain. The men set me down as nearly under the noses of the doctors as could be." Now let the surgeons try to ignore the persistent lieutenant and his injured limb![102]

Even this technique, however, did not secure the treatment Fuller sought. "If something hadn't happened, I presume in a few minutes

99. Muffly, *The Story of Our Regiment*, pp. 331, 325.
100. *Ibid.*, p. 325.
101. Fuller, *Personal Recollections*, p. 100.
102. *Ibid.*

that heretofore good left leg would have made one of the fast growing pile [of amputated limbs]; but about that interesting moment for me, the enemy began dropping shells that exploded in and about the locality." It was just a single Confederate battery throwing random shells at the Union lines, but the range was zeroed in exactly on the hospital. Plans were immediately set in motion to evacuate the hospital again, the second time in less than twenty-four hours. First Division Medical Director R. C. Stiles gave the necessary orders, and Surgeon-in-Charge William W. Potter and his medical teams set about the familiar routine of packing up the hospital.[103]

"It was not a fit place to pursue surgical operations. The doctors knew it, so they hastily gathered up their knives and saws, and moved to a place where those projectiles did not drop. The two friends who had taken me there, picked up my stretcher and started for a like place." For now, at least, Lieutenant Fuller was just going to have to keep on waiting for surgical attention of his damaged limb.[104]

Staff aide Haskell was again serving as traffic director on the crowded crest of Cemetery Ridge. "As early as practicable the lines all along the left are revised and reformed,—this having been rendered necessary by yesterday's battle, and also by what is anticipated to day.... The 2nd and 3rd Divisions of the 2nd Corps are in the positions of yesterday; then on the left come [Maj. Gen. Abner] Doubleday's—the 3rd—Division and Col [George J.] Stannard's brigade of the 1st Corps;—then [Brig. Gen. John C.] Caldwell's—the 1st—Division of the 2nd Corps; then the 3rd Corps, temporarily under the command of Hancock, since Sickle's wound."[105] In spite of all his responsibility, Hancock still managed to dash off a terse telegram to his wife Almira, as was his habit during battle: "I am all right, so far."[106]

About eight o'clock in the morning, Hancock rode along the Second Corps line, and ordered them to fortify their positions.

103. *Ibid.*

104. *Ibid.*

105. Byrne and Weaver, *Haskell of Gettysburg*, pp. 139-40. Hancock himself testified that his command "consisted of the 1st, 2d, and 3d corps, of which I had the general command. I commanded that whole front." Questions still remain as to the actual extent of his authority on July 3. [*Conduct of the War*, General Winfield Scott Hancock, March 22, 1864, vol. 1, p. 407.]

106. Hancock, *Reminiscences of Winfield Scott Hancock*, p. 97.

"Entrenching tool wagons dashed along our lines, and shovels, picks and axes were thrown out while the wagons rushed along the line at a furious speed. We immediately went to fortifying; men never worked harder or faster, or with greater good will than the Second Corps boys under a broiling July sun, from 8:00 to 11:00 A.M., when we called our work finished." By 11:00, the 148th Pennsylvania could boast of "a six-foot breastwork a few feet high and well lined, or backed up with rails, well supported by stakes."[107]

"Eleven o'clock came,—the noise of battle had ceased upon the right,—not a sound of a gun or musket can be heard on all the field,—the sky is bright with only the white fleecy clouds floating over from the West,—the July sun streams down its fire upon the bright iron of the muskets in stacks upon the crest, and the dazzling brass of the Napoleons—the army lolls, and longs for the shade, of which some get a hands [*sic*] breadth, from a shelter tent stuck upon a ramrod,—the silence and sultriness of a July noon are supreme."[108]

The morning had passed quite differently for Jacob H. Cole of the 57th New York Volunteers. Unable to even crawl to the Union picket line from the wheatfield where he had fallen on July 2, the young soldier had laid immobilized, surrounded by the dead and dying, all night long.

"In the morning the rebels carried me from the range of their guns to a small knoll and from where I lay and watched the Confederates moving their artillery along the Emmittsburg [*sic*] road and in the peach orchard to higher ground, for the purpose of obtaining a more commanding position for their artillery and comparatively clear ground for their infantry. I counted nearly seventy-five pieces of artillery near the peach orchard."[109]

Now the young New Englander could only watch, held captive by his own wounded limbs, as the preparations were made by the enemy to shell his friends in the Army of the Potomac. There was nothing he could do except "wait for the coming of the strife that is to decide the battle and the life of the Republic."[110]

107. Muffly, *The Story of Our Regiment*, p. 463.
108. Byrne and Weaver, *Haskell of Gettysburg*, p. 144.
109. Cole, *Under Five Commanders*, p. 204.
110. *Ibid.*

With the entrenchments built along Cemetery Ridge, there was nothing left for the troops to do but sit around and listen to their stomachs rumble and snarl. "We were ready. And our whole line of battle as far as we could see to the right and left were now standing on top of our work watching the enemy locating Batteries along their line on the Emmittsburg Road ridge. We ate a few crackers while we waited; we were hungry."[111]

But the men of the 148th Pennsylvania Pioneers, tough men noted for being wily and resourceful, knew that they could do better than a few dry biscuits. Sgt. Thomas P. Meyer decided to do something about the situation. "I said, 'Boys, watch my outfit while I run down the Taneytown Road for something good to eat. I think I can make the trip before the thing begins again.'"[112]

"I struck out and ran a mile when I came to a farm house. They had just taken a batch of fresh cherry pies from the oven. I bought a number nearly a foot in diameter, 'two for a quarter,' put them on a board and hurried back. I ran out and back, covered the two miles in twenty minutes; returned puffing, overheated and wet with perspiration."[113]

"Sharing with the boys, we had a grand feast and were again standing with the rest on top of our breastworks."[114] Smiling like Cheshire cats, no doubt.

Lunchtime was also approaching at Second Division headquarters, where there was no such deluxe fare as fresh cherry pies; only a few potatoes, some sugar, and a bit of coffee remained in the staff larder. An officer from headquarters, with an associate, had gone on a foraging run for General Gibbon and his staff. The results were several elderly chickens—"'picked up' somewhere (no doubt without due process of law)," suspected Gibbon—a slab of butter, and the remains of a very large loaf of bread, somewhat the worse for wear after being rescued from the jaws of a Pennsylvania hog.[115]

---

111. Muffly, *The Story of Our Regiment*, p. 463.
112. *Ibid.*
113. *Ibid.*
114. *Ibid.*
115. Byrne and Weaver, *Haskell of Gettysburg*, pp. 144-145; John Gibbon, *Personal Recollections of the Civil War* (New York, 1903), p. 146. One of

The poultry was quickly stewed, the few scrubby potatoes from the larder thrown in to boil, and coffee and tea were brewed (some alleged with murky water carried in from a nearby barnyard). Frank Haskell produced a leftover pickle from his saddlebag, and with toasted bread and butter, the repast was ready.[116]

The Second Division commander had invited some of his friends and fellow officers and, one by one, they stopped by to grab a quick bite to eat. No sooner had the meal been laid out on a mess-chest than General Meade and a staff member cantered up, dismounted, and sat down. Generals John Newton (now commanding the First Corps following General Reynolds' death) and Alfred Pleasanton (Chief of Cavalry) next dropped by. Hancock and Gibbon got the camp stools, Meade made do with an empty cracker box, Newton and the cavalry chief got only a roll of blankets, and all the remaining staff simply "sat upon the ground, cross-legged like the picture of a smoking Turk, and held our plates upon our laps."[117]

Dinner was pronounced "large and in good *running* order," and finished in short order. General Meade and his aide soon galloped back to headquarters. Cigars were smoked in the shade of a rather small tree, and the talk turned to the events of yesterday and the prospects of today. "We dozed in the heat, and lolled upon the ground, with half open eyes. Our horses were hitched to the trees, munching some oats. A great lull rests upon all the field. Time was heavy," wrote General Gibbon's aide; "and for want of something better to do, I yawned and looked at my watch;—it was five minutes before one o'clock."[118]

The weary stint of duty on the skirmish line had finally come to an end for the exhausted men of the 111th New York. "After a long tour we were relieved and on going back found our men lying along a stone wall which ran down the hill to General Meade's headquarters. This disposition was made to get cover from a Whitworth gun which was

---

the two foragers was most probably Haskell himself, from the wealth of details he gives of the scavenging run.

116. Byrne and Weaver, *Haskell of Gettysburg*, pp. 144-46; Gibbon, *Personal Recollections*, p. 146.

117. Byrne and Weaver, *Haskell of Gettysburg*, pp. 144-46; Gibbon, *Personal Recollections*, p. 146.

118. Byrne and Weaver, *Haskell of Gettysburg*, p. 147.

throwing bolts about the size and shape of a large seed cucumber, in uncomfortable proximity to our old place." The wall's scant shadow also provided the only local shade from the intense sunshine. "The heat was almost insufferable," recalled Colonel MacDougall of the 111th; "the men . . . were making every effort to keep off the rays of the scorching sun."[119]

"The bummers of our regiment had made use of the quiet morning to forage for coffee and they had begged or stolen enough so that a number of little squads were scattered about building small fires and boiling the coveted beverage in their quart cups. Oh, how delicious was a scalding draught which I received on my return from the hot skirmish line." Rations were still in short supply, but the trip to the lonely picket line out in the grain fields had not been a total waste: "Many of us made breakfast . . . by rubbing ripened wheat between our hands and eating it."[120]

"Our battered little regiment crawled into the shadow of the fence to get some shelter from the burning sun, and Col. McDougal[l] and I discussed the situation. The general humor of our officers and men was doggedness and faultfinding. There was no food, no coffee, no whiskey and tobacco began to fail of its office. How could General Meade expect men to fight under such circumstances[?] We noticed the batteries above us were silent and those of the other side quiet as well. We hoped the enemy might be retreating."[121]

Within moments, Benjamin W. Thompson was about to see his hopes dashed before his very eyes.

---

119. Thompson, *Personal Narrative*, p. 41; *New York at Gettysburg*, vol. 2, p. 800.
120. Thompson, *Personal Narrative*, p. 41.
121. *Ibid.*, pp. 41-42.

CHAPTER 5

FRIDAY, JULY 3: CONFEDERATE CANNONADE

"We were literally shelled out"

Surgeon Justin Dwinelle,
106th Pennsylvania Infantry

The day had passed slowly for Capt. Jack Adams, still stranded along the Taneytown Road with his commandeered Confederate blanket. An endless procession of ammunition wagons, pack mules, limbers, caissons, and ambulances had been traveling the thoroughfare all day, kicking up choking clouds of dust in their passage, yet no Good Samaritan had stopped to help the wounded officer. "The day was fine, only very warm. All was still except an occasional picket shot."[1]

In a single heartbeat, the entire scene was transformed. "The silence was broken by one heavy gun, and the shell went whistling over us, followed by another. Then opened the heaviest cannonading ever heard on earth. Shells burst over me, and on all sides. Solid shot ploughed up the ground and I expected my time had come. Many of the wounded crawled away, but I could not, and must stand it."[2]

Now a new danger appeared. Not only was Adams in jeopardy from the cannonade, but suddenly the possibility of being trampled to death appeared to be a very real threat. "When the shelling opened nearly all the non-combatants were at the front, and they now made the best time possible to get out of danger. I lay near a gate way, where they passed. Down would come a pack mule loaded with cooking utensils sufficient

1. Adams, *Reminiscences of the Nineteenth Massachusetts*, p. 68.
2. *Ibid.*

to start a stove and tin-ware store; then a lot of colored servants, or a runaway horse. I would shout and kick; was sure that I should be either killed by shell or trampled to death. Would beg some skedaddler to get another, and take me away. He would stop, look on me with pity and say he would, but before he could capture another, a shell would come along, and his place would be vacant."[3]

Professor Michael Jacobs of Gettysburg College had been conscientiously maintaining his scientific and weather observations, even with the disrupting presence of two warring armies in his peaceful town. The sudden roar of the cannonade caused him to check his chronometer and jot down the time. It was exactly 1:07 p.m.[4]

All living things in the vicinity of the "protected" rearward Taneytown Road were shocked to find themselves under an astonishing bombardment of rebounding shot and exploding shells.

---

3. *Ibid.*
4. Michael Jacobs, *Notes on the Rebel Invasion of Maryland and Pennsylvania, and the Battle of Gettysburg, July 1st, 2d and 3d, 1863* (Philadelphia: J. B. Lippincott & Company, 1864), p. 41. This would be 2:07 p.m. with our system of Daylight Savings Time. Approximately 1:00 is the most widely accepted time for the beginning of the bombardment; however, the Confederates generally accepted 1:30 as the starting time.

   The time noted down by observers for the onset of this monumental bombardment varied to an astonishing degree. Brig. Gen. Robert O. Tyler, commander of the Army of the Potomac Artillery Reserve, noted that the cannonade began at noon and continued until after 2:00 [*OR*, vol. 27, pt. 1, p. 874]. Capt. Emmanuel D. Roath of the 107th Pennsylvania was sure that the artillery barrage began at 1:30 [*OR*, vol. 27, pt. 1, p. 305]. Col. Thomas A. Smyth of the 1st Delaware, part of Brig. Gen. Alexander Hays' Third Division of the Second Corps, was equally convinced that the shooting commenced at 2:00 and "continued without intermission until 5 p.m." [*OR*, vol. 27, pt. 1, p. 465]. General Hays himself reported the duration of the shelling was from "nearly 2 p.m. . . . uninterupted until 4:30 o'clock." [*OR*, vol. 27, pt. 1, p. 454.]

   Bear in mind that timekeeping was a relative, and not an exact, science for the individual soldier, especially between the Union troops and their Southern counterparts, who set their timepieces to widely divergent chronometers. Jacobs, being a scientist, had timepieces most likely to be set to the correct time, and was a trained scientific observer.

"All in rear of the crest for a thousand yards, as well as among the Batteries, was the field of their blind fury. Ambulances, passing down the Taneytown Road, with wounded men, were struck.—The Hospitals near this road were riddled. . . . Riderless horses, galloping madly through the fields, were brought up, or down, rather, by these invisible horse-tamers, and they would not run any more. Mules with ammunition, pigs wallowing about, cows in the pastures, whatever was animate or inanimate, in all this broad range, were no exception to their blind havoc."[5]

Those that could move made quickly for cover, no matter how slight. Many of the men in the regimental aid stations along the Taneytown Road, however, were so badly wounded that they could not move, or be moved. There was nothing to do but wait and pray that the shells would fall somewhere else. Surgeon Francis M. Wafer, 108th New York, was weathering the storm of shot and shell at the Peter Frey farmhouse, next door to the Widow Leister's home. It was "a place where some Surgeons who were on duty on the field assembled to apply light dressings to the wounded & superintend the removal of the wounded in ambulances to the operating hospital further to the rear.... For a while it seemed here as if a man's being unhurt was perfectly inconsistent with the tremendous shower of iron which fell around, and by their locality."[6]

Troops moving on the Taneytown Road were caught in the deadly cascade of death. Part of the Sixth Corps had been moving all day "from point to point, wherever danger [was thought] to be imminent until noon when we were ordered to report to the line held by [Maj.] Gen [David B.] Birney, [First Division, Third Corps]. Our Brigade marched down the road until we reached the house used by General Meade as Headquarters. The road ran between ledges of rock while the fields were strewn with boulders. To our left was a hill on which we had many Batteries posted."[7]

For Elisha Hunt Rhodes of the 2nd Rhode Island, it seemed as if the sky had opened up and unleashed a deluge of metal. "Just as we reached Gen Meade's Headquarters, a shell burst over our heads, and

---

5. Byrne and Weaver, *Haskell of Gettysburg*, pp. 152, 153.
6. Francis Wafer, original diary, Douglas Library, Queen's University, Kingston, Ontario, Canada, K7L 5C4, copy in the 108th New York Vertical File, Gettysburg National Military Park, p. 47.
7. Elisha Hunt Rhodes, *All for the Union: The Civil War Diary and Letters of Elisha Hunt Rhodes*, ed. Robert Hunt Rhodes (New York: Random House, Vintage Civil War Library Edition, 1992), p. 108.

it was immediately followed by showers of iron. More than two hundred guns were belching forth their thunder, and most of the shells that came over the hill struck in the road on which our Brigade was moving. Solid shot would strike the large rocks and split them as if exploding gunpowder. The flying iron and pieces of stone struck men in all directions."[8]

There was nothing for the men to do but get off the road, seek whatever insufficient shelter they could find, and ride out the storm. "It is said that this fire continued for about two hours, but I have no idea of the time. We could not see the enemy, and we could only cover ourselves as best we could behind the rocks and trees."[9]

Captain Adams, stranded along the Taneytown Road, was experiencing the overflow of mass confusion spilling down the slope from the ridge above. "The storm broke upon us so suddenly that soldiers and officers—who leaped, as it began, from their tents, or from lazy siestas on the grass—were stricken in their rising with mortal wounds and died, some with cigars between their teeth, some with pieces of food in their fingers, and one at least—a pale young German, from Pennsylvania—with a miniature of his sister in . . . [his] hands," reported the New York *World* correspondent to his readers several days later. "The earth, torn up in clouds, blinded the eyes of hurrying men; and through the branches of the trees and among the gravestones of the cemetery a shower of destruction crashed ceaselessly."[10]

The commander of the 111th New York had been chatting quietly with Captain Thompson. "All at once, with the suddenness of the lightning flash, came a crash as of an earthquake and in an instant the whole hill was covered with ploughing shot and bursting shell. For a full minute we were terrified. Col MacDougall rallied first. 'Captain,' he said, 'it won't do for us to lay here; we must get our place in line.'"[11]

But moving a body of troops under these conditions was easier said than done. "We attempted to form our men, but it was impossible. We drove them before us up the hill more like cattle than soldiers. Aides and general officers were dashing in all directions and soon General

8. *Ibid.*
9. *Ibid.*
10. *New York World*, July 7, 1863.
11. Thompson, *Personal Narrative*, p. 42.

Hays, commanding our division (three brigades) joined us in our work of getting the men over the hill. The artillery fire from all of the two hundred and twenty guns of the enemy was continuous and it seemed as if every foot of the hill top was moved with this storm of metal. Just as we reached the brow of the hill a coffee squad of three men was blown to bits by a bursting shell just before our faces, and horses, riders and men on foot were batted to pieces like pith balls by the terrible missiles."[12]

"Most of our men made straight for a designated line in front of our cannon, where, being over the hill and lower than its crest, they would be much less likely to be injured and would be in line for repelling a charge which we felt would follow the cannonade. Some, however, were foolish enough to huddle behind a small house near the line. Seeing them, Gen Hays sent me to drive them out. Returning with them we passed in rear of a small stable and here I got my first knock down.[13] A round shot, going through the stable, brought away a board entire, and this, flying through the air, took me fair upon the nose and laid me flat. This excited a hearty laugh notwithstanding our peril."[14]

Gingerly probing his injured nose, Thompson rousted out the snickering skulkers from the shadow of the small building and brusquely herded them toward the scant cover afforded along the Union line. "As I was last at the line my chances of cover were poor. Our men were laying flat with their heads behind a little stone wall about eighteen inches high, with no cover from the shot and shell that were coming over us as fast as the guns of the rebels could send them. I lay down on a crack between two men—really on them—with my head against a stone as big as a bushel basket that reached through the wall."[15] There Thompson could only huddle, and pray, and wait.

The general staff luncheon had just broken up when "their shells plunged down and exploded all around us.—We sprang to our feet. . . . The wildest confusion for a few moments obtained among us. . . . The servants ran terror-stricken for dear life and disappeared.—The horses, hitched to the trees or held by the slack hands of orderlies,

12. *Ibid.*
13. This was the Bryan house and stable.
14. Thompson, *Personal Narrative*, p. 42.
15. *Ibid.*, p. 43.

neighed out in fright, and broke away and plunged riderless through the fields." "The horses of the ambulance containing the lunch broke away, the driver, an old veteran of the regular service, being killed—altogether creating a scene of such confusion as is seldom seen, even on the field of battle." Alfred Pleasanton had ridden off about fifty yards when the Confederate artillery went off, and, glancing over his shoulder, saw "an indiscriminate mass of sandwiches, cheese, crackers, and stragglers all mixed up together," flying every which direction. One of the first shells had made a direct hit on the improvised table from which they had just been dining.[16]

Winfield Scott Hancock, restive in the afternoon quiet, had taken yet another ride along his lines, "encouraging the men . . . [he] informed us that the enemy was going to make a charge on our line and that he wanted every soldier to stand at his post." Incoming shells abruptly cut short Hancock's remarks.[17]

Gibbon was in the midst of vainly calling for his horse; finally, snatching up his sword, he rushed off for the crest on foot. His staff aide, Lieutenant Haskell, called for his horse as well, likewise with no response. "I found him tied to a tree nearby, eating oats, with an air of the greatest composure, which, under the circumstances, even then struck me as exceedingly ridiculous. . . . Gnl Gibbon's groom has just mounted his horse, and is starting to take the General's to him, when the flying iron meets him and opens his breast,—he drops dead, and the horses gallop away." Another aide finally retrieved the horses; Gibbon and Haskell rode off together to check the disposition of the Second Division troops and batteries. A little more than sixty seconds had elapsed since the shelling began.[18]

Galloping over the crest of the ridge, it at first appeared as if every foot soldier of the Second Corps had magically disappeared. "Where is the Infantry? Has it vanished in smoke? Is this a nightmare, or a juggler's devilish trick?—All too real. The men of the Infantry have seized their arms; and behind their works, behind every rock, in every ditch, wherever there is any shelter, they hug the ground, silent, quiet, unterrified, little harmed." One officer compared the melting away of

16. Byrne and Weaver, *Haskell of Gettysburg*, p. 148; Hancock, *Reminiscences of Winfield Scott Hancock*, p. 207; Hancock Papers, Scrapbook, Pennsylvania State Library.

17. Muffly, *The Story of Our Regiment*, p. 439.

18. Byrne and Weaver, *Haskell of Gettysburg*, pp. 148-49; Hancock, *Reminiscences of Winfield Scott Hancock*, p. 207.

the troops to the effect a torrential downpour has on a crowded city street.[19]

The artillery was answering in kind to the Confederate bombardment, from the heights of Round Top up through the cemetery, but only in a limited fashion. Brig. Gen. Henry J. Hunt, chief of artillery of the Army of the Potomac, had ridden through the gun positions, advising the commanders to conserve their ammunition for the infantry assault he was sure would follow. Pausing on Little Round Top, he watched the Confederate artillery for a moment, describing the shelling with reverential awe, as only a seasoned artillerist could. "From that point the scene was indescribably grand. All their batteries were soon covered with smoke, through which the flashes were incessant, whilst the air seemed filled with shells, whose sharp explosions, with the hurtling of their fragments, formed a running accompaniment to the deep roar of the guns."[20]

The once pastoral serenity of the Evergreen Cemetery was "now trodden down, laid a waste, desecrated," wrote one artilleryman posted there. "The fences are all down, the many graves have been run over, beautiful lots with iron fences and splendid monuments have been destroyed or soiled, and our infantry and artillery occupy these sacred grounds, where the dead are sleeping, engaged in death dealing occupation of warfare. It is enough to make one mourn."[21] In moving the artillery into the cemetery grounds, many markers were run down and crushed, and gun emplacements now sat over the final resting place of some of Gettysburg's most prominent citizens.

As the Southern shelling began to get its stride, only about thirty-five Union guns were replying. More than sixty guns, including all those in the Second Corps, stood silent and waiting.[22]

---

19. Byrne and Weaver, *Haskell of Gettysburg*, p. 149; Stewart, *Pickett's Charge*, p. 130. Many of the men would have undoubtedly questioned Haskell's opinion that they were "unterrified" at that particular moment.
20. Henry J. Hunt, "The Third Day at Gettysburg," in Robert U. Johnson and Clarence C. Buel, eds., *Battles and Leaders of the Civil War*, 4 vols. (New York: The Century Company, 1884-1888; reprint, Secaucus, New Jersey: Castle, a division of Book Sales, Inc., 1956), vol. 3, pp. 372-73.
21. George Breck, letter to Ellen, July 2, 1863, in Blake McKelvey, ed., "Rochester in the Civil War," *The Rochester Historical Society*, vol. 22, (1944): 130-31.
22. Stewart, *Pickett's Charge*, p. 131.

To the men in blue trying to flatten themselves as near the ground as possible, an incredible specter appeared through the smoke, noise, and shrapnel. "I rode along my line to the right of the Second Corps to the [Ziegler's Grove] woods held by General Hays" was General Hancock's understated way of telling it, with the object of letting every one of his men know that "his general was behind him in the storm."[23]

Mounted on his sorrel, with coat buttoned only at the collar and immaculate white shirt gleaming beneath, light rapier belted on beneath the coat, and topped with a stiff black hat decorated with general's cording, Hancock looked every inch a general of generals. As he started out along the line, a nearby regimental band struck up "The Star Spangled Banner," and Hancock doffed his hat, waving it and smiling to the troops as he passed. With all the aplomb of the parade ground he moved past his startled men, seemingly unaware of the deadly storm surrounding him.[24]

Beginning with a cloud of staff and orderlies, Hancock dispatched them one by one until only Pvt. James Wells, "a short, stout Irishman," remained, bearing the Second Corps standard. General Doubleday, who witnessed Hancock's ride, was still awed more than twenty years later: "I can almost fancy I can see Hancock again as he rode past the front of his command, just previous to the assault, followed by a single orderly displaying his corps flag, while the missiles from a hundred pieces of artillery tore up the ground around him."[25]

At one point the incoming fire became so intense that even the seemingly unstoppable Hancock had to rein in until it slacked, his horse balking at the incessant explosions. "Every soldier's heart stopped beating," wrote one observer, "for this seemed certain death for the general." When admonished by one of his men to stop exposing

---

23. Winfield Scott Hancock, letter to artist Peter F. Rothermel, December 31, 1868, Hancock Papers, Pennsylvania State Library.
24. Undated *Philadelphia Times* clipping, Hancock Scrapbook, Pennsylvania State Library; Letter to Peter F. Rothermel, December 31, 1868, Rothermel Papers, Pennsylvania State Library. "The Star Spangled Banner" was not yet the National Anthem in 1863.
25. Hancock Papers, Pennsylvania State Library; Military Service Institute, *Letters and Addresses Contributed at a General Meeting of the Military Service Institute Held at Governor's Island, New York Harbor, February 25, 1886, in Memory of Winfield Scott Hancock, etc.* (New York: Military Service Institute, 1886), p. 21.

himself to the vicious shelling, Hancock retorted: "There are times when a corps commander's life does not count."[26]

When the Second Corps commander's horse finally became totally unmanageable in the plunging fire, he was forced to trade mounts. Turning to Capt. Edward P. Brownson, the Second Corps commissary of musters, Hancock quipped: "You can afford to have a horse of this kind, Captain, on such an occasion as this, but I can not."[27]

Remounted on Brownson's "tall, light bay with a white stripe on its face or nostril," Hancock continued along the lines. Followed by the cheers and huzzahs of his men, Hancock rode on to Ziegler's Grove. Concerned that the effect of the Second Corps artillery's silence would undermine the morale of the troops, he overrode General Hunt's dictates, ordering the gunners to open long range fire on the Confederate batteries. Hancock then cantered back over the crest of Cemetery Ridge on his way to confer with Meade, anxious to discuss some changes in troops placement with the army commander. The echoing thunder of the Second Corps artillery followed him.[28]

After bidding farewell to his lunchtime companions, General Meade had trotted down to the extreme left of the Union line to check out the situation at Little Round Top, then headed back to his headquarters. While the Widow Leister home provided an ideal location for the army commander, with direct line of sight of the signal post on Round Top, and within easy riding distance of the entire Union position, it also carried one grave disadvantage. Nestled as it was behind the center of the convex battle line, any artillery focused on the middle of the northern line, if inadvertently aimed high, was very likely to end up in Meade's lap. And now, with targets obscured by smoke and dust, the

26. Undated *Philadelphia Times* clipping, Hancock Scrapbook, Pennsylvania State Library; Stewart, *Pickett's Charge*, p. 151. While it has become celebrated in print and on film, there is some question as to whether Hancock ever spoke these heroic words.

27. Winfield Scott Hancock, letter to Peter F. Rothermel, December 31, 1868, Rothermel Papers, Civil War Library and Museum, Philadelphia, Pennsylvania.

28. Hancock, letter to Peter F. Rothermel, December 31, 1868; Hancock, *Reminiscences of Winfield Scott Hancock*, pp. 209-10. A controversy arose over the use of the artillery on July 3 and who had the right to command it. For a more detailed coverage of this issue, see Henry J. Hunt, "The Third Day at Gettysburg," *Battles and Leaders*, vol. 3, pp. 369-87.

Rebel shellbursts were gradually walking up Cemetery Ridge, away from the huddled foot soldiers, up through the Union artillery positions, and over the crest into the rear areas.[29]

Shells were beginning to fall thick and fast at army headquarters. One burst in the front yard among the tethered horses with ghastly results; another literally tore an unfortunate orderly serving lunch in half. Two rounds in quick succession almost obliterated the front porch, one demolishing the steps, the other carrying away the porch supports. Soon a door was smashed by incoming fire, then another missile barreled through the garret of the small dwelling. Flying splinters of the disintegrating house made deadly wooden shrapnel. General Meade himself, standing in the doorway, was narrowly missed by an incoming solid shot that buried itself in a box standing by the entrance. It was impossible for the general to receive reports and dispatch aides in this kind of pandemonium, so the army commander and his staff beat a hasty retreat to the leeward side of the house, vainly trying to carry on the business of running an army and dodge incoming artillery fire at the same time.[30]

It soon became evident that nothing was being accomplished by keeping army headquarters at the Leister House; staff officers dispatched from various corps commanders could not even reach the commanding general due to the heavy shellfire, so General Meade and staff reluctantly packed up and moved to a barn several hundred yards down the Taneytown Road. However, the peripatetic firing soon traveled to this location as well, a shell fragment inflicting a debilitating wound to Army Chief of Staff Maj. Gen. Daniel Butterfield. Again the decision was made to evacuate headquarters, this time moving to Maj. Gen. Henry W. Slocum's Twelfth Corps headquarters on Power's Hill. And still the shells continued to fall.[31]

---

29. Stewart, *Pickett's Charge*, p. 122; Bill Cameron, "The Signal Corps at Gettysburg," *The Gettysburg Magazine*, no. 3 (July 1990): 13.

30. Howard Coffin, *Full Duty: Vermonters in the Civil War* (Woodstock, Vermont: The Countryman Press, Inc., 1995), p. 192; Pennypacker, *General Meade*, pp. 188-89; George G. Meade, Jr., *With Meade at Gettysburg* (Philadelphia: John C. Winston Co., 1930), p. 148; George Gordon Meade, *The Life and Letters of George Gordon Meade*, ed. George Gordon Meade, 2 vols. (New York: Charles Scribner's Sons, 1913), vol. 2, p. 106.

31. Stewart, *Pickett's Charge*, p. 134; Meade, Jr., *With Meade at Gettysburg*, p. 150; Meade, *Life and Letters of George Gordon Meade*, vol. 2, pp. 107-8.

Hancock encountered Captain Livermore of the Ambulance Corps as he rode to the rear of the Second Corps on his way to report to Meade. A sudden rush of about fifty men, trying to escape the shelling, streaked by the mounted men. Hancock, furious, shouted "Go after them! Go after them!" to anyone within earshot. Livermore, Second Corps Medical Director Alexander Dougherty on his "very fat and sturdy black horse . . . coat-tails flying, and his elbows out," and a few others headed off the stampede, nipping the beginnings of a rout in the bud. Hancock and Livermore then rode on together, arriving at what was left of army headquarters.[32]

"The projectiles of the enemy mainly flew over our front lines of infantry, who lay flat on the ground, and took effect chiefly among the reserves, who lay in considerable numbers behind the front lines, and the artillerymen and horses, with the limbers and caissons, which, as always in battle, were posted in rear of the pieces," remembered Livermore of that hair-raising ride to the Leister House. "General Meade's headquarters were situated just where many shot and shell struck or exploded, and it was a very uncomfortable place while we were there. After the battle, I saw in the yard of the house a dozen or twenty dead horses, which were a part of those ridden by General Meade and his staff as I believe."[33]

Finding the army headquarters at the Leister Farm deserted, Hancock turned his borrowed horse around and headed back to the crest of Cemetery Ridge. Livermore continued on, riding over the fields, all the while checking how effectively his new ambulance command was operating under the intense Confederate shelling.[34]

Captain Livermore had already had a eventful and significant day before meeting up with Hancock. There had been quite a bit of concern at Second Corps medical headquarters after the First Division Hospital

---

32. Livermore, *Days and Events*, pp. 259-60. There is some question as to whether this incident occurred during the bombardment or the subsequent charge. Even Livermore had a difficult time fitting all the pieces together into a coherent whole [Livermore, *Days and Events*, pp. 263-64]. The author puts this incident here in the narrative as it seems, to him, that most of the pieces of the story belong with the cannonade.
33. *Ibid.*, p. 60.
34. Hancock, *Reminiscences of Winfield Scott Hancock*, p. 210; Livermore, *Days and Events*, p. 263.

had to uproot itself and move the previous afternoon due to shells falling on the backside of Cemetery Ridge. "By direction of Dr. Dougherty, the medical director of our corps, I selected a place removed from the range of projectiles for a [Second Corps] general field hospital, where all the wounded could be carried and provided with shelter and treatment until the battle was over."[35]

After riding the countryside seeking a good location, Livermore found what appeared to be the ideal place. "I selected a spot on Rock Creek about a mile and a half down the stream from the crossing of the Baltimore road, I should think. At this point it was of sufficient volume to afford water for all necessary purposes. The left bank was a hillside, and the right bank was level and low and perfectly accessible from the road leading from the field of battle, and both hillside and level were clothed with trees nearly free from undergrowth. The hillside afforded a fine place for the wounded, being sheltered by the trees and having perfect drainage, and the level was needed for hospital wagons. My selection met with the approval of the medical director."[36] It would certainly prove to be a fateful choice.

With a new site for the Second Corps Hospital picked out, orders came down from the Medical Director's headquarters to start transferring the division hospitals to the Rock Creek location. The individual division hospitals were already packing up for the move when the first shells crashed into the slopes of Cemetery Ridge. "In expectation of an attack on our immediate front to take place in the latter part of the day We determined to move our Hospital into a piece of woods a mile and a half to the rear on the farm of Mr. Geo Bushman," wrote Dr. Justin Dwinelle of that afternoon. "Preparations were being made for the removal when the enemy commenced their attack upon the left centre at one o'clock. We were literally Shelled out and compelled to hurry forward our movements with all possible dispatch."[37]

The thundering herd of fleeing non-combatants that had raced past Jack Adams was not long in reaching the division hospitals. "To add to our other difficulties, for a while we were seriously threatened to be run

35. Livermore, *Days and Events*, p. 258.
36. *Ibid.*, pp. 258-59.
37. Dwinelle, *Medical Report.*

down by a stampede of pack Mules, Saddlehorses, Army Wagons, Prisoners & Stragglers," wrote the surgeon-in-charge of the Second Division. "It required great exertions to render this stampede less dangerous to the helpless wounded than the shells of the enemy."[38]

Following the stampede came the inexorable Southern cannonade, moving up over the crest of Cemetery Ridge and relentlessly advancing into the hospital grounds. One of the very first shells scored a direct hit on a Second Corps field hospital. The capacious barn of William and Lydia Patterson, just to the immediate west of the division hospitals, was filled with wounded from the July 2 clash when a Confederate round came smashing through the structure. The shot tore off the arm of a fourteen-year-old black servant who was attending a wounded New York officer.[39]

"See, there!" wrote one anxious observer from a neighboring corps hospital. "The Second Corps Hospital, between us and Little Round Top, is under fire, and they must move, and that quickly. Men, wounded and otherwise, ambulances, hospital wagons, mules, led horses, servants, surgeons, all come hurrying through the fields under that shell fire. How soon will our turn come?"[40]

For those at the Second Corps Hospitals, it appeared impossible to escape the seemingly omnipresent shells. Mathew Marvin, a member of the 1st Minnesota Volunteers with a crippling foot wound, took it quite stoically: "I thought that if the rebs had a shell for me that it could not kill me any younger & that they can[']t do it but once[.] For about an hour the shell came pretty thick & those that could crawl up near the Tre[e] whare [*sic*] I was. A solled [*sic*] shot came & struck whare a man had just got up not more than ten ft from me[.]" Marvin's situation was complicated by a seriously wounded superior officer who insisted on returning to the firing line. "I was laying by the side of my capt who was wounded in the head the ball going in at the nose & came out back of the left ear. . . . He wanted to go back to the front so I had to hold him most of the time[.] I had got over being faint & could crawl on my hands and kne[e]s[.]"[41]

---

38. *Ibid.*
39. Coco, *A Vast Sea of Misery*, p. 65
40. Samuel Toombs, *New Jersey Troops in the Gettysburg Campaign from June 5 to July 31, 1863* (Orange, New Jersey; The Evening Mail Publishing House, 1888), pp. 326-27.
41. Diary of Mathew Marvin, July 3, 1863, Mathew Marvin Papers, 1861-1863, Minnesota Historical Society.

At the Third Division Hospital, Rev. Thomas G. Murphey, chaplain of the 1st Delaware Volunteer Infantry, was helping the stretchermen and ambulance drivers hurry off the wounded to the new location. "When we were nearly through loading the ambulances and sending off those who could walk, there burst over and around the barn, in which our division wounded were, a terrific storm of shells. Men who had seemed utterly unable to move aroused themselves, and crawled to some other place, as they supposed, of safety, or at least of less danger. Horsemen, footmen, and wagons rushed wildly across the field, or down the road, under cover of the hill in the place of danger, rather than out of it. The confusion, haste, and alarm of each one alarmed the rest, and altogether the scene was both amusing and frightful."[42]

Emergency evacuation, however, was already well under way; Captain Livermore had the ambulance corps in action, transporting the wounded back to the new Rock Creek location. Unfortunately, the small ambulances could only carry a few wounded at a time, so the transfer was going to take quite some time.

Not all the wounded were in stable enough condition to be moved, however. One such case was that of Hiram D. Clark of the 125th New York Infantry. Lying unconscious, under anesthesia, on the operating table of a Second Corps facility along the Taneytown Road when the bombardment began, with his leg just amputated, Clark was unable to be moved. Shells were crashing wildly all around the barn, remembered one eyewitness; the patient finally coming to "from the effects of the chloroform, and with a smile on his lips, remained uncomplainingly there all the terrible afternoon."[43]

At least one seriously injured soldier created his own escape from the incoming shells. Drummer Nathaniel Beerly of Company B, 148th Pennsylvania Volunteers, remembered the almost miraculous recovery of one patient: "While assisting the ambulance corps carrying off the wounded, some of the boys were amazed, after carrying a supposed wounded man to the rear, partly out of danger, yet still under shell fire, while resting, to see the soldier get off the stretcher and run out of

---

42. Thomas G. Murphey, *Four Years in the War. The History of the First Regiment of Delaware Veteran Volunteers*, (Philadelphia: James S. Claxton, 1866), pp. 120-21.

43. Gregory Coco, *War Stories: A Collection of 150 Little Known Human Interest Accounts of the Campaign and Battle of Gettysburg* (Gettysburg, Pennsylvania: Thomas Publications, 1992), p. 63.

danger." Beerly wryly noted, apparently by way of explanation: "Evidently he did not belong to our Regiment."[44]

The ambulance crews, with herculean efforts, were pressing forward the evacuation as rapidly as possible. Marvin would report that "the Ambulances soon came & took us about 2 miles to the rear whar [*sic*] they had established the hospital in a hollow near a creek... we wer[e] all rite [*sic*] at last."[45]

The rush of skedaddlers off the ridge had slowed significantly, and still Captain Adams of the 19th Massachusetts lay by the roadside, wondering if the next shell would land directly on top of him. "At last I saw a staff officer whom I knew riding to the front, and called to him. He heard me, drew his sword, and drove a couple of men to me, who, finding a stretcher, had me carried to the rear of the barn, where an ambulance was found and I was placed in it. My first sergeant, Damon, had been lying near, and I urged that he be taken with me, and my request was granted. Damon was wounded in the leg, the bone shattered, and it was necessary that the leg should be amputated as soon as possible. We started for the rear."[46]

If his ambulance ride of the previous night had been unremarkable for its brevity, the memory of the ride of this afternoon would stay with Adams for the rest of his life. "The driver was anxious for our safety, and it is possible he might have thought of himself," Adams would write years later, when he could look back with humor instead of agony; "at any rate he drove over a corn-field on the jump. Part of the time I was in the top of the ambulance, part on the floor. Damon and I would come together hard enough to drive the breath out of each other; but we were only passengers having a free ride, so we could not complain."[47]

Amazingly, both men survived the traumatic ride. "When at last we reached our destination I expected we were both jelly, and would have to be taken out in a spoon, but we had held together, that is, I had, but Damon's leg was all broken up, and was soon amputated."[48]

---

44. Muffly, *The Story of Our Regiment*, p. 325.
45. Diary of Mathew Marvin, July 3, 1863.
46. Adams, *Reminiscences of the Nineteenth Massachusetts*, pp. 68-69.
47. *Ibid.*, p. 69.
48. *Ibid.*

Unperturbed by the greatest noise ever heard on the continent, Professor Jacobs took his daily two o'clock weather readings on the stroke of the hour. He noted down the fact that it was eighty-seven degrees; "only four-tenths of the heavens are covered, but with cumulus or the massive thunder-cloud of summer." The July atmosphere was brewing up a summer thunderstorm, and the humidity made for a muggy afternoon for everyone in and around the once-sleepy hamlet of Gettysburg.[49]

Back on the ridge top, shells were still falling among the infantry, despite the large number of overshots, and the Second Corps artillery was now lustily returning fire. "The artillerymen were all busily at work at their guns, thundering out defiance to the enemy whose shells were bursting in and around them at a fearful rate, striking now a horse, now a limber box and now a man. Over all hung a heavy pall of smoke underneath which could be seen the rapidly moving legs of the men as they rushed to and fro between the pieces and the line of limbers, carrying forward the ammunition."[50]

"One thing which forcibly occurred to me was the perfect quiet with which the horses stood in their places," noted General Gibbon, himself a seasoned artilleryman. "Even when a shell, striking in the midst of a team, would knock over one or two of them or hurl one struggling in his death agonies to the ground, the rest would make no effort to struggle or escape but would stand stolidly by."[51]

For the poor infantrymen laying below the mouths of the thundering guns, the blast furnace heat of the laboring pieces flowed over the prostrate men in blistering waves with each discharge. "We lay hugging the ground in the rear of our works, the hot July sun blazing down on us; the air above us full of screeching shells and balls from the Rebel lines," remembered one veteran of that terrible shelling. "The shock from our cannon and the bursting of shells from the

---

49. Weather records of Dr. Michael Jacobs of the Pennsylvania College at Gettysburg, Michael Jacobs Vertical File, Gettysburg National Military Park.
50. Gibbon, *Personal Recollections*, p. 147.
51. *Ibid.*, pp. 147-48.

Rebels' guns caused blood to flow from the ears and noses of several members of our company."[52]

The summer sun continued to beat down on the wool-clad soldiers, lying wedged together like sardines behind the scant cover. At least one soldier remembered sweating so much that a muddy spot formed on the dry ground where he was crouched. One of Brig. Gen. William Harrow's men wrote that he longed for relief from the heat as much as from the shelling, possibly even more. Combined with the scarcity of water and the ravenous hunger of most, this was proving to be an extraordinarily uncomfortable afternoon. "I knew of only one word that can describe our position at the time—and that isn't used much except in church and in the army," wrote Captain Thompson of the 111th New York of that miserable afternoon. "The lurid rays of a July sun beating down on us, the appalling roar of at least three hundred pieces of artillery, the stifling fumes of burning sulphur from the exploding shrapnel, all combined to make a heat as unendurable at least as the Valley of the Jordan, not to make any warmer comparison."[53]

Some men made the dash to get water, the nearest source of which was several hundred yards away, totally exposed to shellfire the entire way. A few became heroes to their comrades, many more became casualties. One water runner, on his return from filling as many canteens as he could carry, had a solid shot pass right between his legs. Handing out the canteens to his comrades, he shakily remarked: "The water is cold enough, boys; but it's devilish hot around the spring."[54]

While most were safe behind their slight breastworks and under the muzzles of the cannon, infantrymen in the line were beginning to take some casualties, although most were non-fatal. "I was struck twice," wrote Lt. George Yost the next day, "once on the back of my neck and once in the breast with a ball from a [case]shot. The ball struck me on my tent and rubber blanket which I had rolled up and put over my shoulder. It only knocked me over."[55]

It was not long before Capt. Benjamin W. Thompson took his second "knock down." "Sometime in the cannonade, when I know not, I was knocked endwise out of this line of men by a shell exploding against the stone at my head. So far as any memory of what passed for

---

52. Muffly, *The Story of Our Regiment*, p. 439.
53. Stewart, *Pickett's Charge*, p. 137, Thompson, *Personal Narrative*, p. 43.
54. Stewart, *Pickett's Charge*, pp. 149-50.
55. George Yost, letter to his father, July 4, 1863.

a time, I was entirely unconscious. Yet my Colonel says I came and reported myself wounded, wiping blood from my face, and he told me to go to the rear. My company clerk, who was wounded soon afterward, in passing to the rear found me sitting against the body of an apple tree on the very summit of the hill, and the ground around me literally ploughed with shot."[56]

It did not take long for the wounded men making their way to the rear to discover that Meade had fled his headquarters, and to seek shelter in the vacated buildings. "He led me down the hill to a barn near General Meade's headquarters, and there I fully recovered consciousness." The reason why the headquarters had packed up and left, however, became immediately evident. "We had made a bad selection, for the shells coming over the hill all converged into this vortex and this part of the Taneytown Road was a perfect valley of death. We ran the gauntlet to an old log barn further down the line and got what protection it afforded until the cannonade ceased."[57]

The Confederate shelling continued to play havoc on the Union line, especially riddling the northern artillery. Lt. Alonzo Cushing's Battery A, 4th United States Artillery seemed to be a magnet for the incoming Confederate fire, noted General Gibbon. "Looking . . . at Cushing's Battery, my eyes happened to rest upon one of the gunners standing in rear of the nearest limber, the lid open showing the charges. Suddenly, with a shriek, came a shell right under the limber box, and the poor gunner went hopping to the rear on one leg, the shreds of the other dangling about as he went." Just moments later, "three of Cushing's limber boxes blew up at once, sending the contents in a vast column of dense smoke, and above the din could be heard the triumphant yells of the enemy as he recognized this result of his fire."[58]

Woodruff's 1st United States, Battery I, was fairing no better. "We see the solid shot strike axle, or pole, or wheel, and the tough iron and heart of oak snap and fly like straws. The great oaks there by [Lt. George A.] Woodruff's guns heave down their massy branches with a crash, as if the lightning had smote them. The shells swoop down among the Battery horses, standing there apart,—a half a dozen horses

56. Thompson, *Personal Narrative*, p. 43.

57. *Ibid.*

58. Gibbon, *Personal Recollections*, pp. 148, 149.

start,—they tumble,—their legs stiffen,—their vitals and blood smear the ground. And these shot and shells have not respect for men either. We see the poor fellows hobbling back from the crest, or unable to do so, pale and weak lying on the ground, with the mangled stump of an arm or leg, dripping their life blood away, or with a cheek torn open, or a shoulder smashed. And many, alas! hear not the roar as they stretch upon the ground, with upturned faces, and open eyes, though a shell should burst in their very ears."[59]

Assistant Surgeon Francis Wafer, the Canadian doctor who had come to take part in America's great war, also observed the devastation around Woodruff's guns. "The horses rolled in heaps everywhere tangled in the harnesses with their dying struggles—wheels knocked off, gun capsized and artillerists going to the rear or lying on the ground bleeding in every direction."[60]

"Our artillery . . . is getting roughly handled. A dozen of our caissons have already exploded. Gun after gun is dismounted by the solid shots of the enemy. Here is a battery abandoned because there is not enough men left to work it or horses to take it off. There is a battery of Napoleons in the same situation, because the guns have become so heated that the cartridges explode before they can be rammed home."[61] All along the Second Corps artillery line, gun crews especially were taking a terrible punishment in dead and badly injured.

For the wounded, it was a deadly challenge just getting off the field alive. With the Southern shells falling between the Union line and the regimental aid stations, the men had to run a gauntlet of shellfire just to reach medical help. "Now a wounded man attempts to go back to a hospital and perhaps is cut down before he can gain the rear of the ridge fifteen rods behind us," wrote one veteran to the folks back home. "A case of sunstroke and his comrades start to carry him off; perhaps one of their number is looped [*sic*] off; perhaps all pass uninjured."[62]

After about fifteen minutes, seeing that the shells were mostly "quartermaster hunters," passing overhead with much noise and little

59. Byrne and Weaver, *Haskell of Gettysburg*, p. 151.
60. Wafer diary, p. 43.
61. Alfred Carpenter, letter of July 30, 1863, copy in Minnesota Historical Society.
62. *Ibid.*

danger on their way to the rear, the foot soldiers began to relax a little. Lt. Henry Ropes of the 20th Massachusetts pulled a volume of Dickens out of his knapsack, propped himself up under a tree, and started reading. He was still enjoying the book when killed by the premature detonation of a shell from a Union battery firing behind and above him.[63]

After the massive march of June 29, the rapid push to the battlefield on July 1, and two back-to-back days of grueling battle, the Second Corpsmen were quickly reaching the point of total physical and mental exhaustion. With nerves now pushed nearly to the limit, many of the troops, taking advantage of the forced inactivity, simply snuggled closer to cover and, lulled by the incessant roar, drifted off to sleep.[64]

General Gibbon, commander of the Second Division, closely shadowed by his staff aide Frank Haskell, decided to work his way among the men, and encourage them as he went. "At about two o'clock he and I started," wrote Haskell in a letter to his brother. "We went along the lines of the Infantry; as they lay there flat upon the earth, a little to the front of the Batteries.—They were suffering little, and were quiet, and cool. How glad we were that the enemy were no better gunners, and that they cut the shell fuses too long. To the question asked the men: 'What do you think of this?'—the replies would be: 'O, this is bully,'—'We are getting to like it,'—'O, we don't mind this.' And so they lay under the heaviest cannonade that ever shook the continent, and among them a thousand times more jokes, than heads, were cracked."[65]

After reaching the line, they passed through it, then over the stone wall, and kept on going. "We went down in front of the line some two hundred yards, and as the smoke had a tendency to settle upon a higher plain than where we were, we could see near the ground distinctly all over the field, as well back to the crest where were our own guns, as to the opposite ridge where were those of the enemy. . . . Under the grateful shade of some elm trees, where we could see much of the field, we made seats on the ground, and sat down." When a couple men came down from the line to seek shelter in a nearby excavation, "General Gibbon said to these men, more in a tone of kindly expostulation, than of command: 'My men, do not leave your ranks to

63. Henry Livermore Abbott, *Fallen Leaves: The Civil War Letters of Major Henry Livermore Abbott*, ed. Robert Garth Scott (Kent, Ohio: Kent State University Press, 1991), p. 184.

64. Stewart, *Pickett's Charge*, p. 138.

65. Byrne and Weaver, *Haskell of Gettysburg*, pp. 153-54.

try to get shelter here. All these matters are in the hands of God, and nothing that you can do will make you safer in one place than in another.'"[66]

From their elevated perch, the entire panorama of combat was spread out before them. "No Infantry was in sight save the skirmishers, and they stood silent and motionless,—a row of gray posts through the field on one side, confronted by another of blue."[67]

That row of blue "posts" out by the Emmitsburg Road had been following the events of the bombardment very carefully. When that signal gun went off, "instinct told us at once that the gun had fired a signal," wrote Lt. Thomas Galwey of the 8th Ohio, still out on skirmish duty. "Yesterday afternoon a desperate fight had been waged on our left, which resulted in nothing except carnage. Last night Ewell, with Jackson's old corps, had assaulted our right, with like results. We all felt that *now* they would make a last effort against us, who were at the center. So when the heavy gun had boomed its signal to the enemy's line, a general bucking up could be seen along ours. We had just received fresh ammunition, and our men at once began to arrange their cartridges and caps for the coming 'trouble.' A pause of a few seconds followed the firing of the signal gun, when there broke out on the still air so terrific a cannonade as I had not heard since the morning when our guns bombarded Fredericksburg. From ten minutes to one until half-past two [by Galwey's watch] this cannonade made those Pennsylvania hills vibrate again with its awful sound."[68]

With all possible preparations made to meet any coming assault, the skirmishers could only sit back and watch the show. "We lay on our backs in the ditch, our heads to the enemy. We could see our artillerymen with their jackets off and their sleeves rolled up, at work at their guns. And an inspiring sight it was. . . . Now and again a shell would strike one of our battery ammunition chests, blowing it up with a tremendous detonation. Still our artillery kept at their work, giving out Indian yells whenever they saw that their shots had taken good effect. We were between the fires, but beneath the path of the shells. The infantry on both sides seemed to be letting the artillery on both sides

66. *Ibid.*, pp, 154, 155.
67. *Ibid.*, p. 154.
68. Galwey, *The Valiant Hours*, pp. 112-13.

do the work, knowing that their own more desperate efforts would soon be called for."[69]

The tediousness and exhaustion were beginning to take their toll on the weary men on the picket line as well. "After a while so monotonous became the roar of the artillery that it produced drowsiness among us, and I went to sleep, as I was told later. Most of my regiment did as I did."[70]

Even the advanced position of the skirmish line did not protect the men from the fallout of the cannonade. "Several of our men were hit in the meantime, amongst them Charley Gallagher, who had crossed the road and laid down in the shade of a tree. He was severely wounded while fast asleep. I slept for about ten minutes, then awoke. Shortly afterwards I was struck in the foot by a spent shell fragment. After recovering from the pain of the impact, and whilst laughing at the matter, I was slapped in the thigh by a fragment of an enemy shell. This knocked me over, but I picked myself up, to hear the same melancholy man whom I had helped off [the field] at Antietam, tell me that the next hit would, he feared, be a fatal one. Prophets of evil are always to be found."[71]

So the men of the skirmish line bided their time as best they could, watched the most spectacular show on earth, and waited for the vicious assault they knew must surely follow.

General Hancock was also out in front of the lines, doing some personal reconnaissance work of his own. The general, accompanied by wounded Col. John R. Brooke of the Second Corps, First Division, and a few others rode out several hundred yards in front of the Federal lines to the shelter of a farm house, trying to see how effective the Union artillery fire was on the Confederate gunners. Although the view was obscured by trees, Hancock saw enough to convince him of the reality of a coming infantry attack.

Before returning to the lines, and speaking loudly to be heard over the roar and howl of artillery, Hancock addressed the men in his party. "Gentlemen, after this artillery fire is over it will be followed by an infantry attack upon our lines. This battle is the turning point of the

69. *Ibid.*, p. 113.
70. *Ibid.*
71. *Ibid.*, pp. 113-14.

war; if we win this fight the war is practically over." He then turned retrospective: "We cannot tell where any of us may be before this day is over; before leaving you I wish to say I speak harshly sometimes. If I have at any time ever said anything to offend or hurt the feelings of any one of you I wish now to offer an apology."[72]

After finishing his blanket apology to everyone for everything, the general and his party mounted and rode back to their own lines.

The onset of the artillery bombardment found J. H. W. Stuckenberg still over spectating on the east end of the Union lines, and he hurried back to the First Division Hospital to be ready to assist as he was needed. Struggling through the falling shells and mass mayhem of the rear areas, the chaplain of the 145th Pennsylvania arrived at the location of the hospital. Now the area lay deserted, and the medical facility had left no forwarding address. "My horse had been sent back, as our hospital was again being moved, for fear it would again be exposed, and for hours I searched ineffectually for them. I was faint and sick. The heat was almost insufferable. I walked till I gave out, put wet leaves in my hat and rested—walked on again, obtained somc coffee and a cracker from H. Hays of our regiment, started for our hospital again, which was about two miles further back than it had been."[73]

Stuckenberg finally picked up the trail of the retreating hospital by stumbling across the trail of wounded men leading from the former hospital site. With ambulances at a premium during the enforced withdrawal, any wounded capable of walking were given directions and sent off to the new hospital site. Even with the best intentions, some of these patients lacked the strength, whether from loss of blood or shock, to make it the entire way. The chaplain would stop as he passed these physically and emotionally exhausted men, rendering whatever aid he could. Working his way from patient to patient, Stuckenberg finally managed to trace his way to the new location of the Second Corps Hospital by Rock Creek.

72. Tucker, *Hancock the Superb*, p. 153.

73. Stuckenberg, *I'm Surrounded by Methodists*, p. 80. Pvt. Harrison H. Hays was left behind ill at Gettysburg when the regiment left in pursuit of the Confederates, and died on September 15, 1863. [*Service Records*, National Archives and Records Administration.]

The sheer weight of shot and shell being thrown by Southern artillery was steadily exacting its toll on the Second Corps guns and gunners. "Half past two o'clock, an hour and a half since the commencement, and still the cannonade did not in the least abate; but soon thereafter some signs of weariness, and a little slackening of fire began to be apparent upon both sides. First we saw [Lt. T. Fred] Brown's [1st Rhode Island Light] Battery [B] retire from the line, too feeble for further battle. Its position was a little to the front of the line. Its commander was wounded, and many of its men were so, or worse,—some of its guns had been disabled,—many of its horses killed—its ammunition was nearly expended. Other Batteries in similar case, had been withdrawn before, to be replaced by fresh ones, and some were withdrawn afterwards."[74]

After sitting out on the forward slope of Cemetery Ridge for some time and engaging in a pleasant discussion on God's providential protection, General Gibbon and aide Frank Haskell started back uphill to the Union line. "Soon after the Battery named had gone, the General and I started to return, passing toward the left of the [Second] Division, and crossing the ground where the guns had stood. The stricken horses were numerous, and the dead and wounded men lay about, and as we passed these latter, their low piteous call for water would invariably come to us, if they had yet any voice left. I found canteens of water near,—no difficult matter where a battle has been—and held them to livid lips, and even in the faintness of death, the eagerness to drink told of their terrible torture of thirst."[75]

"Our Infantry was still unshaken, and in all the cannonade suffered very little.—The Batteries had been handled much more severely. I am unable to give any figures. A great number of horses had been killed,—in some Batteries more than half of all. Guns had been dismounted,—a great many caissons, limbers, and carriages had been destroyed,—and usually from ten to twenty-five men to each Battery had been struck, at least along our part of the crest. All together the fire of the enemy had injured us much, both in the modes I have stated, and also by exhausting our ammunition, and fouling our guns, so as to render our Batteries unfit for further immediate use. The scenes that met our eyes on all hands among the Batteries were fearful."[76]

---

74. Byrne and Weaver, *Haskell of Gettysburg*, p. 155.
75. *Ibid.*
76. *Ibid.*, pp. 155-56.

Huddled in the rude log barn against the force of the incoming shells, Capt. Benjamin Thompson and his company clerk got a front row seat to the devastation being done to the artillery and the troops that supported them. "Here we saw something of what it meant to serve the cannons with ammunition. A four or six horse team would come down the hill on a keen run—perhaps one horse would be hit, perhaps two. They would cut them out and dash on. Sometimes they lost a driver and the horses would careen wildly over the field until caught. Just near where we were a team was reduced to one mule, and General Meade, who happened to be passing, dismounted three of his staff and their horses were at once hitched up and helped to take the load of ammunition up the hill."[77]

With very little commanding possible or necessary during the crash and smash of shelling, the Second Corps general staff and their neighboring commanders were enduring the Confederate pounding as best suited their individual personalities. Hancock, still uneasily on the prowl, was riding back up to the Union lines from Meade's shelled-out headquarters. Brig. Gen. William Harrow, commander of the First Brigade, Second Division, was probably the officer one observer mistakenly took to be Gibbon, who "with folded arms and in cool dignity walked up and down in front of the line, apparently indifferent to the rain of shot and shell." Brig. Gen. Alexander S. Webb, head of the Third Brigade, Second Division for only five days, passed the time wreathed in a cloud of cigar smoke as he leaned on his sword, working hard on making a good impression on his new command.[78]

On the other hand, Brig. Gen. Alexander Hays, the six foot tall, sandy-haired commander of the Third Division, affected a fiery bravado in leading his volunteer troops. "Most of the time he was

77. Thompson, *Personal Narrative*, pp. 43-44.

78. Stewart, *Pickett's Charge*, pp. 142-43. "My men did not know me. It was necessary to establish myself," wrote Webb to his wife a few weeks after the battle. "They were to be made to feel that I ordered no men to go where I would not go myself." [Wiley Sword, "Facing the Gray Wave: Alexander Webb at Gettysburg," *Civil War Times Illustrated*, vol. 19, no. 9 (January 1981): 21]

riding up and down the lines in front of us," remembered one soldier, "exhorting the 'boys' to stand fast and fight like men." Always looking for opportunities to focus his men on useful activity, the West Pointer rode by during the height of the bombardment, admonishing his men to gather up all the abandoned rifles and muskets, clean, and load them. Some of the most dedicated troops had four extra weapons ready for use in a short time, many had at least two.[79]

Maj. Gen. Abner Doubleday of the First Corps, whose men had been wedged into an opening in the line of the Second Corps, was grabbing a quick bite to eat. The general was enjoying a sandwich when a shell exploded nearby, spraying him and his lunch with a shower of dirt and gravel. Doubleday glumly surveyed the remnants of his ruined snack for a moment, then quipped: "That sandwich will need no pepper."[80]

Over on Cemetery Hill, Maj. Gen. Oliver O. Howard of the Eleventh Corps had taken up position downhill from one of the batteries. Protected from flying debris from the rear by a stack of cracker boxes, Howard sat in full view of Confederate fire and calmly wrote out a note to Meade on the accuracy of the Rebel bombardment.[81]

Army of the Potomac Chief of Artillery Henry J. Hunt was riding the line of Northern guns, checking the progress of the Union counterfire and the comportment of the individual batteries. "Our fire was deliberate, but on inspecting the chests I found that the ammunition was running low, and hastened to General Meade to advise its immediate cessation and preparation for the assault which would certainly follow."[82]

Like others this traumatic afternoon, Hunt just couldn't seem to find the right person in the right place. "The headquarters building, immediately behind the ridge, had been abandoned, and many of the horses of the staff lay dead. Being told that the general had gone to the

79. W. Scott, "Pickett's Charge as Seen from the Front Line," MOLLUS, California, *War Papers #1;* George T. Fleming, *Life and Letters of Alexander Hays* (Pittsburgh: n.p., 1919), pp. 424, 436; David Shields to John B. Bachelder, August 27, 1884, Bachelder Papers.

80. Stewart, *Pickett's Charge*, pp. 142-43.

81. *Ibid.*, pp. 143-44.

82. Hunt, "The Third Day at Gettysburg," p. 374.

cemetery, I proceeded thither. He was not there, and on telling General Howard my object, he concurred in its propriety, and I rode back along the ridge, ordering the fire to cease."[83]

Riding from north to south along the artillery line, Hunt countermanded Hancock's orders to return fire, and one by one the batteries began to fall silent. On the other hand, Capt. John G. Hazard, commanding the Second Corps artillery, reported that Hancock's guns ceased fire, not because of any order, but simply because they had run out of long-range ammunition.[84]

Hunt found the Union batteries severely mauled, some even incapable of continuing to hold the line. Lt. Alonzo H. Cushing's Battery A of the 4th United States Artillery had a number of ammunition chests exploded, and while three guns remained serviceable, enough uninjured or slightly injured gunners remained to man only two. Cushing himself was horribly wounded in the thighs and genitals, but retained command despite the excruciating pain. The remains of Lt. T. Fred Brown's Battery B of the 1st Rhode Island were just south of the clump of trees. All of its officers were killed or wounded, barely enough men remained to work the remaining three guns, and its ammunition was, most probably, nearly exhausted. There was nothing to do but withdraw it from the line, which, with no officers to oversee it, it did in a piecemeal and posthaste manner.[85]

Hunt rushed off an order for replacement batteries to fill the holes in the line, but the Southern shelling had driven them even further to the rear, and it was going to take time to get them up. The artillery commander finally headed off for the Taneytown Road in person to find them and urge them forward.[86]

As the Union gunners ceased firing, there was a gradual slackening of fire from the Confederate lines. What began with a crash gradually

83. *Ibid.*

84. Stewart, *Pickett's Charge*, p. 156.

85. *Ibid.*, p. 157; Hunt, "The Third Day at Gettysburg," pp. 374-75. Brown's battery had seen severe action on July 2, using all its canister to repel the late afternoon assault. After firing off its long range ammunition in response to the July 3 Confederate shelling, there was nothing left in the chests to fire. [Hancock, *Reminiscences of Winfield Scott Hancock*, p. 208.]

86. Stewart, *Pickett's Charge*, p. 157; Hunt, "The Third Day at Gettysburg," pp. 374-75.

faded away until the last solitary shots soared overhead. "At three o'clock almost precisely the last shot hummed, and bounded, and fell, and the cannonade was over," noted Frank Haskell. He and Gibbon were walking along the Second Division lines, mildly disagreeing over whether there would be an infantry assault. Hancock, always a man devoted to precision, noted that the cannonade had lasted "an hour and forty-five minutes."[87]

Again silence fell over the battlefield, not so much an absence of noise as a palpable presence in itself. One observer called it "a singularly depressing silence." Spontaneously, the whole length of the Union line arose to their feet, and engaged in the greatest mass stretching and scratching scene ever witnessed. The great quantity of smoke generated by the cannon fire was slowing drifting away, leaving a steadily clearing view of the now silent Confederate guns along Seminary Ridge.[88]

The officers rose to their feet also, but with the goal of getting the disorganized battle lines back in shape. "All the officers on our lines, from generals down, set themselves to work repairing the damage caused by the cannonade," wrote one soldier of the post-bombardment activity; "reforming ranks, replacing dismantled guns, rectifying positions, exhorting the men to stand firm, and, in short, themselves offering the best examples of coolness and soldierly conduct."[89]

And then there was excitable General Hays of the Third Division. Hays seemed to be running on pure adrenaline. Instead of acting with the staid dignity and comportment of the average brigadier general as he reformed his troops, he was busy rushing back and forth through his men like an excited schoolboy, calling out, "Now, boys, look out; you will see some fun."[90]

Throughout the Second Corps, there was a general shifting and tightening up of ranks. Hays was arranging and intermixing his Third Division in unorthodox ways, stacking his men four deep in places, and beefing up the fire power. While Generals Hall and Harrow of Gibbon's

---

87. Byrne and Weaver, *Haskell of Gettysburg*, p. 156; *OR*, vol. 27, pt. 1, p. 373.
88. T. W. Osborn, "The Artillery at Gettysburg," *Philadelphia Weekly Times*, May 31, 1879; Anonymous, "The Great Battlefield Forty-Five Years Ago," *Gettysburg Scrapbook*, Gettysburg National Military Park.
89. T. A. Aldrich, *History of Battery A, First Regiment, Rhode Island Light Artillery in the War to Preserve the Union, 1861-1865* (Providence, Rhode Island: Snow and Farnham, 1904), pp. 211-12.
90. Scott, "Pickett's Charge as Seen from the Front Line."

Division moved very little, General Webb's Second Brigade sidestepped to fill the hole around Alonzo Cushing's decimated battery.[91]

Webb was facing an extremely difficult piece of terrain to defend. The Union line along the low ridge suddenly took a right-hand turn, following the helter-skelter meanderings of a low stone wall, veering 155 feet west toward the Emmitsburg Road before continuing south again. The 69th Pennsylvania was in line south of the zigzag along the front section of the wall, extending in front of an innocuous stand of trees, the only regiment along that part of the Union line. The area from the angle in the wall to the right of the 69th was the field of fire for Cushing's mutilated battery. No matter how Webb rearranged his troops, there simply were not enough men to adequately defend this portion of the line. To make matters worse, the rocky soil and lack of tools frustrated any efforts of the men to throw up very much in the way of fortifications along the unimposing line.

Guns were also on the move. Lt. George A. Woodruff's Battery I of the 1st United States Artillery rolled two pieces right into the infantry line, while four others continued to hold the high ground. Lieutenant Cushing reported to General Webb, one hand pressed between his legs in an attempt to stem the flow of blood and case the pain. Instead of asking to be allowed to go to the rear to seek medical aid, he calmly requested permission to move his guns into the infantry line as Woodruff had done, placing them between the 71st and the 69th Pennsylvania. With only enough cannoneers left to service two of the guns, Cushing asked that infantrymen be detailed to move and fire the third piece one last time when the anticipated charge was at point blank range. Webb, himself a former artilleryman, quietly granted the request of his gravely wounded gunner, ordering a detachment of fifty men from the 71st Pennsylvania to service Cushing's last gun.[92]

With the cessation of the shelling came renewed activity behind the lines. Elisha Hunt Rhodes and his Rhode Island compatriots crept out from the rocks and trees along the Taneytown Road and quickly did a

---

91. Stewart, *Pickett's Charge*, pp. 165-66.
92. *Ibid.*, p. 167; *OR*, vol. 27, pt. 1, p. 428; Samuel Roberts, "The 72nd Pennsylvania," *National Tribune*, September 1, 1887.

head count. "About 30 men of our Brigade were killed or wounded by this fire." The road once again became a thoroughfare as traffic and troops started moving in both directions.[93]

The aid stations along the Taneytown Road had weathered the storm of shot and shell, although much the worse for wear. Surgeon Francis Wafer of the 108th New York Infantry surveyed the damage to his facility at the Peter Frey House: "The outbuildings, fences and fruit trees were completely torn to pieces. The roof of the house was torn up & the stone wall broken in one place & the stones thrown upon the floor." The heavy stone construction of the building undoubtedly shielded the medical men and their patients from further injury.[94]

Wounded were quickly gravitating to the shelter of the abandoned corps headquarters at the Leister Farm. If possible, this property had sustained even worse damage than the neighboring Frey buildings. The widow herself related: "I owed a little on my land yit [*sic*], and thought I'd put in two lots of wheat that year, and it was all trampled down, and I didn't get nothing from it. . . . The fences was all tore down, so that there wasn't one standing, and the rails was burnt up. One shell came into the house and knocked a bedstead all to pieces for me. . . . The porch was all knocked down. There was seventeen dead horses on my land. They burnt five of 'em around my best peach tree and killed it; so I ha'n't no peaches this year. They broke down all my young apple trees for me. The dead horses sp'iled my spring, so I had to have my well dug."[95]

It had been a tedious time of waiting for Captain Thompson and his clerk in the old log barn. "As we lay there we suffered very much with the thirst which comes to wounded men, so I took my clerk's canteen and went to a run for water. Here I washed my head and picked bits of stone from my face and decided that my injury was slight, so

---

93. Elijah Hunt Rhodes, *All for the Union*, p. 108.

94. Wafer diary, p. 47.

95. Leister Farm Vertical File, Gettysburg National Military Park. In addition, "I had seven pieces of meat yit [*sic*], and them was all took. All I had when I got back was jest [*sic*] a little flour yit [*sic*]." As a testimony to her incredable industriousness and tenacity, the Widow Leister repaired the house and outbuildings, restoring cash crop farming on the land, and picked up a bit more acreage before she died. Ironically, the only recompense she ever received from the government was payment for the bones of the dead horses, which the United States government bought for fertilizer. [Jack McLaughlin, *Gettysburg: The Long Encampment* (New York: Bonanza Books, 1963), p. 238.]

determined to get back to my regiment as soon as possible." After taking the canteen back to his clerk, Thompson trudged back toward the crest of Cemetery Ridge.[96]

Baltimore, Maryland

Philadelphia Ladies Aid Society Secretary Harris was on her way to the battlefield, unaware of the vast number of men falling wounded even as she stepped off the train in Maryland. "Reached Baltimore at half past one, p.m.; heard conflicting rumors. The atmosphere seems to be loaded with sighs. Wounded are coming in; can only tell that a bloody battle is in progress, and that the 'tide seems to turn in our favor.' Most torturing uncertainty rests upon us."[97]

The fifty-one-year-old volunteer nurse remained undaunted in her decision to take supplies to the battlefield. "I am advised that it is unsafe to venture to the scene of conflict, but must go; the Lord will carry me there safely, if there is work for me. I leave this at five, p.m., carrying some chloroform and a few stimulants. I regret now that I did not bring more without permission. The gentlemen employed here seem to realize the necessity of forwarding such stores at once; but they are not on hand."[98]

Ticket in hand, with her meager collection of medical supplies gathered around her, Ellen Orbison Harris settled back to wait for the five o'clock train.

Gettysburg, Pennsylvania

General Gibbon, accompanied by Lieutenant Haskell, had been surveying the final preparations of their men, still disagreeing over what the Confederates were up to. "We walked slowly along in rear of the troops, by the ridge now cut off from a view of the enemy, or his position, and were returning to the spot where we had left our horses. Gnl Gibbon had just said that he inclined to the belief that the enemy was falling back and that the cannonade was only one of his noisy modes of covering the movement. I said that I thought that fifteen

---

96. Thompson, *Personal Narrative*, p. 44.
97. *Report of the Ladies Aid Society*, p. 12.
98. *Ibid.*
99. Byrne and Weaver, *Haskell of Gettysburg*, p. 157.

minutes would show that, by all his bowling, the Rebel did not mean to retreat."[99]

"We were near our horses when we noticed Brigadier General [Henry J.] Hunt, Chief of Artillery of the Army, near Woodruff[']s Battery, swiftly moving about on horseback, and apparently in a rapid manner giving some orders about the guns. Thought we, what could this mean! In a moment afterwards we met Capt [Francis] Wessels, and the orderlies who had our horses, — they were on foot leading the horses. — Capt Wessels was pale, and he said, excited: 'General, they say the enemy's Infantry is advancing.'"[79]

100. *Ibid.*

Chapter 6

FRIDAY, JULY 3: CONFEDERATE CHARGE

"The muttered thunder of a storm of growls"

Lt. Frank Aretas Haskell

"Our artillery has now ceased to roar and the enemy have checked their fury, too. The time appointed for our charge is come," somberly wrote Confederate Lt. John Dooley on July 3. "I tell you, there is no romance in making one of these charges. You might think so from reading 'Charlie O'Mally,' that prodigy of valor, or in reading of any other gallant knight who would as little think of riding over *gunners and sich like* as they would of eating a dozen oysters. But when you rise to your feet as we did today, I tell you the enthusiasm of ardent breasts in many cases *ain't there*, and instead of burning to avenge the insults of our country, families and altars and firesides, the thought is most frequently, Oh, if I could just come out of this charge safely how thankful *would I be!*"[1]

Dooley, scion of the prominent Dooley clan of Richmond, was the third member of his immediate family to fill the ranks of the Old First Virginia Infantry Regiment. John had enlisted in a company commanded by his father, serving there with his brother. Over time, he had risen to the command of Company C, "The Montgomery Guards." It was this, the most ancient of all American regiments, that was now called upon to prepare for the charge.[2]

---

1. John Dooley, *John Dooley, Confederate Soldier: His War Journal*, ed. Joseph T. Durkin (South Bend, Indiana: University of Notre Dame Press, 1963), pp. 104-5.
2. *Ibid.*, pp. x-xi, xiv-xvi.

"We rise to our feet, but not all. There is a line of men still on the ground with their faces turned, men affected in 4 different ways. There are the gallant dead who will never charge again; the helpless wounded, many of whom desire to share the fortunes of this charge; the men who have charged on many battlefields but who are helpless from the heat of the sun; and the men in whom there is not sufficient courage to enable them to rise,—but of these last there are but few. Up, brave men! Some are actually *fainting* from the heat and dread. They have fallen to the ground overpowered by the suffocating heat and the terrors of that hour."[3]

The grey- and butternut-clad soldiers stepped out of the trees behind the artillery positions and dressed ranks. Final details were attended along the line: one captain led his troops in a hymn, elsewhere a white-haired chaplain offered up prayers for the men. Maj. Gen. George E. Pickett, from the front of the division, made "a brief, animated address," ending with instructions to "charge the enemy, and remember old Virginia!" At least one man at the far end of the long line, a quarter mile away, heard not a single word of Pickett's fiery exhortations.[4]

With the speeches and admonitions, prayers and hymns now all at an end, the command finally rang out: "Forward! Guide Center! March!" Nearly fifteen minutes had passed since the cannonade had ended, and between 10,500 and 12,500 Confederate troops stepped out against the distant fortified heights. "Advance slowly, with arms at will," were the instructions; "no cheering, no firing, no breaking from common to quick step. Dress on the center."[5]

Jacob H. Cole of the 57th New York Volunteers, wounded and stranded behind enemy lines, had grown accustomed to the roar of the nearby Confederate artillery. When it finally ceased, "for a time the stillness was oppressive. Then I suddenly saw what it all meant. Over

3. *Ibid.*, p. 105.
4. H. T. Owen, "Pickett at Gettysburg," *Philadelphia Weekly Times*, May 31, 1879; Stewart, *Pickett's Charge*, p. 170.
5. John H. Lewis, *Recollections from 1860 to 1865: With Incidents of Camp Life, Descriptions of Battles, the Life of the Southern Soldier, His Hardships and Sufferings, and the Life of a Prisoner of War in the Northern Prisons* (Washington, D.C.: Peake and Co., 1895), p. 78; Stewart, *Pickett's Charge*, pp. 172-73, 178, 170. Estimates of Confederate strength vary—possibly as many as 12,000 to 13,000 troops were involved.

the hill came a long line of skirmishers and behind them a line of battle, and behind that line another and then another. I raised on my left elbow and watch eagerly the long lines of the enemy's infantry as they emerged from the woods on Seminary Ridge. It presented one of the finest sights ever witnessed on a field of battle or anywhere else. Its front was nearly a mile in length. With their rifles carried at a right shoulder shift, they moved steadily onward as if on a grand review, marched across the fields, on . . . towards Cemetery Ridge."[6]

On that distant ridge, only about 7,000 infantry were waiting to receive that charge. The wait was an anxious one. At first, the advancing Rebels could not be seen clearly in some places due to inequalities in the gently rolling fields between the two opposing armies.[7]

The men on the picket line were the first to feel the effect of the still-distant Southern advance. "A sharp musketry fire started, beginning on our skirmish line in front," wrote Lieutenant Galwey of the 8th Ohio, still holding down that advanced line. "We sprang to our feet. Just to our left, on the south side of the road, was a poor little farm house. We saw the sharpshooters who had been there all the morning aiming off towards our left front."[8]

This portion of the skirmish line was under the command of Lt. Col. Franklin Sawyer of the 8th Ohio. Sawyer had been instructed on July 2 by his superior, Col. Samuel S. Carroll, to hold the line his skirmishers now occupied; the brigade commander had promised that the rest of the brigade would support the 8th in its advanced position. When Sawyer sent back intelligence reports to his commander, he learned that Carroll had rushed off that evening to help defend Culp's Hill with most of his command. In his absence, Carroll's superior, Brig. Gen. Alexander Hays, sent word back to Sawyer that no reinforcements would be sent to him, and reaffirmed Carroll's instructions to hold on at all costs. Bound by those orders, Sawyer was about to use his 8th Ohio men in a very un-skirmish-line manner.[9]

6. Cole, *Under Five Commanders*, p. 205.
7. Stewart, *Pickett's Charge*, pp. 173-74. Estimates of Union troop strength also vary—some number the defenders as low as 5,750.
8. Galwey, *The Valiant Hours*, p. 114.
9. OR, vol. 27, pt. 1, pp. 456-57; Martin Graham, "A Gallant Defense," *Civil War Times Illustrated*, vol. 25, no. 3 (May 1986): 15-16.

"A staff captain rode down to our regiment with orders to advance. We stepped out of the ditch and moved up on the roadside bank. For a minute we saw nothing but the smoke of our skirmishers in front. Then came a distant murmur from the front, followed by a renewal of our artillery fire, which had slackened for a few minutes. All at once the murmur increased into a prolonged yell, and we saw the enemy with colors flying advancing in columns in mass, to the left of where the [Bliss] barn had been burnt in the morning."[10]

The thin line of skirmishers, drawn out in single rank to make them appear more numerous than they were, and positioned in the shelter of the bank, could do nothing more than grimly wait to single-handedly face off against the oncoming Confederate juggernaut.

Now the troops along Cemetery Ridge could clearly see the enemy. "None on that crest now need be told that *the enemy is advancing.* Every eye could see his legions, an overwhelming, resistless tide of an ocean of armed men, sweeping upon us! . . . More than half a mile their front extends;—more than a thousand yards the dull gray masses deploy, man touching man, rank pressing rank, and line supporting line. Their red flags wave; their horsemen gallop up and down. . . . Right on they move, as with one soul, in perfect order . . . magnificent, grim, irresistible."[11]

"Oh! What a splendid sight," exuded Lt. George Yost of the 126th New York. "You can't imagine how beautiful it looked to see them stretching away across the field in three columns in good line and banners flying." One of his fellow lieutenants, Richard Bassett, thought it was "the grandest sight I ever saw."[12]

General Hancock, riding along the line of the Second Corps, smiled when he spotted the advancing line of Confederates. Turning in his saddle to address his staff, he said: "Gentlemen, that is meant for us."[13]

"All was orderly and still upon our crest,—no noise, and no confusion. The men had little need of commands, for the survivors of a

10. Galwey, *The Valiant Hours*, pp. 114-15.
11. Byrne and Weaver, *Haskell of Gettysburg*, p. 158.
12. George Yost, letter to his father, July 4, 1863, copy in the 126th Vertical File, Gettysburg National Military Park; Willson, *Disaster, Struggle, Triumph*, p. 186.
13. Francis Walker, *National Tribune*, November 28, 1886.

dozen battles knew well enough what this array in front portended; and already in their places, they would be prepared to act when the right time should come. The click of the locks as each man raised the hammer, to feel with his finger that the cap was on the nipple; the sharp jar as the musket touched a stone upon the wall when thrust, in aiming, over it; the clinking of the iron axles, as the guns were rolled up by hand a little further to the front, were quite all the sounds that could be heard. Cap-boxes were slid around to the front of the body;—cartridge-boxes opened;—officers opened their pistol holsters. Such preparation, little more, was needed."[14]

On marched the Southern line, working to keep its alignment as it advanced over the uneven Pennsylvania farmland. "Onward—steady—dress to the right—give way to the left—steady, not too fast—don't press upon the center—how gentle the slope! steady—keep well in line—there is the line of guns we must take—right in front—but how far they appear!" The comments and commands were all that was heard as they came; no yelling now, plenty of time for that later.[15]

"Nearly one third of a mile, off on Cemetery Ridge, and the line stretches round in almost a semicircle. Upon the center of this we must march. Behind the guns are strong lines of infantry. You may see them plainly and now they see us perhaps more plainly."[16]

Brig. Gen. Alexander Webb of Gibbon's Second Brigade was getting more frantic with each approaching step of the Southerners. With the limbering up of Lt. T. Fred Brown's 1st Rhode Island Battery B, Webb was short on firepower and faced a gaping hole in his line. Seeing Capt. Andrew Cowan's unposted 1st New York Independent Battery sitting idle near the Taneytown Road, Webb rushed Assistant Adjutant General Charles H. Banes to Cowan, urging, cajoling, pleading with him to plug the gap in the line. The young captain, under General Doubleday's command, hesitated momentarily, but seeing

14. Byrne and Weaver, *Haskell of Gettysburg*, pp. 158-59.
15. Dooley, *John Dooley*, p. 105.
16. *Ibid.*

Webb frantically waving his hat on the crest of the ridge, Cowan acquiesced. "Limber to the right, forward!" was shouted, and the battery raced off.[17]

Cowan ordered the drivers to lash their horses up to full gallop, even though they only had about three hundred yards to go. The speed of the teams was so great that the first gun overshot the position they were supposed to occupy, dropping trail just south of Cushing's battery, the others setting up battery a little to the rear of the position formerly occupied by Brown's guns.[18]

Captain Cowan could now clearly see the reason for Webb's agitation, and started shouting out distances and fuse settings while his battery was still unlimbering. After a quick ride along his guns to check the readiness of his pieces, Cowan barked out the order to fire.[19]

The area surrounding the remains of Alonzo Cushing's Battery A, 4th United States Artillery was a wasteland of death and destruction. Three batteries had been almost totally destroyed here around this clump of trees. Fragments of exploded ammunition chests, limbers with smashed wheels, dismounted guns and gun carriages with broken axles littered the ground. Intertwined with the flotsam of war were the shredded carcasses of artillery horses and horribly disfigured gunners, living and dead. With the bulk of the ambulances occupied in moving the division hospitals further to the rear, evacuation of the wounded artillerymen was going at a snail's pace, and accomplished largely by stretcher or improvised methods. Most of the wounded would still be on the line when the Southern charge arrived.[20]

Cushing's remaining gunners were working around two of the guns, cleaning and loading the dwindling ammunition. Men from the 71st Pennsylvania hurried to get the other gun ready for one last discharge. With ammunition running low, anything that would fit down the muzzle was stuffed in against the double charge of canister, including pieces of exploded shells, small stones, minie balls, and unused bayonets.[21]

While the massed Southern bombardment had ceased, a covering artillery fire continued to loft over the advancing Confederate columns

---

17. Andrew Cowan, letters of July 2, December 5, and December 10, 1913, Gettysburg National Military Park; *OR*, vol. 27, pt. 1, p. 690.
18. Cowan, letters of July 2, December 5, and December 10, 1913.
19. *Ibid.*
20. Hancock, *Reminiscences of Winfield Scott Hancock*, p. 218.
21. *Ibid.*; Gary G. Lash, "The Philadelphia Brigade at Gettysburg," *The Gettysburg Magazine*, no. 7 (July 1992): 104.

toward the Union lines. Batteries from the heights of Little Round Top to the ravaged grounds of Evergreen Cemetery started long range shelling of the oncoming line; the bulk of the Second Corps guns, however, stood silent and waiting. Nothing was left in the ammunition chests but canister, and that demanded a closeup target. Lt. Tully McCrea of George A. Woodruff's Battery I, 1st United States Artillery, was watching the advancing Rebels from the meager shade in Ziegler's Grove. "We, with the smooth bores, loaded with canister and bided our time," he wrote.[22] There would be plenty of opportunities all too soon.

The Confederates were beginning to take losses as the Union guns acquired the range of the moving line. "To the right of us and above the guns we are to capture, black heavy monsters from their lofty mountain sides belch forth their flame and smoke and storms of shot and shell upon our advancing line; while directly in front, breathing flame in our very faces, the long range of guns which must be taken thunder on our quivering melting ranks. Now truly does the work of death begin. The line becomes unsteady because at every step a gap must be closed and thus from left to right much ground is often lost."[23]

The men on the skirmish line were getting a first-hand view of the effectiveness of the Union gunners on the advancing men. "Our artillery fire that now opened upon the advancing Confederates was such as nothing but the heroic could endure. Before the lines moving against *us* were come within close range, we watched and very anxiously too, that beautiful, terrible mass coming toward our left shoulders. At its head was a mounted officer who rode like a demigod and was worthy by his courage to lead those brave men who followed. We now hear the fearful din of the artillery, the savage, threatening yells of the advancing and now seemingly invincible enemy, of the insulting taunts of the enemy's old skirmish line in our front, who had risen to their feet and were pouring a destructive fire into us. We stood all alone in that open field, waving our colors; in spite of all the threatening advance we took time to praise the valor of the

22. McCrea, *Dear Belle*, pp. 208-9.
23. Dooley, *John Dooley*, pp. 105-6.

Confederate officer who rode ahead, a conspicuous mark for sixty cannon and thousands of muskets."[24]

Brig. Gen. James Johnston Pettigrew's brigade was going to pass safely to the left of Lieutenant Galwey and the men of the 8th Ohio; however, the troops of wounded Maj. Gen. Dorsey Pender (now under the command of Maj. Gen. Isaac Trimble) were on a head-on collision course with this thin line of determined skirmishers. "A few seconds, and a cheer rises to the west of us. Now Pender's line, with colors flying, issues from the trees that cover the crest of the low ridge in our front, and comes right toward us. But from the first it was easy to see the difference between the mettle of these men and those of Pickett's glorious column. Two or three times Pender's line hesitated, whether obliged to reform, because of the irregularity of the ground, or whether owing to a disposition to give way before the effect of our artillery shells exploding right in front of them. These bursts, which occasionally hid them in smoke from us, were now actually tearing their ranks to pieces. The enemy came as far as the fence opposite us, where the Confederate skirmishers had been from the first of the battle, and here they lay down."[25]

The 8th Ohio men could not have imagined a better opportunity. This "single regiment of less than three hundred men, two hundred yards in front of the main Federal position, [in] seemingly a forlorn position" rose up and poured a devastating fire directly into the recumbent enemy immediately to their front, then, incredibly, with fixed bayonets, charged headlong toward the six brigades. This Union fire and screaming attack from where no Northerners should have been was the final straw for this part of the Rebel advance. "We so galled them with our fire that a panic soon took hold of them and they fled, back to the low ridge."[26]

Help for the Buckeye troops was rushing south along the Emmitsburg Road in the person of Capt. Samuel Chapman Armstrong and his 125th New York Infantry skirmish-line reserve. These men also understood this chance of a lifetime, and dashed forward on the double-quick. At this point, every musket would be crucially important.[27]

---

24. Galwey, *The Valiant Hours*, pp. 115-16.
25. *Ibid.*, p. 116.
26. *Ibid.*
27. C. A. Richardson to John B. Bachelder, August 18, 1869, Bachelder Papers; S. C. Armstrong to John B. Bachelder, February 6, 1884

Seeing the impressive fire his men had laid down on Trimble's men, Sawyer now swung his little command around to face south. In a move that some observers on Cemetery Ridge considered the act of a madman or a drunkard, the lieutenant colonel of the 8th Ohio waited until the columns of Pickett's men were exactly opposite his men, at a distance of about one hundred yards, then opened fire. "Every shot was turned on Pickett. On and on came his column, the mounted officer still conspicuous at its head. From time to time the smoke of bursting shells would envelop them for a few seconds, but when the smoke lifted, the gray mass was still coming on, still compact, still orderly, ever and anon raising one of those piercing yelps which had been so terrifying for our new troops to hear."[28]

"The enemy column has now approached the turnpike [Emmitsburg Road] just to the south of us. They seem to pay no attention to us, who are a mere handful. Yet the fire which we pour into their left flank is a deadly one and tells visibly upon them." The hot musketry of the Ohioans was having the same devastating effect on Col. Robert Mayo's brigade that it had on Trimble's men a few minutes earlier, and the deadly fire from the New Yorkers of Captains Armstrong and Morris, shooting from a nearby rail fence, dropped an increasing number of Southerners in their tracks. Already staggered by the accuracy of the Union artillery fire, the unexpected bite of musketry on their flank left the brigade broken and running for cover, exposing in turn the left flank of Brig. Gen. Joseph R. Davis' Mississippi brigade.[29]

The seemingly unstoppable Confederate advance kept on coming, but now pressing increasingly toward the center, away from the galling fire on its left flank. "They are now over the turnpike and begin to ascend the rise to the stone wall. We have entirely recovered from the momentary doubt that had seized us," remembered one of the Ohioans in later years, "and, with the fresh ammunition which a short time ago was issued us, play havoc with them."[30]

With the enemy bearing down directly on his weak position by the angle in the wall, General Webb worked feverishly to fortify his line in

28. Galwey, *The Valiant Hours*, p. 117.
29. *Ibid.*; C. A. Richardson to John B. Bachelder, August 18, 1869, Bachelder Papers; S. C. Armstrong to John B. Bachelder, February 6, 1884, Bachelder Papers.
30. Galwey, *The Valiant Hours*, p. 117.

the few minutes remaining before the Confederates crashed head-on into his position. He ordered the 71st Pennsylvania forward into the corner of the front wall of the angle, to the right of the 69th Pennsylvania. When it became evident that the whole regiment would not fit in the tight spot, part of the regiment continued forward to the front wall, while two companies went back by the rear wall. Col. Richard Penn Smith encouraged the men of the two returning companies to gather up as many loaded and capped muskets as possible; each man collected "three to a dozen guns each," adding to the firepower of the little band of Pennsylvanians. Smith then went with the two companies to the rear wall, leaving orders with Lt. Col. Charles Kochersperger and the front eight companies to withhold fire until the Confederates cleared the Emmitsburg Pike. After the first volley, the men were to reload and fire as rapidly as possible, then to fall back slowly when there was no longer time to reload.[31]

Webb, probably realizing that he had rendered Cushing's artillery largely useless by moving troops into the cannons' field of fire, allowed the wounded gunner to roll his pieces forward, down the slope and into the line of infantry along the front wall. With the bulk of the 106th Pennsylvania not yet returned from detached duty with the Eleventh Corps, the youthful general could do little more than move the 72nd Pennsylvania into support position along the crest of the ridge. And then there was no more time—the Southerners were clambering over the fences bordering the Emmitsburg Pike.[32]

Maj. Gen. Winfield Scott Hancock was a very busy man this afternoon, and seemed to flourish under the intense pressure. With the

31. Robert Penn Smith, letter to Peter F. Rothermel, November 25, 1867; *OR*, vol. 27, pt. 1, pp. 428-29, 431-34; R. Penn Smith, "The Battle. The Part Taken by the Philadelphia Brigade in the Battle," *Gettysburg Compiler*, June 7, 1887; William A. McClean, "The Third Day of Gettysburg. Fight at The Bloody Angle. The Master Report," *Gettysburg Compiler*, February 3, 1891; Nicholson, *Pennsylvania at Gettysburg*, vol. 1, p. 410; James Wilson, Appendix containing testimony from the Court of Common Pleas of Adams County, In Equity. No. 1, January Term, 1889, *Survivors of the Seventy-second Regiment of Pennsylvania Volunteers, Plaintiffs vs. Gettysburg Battlefield Memorial Association, Commissioners appointed by the Governor of the State of Pennsylvania, Defendants*, testimony of Alexander S. Webb and William Stockton, pp. 170, 243.

32. Wilson, *Survivors of the Seventy-second Regiment*, Testimony of Alexander Webb, pp. 169-70; *OR*, vol. 27, pt. 1, p. 428.

wounding of General Sickles on July 2, Meade had given the additional responsibility of commanding the Third Corps to Hancock. Although Gibbon reported that Hancock resumed command of the Second Corps at about one o'clock, Hancock still operated under the impression that he commanded both Second and Third Corps. Running his part of the army from horseback, dealing with a vast array of pressing needs, posting batteries, rotating pickets, overseeing the positioning of specific regiments—Hancock was taking it all in stride as aides and couriers rode in and galloped away carrying his dispatches.[32]

The unusual tactics of the 8th Ohio, in their advanced position on the Union right, especially drew his attention, and he rode to that end of the field to personally check it out. The enemy was within firing range now, and the Confederate skirmishers saw the lathered bay mare, a major general's uniform, and the snowy white shirt-front as the rider dashed by. The men of the 3rd Virginia had Hancock in their sights when Col. Joseph Mayo shouted out: "Don't shoot him! Don't shoot him!" Chivalry still lived on in Southerner hearts, and the conspicuous valor of the Second Corps commander spared him from a fusillade of Virginia bullets.[33]

If the flanks of the advancing columns could be so damaged and deflected by a handful of skirmishers and a few squads of men on the north end of the field, could not the same thing be accomplished on the other flank? Hancock vigorously spurred his mount, heading toward the southern end of the Union line to put that idea into effect.

The commander of the Second Division could see the enemy closing on his position, and was making good use of the remaining time. "Gnl Gibbon rode down the lines, cool and calm, and in an unimpassioned voice he said to the men: 'Do not hurry, men, and fire

32. Coddington, *The Gettysburg Campaign*, pp. 481-82, 783, notes 67-69. It would prove to be an inspired mistake on Hancock's part. He did a brilliant job of marshaling the resources at hand to repulse the Confederate attack.

33. Joseph C. Mayo, "Pickett's Charge at Gettysburg," *Southern Historical Society Papers* (Richmond, Virginia: Published by the Society, 1896), vol. 34, p. 327 (hereafter cited as *SHSP*). General Hancock's incongruous supply of snowy white starched shirts was the result of the tireless efforts of his English valet, Mr. Shaw, who was reputed to spend long hours over the scrubbing board. [Glenn Tucker, "Hancock at Gettysburg," manuscript courtesy of Gettysburg National Military Park.]

too fast;—let them come up close before you fire, and then aim low, and steadily.' The coolness of the General was reflected on the faces of his men."[34]

To the north of Gibbon's position, the hyperactive General Hays employed a different technique to keep his men calm. Standing them up behind their low stone wall, he drilled the troops in the manual of arms, shouting out orders in a booming voice. That finished, he again rode up and down the lines, exhorting the soldiers to stand fast and fight like men. Pointing to Woodruff's battery in nearby Ziegler Grove, he admonished, "'Boys, don't let them touch these pieces,' and in a few minutes more he rode back again laughing, sang out, 'Hurrah, boys, we're giving them hell,' and he dashed up the brow of the hill and cheered our skirmishers."[35]

Gibbon dispatched Lt. Frank Haskell "to ride to General Meade and tell him the enemy was coming upon us in force and we should need all the help he could send us[.] I directed the guns of [Capt. William A.] Arnold's battery [A, 1st Rhode Island light Artillery] to be run forward to the wall loaded with double rounds of canister," continued Gibbon, "and then rode down my line." Haskell headed for the rear at top speed: "To gallop to Gnl Meade's Head Quarters,—to learn there that he had changed them to another part of the field,—to dispatch to him, by the Signal Corps, in Gnl Gibbon's name the message: 'The enemy is advancing his Infantry in force upon my front,'—and to be again upon the crest were but the work of a minute."[36]

Now the skirmishers directly in front of the Confederate advance "open a spattering fire along the front, and, fighting, retire upon the main line,—the first drops, the heralds of the storm, sounding on our windows." The skirmishers of Gibbon's division, mostly from the 19th Maine and the Philadelphia Brigade, put up such a dogged resistance that Brig. Gen. Richard B. Garnett's men were forced to fire, then halted to reload before continuing the advance. Some Southerners actually considered these tenacious pickets the first Union line, and took credit for "having routed the enemy" when the skirmishers retired to the main line.[37]

---

34. Byrne and Weaver, *Haskell of Gettysburg*, p. 159.
35. Fleming, *Life and Letters of Alexander Hays*, pp. 439, 442-43.
36. Gibbon, *Personal Recollections*, p. 151; Byrne and Weaver, *Haskell of Gettysburg*, pp. 160. Haskell would not get back to the line until the Confederate charge had almost arrived. [Byrne and Weaver, *Haskell of Gettysburg*, pp. 161-62.]
37. Byrne and Weaver, *Haskell of Gettysburg*, p. 160; *OR*, vol. 27, pt. 2, p. 386.

As the skirmishers retired firing, "the thunder of our guns—first Arnold's then Cushing's, and Woodruff's and the rest, shake and reverberate again through the air, and their sounding shells smite the enemy."[38]

"When they arrive within five hundred yards, we commence to fire," wrote Tully McCrea of the murderous closeup fire of Woodruff's six Napoleons, "and the slaughter was dreadful. Never was there such a splendid target for light artillery. . . . At the command 'Commence firing' everybody worked with a will and two rounds of canister per minute were delivered from each gun. The slaughter was fearful and great gaps were made in the mass of the enemy upon each discharge."[39]

The effect of the close quarter artillery fire was immediately and horrifyingly evident. The ranks of attacking Confederates "were at once enveloped in a dense cloud of smoke and dust," wrote one spellbound onlooker. "Arms, heads, blankets, guns and knapsacks were thrown into the air. Their track, as they advanced, was strewn with dead and wounded. A moan went up from the field, distinct to be heard amid the storm of battle, but on they went."[40]

Lt. Alonzo Cushing had been wounded three times, but was still at his two remaining guns. The twenty-two-year-old West Pointer was tough as nails, and determined to make every shot count. Though in agony from his wounds, he personally helped load the number four gun; with the leather thumbstall charred into uselessness, and the enemy closing on his pieces, Cushing personally stoppered the gun's vent with his bare thumb, searing it to the bone.[41]

And still the Confederates kept coming up the slope from the Emmitsburg Road, reeling and crouching in the firestorm of cannon fire and small arms projectiles, but moving steadily closer to the Union lines.

38. Byrne and Weaver, *Haskell of Gettysburg*, p. 160.

39. McCrea, *Dear Belle*, pp. 209-10.

40. Franklin Sawyer, *A Military History of the 8th Regiment, Ohio Volunteer Infantry* (Cleveland, Ohio: Fairbanks and Co., 1881), p. 131.

41. Theron Wilber Haight, *Three Wisconsin Cushings: A Sketch of the Lives of Howard B., Alonzo H., and William B. Cushing, Children of a Pioneer Family of Waukesha County* (Madison, Wisconsin: Wisconsin History Commission, 1910), p. 57.

Now the repeated command in the Southern ranks is "Close up! Close up! CLOSE UP!" as swarming canister shot tore huge gaps in the line. "Close up! Close up the ranks when a friend falls, while his life blood bespatters your cheek or throws a film over your eyes!," wrote Virginian John Dooley of that appalling advance. "Dress to left or right, while the bravest of the brave are sinking to rise no more! Still onward! Capt [James] Hallinan has fallen and I take his place. So many men have fallen now that I find myself within a few feet of my old Captain (Norton). His men are pressing mine out of place. I ask him to give way a little to the left, and scarcely has he done so than he leaps in the air, falling prostrate. Still we press on—oh, how long it seems before we reach those blazing guns."[42]

These were seasoned campaigners along the crest of Cemetery Ridge, who knew from experience the value of holding fire until the enemy was in deadly range. While a few isolated units loosed off scattered volleys at a long range of six hundred to seven hundred and fifty yards, the majority of the regiments remained quiet. Now with the Rebel lines approaching a point-blank range of three hundred to four hundred feet, the Union infantry ripped out a devastating opening fire that thundered north along the Yankee line.[43]

"First [Brig. Gen. William] Harrow's breastworks flame,—then [Col. Norman J.] Hall's,—then Webb's. As if our bullets were the fire-coals that touched off their muskets, the enemy in front halts, and his countless level barrels blaze back at us.—The 2nd Division is struggling in battle;—the rattling storm soon spreads to the right, and the blue trefoils are vieing [*sic*] with the white. All along each hostile front, a thousand yards, with the narrowest space between, the vollies [*sic*] blaze and roll; as thick the sound as when a summer hailstorm pelts the city roofs; as thick the fire as when the incessant lightning fringes a summer cloud."[44]

---

42. Dooley, *John Dooley*, p. 106.
43. George J. Stannard diary, July 3, 1863 entry, typescript in the Bachelder Papers; *OR*, vol. 27, pt. 1, pp. 373, 439, 445, 454.
44. Byrne and Weaver, *Haskell of Gettysburg*, p. 161. "Blue trefoils vieing with the white" refers to the colors of the Second and Third Division flags. Although the symbol of the Second Corps was the trefoil, or three leaf clover, the division flags were colored red (First), white (Second), and blue (Third) for quick identification on the battlefield.

The massed volley of Northern lead brought down nearly half of the Confederate flags, and the neat formations began to deteriorate into tattered fragments of lines and groups of individuals. Still they pressed on toward those tantalizing guns at the clump of trees, now shrouded by the drifting clouds of cannon and musket smoke.

"Our men are falling faster now, for the deadly musket is at work. Volley after volley of crashing musket balls sweeps through the line and mow us down like wheat before the scythe," wrote John Dooley of that final approach to the fiery Union crest. "On! men, on! Thirty more yards and the guns are ours; but who can stand such a storm of hissing lead and iron? What a relief if earth, which almost seems to hurl these implements of death in our faces, would open now and afford a secure retreat from threatening death."[45]

"Every officer is in front, Pickett with his long curls streaming in the fiery breath of the cannons' mouth. Garnett on the right, [Brig. Gen. James L.] Kemper in the center and [Brig. Gen. Lewis A.] Armistead on the left; Cols, Lieut Cols, Majors, Captains, all press on and cheer the shattered lines."[46]

Gibbon's Second Division was taking the brunt of the attack this afternoon. The Confederate right flank obliqued in prearranged movements by the left flank, bringing together the sections of the advance into one concentrated strikeforce. In so doing, General Harrow's First Brigade on Gibbon's extreme left was quickly losing targets for their musketry. To Harrow's right, Col. Norman J. Hall's Third Brigade was keeping up a brisk fire on the advancing enemy columns as they sidled to the left. The Southerners, in turn, sought to shelter themselves in the brush and rocks of a stretch of broken ground directly in front of the Union lines.

---

45. Dooley, *John Dooley*, p. 106.
46. *Ibid.* Actually, Pickett stopped in the vicinity of the Codori farmstead to watch the progress of the charge and move reinforcements in where needed. Although this was an appropriate position for a division commander in an operation of this nature, Pickett effectively put himself out touch with his advancing men by staying there.

The 20th Massachusetts were loading and firing to a war chant of their own devising, shouting at the top of their lungs: "Fredericksburg! Fredericksburg! Fredericksburg!" Capt. Henry L. Abbott of the 20th wrote exultantly of that fusillade: "The moment I saw them I knew we should give them Fredericksburg. So did every body. We let the regiment in front of us get within 100 feet of us, & then bowled them over like nine pins, picking out the colors first. In two minutes there were only groups of two or three men running around wildly, like chickens with their heads off."[47]

Further to the north, however, the Second Brigade of General Webb was in real trouble. Only three small regiments and a few companies totaling 375 men and 8 cannon were covering a front of 500 feet, and there were at least 18 enemy regiments bearing down on them. This area near the clump of trees also had that problematic right-hand zigzag in the stone wall which served as the only protection for the men, leaving the 71st Pennsylvania regiment with it's right flank hanging in midair, totally exposed to enfilade fire. To make matters worse, the gunners were ramming home the very last of the ammunition into the smoking barrels of their cannon.

To Webb's right were the men of General Hays' Third Division. The practice in manual of arms was over; now was the time for the troops to check and recheck their weapons with sweaty hands, waiting for the enemy to reach the closest possible range before firing. Suddenly, Hay's shouted out in his great booming voice: "*Fire!*" Forgetting all their orders to stay low, the men leapt to their feet and poured a lethal fire from 1700 muskets into the oncoming Rebel column.[48]

In the Southern ranks, "everything was a wild kaleidoscopic whirl." The Union fusillades of musketry and canister were cutting great bloody swathes through the attacking ranks. "Just here—from right to left the remnants of our braves pour in their long reserved fire; until now no shots had been fired, no shout of triumph had been raised; but as the cloud of smoke rises over the heads of the advancing divisions

47. *OR*, vol. 27, pt. 1, p. 445; Abbott, *Fallen Leaves*, p. 188. The 20th was taunting the Confederates with memories of the battle of Fredericksburg, in which the tables were turned; there it was Union men charging over open ground against the enemy entrenched behind a stone wall.

48. *OR*, vol. 27, pt. 1, p. 454.

the well known battle cry which marks the victory gained or nearly gained bursts wildly over the blood stained field and *all that line of guns is ours*."[49]

But it was not quite that easy. Southern troops were stacking up in front of that thin Federal line, a "mingled mass from fifteen to twenty deep," grinding to a halt a scant twenty yards short, where, virtually toe to toe, the contenders blasted away at each other. If only the longer Union line could be curled around the tightly packed Confederates, they could lay down a converging fire from three sides. Hancock had already grasped that concept and was spurring his mount south along the line; there Brig. Gen. George Jerrison Stannard and his Vermont troops were already preparing to do that very thing.[50]

Gibbon of the Second Division had come to the same conclusion. "To our left of this point was a regiment of the Division, and desirous of aiding in the desperate struggle now taking place on the hill to the right I endeavored to get this regiment to swing out to the front, by a change front forward on the right company, take the enemy's line in flank to sweep up along the front of our line. But in the noise and turmoil of the conflict it was difficult to get my orders understood." Driven to desperation by the swelling mass of Confederates bearing down on his right, "I spurred my horse in front of [the regiment] and waved forward the left flank. I was suddenly recalled to the absurd position I had assumed by the whole regiment opening fire! I got to the rear as soon as possible."[51]

If this regiment could not be moved out from the wall, maybe the next in line could be persuaded to action. "Looking to my left to see if I could find troops there likely to be induced to follow out my orders[,] I saw a command lying behind a small breastwork I had, myself, caused to be erected the day before[,] and putting spurs to my horse, I rode toward it. Just before I reached the position[,] to my amazement, the men commenced to break to the rear, though there was no fire whatever to amount to anything in their front. With some difficulty I induced the command to return to their breastwork. . . . Satisfied that I could derive

49. Dooley, *John Dooley*, pp. 106-7.
50. Owen, "Pickett at Gettysburg"; *OR*, vol. 27, pt. 1, pp. 349-50.
51. Gibbon, *Personal Recollections*, pp. 151-52.

no benefit from that command, I galloped back to my own division and again attempted to get the left of that to swing out."[52]

Gibbon had been making a conspicuous target of himself as he galloped about from regiment to regiment, in some places scant yards from the attacking troops. No mounted man could last long in those circumstances. "Whilst so engaged [in attempting to swing out the left of the 19th Maine], I felt a stinging blow behind the left shoulder." There was still much to do, so the Second Division commander kept on feverishly working to get his men to wheel to the right and open an enfilade fire; however, "I soon began to grow faint from the loss of blood which trickled from my left hand [pressed over the wound]. I directed Lt [Edward] Moale, my aide, to turn over the command of the Division to Gen Harrow[,] and in company with another staff officer, Capt Francis Wessells, 106th Penn, Division J[udge] A[dvocate], left the field, the sounds of the conflict on the hill still ringing in my ears."[53]

General Armistead, old felt hat perched on his sword like a personal battle flag, pushed his way through the mass of men stalled before the Union line. Banner-like, his black hat had been struck and run up again and again as the sharp sword pierced the fabric and the hat slid down to the hilt. Now it was again proudly perched on the tip of the weapon as he pushed forward, the battle flag of the 14th Virginia in tow, and other flags struggling to keep up.[54]

The Southerners desperately needed a leader to carry them forward over that last deadly space. General Garnett had been fatally shot from horseback while trying dress on Col. Birkett Fry and his 13th Alabama. "A moment later, . . . a shot through the thigh prostrated me," recalled Fry fifteen years later. "I was so confident of victory that to some of my men who ran up to carry me off I shouted: 'Go on; it will not last five minutes longer!' The men rushed off into the smoke, which soon became so dense that I could see little of what was going on before me."[55]

52. *Ibid.*, p. 152.
53. *Ibid.*, pp. 152-53.
54. Lewis, Recollections from 1860-1865, p. 79; Rev. James E. Poindexter, "Address on the Life and Services of Gen. Lewis A. Armistead Delivered . . . Before R. E. Lee Camp, No. 1, Confederate Veterans," Richmond, Virginia, January 29, 1909.
55. Birkett D. Fry, "Pettigrew's Charge at Gettysburg," *SHSP*, vol. 7, p. 93.

Now it was General Kemper that had fallen, gravely wounded; colonels, lieutenant-colonels, and majors were toppling in the swirling battle smoke as the firestorm of musketry and artillery continued from Cemetery Ridge. Armistead, coming to the front on the southern end of the narrow Confederate front, grasped the opportunity, and started trotting diagonally north across the front. He ended up just north of Cushing's guns, and the men, inspired by his example, pressed on.[56]

A few quick steps, taking an eternity of musket fire and canister to cover, brought Armistead to the low wall sheltering the Union troops. Turning to Lt. Col. Rawley Martin of the 53rd Virginia at his side, he shouted: "Martin! We can't stay here; we must go over the wall!" Martin jumped over the wall, crying out to his men: "Forward with the colors!" then fell with a shattered thigh. Just to the north, the Confederates already held the wall; Armistead jumped up, hat-tipped sword held high, and shouted back to the men behind him: "Come on, boys, give them the cold steel! Who will follow me?" With one large step, he was over the low stone barrier, heading toward the prize of those coveted Union guns; a mob of men, mostly Virginians, and flags followed him into that deadly zone.[57]

One by one, the Second Corps cannons fell silent as the last few rounds of canister were quickly exhausted. Now the gunners were being specially targeted as Southerners closed in on the artillery pieces.

Lieutenant Cushing, still at his post at Battery A, 4th U.S. Artillery, in agony and faint from loss of blood, asked for double canister. One gun was forced to improvise with a makeshift load of cartridges, shell fragments, rocks and a spare bayonet stuffed unceremoniously into the muzzle. Cushing, peering through field glasses, waited for a seeming eternity before ordering his pieces to fire. As they bucked in recoil, the lieutenant himself lunged violently. A bullet had caught him just below the nose, and penetrated directly to the brain. He was dead before he hit the ground. Command passed to his sergeant, Frederick

56. Dr. R. W. Martin, "Armistead at the Battle of Gettysburg," *SHSP*, vol. 39, pp. 186-87.

57. *Ibid.*

Fuger, who immediately ordered "treble canister" as the Rebel attack closed to within fifty yards of the Union lines.[58]

Similar scenes were found in each battery. Capt. James McKay Rorty, commanding the 1st New York Light, Battery B, was dead, shot through the head while helping his men replace a damaged wheel. Lieutenant Miller of Arnold's Battery A, 1st Rhode Island Artillery, was felled with a mortal wound. Lt. George A. Woodruff of Battery I, 1st U.S., was also down and dying, his life oozing out of a gaping wound as he lay sheltered behind a small tree; his command had devolved to Lt. Tully McCrea.[59]

Capt. Andrew Cowan, the late arrival from Doubleday's command, was facing an open space of wall with no infantry support whatsoever. A Confederate major, leading a small band of men, waited until the discharge of Cowan's battery before making a wild dash for the artillery. From 200 feet away they raced full tilt toward the pieces, screaming: "Take the guns! Take the guns!!" Captain Cowan calmly ordered his guns double-shotted with canister as his lieutenant went down beside him. Pvt. Jake McElroy shouted back, "Captain, this is our last round!" Cowan replied "I know it, Jake" as McElroy took three bullets in the face and dropped. Private Gates rammed the charges home, then fell, shot through both legs. The Confederates were over half way to the pieces.[60]

Artillery Chief Henry J. Hunt had ridden up to the battery; grasping the situation, and overcome by the moment, he squeezed off round after round from his service revolver while shouting at the top of his lungs: "See 'em! *See 'em!* SEE 'EM!"[61]

---

58. Frederick Fuger, *Family History* (Detroit: Privately Published, 1904); Frederick Fuger, "Cushing's Battery at Gettysburg," *Journal of Military Service Institution of the United States*, vol. 41, (November-December 1907): 408-9; W. H. Morgan, *Personal Reminiscences of the War of 1861-5* (Lynchburg, Virginia: J. P. Bell Co., 1911), p. 212; John J. Bachelder, "Notes Relating to the Services of the Troops at Gettysburg, 1863," manuscript in the Nicholson Collection, Huntington Library; *Fredonia Censor*, July 11, 1900; *Buffalo Evening News*, May 29, 1894.

59. Byrne and Weaver, *Haskell of Gettysburg*, p. 161; Hancock, *Reminiscences of Winfield Scott Hancock*, pp. 217-18; McCrea, *Dear Belle*, p. 210.

60. Andrew Cowan, letters of July 2, 1913, December 5, 1913, December 10, 1913, Gettysburg National Military Park; Anonymous, *In Memoriam Alexander Stuart Webb* (Albany, New York: 1916), sections 3 and 5; *New York at Gettysburg*, p. 82.

61. Andrew Cowan, letters of July 2, 1913, December 5, 1913, December 10, 1913, Gettysburg National Military Park; *New York at Gettysburg*, p. 82.

The Southerners were a mere ten paces away now. Gunner MacKenzie raised his hand for the signal to fire, then collapsed wounded across the trail of his gun. In falling, the signal was given; five guns roared out a shotgun blast of iron balls at point blank range. When the smoke cleared, no Confederates were left standing, only a twisted mass of dead bodies and screaming, writhing wounded.[62]

Surveying the carnage before them, the gunners heard the general's shouts for help. Prying him out from under his dead horse, they remounted him on a sergeant's mount, and saw him safely on his way. By way of thanks for a job well done, Hunt shouted back: "Look out or you will kill our men!"[63]

Looking after the receding figure of Hunt, Cowan shook his head and then got back to work. With all its canister exhausted, and most of the battery teams dead or fatally wounded, Cowan and his remaining men uncoiled the prolonges and laboriously dragged the decimated battery to the rear.[64]

Over at Cushing's battery, First Sgt. Frederick Fuger ordered the body of his commander sent to the rear while keeping up the intense canister fire over the ever-decreasing distance between the two opposing forces. "When the enemy was almost on top of us, I ceased firing and told the men to pitch in with anything they had in their hands, such as pistols, sabres, sponge-staves, and handspikes." The young German then pulled out his own service revolver, drew bead on the closest Confederates, and fired.[65]

Finally, overwhelmed by the sheer number of attackers, Cushing's last few artillerymen grudgingly headed for the rear, followed by a chorus of "stop you Yankee devils" and a shower of hot lead.[66]

---

62. Cowan, letters of July 2, 1913, December 5, 1913, December 10, 1913; *In Memoriam Alexander Stuart Webb*, sections 3 and 5.
63. Cowan, letters of July 2, 1913, December 5, 1913, December 10, 1913; *In Memoriam Alexander Stuart Webb*, sections 3 and 5.
64. Cowan, letters of July 2, 1913, December 5, 1913, December 10, 1913; *In Memoriam Alexander Stuart Webb*, sections 3 and 5.
65. Henry S. Stevens, *Souvenir of Excursion to Battlefields by the Society of the Fourteenth Connecticut Regiment and Reunion at Antietam, September 1891; with History and Reminiscences of Battles and Campaigns of the Regiment on the Fields Revisited* (Washington, D.C.: Gibson Brothers, Printers and Bookbinders, 1893), p. 36; typescript statement of Thomas Moon, June 23, 1913, Gettysburg National Military Park; Fuger, "Cushing's Battery at Gettysburg," pp. 408-9.
66. Thomas Moon statement; Fuger, "Cushing's Battery at Gettysburg," p. 409.

Still the Confederates pushed forward after Armistead, finding a gap in the Union line and fighting to wedge their way through. The 71st Pennsylvania, with its right flank hanging in midair at the right-hand angle in the wall, was unable to stand the assault and fell back toward the crest of Cemetery Ridge. To their left, the 69th Pennsylvania refused their right flank, bending back to keep their front to the enemy. The door stood open to a strong Southerner push.[67]

Virginian John Dooley was pressing toward that opportunity when a massive blow dropped him in his tracks. "Shot through both thighs, I fall about 30 yards from the guns. By my side lies Lt Kehoe, shot through the knee. Here we lie, he in excessive pain, I fearing to bleed to death, the dead and dying all around, while the division sweeps over the Yankee guns. Oh, how I long to know the result, the end of this fearful charge! We seem to have the victory in our hands; but what can our poor remnant of a shattered division do if they meet beyond the guns an obstinate resistance?"[68]

Staff aide Frank Haskell was up on the ridge again, after seeing Gibbon's message transmitted to Meade by wigwag signal, searching in vain for his general; in fact, for *any* general. Finally, "I gave up hunting as useless,—I was convinced Gnl Gibbon could not be on the field,—I left him mounted,—I could easily have found him now had he so remained,—but now, save myself[,] there was not a mounted officer near the engaged lines,—and [I] was riding towards the right of the 2nd [Gibbon's] Division with purpose to stop there, as the most eligible position to watch the further progress of the battle, there to be ready to take part, according to my own notions, whenever and wherever occasion was presented."[69]

"The conflict was tremendous, but I had seen no wavering in all our line. Wondering how long the Rebel ranks, deep though they were,

67. Philadelphia Times, May 28, 1887; Charles H. Bane to Alexander S. Webb, August 9, 1887, Alexander S. Webb Collection, Yale University Library; A. W. McDermott to John B. Bachelder, October 21, 1889, Bachelder Papers; Richard Penn Smith to Peter F. Rothermel, November 25, 1867, Peter F. Rothermel Collection, Pennsylvania Division of Public Records; *OR*, vol. 27, pt. 1, pp. 428, 439-40.

68. Dooley, *John Dooley*, p. 107. Southern Irishman John Dooley fell before the guns of Northern Irishman James McKay Rorty, captain of the 1st New York Light Artillery, Battery B. It was that kind of war.

69. Byrne and Weaver, *Haskell of Gettysburg*, pp. 161-62.

could stand our sheltered vollies, I had come near my destination." Gazing at the action playing out directly ahead of him, Haskell spotted the 71st Pennsylvania as it began to fall back under the weight of the Confederate push. The enemy was now within feet of their line, and there was no longer time to reload and fire; complying with their colonel's orders, they began to drop back from the wall in a fairly orderly manner. Those unwilling to fall back continued to fight on alone and in squads; the detail of infantrymen manning Cushing's last gun, after pulling the lanyard on the charge of canister and battlefield scrap, fought on with artillery tools. The two companies by the rear wall, under the direct command of Colonel Smith, slackened their fire to let their comrades fall back safely; once the other companies were clear, the two right wing companies picked up their collection of muskets and fired a lethal sustained volley into Armistead's advancing men.[70]

For Frank Haskell, however, just returning to the field, and knowing nothing of Colonel Smith's orders to his men, it looked like the beginnings of an enemy breakthrough. "Great Heavens!—Were my senses mad! —the larger portion of Webb's brigade,—my God, it was true,—there by the group of trees and the angles of the wall, was breaking from the cover of their works, and without orders or reason, with no hand lifted to check them, was falling back a fear-stricken flock of confusion!"[71]

Staff aides to generals, despite their lesser rank, held special privilege to act in their general's behalf. With one last look around for any general officers, Haskell spurred forward and rode into the retreating meleé, ceremonial sword gleaming in his hand.[72]

---

70. *Ibid.*, p. 162; *OR*, vol. 27, pt. 1, p. 428; Smith, "The Battle,"; McClean, "The Third Day of Gettysburg."

71. Byrne and Weaver, *Haskell of Gettysburg*, pp. 161-62. It was not "the larger portion of Webb's brigade" that Frank Haskell saw falling back, only portions of the forward eight companies of the 71st Pennsylvania. After dropping back, they reformed on the right two companies of the 71st, some intermixing with the line of the 72nd Pennsylvania along the crest. The remaining troops of the 71st that did not drop back, as well as the two rear companies, held fast, even to the point of decimation, while the 69th Pennsylvania posted to their immediate left hinged back to keep their front to the enemy. The 72nd Pennsylvania, bolstered by a section of the 106th Pennsylvania, posted on the slope behind the 71st, remained firm. [For an excellent discussion of Frank Haskell's part at the Angle, see Daniel Bauer, "The Long Fight over the Bloody Angle," *Civil War*, vol. 17 (April 1989): 39-43.]

72. Byrne and Weaver, *Haskell of Gettysburg*, pp. 161-62.

Second Corps commander Hancock was still mounted, but hidden from Haskell by the mass of men and the roll of the landscape off to the south. Galloping toward the Union left, he encouraged the troops and spoke briefly with several of their commanders as he sped past Harrow's and Hall's brigades.[73]

General Doubleday's division of the First Corps lay wedged in next to the left of Hancock's Second Corps, and Hancock had to ride through Doubleday's position to reach General Stannard and his nine-month Vermont brigade. Stannard's position was forward of the main Federal line, and Hancock guided his mount out over the crest of the ridge, away from any shred of cover for a horseman, "a place where no mounted man had for hours been seen," to reach the Green Mountain troops.[74]

Riding along the length of the Vermonters, Hancock quickly surveyed the situation and located their commander. Stannard already had his men in motion as Hancock rode up, but apparently the arrangements were not to the general's liking; as he reined to a halt, Hancock shouted out to Stannard that he had "gone to H--l." The Vermont commander coolly replied: "To Hell it was then, as it was the only thing that could possibly save the day!" Realizing that both of them had similar ideas, Hancock quickly issued orders to alter the present disposition of the Vermont troops. Orders rang out, and the New Englanders promptly began to rearrange their lines, preparing for the coming movement.[75]

Hancock paused to let his winded horse cool down; General Stannard had also mounted up to survey his troops, and the two now sat side by side, conversing about the pending swing against the Confederate flank. Lt. George G. Benedict, Stannard's aide, stood looking on, admiring Hancock as "the most striking man I ever saw on horseback, and magnificent in the flush and excitement of battle—when he uttered an exclamation and I saw he was reeling in the saddle."[76]

---

73. Winfield Scott Hancock, letter to Peter F. Rothermel, January 21, 1869, Hancock Papers, Pennsylvania State Library.

74. Francis A. Walker, Paper, MOLLUS Mass. Papers, X, p. 49.

75. George G. Stannard, letter to Abner Doubleday, September 3, 1865, Abner Doubleday Papers, Baseball Hall of Fame, Cooperstown, New York.

76. George G. Benedict, *Army Life in Virginia*, pp. 182-83. "Major General Hancock rode down to speak to Gen. Stannard, and fell, while addressing him, close to the front line, just after the flank attack had been ordered." [George G. Benedict, *Vermont At Gettysburg* (Burlington, Vermont: The Free Press Association, 1870), p. 21.]

Benedict, along with staff aides Lt. Sidney S. Morey of the 13th Vermont, and Lt. George W. Hooker of the 12th Vermont, caught the wounded Hancock as he toppled from his horse. Carrying him a few yards to a crumbling stone wall, they laid the wounded general gently down with his head facing south, feet to north. "General Stannard bent over him as we laid him upon the ground, and opened his clothing where he indicated by a movement of his hand that he was hurt, a ragged hole, an inch or more in diameter, from which the blood was pouring profusely, was disclosed in the upper part and on the side of his thigh. He was naturally in some alarm for his life."[77]

Lieutenant Morey saw the seriousness of the wound and ran over to Pvt. Clark H. Butterfield of the 13th, asking to borrow the tourniquet he knew Butterfield carried with him at all times. Dashing back to the fallen general, it was discovered the wound was too close to the body to get the tourniquet around. "Don't let me bleed to death," hissed Hancock through gritted teeth. "Get something around it quick."[78]

There was no time to be wasted, so Stannard improvised. Reaching into his pocket, the Vermont general pulled out his oversized handkerchief to use as a emergency tourniquet. Lieutenant Benedict helped his general get the bandanna in place, and studied the wound

---

The origin of the bullet that felled Hancock, long thought to have come from the attacking Confederates, has been called into question by A. M. Gambone. "It is generally assumed, and Hancock himself assumed, that he was hit by Rebel fire. However, when we look closely at his reported position and southerly vector, it becomes increasingly possible that he was hit by one of the volleys fired by the Vermont regiments or some other unidentified Union soldier. The precise timing of those volleys is not exactly clear. This possibility is furthered when we consider that the bullet which hit the general had to penetrate his wooden saddle tree, remove a hand wrought nail that had been peened into rivet form, exit the saddle tree while carrying the bullet, and enter Hancock's groin. All of that demanded energy indicates a missile fired from a close range with a direct northerly path. Shots from the attacking Rebels would have been to Hancock's right flank, most likely. Unfortunately, we will probably never know for certain." [A. M. Gambone, *Hancock At Gettysburg . . . and Beyond.* (Baltimore: Butternut and Blue, 1997), p. 268, n. 97.

77. Ralph O. Sturtevant and Eli N. Peck, *Pictorial History of the Thirteenth Vermont Volunteers, War of 1861-1865* (Burlington, Vermont: Regimental Association, 1910), pp. 703, 717; Winfield Scott Hancock, letter to Francis A. Walker, December 12, 1885, Sessler Collection, Civil War Library and Museum, Philadelphia, Pennsylvania; Benedict, *Army Life in Virginia*, p. 183.

78. Sturtevant and Peck, *Pictorial History of the Thirteenth Vermont*, p. 717; Benedict, *Army Life in Virginia*, p. 183.

as he worked. "As I helped to pass it around General Hancock's legs I saw that the blood, being dark in color and not coming in jets, could not be from an artery, and I said to him: 'This is not arterial blood, General; you will not bleed to death.' From my use of the surgical term he took me for a surgeon, and replied, with a sigh of relief: 'That's good; thank you for that, Doctor.' We tightened the ligature by twisting it with the barrel of a pistol, and soon stopped the flow of blood."[79]

Col. Wheelock G. Veazey of the 16th Vermont offered to have Hancock carried from the field, but the wounded commander preferred to remain where he could watch the progress of the Vermont troops, and be in a position to order up support if necessary. "No, I thank you, Colonel," replied Hancock to Veazey's offer. "Attend to your commands, gentlemen. I will take care of myself."[80]

Stannard's troops had been pulling garrison duty for many months, with plenty of time for drill, and now those long sweaty hours of tedious practice were paying off. The 13th Vermont led out, reforming from double-rank line to columns of four; then the crucial order rang out: *"Change front forward on first company!"* The Union infantry began to swing, wheeling ponderously perpendicular to the side of the attacking Confederate column, the entire command pivoting on First Sgt. James B. Scully of Company A.[81]

Propping himself up to see as well as possible, Hancock spent the time waiting for medical help by cheering on the troops as they manuevered into position against the Confederate right. Colonel Veazey, a comrade of Hancock's from the old prewar army, was leading the 16th Vermont. "As Veazey passes by with his gallant regiment, [Hancock] calls him to himself, clasps his hands as in the old days, and, in a voice still martial and stirring, cries, 'Go in, Colonel, and give it to them on the flank.'"[82]

---

79. Benedict, *Army Life in Virginia*, pp. 183-84.
80. Chaplain C. W. Denison and Capt. G. B. Herbert, *Hancock "the Superb," The Early Life and Public Career of Winfield Scott Hancock* (Detroit and Chicago: 1880), p. 204.
81. George G. Benedict, *Vermont in the Civil War: A History of the Part Taken by the Vermont Soldiers and Sailors in the War for the Union, 1861-5*, 2 vols. (Burlington, Vermont: Free Press Association, 1886-1888), vol. 2, pp. 468-69, 469 note.
82. Francis A. Walker, *General Hancock* (New York: D. Appleton and Co., 1895), pp. 143-44.

Up by that angle in the wall, as the 71st Pennsylvania fell back, it exposed the right of the 69th Pennsylvania. The Confederate thrust caromed into the 69th, and the fighting went hand-to-hand. Orders were shouted for the Pennsylvanians to fall back and change front, but in the wild meleé, some never got the word. Col. Dennis O'Kane of the 69th was down with a mortal wound; Lt. Col. Martin Tshudy, already wounded on July 2, fell dead. The Confederates grappled with the Keystone State men, who, intermingled with the remnants of Cushing's gunners and scattered knots of the 71st, put up a white-knuckled, determined resistance. The artillerymen were "fighting with handspikes and rocks and anything we could get our hands on." The right of the 69th was gradually being twisted back by the sheer weight of the massed Confederates, forming a new front. It wasn't neat, or by the book, but the 69th obstinately stood its ground, their state-issued Stars and Stripes and the kelly green regimental flag snapping defiantly in the hot breeze issuing from thousands of overheated muzzles.[83]

General Webb was working to move reinforcements into the extended breach by the wall. The 72nd Pennsylvania "Fire Zouaves" were formed on the crest behind the men of the 71st, but, try as he might, Webb could not get them to advance. In his excitement, Webb did not think to issue orders through their colonel, but stood shouting in person at the men. The brigade commander, appointed to that post only days before from a staff position, was so new to his command that most of the men had no idea who he was. Webb shouted again, then waved his sword toward the enemy. Finally, in a last ditch effort to force the regiment to advance, the brigadier tried grabbing the regimental flag, but the husky color-bearer wrested it away from him.[84]

Men of the 71st Pennsylvania were still moving to the rear, working on reestablishing their own line in a less vulnerable position. Into these reforming companies rode a mounted officer, waving his ceremonial sword, attempting to rally the already steadying Keystone line. "I ordered these men to '*halt*,' and '*face about*,' and '*fire*,'" wrote Frank

---

83. Stewart, *Pickett's Charge*, pp. 217-18.

84. Alexander S. Webb, letter to his wife, July 6, 1863, copy in the Bachelder Papers; A. W. McDermott, letters to John B. Bachelder, September 17, 1889, and October 21, 1889, Bachelder Papers; A. F. Devereux, letter to John B. Bachelder, July 22, 1889, Bachelder Papers; Alexander S. Webb, letters to John B. Bachelder, November 25, 1869, and June 16, 1888, Bachelder Papers; Alexander S. Webb, letter to his father, July 17, 1863, Webb Collection; Alexander S. Webb, letter to his wife, July 27, 1863, Webb Collection.

Haskell, "and they heard my voice, and gathered my meaning, and obeyed my commands. On some unpatriotic backs, of those not quick of comprehension, the flat of my sabre fell, not lightly; and at its touch their love of country returned; and with a look at me as if I were the destroying angel, as I might have become theirs, they again faced the enemy." Webb and Haskell, working separately, realigned the retreating fragments of the 71st behind its sister regiment. The two Pennsylvania regiments, along with a few companies of the 106th Pennsylvania, were now somewhat protected by the abrupt crest of the ridge, and returned a lively fire on the Southerners coming over the wall.[85]

This was not a solution, only a stopgap measure; more troops were going to be needed to throw back the persistent Confederate attack. Haskell, looking left along the line toward the Round Tops, but could see and hear little firing in that direction. With one last look around the field for General Gibbon, Haskell hurriedly spurred off for reinforcements. Webb, on foot, headed forward to check on the 69th Pennsylvania, still stubbornly holding their position at the front part of the wall. The general stolidly plowed his way through the struggling men and flying lead; a bullet "from a Mississippi rifle" tore a burning hole through the inside of his thigh, but still he pressed on.[86]

---

85. Byrne and Weaver, *Haskell of Gettysburg*, p. 162. It is interesting to note that Webb makes no mention of Haskell's part in "rallying" the 71st Pennsylvania in his report [*OR*, pt. 1, pp. 428-29.] In later years, when Webb was serving as president of City College of New York, he read through Haskell's Gettysburg letter and voiced no disagreement. He went so far as to write Haskell's brother that Frank Haskell "was one we all respected & liked and any document bearing his name will carry great weight in the 2d Corps." [Alexander S. Webb, letter to H. M. Haskell, Haskell Papers, Pennsylvania Historical and Museum Commission.] [See footnote 116 for Webb's later change of opinion.]

86. Byrne and Weaver, *Haskell of Gettysburg*, pp. 164-65; Alexander S. Webb, letter to his wife, July 6, 1863, copy in the Bachelder Papers; A. W. McDermott, letters to John B. Bachelder, September 17, 1889, and October 21, 1889, Bachelder Papers; A. F. Devereux, letter to John B. Bachelder, July 22, 1889, Bachelder Papers; Alexander S. Webb, letters to John B. Bachelder, November 25, 1869, and June 16, 1888, Bachelder Papers; Alexander S. Webb, letter to his father, July 17, 1863, Webb Collection; Alexander S. Webb, letter to his wife, July 27, 1863, Webb Collection; Wiley Sword, "Facing the Gray Wave: Alexander Webb at Gettysburg," *Civil War Times Illustrated*, vol. 19, no. 9 (January 1981): 22.

General Armistead was over the wall, heading toward Cushing's guns, four of his men clustered close. Sergeant Fuger of Cushing's battery saw him coming, and turned his service revolver on the advancing general. "I fired at Armistead with my pistol several shots; if he was hit by it I do not know. I fired my pistol after he got seven or eight feet in rear of the gun (Number 3)."[87]

Suddenly, the odds caught up with the venerable Southern commander. Within feet of Cushing's guns, one shot caught Armistead in the leg, another took him in the arm, apparently almost simultaneously. "When Armistead was shot, he tottered two or three paces and fell," wrote Pvt. Anthony W. McDermott of the battered 69th Pennsylvania. "He thought he was only two or three steps from the muzzle of a gun, and he tried to catch it to break his fall, but he could not reach it."[88]

Lying in the scant shade of the gun, the fallen Confederate commander looked on as the colors of the 53rd Virginia passed him, and were planted on the slope of Cemetery Ridge. Lt. Hutchings Carter, the eleventh man to bear the Virginia colors that afternoon, was promptly taken captive. Armistead, meanwhile, gave the Masonic distress signal, and called out for help "as the son of a widow." Some of the men of the 72nd Pennsylvania heard his cry, and, understanding its significance, immediately came up to assist him.[89]

---

87. Frederick Fuger, *Family History* (Detroit: Privately Publihed, 1904); Frederick Fuger, "Cushing's Battery at Gettysburg," *Journal of Military Service Institution of the United States*, vol. 41, (November-December 1907): 408-9; Wayne Motts, "If Mortal Man Can: Lewis Armistead at Gettysburg," *Blue & Gray Magazine*, vol. 5, no. 6 (July 1988): 46, sidebar. As Webb was heading toward the front, he walked within a few paces of Armistead, who "passed me with four of his men. . . . This is the only case I have known of the two commanding officers (Generals) passing each other in front. I wish Armistead had lived," added Webb wistfully; "I would like to know him as a gallant man." Webb, for his determined effort under fire to stop the Confederate attack and push in reinforcements, was awarded the Medal of Honor in 1891. [W. F. Beyer and O. F. Keydel, eds., *Deeds of Valor: How America's Civil War Heroes Won the Congressional Medal of Honor* (Detroit: Perrien-Keydel co., 1901; reprint, Stamford, Connecticut: Longmeadow Press, 1991), pp. 224-25.] For his part in heroically defending Cushing's guns in the face of overwhelming odds, Sgt. Frederick Fuger was given the same award in 1897. [Beyer and Keydel, *Deeds of Valor*, p. 232.]
88. A. W. McDermott, letters to John B. Bachelder, September 17, 1889, and October 21, 1889, Bachelder Papers.
89. Motts, "If Mortal Man Can," p. 46, text.

Capt. Henry H. Bingham, staff aide to General Hancock and fellow Mason, happened to be passing by, and asked the identity of the downed Confederate officer. Informed that it was Lt. Gen. James Longstreet, Bingham sent the Pennsylvania troops back to their regiment, promising that he would care for the wounded officer. Armistead introduced himself to Captain Bingham, who in turn revealed that he was on General Hancock's staff.[90]

Armistead asked that General Hancock, his close friend from antebellum days, be called to his side. When informed of Hancock's serious condition, Armistead replied: "Tell General Hancock for me that I shall regret or repent (I forgot the exact word) the longest day I live."[91]

The two talked briefly, and then Captain Bingham offered his help to the downed man. "If you have anything valuable in your possession which you desire to be taken care of—I will take care of it for you." After receiving Armistead's spurs, watch, chain, seal, and some personal papers to be given to Hancock, the captain had the wounded general carried from the field.[92]

Meanwhile, the Confederates were finding the Union side of the wall a very inhospitable place. After the initial thrust into the Northern

---

90. Henry H. Bingham, letter to Winfield Scott Hancock, January 5, 1869, Gettysburg National Military Park. Oddly, there is no known record that Bingham ever realized that General Armistead was a Mason.

91. *Ibid.*; Motts, "If Mortal Man Can," p. 46, sidebar; *SHSP*, vol. 10, p. 428; Ladd, *The Bachelder Papers*, vol. 3, pp. 1494-97. There is some serious doubt that Armistead actually spoke these words, however legendary they have since become.

92. *Ibid*; Tucker, *Hancock the Superb*, p. 161. Armistead was carried to the Eleventh Corps Hospital at the George Spangler Farm, located between the Taneytown Road and Baltimore Pike, just south of the Granite Schoolhouse Road. Carried into the kitchen, he was placed on the floor with the other wounded. Surgeon H. C. Hedrick, 157th New York Volunteers, and Dr. Daniel G. Brinton examined and dressed his injuries. "His prospects of recovery seemed good," recalled Brinton. Although neither wound was mortal in nature, the general had lost a massive amount of blood, and was not able to recover from the resultant shock. The forty-six-year-old warrior died at the Spangler Farm at 9:00 a.m. on July 5, never having the opportunity to see his old friend General Hancock one last time. [Coco, *A Vast Sea of Misery*, pp. 105, 107; Gary Gallagher, ed., *The Third Day at Gettysburg and Beyond* (Chapel Hill: The University of North Carolina Press, 1994), pp. 121-22; Wayne E. Motts, *Trust in God and Fear Nothing: General Lewis A. Armistead, C.S.A.* (Gettysburg, Pennsylvania: Farnsworth House Military Impressions, 1994), p. 49.]

lines, most of those Rebels not at once shot down or captured found it expedient to fall back to the scant shelter of the low wall, using it as a meager breastwork as the firefight intensified.

Further to the north, between the angle and Ziegler's Grove, the command structure of the Third Division under General Hays was taking a dreadful beating. Col. Eliakim Sherrill of the 126th New York, now commanding the Third Brigade after Colonel Willard's death yesterday, was carried off the field with a gaping abdominal wound that would end his life. Col. Clinton D. MacDougall of Captain Thompson's 111th New York took over for Sherrill, only to be incapacitated a few moments later. Then the command moved on to the next most senior man, this time Lt. Col. James M. Bull of the 126th. And so it went. Col. Thomas A. Smyth, heading the Second Brigade, still kept his command despite a nasty facial wound, blood dripping off the end of his chin and onto his uniform.[93]

General Hays had been following the plucky initiative of the lonely 8th Ohio skirmishers, bolstered by the few guns of the 125th New York, as they attacked the Confederates from the flank. Inspired by what he saw, he swung out the unengaged 126th New York Regiment to link up with the Ohioans. To strengthen the impact of the enfilade fire, two of Woodruff's Napoleons focused a sustained destructive fire into the Southern ranks. About 450 Ohio and New York muskets joined the artillery pieces in the deadly work.[94]

Hancock watched from the ground as the Vermonters swung into position. The 13th Vermont came around first, took calculated aim as the enemy passed by not more than sixty yards away, and fired, shooting from south to north into the charging columns. At that range, it was virtually impossible to miss. "The effect upon the rebel lines was

---

93. Stewart, *Pickett's Charge*, p. 225.

94. R. L. Murray, The Redemption of the "Harpers Ferry Cowards": The Story of the 111th and 126th New York State Volunteer Regiments at Gettysburg (Published privately by the author, 1994), pp. 137-39; Stewart, *Pickett's Charge*, pp. 225, 233.

instantaneous. . . . For a moment they crowded together in bewilderment, falling like wheat before a reaper."[95]

Each company, as it came into line, loosed a lethal volley at the attackers, causing great consternation among the Confederates. Southern officers desperately tried to get their men to change front to face the new attack. Then the 16th Vermont advanced from behind its sister regiment, with parade ground precision, coolly leveled their weapons, and mowed down still more attackers.[96]

General Doubleday, looking down on the movement from the slope of Cemetery Ridge, was shouting himself hoarse and waving his hat. "Glory to God, glory to God!" he cheered as he watched his own men step out. "See the Vermonters go it!" Close to 900 Vermont muskets were cutting ragged, bloody gashes into the attacking formations.[97]

By the time Hancock reached the Vermont troops, all his staff had departed on various errands for the general; only Private Wells accompanied him, still carrying the blue swallowtail flag of the Second Corps command with a white Maltese cross in its center.[98] Maj. William G. Mitchell of Hancock's staff soon rode up in search of his commander; not seeing the fallen general, he ordered an officer of Stannard's brigade, in Hancock's name, to swing his men out to attack the Confederates as they passed by. The officer declined without specific instructions from his colonel, and it was then that Mitchell spotted Hancock, laying prostrate in the grass with one hand clutching the revolver and bandanna tourniquet. Shocked, Mitchell rushed to Hancock's side.[99]

Seeing the Confederate lines start to disintegrate under the flank fire of the Vermonters, Hancock brushed off Mitchell's torrent of concerned questions and news of General Armistead's wounding, and

95. Ralph Orson Sturtevant and Carmi Lathrop Marsh, *History of the 13th Regiment, Vermont Volunteers* (Burlington, Vermont: Regimental Association, 1910), p. 305.

96. *Ibid.*, pp. 232-33; Coffin, *Full Duty*, pp. 194-95; H. T. Owen, *Philadelphia Weekly Times*, March 26, 1881.

97. Benedict, *Vermont in the Civil War*, vol. 2, p. 478.

98. The trefoil had been recently adopted by the Second Corps as its symbol, but a new corps flag had not yet been issued. [Hancock to Peter F. Rothermel, December 31, 1868, Hancock Papers, Pennsylvania State Library.]

99. Hancock, *Reminiscences of Winfield Scott Hancock*, p. 214.

instead dispatched him with a verbal message to army commander Meade. "Tell General Meade that the troops under my command have repulsed the enemy's assault and that we have gained a great victory. The enemy is now flying in all directions in my front."[100]

With a last look at his wounded commander, Mitchell threw himself into the saddle again, and dashed off in search of Meade. Unlike so many others this afternoon, the senior staff aide promptly located the army commander, riding toward the crest of Cemetery Hill from the Taneytown Road area. Quickly reciting Hancock's words, Mitchell added that his chief was lying further down the ridge, severely wounded in the thigh. Meade sent back a oral communiqué of his own: "Say to General Hancock that I regret exceedingly that he is wounded and I thank him for the country and for myself for the service he has rendered today."[101]

Back in the saddle again, Mitchell spurred back to Hancock, and dutifully delivered the return message; only then did Hancock allow his aide-de-camp to go off in search of medical assistance. "Major Mitchell of Hancock's staff rode up as we were at work over the general," wrote Lieutenant Benedict, "and uttering an exclamation of pain as he saw the condition of his chief, turned and darted away after a surgeon."[102]

Haskell reined in directly in front of Norman J. Hall, commander of the Third Brigade of Gibbon's Second Division. "Col Hall I found just in rear of his line, sword in hand, cool, vigilant, noting all that passed, and directing the battle of his Brigade. The fire was constantly diminishing now in his front," as the enemy moved obliquely away from them toward the Union center, away from General Stannard's enfilade musketry.

"How is it going," asked Hall, looking up at the sweaty, balding middle-aged lieutenant on the lathered horse.

"Well, but Webb is hotly pressed, and must have support, or he will be overpowered. Can you assist him?"

---

100. Hancock papers, Pennsylvania State Library.
101. Winfield Scott Hancock, letter to Peter F. Rothermel, December 31, 1868, Hancock Papers, Civil War Library and Museum, Philadelphia, Pennsylvania.
102. Tucker, *Hancock the Superb*, p. 157; Benedict, *Army Life in Virginia*, p. 184.

"Yes."

"You cannot be too quick."

"I will move my Brigade at once."

"Good," replied Gibbon's staff aide with obvious relief.[103]

"He gave the order," wrote Haskell, "and in briefest time I saw five friendly colors hurrying to the aid of the imperiled three [regiments at the angle]; and each color represented true, battle-tried men, that had not turned back from Rebel fire that day nor yesterday." It was not far to Webb's embattled man, and Colonel Hall personally supervised the hurried flank march of his Third Brigade.[104]

Hall's officer corps had already taken a beating this hot afternoon. Maj. Edmund Rice of the 19th Massachusetts was bleeding from a serious wound. The 20th Massachusetts had lost their colonel, Paul J. Revere, yesterday; today, Lt. Col. George N. Macy had just had his left hand shot clean away. The regiment then passed to Capt. Henry L. Abbott, who also was soon wounded, but retained command. Lt. Col. Amos E. Steele, Jr. of the 7th Michigan had been killed a short time earlier by enemy fire, and the midwestern regiment headed towards the angle under the command of its major. Only the 19th Massachusetts and the 42nd New York were still led by their colonels. These four regiments, accompanied by four companies of the 59th New York under the direction of a captain, were now double-timing toward Cushing's contested guns as Haskell headed further to the left to General Harrow's brigade.[105]

The lieutenant pulled up at Harrow's First Brigade, but was never able to find the general. Hall's men were already beginning to engage the enemy, so Haskell turned in his saddle, pointing to them, and shouted at the most senior officer he could find: "'See,' I said to the men, 'see the *"chivalry,"* See the graybacks run!'" Indeed they did see, and soon four more regiments were dashing to the aid of the struggling Pennsylvanians by the wall, included the shattered remnants of the 1st Minnesota. These were all seasoned veterans, and knew what they were running into; nevertheless, "as they swept to their places by the side of Hall's [troops] and opened fire, they roared."[106]

---

103. Byrne and Weaver, *Haskell of Gettysburg*, p. 166. Colonel Hall cited Lieutenant Haskell for bravery in leading regiments into battle, but reported that he himself, not Haskell, had seen Webb's predicament and ordered his men forward. [OR, vol. 27, pt. 1, pp. 439-40.]

104. *Ibid.*

105. *Ibid.*, pp. 166-67.

106. *Ibid.*, p. 167.

General Gibbon's aide paused for a second to catch his breath. His task was accomplished—eight bloodied regiments and a fragment of another were already in motion, rushing to shore up the breach by the clump of trees. There was nothing left to do here; Frank Haskell turned his horse's head back toward the sound of battle, and put in the spurs.

At the angle, the Confederate assault was still at a bloody standstill. The Southerners, using the low wall as a breastworks of sorts, lay down a deadly fire on the enemy, dimly seen in the swirling gunsmoke. Riflemen were pressed up to the wall three and four deep just south of the angle. Of the pockets of Rebels that had clambered over the wall with Armistead, those still on their feet were struggling furiously at close quarters in the little copse of trees. The remainder of the arriving Rebels seemed content to enjoy the scant cover afforded by the backside of the little wall.[107]

For their part, the Yankees were using the abrupt break of the crest of Cemetery Ridge to shield themselves, rising above its safety only to fire at the attackers. In doing so, however, they presented a silhouetted target against the skyline. Marooned between the two hostile forces stood the shattered remains of Cushing's guns, ripped and torn by the deadly fusillades of both armies, standing silent now, unmanned and alone except for the wounded and dead sheltered there.

Hall's men had already arrived, with Harrow's close behind, all hopelessly intermingled in the pellmell push to reach the Union center. Minnesotans, New Yorkers, and Michiganders fought side by side with Bay Staters and men from Maine, adding stability to the embattled lines of the Pennsylvanians. The northerners crammed together five and six deep; those wanting to fire their weapons would push and shove to the front, discharge their piece, then drop back into the milling crowd to reload.[108]

---

107. Owen, "Pickett at Gettysburg."

108. *OR*, vol. 27, pt. 1, pp. 373-74, 417-18, 420, 425, 426, 428, 431, 439-40, 443-46, 448-51; George N. Macy, letter to John B. Bachelder, May 12, 1866, Bachelder Papers; A. W. McDermott, letter to John B. Bachelder, October 10, 1889, Bachelder Papers; E. Wise, letter to Alexander S. Webb, August 1, 1887, Webb Collection.

Sometimes, the sheer press of men would sway the two lines into each other, precipitating a swirling free-for-all, muskets swinging, fists flailing, artillery tools, bayonets, knives all pressed to the deadly work. The color-bearer of the 19th Massachusetts was pushed face to face with his opposite of the 14th Virginia; the Yankee promptly felled his opponent by an vicious uppercut with his flag staff, grabbed the Virginia banner, and bore it triumphantly off the field. Those in the rear lobbed cobblestones scooped up from the field onto the heads of their adversaries. One participant's description of the fight sounds like a scene straight from Hell: Union men "shouted and killed—hatless, coatless, drowned in sweat, black with powder, red with blood, stifling in the horrid heat, parched with smoke and blind with dust, with fiendish yells and strange oaths they blindly plied the work of slaughter."[109]

"Now it was as if a new battle, deadlier, stormier than before" was raging. "All depths of passion are stirred, and all combattive [*sic*] fire, down to their deep foundations. Individuality is drowned in a sea of clamor; and timid men, breathing the breath of the multitude, are brave. The frequent dead and wounded lie where they stagger and fall;—there is no humanity for them now, and none can be spared to care for them. The men do not cheer, or shout,—they growl; and over that uneasy sea, heard with the roar of musketry, sweeps the muttered thunder of a storm of growls." Reinforcements rushing into Ziegler Grove heard a noise "strange and terrible, a sound that came from thousands of human throats, yet was not a commingling of shouts and yells but rather like a vast mournful roar."[110]

Thoughts of personal safety were suddenly overwhelmed by the excitement and fever pitch of the battle. "Lieutenant John Tibbetts stands up yelling like mad, 'Give it to 'em! give it to 'em!,'" recalled a 14th Connecticut veteran of one comrade. "A bullet enters his arm—that same arm in which he caught two bullets at Antietam; Johnny's game arm drops by his side; he turns quickly to his first lieutenant,

---

109. Byrne and Weaver, *Haskell of Gettysburg*, p. 168; Stewart, *Pickett's Charge*, pp. 236-37; John Edward Pierce, "The Civil War Career of Richard Brooke Garnett: A Quest for Vindication" (M.A. dissertation, Virginia Polytechnic Institute, 1969).

110. Byrne and Weaver, *Haskell of Gettysburg*, pp. 168-69; Abner Small, *The Road to Richmond: The Civil War Memoirs of Major Abner Small of the 16th Maine Volunteers*, ed. Harold Adams Small (Berkeley: University of California Press, 1939), p. 106.

saying, 'I have got another bullet in the same old arm, but I don't care a d--n!"[111]

Yet, in spite of the bold and reckless daring evidenced on both sides, the opposing forces seemed to instinctively hold off crossing that deadly parcel of ground, the space which had to be traversed in order to grapple with the enemy. A member of the 19th Maine remembered the continued firestorm, with the opposing sides "in some places within rifle-length of each other and other places hopelessly mingled." It seemed to Col. Arthur F. Devereux that "whichever side could get a motion forward must surely win."[112]

Lieutenant Haskell was back at the Union center again, trying one more time to get the Keystone State troops to advance on the enemy. "These men of Pennsylvania, on the soil of their own homesteads, the first and only to flee the wall, must be the first to storm it," he reasoned.[113]

Working down the chain of command, orders were being given to advance. The major of the 72nd Pennsylvania politely refused to lead such an advance, because he felt that his proper place was in the rear of the troops. In response to the order to spearhead the counterattack, a captain declined for fear of being shot down from the rear by the massing Union troops. The command to move forward finally came to the color-bearer.[114]

Sergeant Murphy was the latest man to bear the colors that day; six men had fallen already—men with fine Scotch-Irish names like Wills, and O'Donnell, and Finnessey. The flag was the Stars and Stripes, for the 72nd Pennsylvania carried no regimental colors. The staff was

---

111. Joseph W. Morton, Jr., ed., *Sparks from the Camp Fire. Or Tales of the Old Veterans. Thrilling Stories of Heroic Deeds, Brave Encounters, Desperate Battles, Bold Achievements, Reckless Daring, Lofty Patriotism, Terrible Suffering and Wondrous Fortitude. As Retold To-day Around the Modern Camp Fire. New and Revised Edition with Contributions from One Hundred and Fifty Comrades* (Philadelphia: Keystone Publishing Co., 1893), p. 232.
112. John Day Smith, *History of the 19th Regiment of Maine Volunteer Infantry* (Minneapolis: The Great Western Printing Company, 1909), p. 82; J. F. Devereux, "Some Account of Pickett's Charge at Gettysburg," *Magazine of American History* (July 1887): 17.
113. Byrne and Weaver, *Haskell of Gettysburg*, p. 169.
114. *Ibid.*

splintered and broken by shot, with only a short piece still left holding the banner. This time there would be no polite refusals, no declining for fear of being gunned down from behind; the order came clear and implacable: "Sergeant forward with your color. Let the Rebels see it close to their eyes once more before they die."[115]

"The Color Sergeant of the 72nd Pa[,] grasping the stump of the severed lance in both hands, waved the flag above his head, and rushed toward the wall. The question is shouted out to be heard over the rattling musketry and the roar of men grappling in mortal combat: 'Will you see your colors storm the wall alone!' One man only starts to follow."[116]

---

115. *Ibid.*; Stewart, *Pickett's Charge*, p. 244.

116. Byrne and Weaver, *Haskell of Gettysburg*, p. 169. The words of Frank Haskell would come under heavy attack in later years. Had he survived the war, the aide might have softened his harsh language concerning the activity of the 71st Pennsylvania on July 3. Decades later, Haskell's voluminous letter was scathingly attacked by General Webb, who caustically stated that Haskell had "paraded with the stragglers and prisoners." [Alexander S. Webb, letter to Frazier, September 7, 1909, in Philadelphia Brigade Association, *Reply of the Philadelphia Brigade Association to the Foolish and Absurd Narrative of Lieutenant Frank Haskell* (Philadelphia: Bower Printing Co., 1910), pp. 34-35.]

Members of the Philadelphia Brigade went so far as to publish a vindictive tract against Haskell's narrative, which was long on rhetoric but short on any fresh evidence for their case. [Philadelphia Brigade Association, *Reply of the Philadelphia Brigade Association*] The actions of Frank Haskell that afternoon, however, met with the full approval of his commander, although not seen firsthand. "From others I learned of Haskell's distinguished conduct on that day, and I have always thought that to him, more than any one man, are we indebted for the repulse of Lee's assault," wrote Gibbon. "His personal gallantry in aiding the officers in reforming their overpowered troops was seen and commented upon by many, whilst his quick judgment in using his authority as a staff officer of his absent general in moving assistance to the critical point, was admirable, and, from all I could learn, undoubtedly assured our success there." [Gibbon, *Personal Recollections*, p. 153.]

Those "others" who had "seen and commented" included Third Brigade commander Col. Norman J. Hall, who wrote of Haskell's "magnificent conduct" on the field "in the highest terms." General Harrow, whom Haskell had not been able to locate when searching for reinforcements, had taken over command of the Second Division after the wounding of General Gibbon. Harrow commented in his official report of the afternoon's battle that Haskell had "greatly distinguished himself by his constant exertion in the most exposed places. [*OR*, vol. 27, pt. 1, pp. 376, 418, 421, 440.] C. H. Morgan, inspector-general of Hancock's staff, also spoke in the highest terms of Haskell's work on July 3. [Hancock, *Reminiscences of Winfield Scott Hancock*, pp. 213, 221-22.]

Up at Ziegler Grove, to the right of the zigzag stone wall, the men of General Hays had successfully weathered three separate waves of Confederate attackers. With the repulse of the final onslaught, additional men from the Third Division came across the wall, swung around to the left, and joined the Ohioans, the New Yorkers, and the two cannon in tearing into the Confederate left flank. The Union forces now had a concave line, wrapping around the front and sides of the Southerners, from the tenacious 8th Ohio on the extreme right to the Vermont troops fully deployed on the left. The Rebels were taking a devastating fire from three sides, and the glorious charge of thirty minutes ago was facing the very real threat of total annihilation.[117]

With the wounding of Southern General Armistead, the Confederate fire near Cushing's ruined battery had slackened noticeably, and some of the most advanced enemy troops were throwing down their weapons. The 72nd Pennsylvania opened ranks to let surrendering soldiers pass to the rear.

General Webb, blood running down his right leg from a painful flesh wound, had made it up to the front part of the angle where the tenacious 69th Pennsylvanians were doggedly hanging on to their fragment of stone wall; the twenty-eight-year-old brigadier, shouting at the top of his lungs to be heard over the musketry, told the 69th to keep up a hot fire to the front *and* rear as Confederates penetrated the Union line. "To a man they replied that I could count on them." Satisfied, the plucky West Pointer turned and hobbled back to the rest of his swaying line, determined to try one last time to get the 72nd Pennsylvania to move forward. "Come up, boys," he bellowed at the top of his lungs, "the enemy is running." Up by the front stone wall, the portion of the 69th which had bent back started to swing out again, slowly at first, then picked up momentum.[118]

---

117. Stewart, *Pickett's Charge*, p. 238, 243.

118. Wilson, *Survivors of the Seventy-second Regiment*, Testimony of James C. Lynch, Anthony W. McDermott, Charles H. Banes, Joseph W. Garnett, Alexander S. Webb, Arthur Devereux, Frank Weible, Samuel Roberts, Henry Russell, Elwood N. Hamilton, Robert McBride, James R. Johnston, pp. 71, 101, 108, 125, 146, 151, 174, 185, 187, 220-21, 252, 272, 275, 283, 305; Sword, "Facing the Gray Wave," p. 22.

About halfway to the stone wall, Color Sergeant Murphy of the 72nd fell, riddled with bullets. The national flag drifted down, its folds gradually settling around his body. But something about that banner fluttering to the ground sparked these soldiers in a visceral way that neither Haskell or Webb were able to accomplish; with a spontaneous roar of rage and blood, the 72nd bolted forward, drawing along some of the 71st Pennsylvania in its wake. "Boys, the enemy are ours," screamed out Webb as the blue lines surged past him toward the bloody wall and Cushing's ravaged guns. "A strange resistless impulse," one soldier called it.[119] The fragmentary 106th Pennsylvania rushed forward as well.

To their left, the intermingled troops of Col. Norman J. Hall's Third Brigade and Brig. Gen. William Harrow's First Brigade, in response to Lieutenant Haskell's call for help and on their own initiative, surged toward the wavering Confederate assault. Time seemed to slow to an incongruous crawl for some of the participants, "measurable by seconds. The men near seemed to fire very slowly. Those in [the] rear, though coming up at a run, seemed to drag their feet. Many were firing through the intervals of those in front, in their eagerness to injure the enemy."[120]

Dashing down the slope, the Northerners vaulted the wall and were into the Confederates. "Thrusts, yells, blows, shots, and undistinguishable conflict" was how one soldier described it. Muskets were rammed against men's bodies and the triggers pulled. Bayonets were driven home to the hilt and twisted. Some men were slugging it out with bare fists, others rolling on the ground, wrestling and gouging. In the confusion, Rebels fighting to the last cartridge stood side by side and intermixed with Southerners throwing up their hands in surrender.[121]

---

119. Byrne and Weaver, *Haskell of Gettysburg*, pp. 169-70; William Lochren, "The First Minnesota at Gettysburg," *Glimpses of the Nation's Struggle*. Papers read before the Minnesota Commandery. MOLLUS (Series 3), New York, St. Paul, Minneapolis, 1892, Number 42, p. 54; Sword, "Facing the Gray Wave," p. 23. As a personal souvenir of the battle, Webb sent the shattered flagstaff of the 72nd Pennsylvania by express to his father after the battle. [Sword, "Facing the Gray Wave," p. 24.]

120. Edmund Rice, "Repelling Lee's Last Blow at Gettysburg," *Battles and Leaders*, vol. 3, pp. 388-89.

121. Byrne and Weaver, *Haskell of Gettysburg*, p. 170; Rice, "Repelling Lee's Last Blow at Gettysburg," p. 389.

Other regiments ran to the aid of the embattled Pennsylvanians. "Closing on them with a rush and a cheer," wrote one Minnesotan tersely; "there was shooting stabbing and clubbing, for there was no time to reload." "If men ever become devils, that was one of the times," added another 1st Minnesota veteran. "We were crazy with the excitement of the fight. We just rushed in like wild beasts. Men swore and cursed and struggled and fought, grappled in hand-to-hand fight, threw stones, clubbed their muskets, kicked, yelled and hurrahed." "Every foot of ground was occupied by men engaged in mortal combat, who were in every possible position which can be taken while under arms, or lying wounded or dead," wrote yet another participant of the moment just before he was shot twice and fell.[122]

Suddenly, the breaking point of Southern endurance was reached and passed. It seemed as if the field were suddenly blossoming white as handkerchiefs, white shirts, papers, anything close to being white was waved and fluttered, and Southerners were dropping their weapons, shouting out: "Don't shoot! Don't shoot!"[123]

"Those who were not wounded threw down their arms," wrote one Union soldier. "I remember that a Conf officer . . . gathered himself up as our men swept by and coolly remarked, 'You have done it this time.'"[124]

Col. Birkett Fry of the 13th Alabama Infantry lay bleeding on the field, straining to see through the thick fogbanks of smoke from Federal cannons and muskets, but unable to make anything out through the choking sulfurous cloud. "The roll of musketry was then incessant, and I believe the Federal troops—probably blinded by the smoke—continued a rapid fire for some minutes after none but dead and wounded remained in their front. At length the firing ceased, and cheer after cheer from the enemy announced the failure of our attack. I was of course left a prisoner."[125]

John Dooley of the 1st Virginia Infantry also lay incapacitated where he had fallen, just short of the Yankee lines; he too was

122. James A. Wright, *Story of Company F*, unpublished manuscript, Minnesota Historical Society; William Harmon, "Co. C at Gettysburg," *Minneapolis Journal*, June 30, 1897, copy at Gettysburg National Military Park; Rice, "Repelling Lee's Last Blow at Gettysburg," p. 389.

123. Stewart, *Pickett's Charge*, p. 245.

124. Harmon, "Co. C at Gettysburg."

125. Fry, "Pettigrew's Charge at Gettysburg," p. 93.

struggling to plot the course of the attack solely by the sounds reverberating hollowly through the dense overcast. "There—listen—we hear a new shout, and cheer after cheer rends the air. Are those fresh troops advancing to our support? No! No! That huzza never broke from southern lips. Oh God! Virginia's bravest, noblest sons have perished here today and perished all in vain!"[126]

---

126. Dooley, *John Dooley*, p. 107.

Part 3
The Aftermath

They are coming—they are coming—A band of saddened men,
To look for graves on hillsides, In valley and in glen.
We see them 'neath the oak tree, And near the bending corn;
We see them in the fading light, And in the early morn.

Oh! mournful are the stories That we gather day by day,
Of those who fought and those who fell In that long, bloody fray;
And mournful are the daily scenes That greet the roving eye,
Of mothers sitting near the tent To see their brave sons die. . . .

Pilgrimage to Gettysburg
Emily Bliss Souder

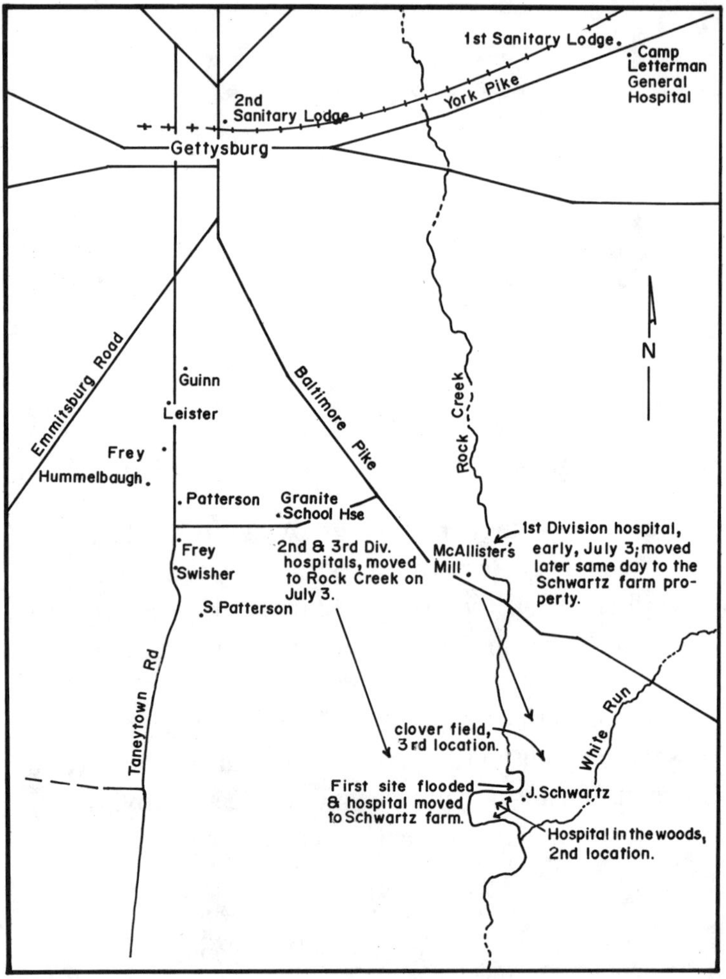

Map by John Heiser

Second Corps hospital sites at Gettysburg.

CHAPTER 7

FRIDAY, JULY 3: LATE AFTERNOON—SATURDAY, JULY 4: 4:00 A.M.

"The wounded began to arrive in vast numbers."

Assistant Surgeon Francis Moses Wafer, 108th New York Volunteers

Once the tide of battle turned, there was no swinging it back. As the Confederate lines fluttered with white tokens of capitulation, those not willing to surrender began the long, dangerous trip back to the main Southern lines. Maj. Thomas W. Osborn, looking from the top of Cemetery Hill, saw "no two men together, but each man was running by himself to gain the cover of the hills within his own lines." Some, fearful of being shot in the back, retired backwards, a few loosing off sullen parting shots as they withdrew.[1]

The men of the 8th Ohio, with ragtag bits and pieces of other regiments that had now pitched in by their side, kept hammering away at the sides of the wavering Southern assault. "From our position on the flank, we and other troops off on the Confederate right (south) flank [Stannard's Vermonters], have not ceased to pour a devastating fire into their masses. Now at last they begin to melt. . . . They threw away everything—cartridge boxes, waistbelts, and haversacks—in their stampede. We dashed in amongst them, taking prisoners by droves. One man of my company, a corporal, took fifteen prisoners including two officers as well as a stand of colors. They all seemed to extend their arms in their flight, as if to assist their speed," wrote Thomas Francis Galwey of the culmination of that afternoon's work.[2]

---

1. Osborn, "The Artillery at Gettysburg."
2. Galwey, *The Valiant Hours*, p. 118.

The area by the hotly contested stone wall was still being swept by a deadly musket fire; to fall back was almost certain death for the Confederates trapped there. One New York captain wrote that "most of those near our line sank to the ground and gave up the attempt to get away. Our men shouted to them to come in and promised not to hurt them, and at the words hundreds rose up and came into our lines, dropping their arms and crouching to avoid the fire of their own artillery which was pouring upon our position." The musketry dropped off noticeably as many Federal troops turned their weapons to guard the influx of surrendering soldiers.[3]

Northerners, many with bloody uniforms and hastily bound up wounds, were also beginning the daunting task of gathering up the vast number of enemy wounded from the field and assisting them over the wall and through the battle lines toward the rear. As Colonel Fry of the 13th Alabama was brought into Union lines, he was struck by a distinctive wound suffered by one of his Northern captors. "As evidence of how close was the fighting at that part of the line, I saw a Federal soldier with an ugly wound in his shoulder which he told me he received from the spear on the end of one of my regimental colors; and I remembered having that morning observed and laughingly commented on the fact that the color-bearer of the Thirteenth Alabama had attached to his staff a formidable looking lance head."[4]

A scattered Southern artillery shelling, ostensibly to provide a covering fire for the retiring soldiers, had begun to drop indiscriminately among prisoners and captors, wounded and unwounded alike, and the surrendering Confederates needed no prompting to hurry off toward the Union rear. This precipitate rush convinced Assistant Surgeon Francis M. Wafer at the Peter Frey Farm aid station that the enemy forces had once again staged a major breakthrough. "A large & quite regular column of the enemy emerged from the thickest cloud of smoke & moved rapidly down the road toward our rear. I for the moment believed with others that our line was penetrated & am not sure but that the exclamation escaped me aloud 'Are they invincible,' knowing the tenacity with which our men were fighting. My first impulse was for to escape, but after a moment's reflection I decided on remaining a prisoner, in hopes that I might

3. J. D. S. Cook, "Personal Reminiscences of Gettysburg." MOLLUS, *War Talks in Kansas* (Kansas City, 1906), p. 320.
4. Fry, "Pettigrew's Charge at Gettysburg," p. 93.

possibly be able to render some assistance to the numerous wounded that would be left of ours."[5]

The truth of the situation was soon revealed, however. "I was about to tell my orderly to make his escape when I caught sight through the smoke, as the column came nearer, of a few blue uniforms. A second look revealed almost a whole Brigade of prisoners taken from Longstreet's Corps being sent to the rear under a very light guard. The knowledge of this column being prisoners with the tremendous cheering of our men in the line now told the true state of affairs." Reassured, Wafer went back to examine his next patient.[6]

The artillery fire was also falling on the exposed line of the 8th Ohio as they continued pouring their deadly lateral fire into the retreating Confederates. Ohioan Azor H. Nickerson was down, wounded in the fierce musketry of the preceding hour. Now the distant artillerists were zeroing in on the wide-open Union line; "the shells coming from the right rear and front enfiladed the position and appeared to cover every foot of ground. Men lying near me were cut in two and others torn in pieces by the jagged missiles."[7]

Despite his serious wounds, Nickerson could see his only hope was to make his way toward the rear. "I thought a change of location, no matter how slight, might take me out of their range. Certainly it could not be worse, so I dragged myself a short distance only to find that I was in a worse place, if possible, than where I had been. Then, by a supreme effort, for I had been shot through one arm and through the lungs, I struggled to my feet and started to run. I had taken but a few steps when the blood gushed from my mouth in a torrent, and I fainted and fell."[8]

Somehow, one of the few ambulance teams on the artillery-swept field found the badly wounded captain. "When consciousness returned, an ambulance attendant was bathing my face, and as soon as I opened my eyes he, with the aid of the driver, placed me in his ambulance. Even while they were doing this a conical shell went crashing through one of the wheels of the vehicle. The driver very

5. Wafer diary.
6. *Ibid.*
7. Nickerson, "Personal Recollection of Two Visits to Gettysburg," p. 21.
8. *Ibid.*

properly did not wait to see whether his wheel could hold together, or if the shell exploded, but went tearing over the ground at full speed. The ground was awfully rough and covered with *debris*, but he turned out for nothing. There were two of us in the ambulance, but how we remained there is, to this day, a mystery to me. In the mad fury of that drive we were dashed together against each other until the awful torture made us both unconscious."[9]

With the Confederates falling back from their catastrophic attack, the appalling extent of three days of single-minded carnage was finally beginning to be seen. Realizing the ultimate extent of the damage would take much longer.

More than 14,500 Union wounded were scattered over the battlefield, and in Union and Confederate hospitals. Regiments were decimated; the command structure shattered. Some units had lost all of their field grade officers.

The Confederates would evacuate their wounded, somewhere in the vicinity of 8,000 men, in a 17-mile-long wagon train of misery and death. But some 5,500 Southerners, too critical to be moved, were left behind. This was in addition to more than 1,800 wounded Rebels already captured by Union forces.

There were literally dead men everywhere. In the streets of Gettysburg, bloated bodies from both sides were "all lying in the streets, so far as we could see, either up or down."[10] Files of corpses were lined up beside each field hospital, awaiting burial. Desperately wounded men had crawled off to find a spring or creek, or to find shade, or medical help, and had died on the way. Dead men in the bushes; dead men in farm buildings; dead men in the rocks; dead men under fences; sitting up; laying down; some whole and some disintegrated. Many still lay where they had fallen, in the deadly no-man's-land between the two armies. About 7,000 were dead in and around Gettysburg, and few of the nearly 4,000 Confederate fatalities had yet been buried.

9. *Ibid.*
10. Fannie J. Buehler, *Recollections of the Rebel Invasion and One Woman's Experience During the Battle of Gettysburg* (Gettysburg, Pennsylvania: n.p., 1896), p. 64.

An often overlooked group of fatalities were also strewn over the countryside. Somewhere between 3,000 to 5,000 horses and mules lay dead in the fields around the town. Most silently marked the location of now-vacant artillery positions, or roads that had been swept by heavy artillery fire. Many more hundreds suffered intensely in the aftermath: galloping lopsidedly around the battlefield on three legs, or standing with intestines protruding from abdomens ripped wide open, or staring mutely, pleadingly, with almost-human eyes, as blood ran down their sides from gaping wounds. Isolated shots would continue to ring out for days after the battle, as compassionate soldiers and details assigned to clear the battlefield put the unoffending creatures out of their misery. They were then dragged by surviving teams of horses onto mounds, where they were cremated.[11]

With the Confederate assault repulsed, men in the Second Corps turned their attention to the treatment of wounds, whether their own or those of a friend. Ambulances and stretchermen loaded up their bloody cargo, and rushed to the rear. In the meantime, the area behind the battle lines was swiftly transformed into a giant transit hospital. "Immediately after the firing ceased, two large haystacks in the rear of our [148th Pennsylvania Volunteers] Regiment were torn down, the hay scattered over the ground, and long rows of wounded men were laid side by side."[12]

Ambulances and stretchers were now at a premium on the crest of Cemetery Ridge; with so many fallen men to evacuate, and hindered by the littered and devastated landscape, many men devised makeshift methods to get their wounded friends to desperately needed medical care. "Lannegan, my lead driver, was holding his horses when shot," wrote Gunner Thomas M. Aldrich of Battery A, 1st Rhode Island Light Artillery. "As our battery was being relieved at that time, and just as the enemy were retreating down the hill, Lannegan begged me to take him from the field."[13]

---

11. Blake A. Magner, *Traveller and Company: The Horses of Gettysburg* (Gettysburg, Pennsylvania: Farnsworth House Military Impressions, 1995), p. 47.
12. Muffly, *The Story of our Regiment*, p. 440.
13. Aldrich, *The History of Battery A*, p. 220.

With the battery falling back, and not even a blanket or poles to improvise a stretcher, Aldrich had to come up with a split-second solution. "Lieutenant Lamb put a man in charge of my horses, and I took Lannegan on my back and carried him to the hospital, remaining with him until I had placed him on the operating table. When it was found that his stomach refused whisky the surgeons would not operate upon him, and he was laid out to die. I entreated the surgeons to give him proper treatment, but it was of no avail. The Sisters of Mercy, who were at the hospital, took charge of him."[14]

Unable to do any more for his badly wounded driver, "I gave Sergt Benjamin H. Child, and other comrades who had been wounded, all the assistance in my power, and then returned to the battery."[15]

As artilleryman Aldrich was heading toward the rear, Capt. Benjamin Thompson of the 111th New York was on his way to the front to rejoin his company, slogging his weary way from the spring toward the backside of Cemetery Ridge. He was still wiping blood and rock chips from his lacerated face, and looked up to see a "regular column of the enemy" rushing over the crest. "The first intimation we had of the outcome of the fight was a great crowd of men coming over the hill. For

---

14. The Sisters of Mercy were one of twelve orders of Catholic sisters specializing in medical care. As the only formally trained corps of female medical personnel in the country at that time, the services of these orders were greatly appreciated by wounded and surgeons alike. The nearest order was the Daughters of Charity of St. Vincent de Paul at Westminster, Maryland, and they assisted in many of the hospitals at Gettysburg. It is uncertain whether Aldrich was referring to the specific order, or using the term "Sisters of Mercy" to describe the sisters in general. [Jeane Heimberger Candido, "Sisters and Nuns Who were Nurses during the Civil War," *Blue and Grey*, volume 11, no. 1 (October 1993): 30-35; Karen Hurley, Letter, *Blue and Grey*, vol. 11, no. 3 (February 1994): 6.] If this aid station was one belonging to the Second Corps, it is the only recorded instance of any of the orders assisting at the Second Corps Hospitals.

15. Aldrich, *The History of Battery A*, p. 220. Artillery batteries usually did not have a surgeon and assistant surgeons accompanying them as did the infantry regiments they supported. The wounded gunners were normally taken to the nearest hospital to await treatment. [For an example of this practice, see Richard Hall, *Patriots in Disguise—Women Warriors of the Civil War*. (New York: Paragon House, 1993), pp. 41-42.]

a moment our hearts sank as we felt our line had been broken; but in a second I saw they had no guns and our spirits rose very rapidly."[16]

After dropping off a filled canteen for his clerk at the log barn, and stopping by Meade's abandoned headquarters to check on the wounded from his company, Thompson finally located what was left of his decimated command. "The saddest moment of all was when I reached my company. There was only a pitiful remnant. [John H.] Drake, my only Lieutenant, was killed. He had been a tent mate and companion for nearly a year. A perfect gentleman, a consistent Christian, and a most faithful officer, his loss was to me a personal bereavement. Of the forty seven men we led into the fight, twenty five were killed or wounded. Of the color guard attached to my company, and in my command, two were killed and four were wounded out of the eight, and two of the wounded lost a leg apiece. My whole command, officers and men, numbered fifty seven, and the loss was thirty two."[17]

Despite the high number of casualties, it was a day of rejoicing in the Union lines. "After the fight was over, these troops went in and a hurrah went up," testified one private of that exciting moment, "and they were in front and we were hurrahing and some of them held up their hands and we were all hollering at them." One of Stannard's men laconically noted: "I forgot all about the danger. Must have been excited." Northerners were even cheering Southerners as they stepped over the wall in defeat, offering them the contents of canteens and haversacks. One Confederate commented: "Many of them were taking off their hats as we went to the rear, and remarking that we had 'done well,' 'No troops could have done more,' and then offering us a part of their rations."[18]

There was a special bittersweet satisfaction in the victory for the men of Thompson's regiment. "The triumph of our brigade was one of the many wonderful retributions of the war. We were all surrendered at Harper's Ferry by Col [Dixon] Miles, and in this charge we fought the very men who captured us, and we took from them fourteen stands of

---

16. Thompson, *Personal Narrative*, pp. 45-46. Lieutenant John H. Drake was a native of Auburn, New York.
17. *Ibid.*, p. 46.
18. Supreme Court of Pennsylvania. May Term, 1891. #20, 30. Middle District. *Appeal of the Gettysburg Battlefield Memorial Association from the Decree of the Court of Common Pleas of Adams County. Paper Book of Appelants.* Testimony of Private Joseph McKeever; Sturtevant and Peck, *Pictorial History of the Thirteenth Vermont Volunteers*, p. 506; Stewart, *Pickett's Charge*, p. 250.

colors with 'Harper's Ferry' inscribed upon them, and several thousand of our own Springfield rifled muskets with full suits of accouterments, even to the belt plates with 'U.S.' on them. As they passed through our lines they recognized our regiment, and as they threw down their arms and accouterments they would say: 'There's what we got from you'uns at Harper's Ferry. We'uns have had 'em long enough.'"[19]

Division commander Alexander Hays was even more demonstrative in his celebration. The impetuous general had had two horses shot out from under him during the attack, and sixteen of his twenty staff members had fallen in the last several hours. But Hays was still giddy over the Cofederate repulse; after planting a big kiss on the young aide still by his side, he shouted out to the rest of his staff: "Boys, give me a flag! Get a flag, Corts; get a flag, Dave, and come on!" Riding side by side, the division chief and his men dragged captured Confederate flags behind them. "General Hays seized a battle flag marked 'Harper's Ferry,' rode up and down our line trailing the flag in the dirt and blood and shouted—'So we wipe out Harper's Ferry.' This raised rousing cheers from our brigade, and, for a time, made us the lions of our Corps."[20]

New Yorker Jacob H. Cole, wounded in the arm and leg in the vicious Wheatfield fighting of July 2, still lay behind enemy lines, in a torment of doubt and speculation over the outcome of the heavy firing he could hear on the distant slope of Cemetery Ridge. "The smoke after a while became so dense that I was unable to see anything further." It was his ears that finally told him of the ultimate outcome. "At last I heard the Union band play the 'Star Spangled Banner.' Then I knew that Pickett's grand charge at Gettysburg had failed and that the Union troops had won the victory." Relieved, the wounded soldier lay back to wait for someone—someone in blue—to carry him off to an aid station.[21]

19. Thompson, *Personal Narrative*, p. 45.
20. David Shields, "Capt. David Shields' Story," Section III, Fleming, *Life and Letters of Alexander Hays*, p. 464; Thompson, *Personal Narrative*, p. 45.
21. Cole, *Under Five Commanders*, pp. 205, 206.

Maj. William G. Mitchell, senior aide-de-camp and acting assistant adjutant general for General Hancock, was trying to make a swift ride for medical assistance for his downed chief, but the going was rough. Detouring around smoking shell craters and destroyed equipment, dodging downed tree limbs, swerving around knots of wounded men and prisoners making for the rear, Mitchell finally reached the Federal aid stations situated along the Taneytown Road.

Mitchell undoubtedly worked his way from station to station, looking for a surgeon and an ambulance to meet Hancock's needs. Assistant Surgeon Wafer at the Peter Frey regimental depot remembered Mitchell's visit very well, at least in retrospect: "An orderly came to the house in search of a Surgeon for Genl Hancock. I did not hear this, but my orderly told me afterwards that one surgeon refused to go out, and that the man went away threatening to report all those surgeons present." This concerned Wafer, a conscientious Canadian doctor serving with the 108th New York Volunteer Infantry. "I have always much regretted that I did not properly understand how matters stood with the Genl then, not only because my name might be mentioned among those who refused to go out, but because I would have been glad to have an opportunity to render a service to the gallant leader of the 2nd Corps."[22]

Success in finding transportation to move Hancock off the field proved to be just as unrewarding as the search for a surgeon. With most of the corps ambulances still busy moving the division hospitals to the new Rock Creek location, every vehicle the major encountered was already fully loaded, and heading to the rear. Second Division commander John Gibbon wrote that "after making my way off the field, I got into an ambulance and was about to start for the hospital, when Capt [*sic*] Mitchell, aide to Gen Hancock, rode up in search of one for the General, who had been wounded." Unfortunately, this transport was already filled to capacity, but Mitchell paused long enough to bring Gibbon up to date on the situation. "He informed me the enemy had been completely repulsed, and I drove to the hospital on Rock Creek greatly relieved in mind."[23]

Unable to find any help along the Taneytown Road, Mitchell finally spurred his horse along the trail of shattered men and hospital transports heading for the division medical facilities. The aide-de-camp

22. Wafer diary.
23. Gibbon, *Personal Recollections*, p. 168.

finally found Surgeon Alexander N. Dougherty, medical director of the Second Corps, overseeing the transportation of the wounded from the cluster of hospitals along the Granite School House Road back to the new Rock Creek site. The major quickly filled in Dougherty on the details, as he knew them, of Hancock's wound, then headed back for the field, picking up an ambulance on the way.

The Medical Director at once turned over the supervision of the evacuation to someone else, most likely to his assistant, Dr. LeBaron Monroe. Mounting his fat little horse, with another ambulance in tow, the surgeon galloped off after Mitchell.[24]

Frank Haskell still sat mounted on the ridge, surveying the carnage and destruction around him. In fact, he was almost unable to dismount. "I had been struck upon the thigh by a bullet, which I think must have glanced, and partially spent its force, upon my saddle. It had pierced the thick cloth of my trowsers, and two thicknesses of underclothing, but had not broken the skin; leaving me with an enormous bruise, that for a time benumbed the entire leg. At the time of receiving it, I heard the thump, and noticed it and the hole in the cloth, into which I thrust my finger; and I experienced a feeling of relief I am sure, when I found that my leg was not pierced."[25]

General Meade was riding up the rearward slope of Cemetery Ridge, accompanied only by his son who served as his aide-de-camp, heading for the lone mounted officer on the crest. A good bit of firing was still going on, and it was not readily evident to the new arrivals as they rode up the back side of the ridge that the Union had gained the advantage and repulsed the attack.

> As he arrived near me, coming up the hill, he asked in a sharp, eager voice: "How is it going here?"
>
> "I believe, General, the enemy's attack is repulsed:" I answered.
>
> Still approaching, and a new light began to come in his face, of gratified surprise, with a touch of incredulity, of which his voice was also the medium, he further asked:

24. Tucker, *Hancock the Superb*, p. 157; Hancock, *Reminiscences of Winfield Scott Hancock*, p. 21.
25. Byrne and Weaver, *Haskell of Gettysburg*, p. 189.

"*What? is the assault entirely repulsed?"*—his voice quicker and more eager than before.

"It is, Sir:" I replied.

By this time he was on the crest; and when his eye had for an instant swept over the field, taking in just a glance of the whole,—the masses of prisoners,—the numerous captured flags, which the men were derisively flaunting about,—the fugitives of the routed enemy, disappearing with the speed of terror in the woods,—partly at what I had told him, partly at what he saw, he said impressively, and his face was lighted: "*Thank God.*" And then his right hand moved as if it would have caught off his hat and waved it; but this gesture he suppressed, and instead he waved his hand and said, "Hur-rah." The son, with more youth in his blood, and less rank upon his shoulders, snatched off his cap, and roared out his three "hurrahs," right heartily.[26]

After surveying the field for several minutes, Meade passed on his orders to Haskell, charging the lieutenant to deliver them to the ranking officer on the field, then rode away with his son to see to the situation elsewhere on the field.[27]

The exertion, fatigue, and wound of the afternoon were beginning to be felt by Haskell, and he noted with distress the condition of his faithful mount. "My brave horse, *Dick,*—poor creature[,] his good conduct in the battle that afternoon had been complimented by a Brigadier,—was a sight to see. He was litterally [*sic*] covered with blood. Struck repeatedly, his right thigh had been ripped open in a ghastly manner by a piece of shell, and three bullets were lodged deep in his body; and from his wounds the blood oozed and ran down his sides and legs, and with the sweat formed a bloody foam. . . . I think, when I dismounted from my horse after the fight, that I was no very comly [*sic*] specimen of humanity. Drenched with sweat, the white of battle, by the reaction, now turned to burning red, I felt like a boiled

26. *Ibid.*, pp. 173-74. Meade had already heard of the repulse of the Confederate assault from Lt. John Egan of Woodruff's battery, just before riding up to Haskell. What he now was able to actually see from Haskell's position confirmed the earlier report, and gave the Union commander the proof he needed to celebrate. [George Meade, Letter to John Bachelder, May 6, 1882, Bachelder Papers; John Egan, Letter to George Meade, February 8, 1870, Copy in the Peter F. Rothermel Collection, Pennsylvania Division of Public Records.]

27. There has been some questions as to the veracity of this episode.

man; and had it not been for the exhilaration at results, I should have been miserable." Haskell hobbled about the crest, looking for someone to help him transfer his saddle to another horse; Dick, weak from loss of blood and exhaustion, was interested only in lying down.[28]

General Hancock still lay by the crumbling stone wall, keeping a tight hold on the pistol grip, maintaining the pressure on the handkerchief knotted around his thigh. Aide-de-camp Lt. J. B. Parker soon arrived; and as he bent over his commander, Henry H. Bingham, Hancock's judge-advocate, galloped up. Bingham's head had been grazed in the closeup fighting by the angle and the clump of trees, and now the captain, a bandage wrapped around his head, dismounted to assist Parker in attending the general. Stooping over his chief, Bingham related Confederate General Armistead's words and passed along the Southerner's personal papers and watch. Although Hancock grieved at the wounding of his old friend, he now knew with certainty that the attack had been decisively thrown back along his entire front.[29]

Major Mitchell, having been gone about fifteen to twenty minutes, now reined up with an ambulance, closely followed by Surgeon Dougherty and his ambulance. Dougherty remembered his first impression of General Hancock "lying on the hill slope, under a tree and facing the enemy. There was a deep, wide gash in his leg, near the groin." Surrounding Hancock were members of his staff, several of whom were wounded as well, including the Private Wells, his devoted standard-bearer.[30]

Dougherty quickly set about examining the general as best as he could under the existing field conditions. The wound was a severe puncture to the upper inner thigh, "an ugly one and ghastly to see. An

28. Byrne and Weaver, *Haskell of Gettysburg*, pp. 188, 189.
29. Hancock, *Reminiscences of Winfield Scott Hancock*, pp. 214-15; Tucker, *Hancock the Superb*, p. 156. Years later, Bingham wrote to his old commander that ". . . about fifteen minutes after I got Armistead's message and effects . . . I rode up to you in company with General [at that time Major] Mitchell. . . ." [Henry H. Bingham to Winfield Scott Hancock, January 5, 1869, Gettysburg National Military Park Library; Letter of Winfield Scott Hancock to Peter F. Rothermel, December 31, 1868, Civil War Library and Museum, Philadelphia, Pennsylvania.]
30. Alexander N. Dougherty, The *Washington D.C. Sunday Herald*, July 4, 1880; Henry H. Bingham to Winfield Scott Hancock, January 5, 1869.

onlooker has compared it to the stab of a butcher's knife." After loosening the makeshift tourniquet, the Second Corps Medical Director "thrust his forefinger to the knuckle into the wound and brought out from it an iron nail bent double." The initial probing of the gaping injury also brought out several splinters of wood, and a few small pieces of lead.[31]

The surgeon held up the trophies for the general to see: "This is what wounded you, General," said Dougherty; "and you are not so badly hurt as you think." Subsequent investigation would show that a minié ball had passed through the pommel of the general's saddle, carrying the wood and nail with it into Hancock's lower groin area. The fragments of lead doubtlessly chipped off the bullet as it contacted the saddle and the nail, and were carried by momentum into the wound. Dougherty's hasty probing, however, did not succeed in extracting the ball from the wound.[32]

The Second Corps commander assumed that the nail was the actual projectile that had wounded him. "They must be hard up for ammunition when they throw such shot as that," he quipped to the group gathered around him.[33]

Dougherty, despite his encouraging words, knew very well the seriousness of a wound this close to the torso; after replacing thc

---

31. Hancock, *Reminiscences of Winfield Scott Hancock*, p. 215; Benedict, *Army Life in Virginia*, p. 184.
32. Hancock, *Reminiscences of Winfield Scott Hancock*, p. 215; Benedict, *Army Life in Virginia*, p. 184. Surgeon Dougherty apparently tossed the nail aside after showing it to Hancock, since there is no further record of it.
33. Benedict, *Army Life in Virginia*, p. 184; Walker, *General Hancock*, pp. 144-45; W. G. Mitchell, Letter to Dr. L. W. O'Neal, September 20, 1880, Winfield Scott Hancock Vertical File, Gettysburg National Military Park Library; A. T. Freed, *The Life and Public Services of Winfield Scott Hancock* (Chicago: Henry A. Sumner and Co., 1880), p. 44. For years, there has been some question as to where the nail came from. Although it passed through the saddle, a superior quality saddle of the type used by Hancock should have had no nails in it. [George R. Stewart, Letter to Glenn Tucker, July 3, 1959, in the possession of Glenn Tucker.] However, during his ride along Union lines during the early afternoon bombardment, Hancock's mount became totally unmanageable. "The General was, therefore, obliged to borrow a horse from one of his staff—Captain Brownson [the Second Corps commissary of musters]. This was the horse, a very tall, light bay with a white nose, the General was riding when he was wounded." [Hancock, *Reminiscences of Winfield Scott Hancock*, p. 209.] The nail came from Brownson's saddle. For a more detailed discussion of the nail, see Gambone, *Hancock At Gettysburg*, pp. 271-72, n. 117.

tourniquet, the medical director made immediate preparations to transport the Second Corps commander to the division hospitals at Rock Creek. Before leaving, Hancock, his mind still on the battle, set off word with the ubiquitous Captain Bingham to Brig. Gen. John C. Caldwell, commanding the First Division of the Second Corps, informing him that he was now in charge of the entire corps. With that detail cared for, the wounded general was gently lifted into Mitchell's ambulance, the surgeon got in with Hancock, and the vehicle started off for the rear.[34]

Just as the ambulance was approaching the Taneytown Road, they met Captain Livermore, Second Corps ambulance chief. Livermore was riding along the lines, carefully supervising the evacuation and transportation of the wounded from the field. "Soon after the charge had been made, I met an ambulance between the Taneytown road and our line of battle coming off the field with General Hancock wounded, and this was the first I knew of that misfortune, I think."[35]

Hancock, however, was not quite content to stop being a general just yet. "When we had reached the vicinity of the Taneytown road, the general, who was somewhat excited, insisted upon halting for some purpose—I think to write a dispatch." Hancock dictated a somewhat rambling and disjointed message to Meade, urging the army commander to follow up the repulse by throwing the two relatively fresh corps at his disposal against the shattered Confederates. Surgeon Dougherty took it all down, scribbling furiously on a scrap of paper with a lead pencil he had pulled from his pocket.[36]

---

34. Tucker, *Hancock the Superb*, p. 157; Meade, *The Life and Letters of George Gordon Meade*, 2:134; Henry H. Bingham to Winfield Scott Hancock, January 5, 1869.
35. Livermore, *Days and Events*, p. 264.
36. *Ibid.*; Hancock, *Reminiscences of Winfield Scott Hancock*, pp. 215-16. The message read: "HEADQUARTERS, SECOND CORPS, July 3, 1863. Although I repulsed a tremendous attack, yet on seeing it from my left and advancing to the right, much to my sorrow, I found that the twelve guns on my salient had been removed by some one, whom I call upon you to hold accountable, as without them, with worse troops, I should certainly have lost the day. I arrived just in time to put a small battalion of infantry in the place occupied by those two batteries. I have never seen a more formidable attack, and if the Sixth and Fifth Corps [on the Union left at Cemetery Ridge and the Round Tops] have pressed, the enemy will be destroyed. The enemy must be short of ammunition, as I was shot with a tenpenny nail. I did not leave the field till the victory was entirely secured and the enemy no longer in sight. I am badly wounded, though I trust not seriously. I had to break the line to attack the enemy in flank on my right, where the enemy was most persistent

The party was now exposed to a new danger as it sat stationary on the road. "At this time the rebels had a piece of artillery posted in the vicinity of Gettysburg with which, at intervals of three or four minutes, they threw shot or shell down the Taneytown road which must have gone as far as Weed's Hill [Little Round Top], and it was directly in the range of those shots that the general caused the ambulance to halt." Livermore was anxious to get his important patient to the hospital safely, and recommended with some urgency that the party continue on. "I suggested to him that he had better move on a little, as the rebels were enfilading our line with their shots and we were directly within their range."[37]

Even though severely wounded, Hancock had not lost his short fuse or salty vocabulary. At Livermore's suggestion, he snapped back: "'We've enfiladed them—d--n them!'—and added that we had so completely beaten them that if other troops were only now sent in, we could rout them." Finishing the dispatch, Hancock spoke a few quiet words with his brother, Col. John Hancock, and then asked him to personally deliver the memo to Meade. (The colonel, assistant adjutant general of Caldwell's First Division, had heard of his brother's wounding, and ridden as quickly as possible to his side). Only when the colonel had disappeared in a cloud of dust, the message safely in his possession, did the general allow the ambulance to resume its course.[38]

Hancock's ambulance finally jostled into the Second Corps Hospital along Rock Creek. Even though in shock from loss of blood, Hancock was adamant that he be allowed to dictate a telegram to his

---

after the front attack was repelled. Not a rebel was in sight upright when I left. The line should be immediately restored and perfected. General Caldwell is in command of the corps, and I have directed him to restore the line. Your obedient servant, WINF'D S. HANCOCK, MAJOR-GENERAL. By A. N. Dougherty, Surgeon, and Medical Director Second Corps. General Meade." [*OR*, vol. 27, pt. 1, p. 366; Winfield Scott Hancock, Letter to Peter F. Rothermel, December 31, 1868; Alexander N. Dougherty, Letter to W. G. Mitchell, January 2, 1869 (copy attested by Winfield Scott Hancock); Winfield Scott Hancock, Letter to Peter F. Rothermel, January 9, 1869, Rothemel Papers, Pennsylvania Historical and Museum Commission, Division of Archives and Manuscripts.]

37. Livermore, *Days and Events*, p. 264; Letter of Winfield Scott Hancock to Peter F. Rothermel, December 31, 1868, Civil War Library and Museum, Philadelphia, Pennsylvania.

38. Livermore, *Days and Events*, p. 264; Tucker, *Hancock the Superb*, pp. 157-58.

wife Almira, who was spending some time at her mother's home in St. Louis. The general was in the habit of wiring her frequently when in action, and had sent her a message just that morning: "I am all right, so far." Now he dictated a message reading: "I am severely wounded, not mortally. Join me at once in Philadelphia. Parker and Miller, I fear, are gone up." Surgeon Dougherty advised that the critical nature of the wound should be mentioned, but Hancock refused, knowing the length of the trip that lay ahead of her. With the dispatch to his wife safely on its way to the military telegraph office, Hancock lay back in the ambulance to rest.[39]

Thomas Galwey and his intrepid party of 8th Ohio skirmishers were finally being allowed to retire from their advanced post. It was a sobering return trip. "When we reached the ditch of the Emmitsburg Pike on our way back, we beheld a sorry sight. Many of the wounded had been carried back to it during the fight. Others hobbled and crawled into it, some dying after reaching it. It was full of pools of blood, and the grass for some distance in front was saturated with blood. In the ditch along with many others in like condition, lay two of our sergeants, [John G.] Fairchild (Orderly) [Sergeant,] and [James] Kelly (Second) Sergeant; each with the lower part of the leg hanging by a piece of flesh to the rest of the limb. This brought the tears to my eyes, for they were both good men, brave soldiers, and favorites with everyone."[40]

"But we were only allowed to remain a few minutes with our poor wounded fellows, when we re-formed our badly shattered line, and as we ascended the hill down which we had come yesterday in gallant array, the artillery, who had seen us through all the fight, cheered us and spoke flattering words to us as we passed them." At last the bone-

39. Hancock, *Reminiscences of Winfield Scott Hancock*, p. 97. Another Hancock aide-de-camp, Capt. W. D. W. Miller, was "twice severely wounded on the 2d. . . ." [*OR*, vol. 27, pt. 1, p. 376.] Whether as surgeon, stenographer, or advisor, Doctor Dougherty was greatly appreciated by his commander. In his official report, Hancock singled out the easy-going doctor for special commendation. "Surg A. N. Dougherty, medical director of the corps, in the performance of his duties gave me entire satisfaction. No matter whether under fire of the enemy or not, he was always at his post." [*O.R.*, vol. 27, pt. 1, p. 376.]

40. Galwey, *The Valiant Hours*, p. 119.

tired Buckeye troops could relax a little. "We passed on, back over the Baltimore pike, down into a hollow, where we stretched ourselves out on the grass to rest. A detachment of the Provost Guard soon came and relieved us of our prisoners and captured colors."[41]

After seeing to the gathering together and situating of his fractured little command, and attending to some basic paperwork, Captain Thompson went off to see for himself the aftermath of the massive charge. "Just as the sun was setting, I went to the crest of the hill and took a look at the field. No words can depict the ghastly picture. The track of the great charge was marked by bodies of men in all possible positions, wounded, bleeding, dying and dead. Near the line where the final struggle occurred, the men lay in heaps, the wounded wriggling and groaning under the weight of the dead among whom they were entangled. In my weak and exhausted condition I could not long endure the gory, ghastly spectacle. I found my head reeling, the tears flowing, and my stomach sick at the sight."[42]

In the growing twilight, Thompson worked his way back to his company of the 111th New York, and made ready for the coming night. The 111th was a mere shadow of its former self—every field officer had fallen in the battle. "I had just nine men in line and the two color corporals with their colors that night. The rest of my regiment were all busy in the care of prisoners, removing the wounded, or burying the dead." In some regiments, however, the care of the wounded was left solely to the ambulance men and stretcher-bearers. "Can we not go and care for the wounded?" lamented Sgt. Alfred Carpenter of the 1st Minnesota in a letter home. "No, another attack is expected, and every man must be in his place. Hospital attendants must take care of the wounded till darkness closes down upon us."[43]

41. *Ibid.*

42. Thompson, *Personal Narrative*, p. 46. The captain wrote in 1910: "For months the spectre haunted my dreams, and even after forty seven years it comes back as the most horrible vision I have ever conceived." [*Ibid.*]

43. *New York at Gettysburg*, 1:143, 285; Thompson, *Personal Narrative*, pp. 46-47; Willson, *Disaster, Struggle, Triumph*, p. 188; Alfred Carpenter, Letter to his brother, July 30, 1863, copy at Minnesota Historical Society.

The ambulances were hard at work in the failing light, and the sudden surge of wounded at the primary stations along the Taneytown Road following the attack was creating a serious backlog of patients. "As soon as the firing had abated a little, the wounded began to arrive in vast numbers," wrote Assistant Surgeon Francis Wafer at the Peter Frey station. "In the course of an hour fully a quarter of an acre about the house where I was was pretty thickly covered with victims of the struggle, the greater number of the enemy, many of these officers of high rank."[44]

"The enemy were loudest by far in their outcries for help. I have found this to be invariably the case on subsequent occasions. This I am not prepared to explain unless it be that they had no confidence in our humanity & dread willful neglect—but I can confidently and earnestly assert that I have never seen any distinction in their treatment—more than attending to our own first, which is our duty."[45]

The sky was clouding up now, and a moderate rain slanted down over the battlefield, settling the dust on the roads, and bringing down the temperature. For the multiple thousands of wounded clustered shelterless around the hospitals and aid stations, or still laying helpless on the field, the slow steady rainfall soon drenched their wool uniforms, at first cooling their feverish wounds, then leaving them chilled and shivering as night came on. Countless rivulets and rills carried the runoff of battlefield blood and putrefying bodies into the local streams and ponds.

Lt. Frank Haskell had finally found someone to help him transfer his saddle to another horse. After seeing that Meade's orders were passed on to the senior field commander, the bruised lieutenant set off on foot through the tangled confusion of the backside of Cemetery Ridge, heading toward the Taneytown Road in search of his commanding officer. "I hobbled on among the Hospitals in search of General Gibbon. . . . To find the General was no easy matter. I inquired for both Gnls Hancock and Gibbon—I knew well enough that they would be together,—and for the hospitals of the 2nd Corps."[46]

44. Wafer diary.

45. *Ibid.*

46. Byrne and Weaver, *Haskell of Gettysburg*, pp. 189, 190.

It had been difficult enough to find the hospitals yesterday; today it was much worse to find one *particular* hospital. The rearward slope of Cemetery Ridge and the Taneytown Road area was clogged with a vast conglomeration of prisoners, the wounded of both armies, teamsters, provost guards, couriers, generals with their staffs, stragglers, ambulances, forage wagons, ammunition wagons, forge wagons, and batteries.

There seemed to be nothing left to do but ask passersby as he painfully limped along. Yet the responses he received to his questions only muddied an already confusing situation.

> My search was attended by many incidents that were provokingly humorous. The stupidity of most men is amazing. I would ask of a man: "Do you know, sir, where the 2nd Corps hospitals are?"
>
> "The 12th Corps Hospital is there!"
>
> Then I would ask sharply: "Did you understand me to ask for the 12th Corps hospital?"
>
> "No!"
>
> "Then why tell me what I do not ask or care to know." Then stupidity would stare, or mutter about the ingratitude of some people for kindness. Did I ask for the Generals I was looking for, they would announce the interesting fact, in reply, that they had seen some other Generals. Some were sure that Gnl Hancock, or Gibbon, was dead. They had seen his dead body.—This was a falsehood, and they knew it.—Then it was Gnl Longstreet.—This was also, as they knew, a falsehood.[47]

Never before in the war had such an enormous host of wounded soldiers been packed together so tightly into one narrow strip of land.

> The whole neighborhood in rear of the field became one vast hospital, of miles in extent. Some could walk to the hospitals, such as could not, were taken upon stretchers from the places where they fell, to selected points, and thence the ambulances bore them, a miserable load, to their destination. Many were brought to the buildings along the Taney town [*sic*] road and too badly wounded to be carried

47. *Ibid.*, p. 190.

> further, died and were buried there, Union and Rebel soldier together. At every house, and barn, and shed the wounded were; by many a cooling brook, or many a shady slope, or grassy glade the red flags beckoned them to their tented asylums; and there they gathered, in numbers a great army, a mutilated, bruised mass of humanity.[48]

The attitude and morale of the men varied greatly, but was mostly upbeat—the rush of adrenaline produced by the charge and repulse of the Confederates had not yet totally worn off.

> The men are generally cheerful, and even those with frightful wounds, often are talking with animated faces of nothing but the battle and the victory; but some are downcast, their faces distorted with pain. Some have undergone the Surgeon's work; some, like men at a ticket office, await impatiently their turn,—to have an arm or leg cut off. Some walk about with an arm in a sling; some sit idly upon the ground; some at full length lie upon a little straw, or a blanket, with their brawny, now bloodstained, limbs bare, and you may see where the minie bullet has struck, or the shell has torn.[49]

"Such things I saw as I rode along," continued Haskell, who had apparently mounted up somewhere along the way. Finally, all the questions paid off. "At last I found the Generals.—Gnl Gibbon was sitting in a chair that had been *borrowed* some where, with his wounded shoulder bare, and an attendant was bathing it with cold water.—Gnl Hancock was near by in an ambulance.—They were at the tents of the 2nd Corps hospitals, which were on Rock Run [*sic*]."[50]

Gibbon had been brought to the hospital by ambulance shortly after the repulse of the Southern charge. "Soon after my arrival at the hospital Gen Hancock reached there with a very ugly wound in his thigh," remembered Gibbon in later years. Surgeons were soon at work examining each general, Gibbon as he sat in his pilfered chair, Hancock while stretched out recumbent in the ambulance. Gibbon was greatly relieved to learn that he had been shot from the front, not the back. He

---

48. *Ibid.*
49. *Ibid.*, p. 191.
50. *Ibid.*, pp. 191-92.

was concerned that his riding in front of some of the Union troops, while attempting to get them to advance on the enemy, may have led to his injury. Nearby, Chaplain William Henry Stevens of the 148th Pennsylvania Volunteers was at Hancock's side as his wound was further probed and more debris removed. "The remarks made by the General when told of the discovery were not exactly religious," noted Stevens rather astringently.[51]

For the common foot soldiers laid out nearby, there was often a long wait for medical care, even after reaching the hospital. Generals and higher echelon officers always rated better care—it was an unwritten rule of the military that the men knew all too well. "Those seriously hurt merely looked around with a quiet beseeching look, following the movements of the busy surgeons with the hope that their turn will come next," wrote an officer of his visit to a division hospital on July 3:

> those slightly wounded talked pleasantly & even cheerfully bantering each other on the extent of the leave of absence likely to send them home.
>
> How many days have you got, John?
>
> Oh, only twenty days in the arm? but I guess I can keep it sorc ten days more.
>
> Mine's a sixty day fellow just below the hip.[52]

So frequent and common had wounds become that the average soldier could accurately grade them by the amount of furlough he could expect to receive.

"As I approached Gnl Gibbon, when he saw me he began to 'hurrah' and wave his right hand,—he had heard the result," continued his staff aide. "I said: 'O, General, long and *well* may you wave,'—and he shook me warmly by the hand. Gnl Gibbon was struck by a bullet in the left shoulder, which had passed from the front, through the flesh, and out behind, fracturing the shoulder blade, and inflicting a severe, but not dangerous[,] wound. He thinks he was the mark of a sharp shooter of the enemy, hid in the bushes, near where he and I sat so long during the cannonade. . . ."[53]

---

51. Gibbon, *Personal Recollections*, pp. 168, 170; Muffly, *The Story of Our Regiment*, pp. 198.
52. Adolfo F. Cavada, Diary, July 3 entry, copy in Adolfo F. Cavada Vertical File, Gettysburg National Military Park Library.
53. Byrne and Weaver, *Haskell of Gettysburg*, p. 192.

"And then at Gnl Gibbon[']s request, I had to tell him, and a large voluntary crowd of the wounded who pressed around, now, for the wounds they showed, not rebuked for closing up to the Generals, the story of the fight. I was nothing loth; and I must say, though I used sometimes before the war, to make speeches, that I never had so enthusiastic an audience before. Cries of 'good,' 'glorious,' frequently interrupted me, the storming of the wall was applauded by enthusiastic tears and the waving of battered, bloody hands." Men who had followed ineffectual and incompetent leaders for two years could not restrain their emotions, and, at least for now, the wounds did not seem quite so serious, or the pain nearly as severe.[54]

It was a time of celebration and rejoicing, and the men turned to Hancock, asking him to deliver some appropriate remarks. Over Surgeon Dougherty's vehement protests, the Second Corps commander struggled out of the ambulance, and rose unsteadily to his feet to say a few words. After a sentence or two, however, the shock and loss of blood caught up with the general, and he slowly toppled backwards into the arms of his aides. His men tenderly laid him back in the ambulance, and there he stayed, effectively ending any further speechmaking for the day. One witness vividly remembered the scene, and "the blood from his [Hancock's] wound as it dripped from the wagon to the ground." [55]

Not all of the wounded from the division hospitals on Granite School House Road had made it back to the new Rock Creek location when the medical facilities were evacuated during the midday shelling. Instead of following the caravan of Second Corps ambulances east to the creek, Lt. Charles Fuller of the 61st New York was still waiting to have his shattered leg removed. When ambulance after ambulance had passed him by, he was finally picked up and manually carried south by his friends. "The boys who were toting me came to a stone house with a wide piazza clear around it [probably the eight-room house of Jacob Weikert, on the Taneytown Road behind the Round Tops, which had

54. *Ibid.*

55. J. T. Riemer, "General Hancock and Dr. Read," *Bulletin of the Historical Society of Montgomery County, Pennsylvania*, (Spring 1972): 173; Walker, *General Hancock*, pp. 144-45; C. A. Richardson, Letter to John Bachelder, May 8, 1868, Bachelder Papers; Muffly, *The Story of our Regiment*, p. 332.

been evacuated earlier in the day by the Fifth Corps medical department]. I was laid on the floor of it, which made a hard bed. I ached in every bone, but there was nothing to do but 'grin and bear it.'"[56]

Other soldiers of the Second Corps were soon carried in to this way station for evacuating of the wounded. "After a while Frank Garland of Co G was brought and laid on the floor near me. He could raise upon his elbow, but his breathing was painful to hear. A bullet had gone through his lungs and every time they filled a portion of the air went through the wound with a ghastly sound. I said to him, 'Are you badly wounded, Frank?' He replied, 'Oh, yes!'"[57]

Somehow, Fuller had been passed over during the morning meal at the First Division hospital, probably when he had gotten himself carried up to the very edge of the operating tables. Now the lack of food was starting to catch up with the weakened officer. "I had eaten nothing since the morning of the day before, and was faint. Some of our drummer boys found a bin of ground oats, and they made a gruel that tasted good, and I made quite a meal of it."[58]

Although well to the south of the incoming artillery shells of the afternoon bombardment, the wounded men at the Weikert House could not escape the rumble and crash of the cannonade. "We were out of range of it, but we could not hide from the tremble of the ground—the surface of the earth at that place shook and quivered from the terrible concussion of the artillery. The roar was enough to deafen one, and inspire the dread that no one would be left alive and unhurt."[59]

Now as the tedious afternoon gradually turned into dusk, the New Yorker was still waiting—this time for transportation to the division hospitals on Rock Creek, where he could finally get his wounded leg amputated. "During the day friends occasionally poured water on my wounds, which, doubtless, kept the swelling down."[60]

The Second Corps hospitals at Rock Creek were growing by leaps and bounds with each passing minute. Ambulances were running

---

56. Fuller, *Personal Recollections of the War of 1861*, p. 101; Coco, *A Vast Sea of Misery*, pp. 68-70.
57. Fuller, *Personal Recollections of the War of 1861*, pp. 101, 100.
58. *Ibid.*
59. *Ibid.*, p. 100.
60. *Ibid.*

instead relays from the battlefield now that darkness had fallen, heading down the Taneytown Road to the Granite School House Road where the hospitals had recently been located. Turning east, they hurried down the short road past the artillery reserves, then turned south to the George Bushman Farm. The Twelfth Corps hospitals had set up at the Bushman Farm, with some wounded occupying the house and barn; most of the patients, however, were under shelter in hospital tents. The Second Corps ambulances turned in at the Bushman Farm lane, heading eastward past the farmstead and through the property to the site on Rock Creek that ambulance chief Livermore had selected. With at least three right-hand turns and the rugged trip over Bushman's farmland, the agonizing ambulance ride must have been one that few of the wounded ever forgot.[61]

The Rock Creek hospital was located in a marked convolution in the course of the local waterway. The creek, after flowing in a roughly southward fashion, suddenly snaked east above the hospital site, swinging again to the south for a short space, then turning unexpectedly westward toward the battlefield. After flowing past the expanding Second Corps hospitals for several hundred feet, it cut to the south, then abruptly veered back to the east. After another short stretch, the run turned to continue it's mostly southerly heading. The hospitals were set up in the middle of this reverse "S," at the two peninsulas of land jutting out from opposite banks.

As the ambulances completed their trip, they were directed onto the level north bank of Rock Creek, on the western peninsula bordered by the zigzag watercourse. Stretcher-bearers and aides quickly unloaded the stretchers and helped the walking wounded out of the vehicles. The drivers promptly whipped up their horses and clattered away for another trip.

Livermore had originally intended that the wounded would then ford or be carried over the creek and situated as comfortably as possible on the hillside bank of the eastern jut of land, "sheltered by the trees and having perfect drainage." However, the massive influx of

---

61. Coco, *A Vast Sea of Misery*, p. 102. It must have been frustrating to the Second Corps medical people to pass the Twelfth Corps Hospitals, which had somehow managed to be the only corps that successfully brought all their hospital equipment with them (in spite of army orders specifically to the contrary). With ample supplies and under shelter of a colony of roomy hospital tents, the wounded must have wondered why they passed by this picture-perfect hospital only to end up in a dismal creek bottom with almost no shelter.

wounded quickly swamped the newly located hospitals and any elaborate plans for placement of the wounded. While much of the Third Division wounded were moved to the hillside on the south bank of the stream, the majority of the Second Division casualties were laid out on the low flat northern bank of Rock Creek.[62]

Another unexpected development was the detour taken by the First Division when it evacuated its wooded camp near the Granite School House. Probably seeking room to expand and another source of fresh water, it headed northeast, away from it's sister divisions, ending up "near the sawmill on the Baltimore Pike." This was the William McAllister Mill, a local landmark that had been serving as an underground railroad station, just north of the bridge over Rock Creek. The location was ideal except for one problem—by the time the First Division arrived, the building was already being used as a hospital by the Twelfth Corps. Reluctantly, Medical Director R. C. Stiles turned his entourage around and headed south along Rock Creek, pulling up by the other two divisions shortly before midnight. There they added their own collection of wounded to the rapidly growing number of incapacitated troops on the level bottomland of the northern creek bank.[63]

The surgical staff of the divisional hospitals had accompanied the first load of wounded when the hospitals started their move; they immediately set up the operating tables, laid out their instruments, and went to work, scarcely slowed by the unexpected move. The commissary departments remained on Granite School House Road until the afternoon meal had been distributed, then packed up their borrowed pots, pans, and utensils, and headed out for the new location. Within two hours of the move, they were fully operational again, and supper was passed out as quickly as possible to the swelling ranks of the wounded.[64]

As darkness fell, the amputating tables continued their gruesome task unabated, dimly illumined by the flickering light of lanterns and lamps hanging on poles around the doctors. Without the medical wagons and their stores, even the surgical tents were little more than improvised affairs, cobbled together from whatever supplies came readily to hand. "Our temporary hospital consisted of just a frame-work constructed of wooden posts and cross pieces with a fly, and a tent used as a covering," wrote one First Division surgeon. The surgical

62. Livermore, *Days and Events*, pp. 258-59; Dwinelle, *Medical Report*.

63. Dwinelle, *Medical Report*; Coco, *A Vast Sea of Misery*, pp. 76-77.

64. Dwinelle, *Medical Report*.

team used this meager shelter to keep the increasingly heavy rainfall from interfering with their work; even something as simple as moving freely around the operating table became increasingly difficult as bloody mud caked their shoes.[65]

The rest of the expanding hospital complex was shrouded in darkness. Occasional pinpricks of light floated through the gloom as dressing surgeons moved through the mass of men on the ground, examining and dressing wounds, or sadly shaking their heads over injuries that could not be fixed. It was a challenge just to keep from stepping on the casualties, so tightly were their bodies laid together.[66]

Men shouted and bellowed out to each other in the darkness, their hearing dimmed temporarily by the high decibel roar of the afternoon artillery. The wooded slope of Rock Creek was abnormally still, no birds calling or insects shrilling. All animal life had seemingly fled from the unearthly sounds of the cannon, and the groans of pain, the cries of fear, the screams, hysteric babbling, and murmured prayers of the growing community of wounded only accentuated the awesome hush of nature.[67]

For Capt. Jack Adams, after being abandoned by the road and then subjected to a wild ambulance ride, arriving at the hospital had done little to reassure him. "They laid us on the ground on the side of the hill, near a stream called Cub Run [*sic*]. This was the field hospital of the 2d corps, Dr. [J. Franklin] Dyer, my regimental surgeon, in charge. He soon visited me, and found that one bullet had entered my groin and had not come out, the other had passed through my right hip. I asked him what he thought of it and he said, 'It is a bad wound, John, a very bad wound.'"[68]

Adams soon had other acquaintances to keep him company; though certainly not in the best of circumstances, they quickly brought him up to date on the battlefield action he had missed.

---

65. Albert Vander Veer, Vander Veer Papers, DB 560, Albany Institute of History and Art, Albany New York; transcribed copy in the 66th New York Infantry Vertical File, Gettysburg National Military Park Library.

66. *Ibid.*

67. Dwinelle, *Medical Report*; Coco, *A Vast Sea of Misery*, p. 189; Coco, *On the Bloodstained Field II*, pp. 86-87.

68. Adams, *Reminiscences of the Nineteenth Massachusetts*, p. 69. Dyer was surgeon of the 19th Massachusetts, and Second Division Medical Director. He would add Surgeon Dwinelle's duties as surgeon-in-charge of the Second Division Hospital to his own responsibilities when Dwinelle became surgeon-in-charge of all Second Corps Hospitals on July 7. [Dwinelle, *Medical Report.*]

"Officers of the regiment began to come in, and soon there were seven of us lying side by side. They told the story of the battle. Lieutenants [Sherman S.] Robinson and [Herman] Donath had been killed, also many of our bravest and best men. My company the day before had numbered fifteen, officers and men. Only Lieutenant [Edmund] Rice and five men remained. They also told me how well our boys had fought; that at last they had met the rebels in an open field and had won a substantial victory. . . . It was glorious news," wrote Adams exultantly; "it revived me, and my wounds pained me less than before."[69]

Sometime after dark, General Gibbon, his shoulder wound neatly bandaged, and General Hancock, still weak from shock and loss of blood, were evacuated from the Second Corps hospitals. "After remaining there for several hours during which authentic reports were received together with various details of the fight," wrote Gibbon in later years, "I left the hospital in an ambulance for Westminster, thirty miles distant." Westminster was the nearest railhead known to have been unaffected by the Confederate invasion, and some wounded, especially senior officers, were already heading out the rain-drenched road to Maryland.[70]

"By the custom of the service the General [Gibbon] had the right to have me along with him while away with his wound," wrote Lieutenant Haskell; "but duty and inclination attracted me still to the field, and I obtained the General's consent to stay." The staff aide did go along as far as Westminster, however, just to see his commander safely on board the train. As they had on the battlefield, the two men, general and aide, soldiers by profession and friends by choice, rode side by side as the ambulance rattled away into the night.[71]

---

69. Adams, *Reminiscences of the Nineteenth Massachusetts*, pp. 69-70. Lt. Sherman Robinson had shouted: "We are in for it" to Adams when he saw Sickles' line buckle on July 2. This proved to be the last words Adams was to hear from his friend's lips. [*Ibid.*, p. 66.]

70. Gibbon, *Personal Recollections*, p. 170. General Sickles had already evacuated to Westminster, heading out of town about 11:00 p.m. on July 2. Too unstable to be moved by ambulance, he was hand-carried by a forty-man stretcher team to the distant railhead. [Potter, *Three Years with the Army of the Potomac*, p. 60.]

71. Byrne and Weaver, *Haskell of Gettysburg*, pp. 192-93.

With medical care well under way at the new facility, several surgeons were sent back to the barns and woods around the Granite School House. Some wounded had been left behind when the hospital evacuated to the rear, so critically injured that they were incapable of surviving the bumpy ambulance journey to the new hospital site. The surgeons checked in with those monitoring their progress, arranged transportation for the ones stable enough to now be moved, and cared for any newly arrived wounded seeking shelter from the rain.[72]

"The most profound calm reigned now, where a few hours before so furious a tempest had raged," wrote one general officer, looking out across the field of carnage. "The moon, with her smiling face, mounted up in the starry heavens, as at Chancellorsville. Her pale light shone equally upon the living and dead, the little flowers blooming in the grass as well as on the torn bodies lying in pools of clotted blood. Dead bodies were everywhere. On no field of battle have I ever seen them in such numbers."[73]

"Beyond the line of advanced sentinels, the wounded still lay where they had fallen, calling for assistance or asking for water. Their cries died away without any reply in the silence of the night, for the enemy was close by, and it was a dangerous undertaking to risk advancing into the space which separated us. In making an attempt, an officer of my staff drew three shots, which whistled unpleasantly near his ears. All labors of charity were necessarily put off till the next morning. It is sad to think that this was a sentence of death to numbers of the unfortunate," somberly noted the general, pronouncing a memoriam on the many that would not see the light of another sunrise.[74]

"Night came on, and then the only sounds to be heard were the groans of the wounded, the prayers of the dying, and the strident noise of shelter tents and clothes of all sorts being torn up for bandages," remembered Thomas Galwey of that gruesome night. "After doing all I

72. Dwinelle, *Medical Report.*

73. P. Regis de Trobriand, *Four Years with the Army of the Potomac*, trans. George K. Dauchy (Boston: Ticknor and Company, 1889), p. 512.

74. *Ibid.*, pp. 512-13.

could for such of my own wounded as I could find, I lay down and slept."[75]

Ambulance traffic continued to roll throughout the night between the battlefield and the Seconds Corps hospitals, and the heavy travel over saturated terrain soon turned the farm lanes and market roads into a muddy, rutted morass. Captain Thomas Livermore rode from place to place on the littered field, encouraging his weary ambulancemen as they gathered the wounded from the field. Even those herculean efforts did not satisfy everyone. "Before nine o'clock I think we had collected all our wounded, but General Webb complained to the authorities at headquarters that his wounded were not collected," wrote Livermore of that grueling night's work. "I, upon being informed of this, asserted that all were collected that we could find, and I believe that a renewed search in the places indicated by General Webb confirmed my statement. I am inclined to think that General Webb had heard of wounded whom we had taken up after he had heard of them, or else referred to men who upon search proved to be outside our skirmish lines, but whose groans and calls could be heard through the darkness."[76]

For the stretcher-bearers and ambulancemen, these unreachable sufferers were the hardest to bear; so close, and yet so entirely out of reach. "We ventured out, I believe, beyond our skirmish lines, but as the rebel skirmishers a few yards in front fired at every one they could see, we could not get to those wounded who were within sight of them." Even though severely disappointed, the ambulancemen escaped serious injury because "the darkness favored us very much."[77]

"After we had cleared the field of the wounded, we took those who had been carried to the houses and barns along the Taneytown road." Horrifying and bloody sights appeared at each location, some so ghastly and inconceivable that they almost beggared description. "One poor fellow I found in a cow shed lying on his face. A cannon shot had carried away all the flesh of his hams so that his bones were visible. He was not complaining in the least. I asked him if he desired to be moved. He said in a calm tone that he did; that if he lay there he

75. Galwey, *The Valiant Hours*, p. 120.
76. Livermore, *Days and Events*, p. 266.
77. *Ibid.*

should surely die, and that if he got to a hospital he might live. He told me that he was an artilleryman, and that his position in the battery caused him to stand with his side toward the enemy, and that a shot coming from the front had gone through his hams from side to side. He said he hated to be shot in the rear, and seemed to care more for that than for being so grievously hurt."[78]

Captain Livermore immediately summoned his nearest stretcher crew. "I had some men lift this poor fellow in an ambulance, and neither while they did so nor as the train moved away over the rough road did I hear a complaint from the brave man." With that primary station cleared of transportable wounded, the ambulance chief and his men wearily moved down the road to the next aid station. The twinkle of sperm lamps and the moans of the sufferers made them easy enough to find in the darkness. The job seemed to be endless one, with new wounded constantly arriving to take the place of the ones Livermore and his crews were hauling away.[79]

Night after night of strenous activity was beginning to take a toll on the young ambulance chief. "Having very little sleep for three nights, I found myself so sleepy that I was obliged to keep my horse trotting, for when he walked I fell asleep. I found also during the day and night that it was necessary for me to drink whiskey to keep myself up, and it was astonishing to see how much of it without water or sugar I drank without feeling it."[80]

It was dangerous work evacuating the wounded from the field, and the Second Corps ambulances and crews were not escaping unscathed. "The losses from my ambulance corps were six or seven horses shot, six or seven men shot, and three ambulances struck by cannon shot," continued Livermore, obviously deeply concerned with the performance of his new command, "and I believe that this list of casualties was taken at headquarters as a guaranty that my command had been under fire to the full extent required by its duties."[81]

No Union ambulances were going to reach Jacob H. Cole of the 57th New York this night, still lying wounded on the field, out beyond the

78. *Ibid.*, pp. 266-67.
79. *Ibid.*, p. 267.
80. *Ibid.*
81. *Ibid.*

Emmitsburg Road. "In the early part of the night the moon shone very bright, and as I lay within the rebel lines I ascertained that the rebels were about to retreat. This I learned by overhearing General Lee order General Longstreet to leave a strong picket force and to withdraw the troops under cover of the darkness." As threatening clouds began to obscure the moon, the dim flickering lanterns of the Northern ambulances could be seen bobbing and swaying on the distant slopes of Cemetery Ridge, the vehicles jarring and jouncing over the rough terrain of that vast bloody field.[82]

Livermore's ambulances rolled into the Jacob Weikert farmyard well after dark, looking for any Second Corps wounded to transport to the Rock Creek divisional hospitals. By now, the property that had been abandoned by the Fifth Corps in the afternoon was filled again with wounded from the Second, Third, and Fifth Corps, carried in and laid intermingled in any and every available space. "The approaches [to the house] were crowded with wounded, dying and dead," wrote a young girl from town, who stopped by to check on her friends on her way back to Gettysburg. "The air was filled with moanings, and groanings. As we passed on toward the house, we were compelled to pick our steps in order that we might not tread on the prostrate bodies."[83]

For the civilian population, the utter disbelief and shock of having their property, their barns, even their very homes brusquely invaded by bleeding men and gruff strangers with dirty boots was forcefully brought home to young Tillie Pierce. "When we entered the house we found it also filled with the wounded. We hardly knew what to do or where to go. They, however, removed most of the wounded, and thus after a while made room for the family."[84]

Moved with compassion by the plight of these shattered soldiers, Tillie and her hosts set about trying to be of help to these unexpected houseguests. "As soon as possible, we endeavored to make ourselves useful by rendering assistance in this heartrending state of affairs. I remember that Mrs. Weikert went through the house, and after searching awhile, brought all the muslin and linen she could spare.

---

82. Cole, *Under Five Commanders*, p. 206.
83. Tillie Pierce Alleman, *At Gettysburg: Or What a Girl Saw and Heard of the Battle. A True Narrative.* (New York: W. Lake Borland, 1886), p. 72.
84. *Ibid.*

This we tore into bandages and gave them to the surgeons, to bind up the poor soldier's wounds."[85]

Some surgeons had finally arrived at the house, and "amputating benches had been placed about the house." Such a sight as this had never been witnessed in Gettysburg before, and young Tillie was stunned by what she saw. "I was looking out one of the windows facing the front yard. Near the basement door, and directly underneath the window I was at, stood one of these benches. I saw them lifting the poor men upon it, then the surgeons sawing and cutting off arms and legs, then again probing and picking bullets from the flesh."[86]

No matter how fast the surgeons worked, the backlog of mangled bodies kept increasing. "Some of the soldiers fairly begged to be taken next, so great was their suffering, and so anxious were they to obtain relief. I saw the surgeons hastily put a cattle horn over the mouths of the wounded ones, after they were placed on the bench. At first I did not understand the meaning of this[,] but upon inquiry, soon learned that that was their mode of administering chloroform, in order to produce unconsciousness. But the effect in some instances was not produced; for I saw the wounded throwing themselves wildly about, and shrieking with pain while the operation was going on." Rushed by the relentless influx of the wounded, some of the doctors apparently were not being careful to make sure that full unconsciousness was achieved before beginning their surgery.[87]

"To the south of the house, and just outside of the yard, I noticed a pile of limbs higher than the fence. It was a ghastly sight! Gazing upon these, too often the trophies of the amputating bench, I could have no other feeling, than that the whole scene was one of cruel butchery." For at least one young girl, the innocence of youth came to an abrupt, screaming end on this muggy Friday night in July.[88]

It had been a thirsty and inhospitable stay at the Weikert Farm since midday for Lt. Charles Fuller of the 61st New York. A Union lieutenant, Ziba Graham of the 16th Michigan, on his way back to the line after having a tooth pulled at a divisional hospital, discovered the problem

85. *Ibid.*
86. *Ibid.*, pp. 72-73.
87. *Ibid.*, p. 73.
88. *Ibid.*, p. 74.

at the Weikert barnyard. "I called at a large house for a drink of water; I saw that the well crank had been removed. I turned to a rebel captain who was lying on the grass and asked him if he knew where it had gone to; he said that but a few moments before the owner of the house had taken it off, declaring he was not going to have his well pumped dry by rebel soldiers, and that they wasted the water. This captain begged that I might get it again."[89]

Graham looked around the farmyard, pondering what to do. "There were some fifty rebel wounded in the yard, beside a few of our own men. The surgeons who had been with them, and who had partially gone around in their first examination, had cleared out and left them on the commencement of the firing, and with the fever of their gunshot wounds they were thirsting for water."[90]

The Michigan lieutenant had already seen enough needless suffering for one day. Incensed at the callousness of farmer Weikert toward these desperately wounded men, Graham set out to find the ungracious host. "I went into the house, found this man, a mean Dutchman, buried in the bosom of his family, and his family buried in the bowels of the cellar, they having taken safe refuge from the hail of iron which was bursting in every direction. I ordered him to give me the well crank. He first refused. Just at that time a shell struck his chimney, and the noise and rattle of the falling brick nearly frightened him to death. I threatened to shoot him if he did not give me the crank; this brought it out of its hiding place back of the stairway."[91]

Graham lost no time in making use of the recovered pump handle. "I went out, watered the boys, put two of the least wounded in charge of it and then left, receiving the thanks of all." Lieutenant Fuller and his gravely wounded companion could now have at least a cool drink of water while waiting for surgical care.[92]

---

89. Ziba B. Graham, *On to Gettysburg: Ten Days from My Diary of 1863.* (Detroit: Winn and Hammond, Printers and Binders, 1893), p. 13.
90. *Ibid.*
91. *Ibid.*
92. Ziba Graham added a short postlude to this story in later years: "Every visit I have since made to Little Round Top, I have seen 'old Wikert's' [*sic*] son—his father is now dead—telling interested hearers of 'the wonderful acts of heroism' his father and he did in taking care of the wounded in their yard that fearful day, and how kind the government was to recognize their services."

"That evening about 10 o'clock, an ambulance came for me," wrote Fuller, "and I was taken to the ground selected for the 2d Corps hospital. It was another rough ride across lots. Once there I was taken out of my stretcher, the one Phil Comfort took me off the field on, and taken at once to the operating table."[93]

At long last, after being trapped on the battlefield, after attempts to transport by hand, by back, by stretcher and by ambulance, after promises of treatment and forced evacuations, after being shunted off to another hospital, the New York lieutenant's wounds were finally going to receive medical treatment. "A napkin was formed into a tunnel shape, a liberal supply of chloroform poured into it and the thing placed over my nose and mouth. I was told to take in long breaths. To me it seemed a long time before the effects came, probably it was a short time, but at last my head seemed to grow big and spin around. At this stage I remember a doctor had his fingers in the wound in the shoulder and said to the others 'Here is a fine chance for a resection.' I did not know what that meant, but learned afterwards." With that, Fuller sank into welcome unconsciousness as the surgeons set to work.[94]

Capt. Azor H. Nickerson of the 8th Ohio struggled back to consciousness, images of the agonizing ambulance ride still fresh in his mind. The two-story log house of the Widow Guinn was dimly visible outside as

> . . . the nurses, at the barn where we next found ourselves, revived us with brandy.
>
> Here I found that the attending surgeon [Harry McKindree McAbee] was an old friend from my native State, and I felt that he would not hide the truth of my condition from me. When he came to examine me, I remarked that it looked very badly for me.
>
> "Very badly," said he, sententiously; as his hand came to the great jagged hole made by the bullet in its exit.
>
> "You know," said I, "I am not afraid to hear the worst; is there any hope for me, doctor?"

93. Fuller, *Personal Recollections*, p. 101.
94. *Ibid.*

> "No," said he, very kindly, as he patted me gently on the forehead, and looked away; "no, my boy, none whatever."[95]

Surgeon McAbee moved on to attended to another bleeding man, and Captain Nickerson, now under sentence of death, lay back on the cold barn floor to consider the surgeon's parting words.

Assistant Surgeon Francis M. Wafer was literally ransacking the Peter Frey farmhouse in an effort to keep up with the continual arrival of more wounded. "It soon became impossible to do much for this large & hopeless mass. The few bandages in our medical knapsacks were already exhausted. We found many homespun linen sheets in the house; these were torn into strips & made a good substitute while they lasted. Our assistants exhausted the only well there giving them water, as that & some morphia to those who were in much pain was all we could do for them until [they were] removed to the large field hospital. This could not be done that night, although the ambulance train worked unceasingly all night through a violent storm of rain that set in at nightfall."[96]

After doing all that was possible to aid the wounded in and around the Frey homestead, the Canadian surgeon tried to find some unoccupied place to get some sleep. "I sought for a place to rest being completely exhausted & being thankful as well as surprised to find myself alive & uninjured amongst the tons of iron thrown around me. Climbing into the garret of the house & finding in a corner under a part of the roof not so badly torn up as to let the rain through a bedstead & tick upon which a pile of dried apples had been emptied. Scraping a trench through the apples with my hands & laying myself in this, I slept soundly until sunrise next morning, July 4th."[97]

If possible, the Jacob Hummelbaugh primary station, just to the south of the Peter Frey Farm, was even more swamped with walking wounded and the ongoing arrival of stretchers. "The wounded were

95. Nickerson, "Personal Recollections of Two Visits to Gettysburg," p. 21.
96. Wafer diary.
97. *Ibid.*

carried in during the night of the 3d in such numbers that they filled the barn floor and open space surrounding it," wrote Assistant Surgeon Alfred T. Hamilton of the 148th Pennsylvania Volunteers. "The wounded received all the care my attendants could give."[98]

Of all the people to filter through the primary aid station, one patient stood out vividly in the young surgeon's memory. "One poor fellow who was badly wounded seemed to be in the way of those moving among the wounded and, pained by being knocked about, got into the hopper of an old wind mill after dark, hoping to be undisturbed. A shell struck him and tore him to pieces as he lay coiled in the hopper."[99]

After a full day of operation and two pitched battles, the aid station at the farm of the Gettysburg shoemaker resembled nothing so much as a giant waterlogged morgue. "Several hundred steps to the rear of our Regiment was a dwelling house with some outbuildings. These were crowded with wounded soldiers. A small orchard of about an acre in extent, near by, was literally covered with the dead; they presented a ghastly sight, some being covered with rubber blankets, or parts of shelter tents, lying there in the rain and mud. Close by was a small spring in a swampy place where the boys used to get their water while occupying their position in that part of the field. During the rain, surface water carried blood from the field into the spring, but water being scarce in the locality, the boys were obliged to fill their canteens with the tainted liquid."[100]

Still the wounded kept pressing up to the aid depots along the Taneytown Road; the weary medical men dug deeper into their medical knapsacks, often coming up empty-handed. Outside, the drizzle was turning into a steady downpour.

Men of both sides also continued to pour into the three divisional hospitals back by the meandering Rock Creek. One of the new arrivals was Capt. Azor Nickerson, still shocked by his doctor's grim diagnosis of his wound. Shot through one arm and a lung, his condition was serious enough to warrant swift removal from the Widow Guinn aid

98. Muffly, *The Story of Our Regiment*, pp. 172-73.
99. *Ibid.* "Strange to say I saw the same old mill many years afterward at the same barn," wrote Hamilton after the war, "having been patched up and used."
100. Muffly, *The Story of Our Regiment*, pp. 542-43.

station to the more medically-advanced division hospitals. In shock from his wound and a brutal ambulance ride, Nickerson was semi-conscious of the dark trip to the Rock Creek hospital. "What took us from this barn hospital, which was near Meade's headquarters, I do not know. I have an indistinct remem-brance of another ambulance ride across fields, another jolting and banging, and finally being laid not too tenderly on the ground. . . ."[101]

"There were no less than two thousand companions in misery, Union and Confederate, and all the worst character of wounds. The location was in a bend of Rock Creek; the ground was very low and spongy, and, in accordance with the usual custom after a heavy cannonade, it commenced to rain soon after we got there and continued to do so all night."[102]

Lieutenant Fuller struggled back to wakefulness from the giddy effects of the chloroform. "When I came to myself, I looked down far enough to see a quantity of bandage wound around a stump of a leg eight inches long. My shoulder was bound up, but otherwise not operated on. Failure to resect may have been due to the great amount of work pressing upon the surgeons. They were worked as many hours continuously as they could stand, and still many a man had to be neglected. . . . As I was taken from the table one of my doctors said, 'Fuller, you may drink all the whiskey you can get, and want.'"[103]

"I was taken off the table and put back on my stretcher, which was set down in a wall tent, this tent was as full as it well could be of amputated cases.[104] For the most part the men bore their sufferings without a groan. Among the number was a young Confederate officer, that had lost an arm. He probably felt that he was a good way from home, and he 'took on,' bemoaning his fate as a cripple and a sufferer. He wore out the patience of every other man in the tent. At last I yelled

101. Nickerson, "Personal Recollections of Two Visits to Gettysburg," p. 21.

102. *Ibid.* "Many years have passed since then," continued the Ohio captain, "and yet the recollection of the horrors of that awful night almost wrench a groan from me now."

103. Fuller, *Personal Recollections*, pp. 101-2

104. With the medical supply wagons far to the rear, the very few walled hospital tents that the hospital managed to scrounge up were reserved for the most serious amputation cases and those with extremely dangerous wounds. All others were forced to lay outside in the rain.

out to him to shut up, or I would get up and kick him out doors. My bark was effective, we heard no more from him."[105]

"All of us were amputates [*sic*], or seriously wounded. During the night a doctor came, and gave every man a dose of morphine, which produced a happy state of mind and body." Lulled by the effects of the painkiller and the soporific sounds of the rain on the canvas ceiling, Fuller and his companions drifted in and out of drug-induced sleep.[106]

For the exhausted infantry and artillerymen posted along the crest of Cemetery Ridge, the cloudburst seemed like one more wearisome burden to be borne. No food, no relief, no shelter, no fires, tobacco running short, and now a torrential downpoor of rain. One soldier asserted that "the downpour was in proportion to the violence of the cannonade. . . . Everyone was drenched to the skin in a minute. Floods of water swept down the slopes of the hills and in some places almost submerged the weary sleepers who could scarcely be roused to the danger of their situation." At least one soldier slept soundly through the storm, "not aware until he awaked at daylight that he was lying in a pool of muddy, bloody water which had backed up from the slope of [the] rifle pit." Try as he might, he was never able to remove the bloody water stains from his uniform.[107]

Even in the midst of such suffering, men still found humor to be a wonderful relief from the overwhelming strain of battle. Captain Thompson of the 111th New York spent the cheerless night in line on the slope of Cemetery Ridge with the remnant of his command. "During the night we had one of those drenching rains that are said always to follow a great battle. But we were too tired and sleepy to think of shelter. I was waked in the midst of it by a prank of the boys, who lay close and dammed back the water until they had a flood, then all rose at once and gave me a thorough sousing." The hearty laugh that followed temporarily pushed aside the specter of sudden and violent death that had loomed so large for the past three days.[108]

One last individual fell in the confusion and misery of that rain-soaked night. "A number of shots were heard in quick succession from

105. Fuller, *Personal Recollections*, p. 102.
106. *Ibid.*
107. Stewart, *History of the One Hundred and Fortieth Pennsylvania*, p. 127.
108. Thompson, *Personal Narrative*, p. 47.

our picket-lines," wrote a Connecticut soldier, "the men hastily aroused took their places at the wall and waited patiently for orders. Intently they held themselves in readiness to meet the approaching foe, peering into the darkness, with their weapons in their hands. Several volleys were fired and when morning came, it was found that a white cow had been the cause of all the trouble. This was the last foe met on the battle-field of Gettysburg."[109]

Throughout the long weary hours of night, one at a time, or two unsteadily supporting each other, or foursomes carrying an individual on a blanket held at each corner, or carried on another's back, by stretcher, by ambulance, the wounded continued to irresistably flow into the already packed aid stations and division hospitals. Like the rain, this flood also showed no signs of stopping.

109. Page, *History of the Fourteenth Regiment*, p. 167.

CHAPTER 8

SATURDAY, JULY 4: 4:00 A. M.—SUNDAY, JULY 5: PRE-DAWN

"The whole ground around us is a great hospital."
Thomas Francis Galwey

Gettysburg, Pennsylvania

The soaking rain finally slacked off in the early morning hours, only to pick up force again. New Yorker Jacob H. Cole, lying awake behind enemy lines, listened to the stealthy sounds of movement through the drumming downpour. "About four o'clock in the morning it commenced to rain. The rebels were retreating; in fact, they have been retreating since midnight. This did not carry out what the rebels had told me on the morning of the 3rd. On that day they very boastingly said to me, 'Well, Yank, we expect to eat our Fourth of July dinner in Harrisburg,'" noted the injured infantryman. He wryly continued: "This was said before Pickett made his charge."[1]

Cole shifted painfully in the dark, favoring his wounded arm and leg. As the rain continued its dreary pouring, the sounds of movement gradually faded, then ceased altogether.

Westminster, Maryland

"Westminster, four o'clock, a. m.," wrote Ellen Orbison Harris, secretary and field representative of the Philadelphia Ladies Aid Society, to the members back home. "Spent the night on the cars, being

1. Cole, *Under Five Commanders*, p. 206.

ten hours, the only woman." Once she reached her destination, she, along "with a kind-hearted baker and his wife, had an opportunity of comforting some of our wounded with pies and cakes of their manufacture."[2]

The small railhead community of Westminster, already serving as an army supply depot, was rapidly becoming a major evacuation point and emergency transit hospital for the Army of the Potomac. "Large numbers are coming in, all giving the most frightful accounts of the fearful losses on both sides. Have seen hundreds of wounded soldiers from the battles of Wednesday and Thursday [July 1 and 2], whom I cannot name, who greet me with the kindest expressions. Many of them severely wounded, but all cheerful."[3]

The early morning hours also saw the arrival of the wounded Second Corps commanders in Westminster. "Generals Hancock and Gibbon have just arrived, wounded on the 3d; report favorably of our position; speak of the admirable handling of the troops on our side," tersely reported the Philadelphia volunteer. "Brave men, they lose sight of their own sufferings in their zeal for their country."[4]

As soon as all available wounded soldiers and any passengers were on board, the train on which Mrs. Harris had arrived immediately pulled out for the return trip to Baltimore, leaving just before the ambulances bearing Hancock and Gibbon reached the depot. The vehicles and their jostled passengers pulled up at Westminster "just at daylight to learn that no train would leave for Baltimore till late in the day. It is needless to detail the sufferings of a bullet wound," wrote General Gibbon somberly, "sufferings which in those sad days, were brought to nearly every home in the land."[5]

---

2. *Report of the Ladies Aid Society*, p. 12.
3. *Ibid.*
4. *Ibid.*
5. Gibbon, *Personal Recollections*, p. 170. According to a Sanitary Commission worker, twice daily, at 10:00 a.m. and 5:00 p.m., long trains of baggage cars, with straw scattered on the floors and each car open on both ends, pulled out of Westminster. Gibbon and Hancock arrived just after the morning train left, but were evacuated to Baltimore on the second. [Wormeley, *The United States Sanitary Commission*, pp. 128, 130, 145.] Herman Haupt, the Union general officer overseeing the operation of the military railroad, was actually running three rail convoys into and out of Westminster daily, "at intervals of eight hours." As fast as all the carloads of supplies were unloaded and the wounded soldiers loaded in, the trains steamed back to Baltimore. Haupt stressed in a communiqué to the regional commander at Westminster that "it will be all-important, on the arrival of

Fortunately, the Second Division commander had a relative living in town, and his ambulance forced its way through the crowded streets to the address. "I was tenderly cared for at the house of my wife's aunt, Mrs. Neal, who, poor lady, was torn with anxiety for one of her sons serving in the Rebel army, from whom she had had a visit only a few days before. For all she knew, he might now be lying dead or wounded on the battlefield of Gettysburg. Our Civil War was full of such cases. We were a band of brothers fighting."[6]

General Hancock, with no relations or acquaintances in town, apparently spent the entire morning resting in his ambulance.[7]

Between Baltimore and Westminster, Maryland

It had been a long and uncomfortable night for Andrew Cross and the delegation of men from the Christian Commission. Confusion had plagued the military railroad convoy every step of the way. There had been unexplained delays even before leaving the junction at Baltimore. Then there was confusion over whether the train that Ellen Orbison Harris had ridden to Westminster was on its way back along the single track from Westminster. Lack of telegraph lines along this particular stretch of track cut off any way to confirm what was happening on the twenty-nine miles between Baltimore and Westminster. A rail line that had been laid out for market and casual passenger service had suddenly skyrocketed in importance into the only undamaged railroad that could carry supplies to the Army of the Potomac. The transition was not an easy one.

The railroad convoy of five trains had labored throughout the day and on into the night, making the best speed possible along the second-rate Western Maryland Railroad. It was necessary to slow down for each wobbly bridge along the way, and civilians peered in amazement as train after train rumbled past. Brig. Gen. Herman Haupt, the commander of the military railroad system, had rushed in a trainload of cut and split wood for the fireboxes, buckets to dip water out of the streams for the boilers, and lanterns to carry on the necessary watering

---

the convoy, to unload each and every car on the main track and send back immediately. . . . The rapidity with which cars can be unloaded will measure the capacity of this road to supply the army." Allowing for delays, the last convoy of the day must have arrived at Westminster no later than midnight or 1:00 a.m. [Haupt, *Reminiscences of General Herman Haupt*, p. 216.]

6. *Ibid.*

7. *Report of the Ladies Aid Society*, p. 12.

and refueling in the middle of the night along the isolated Maryland tracks.

Now the lightening skies in the east found the Christian Commission delegation still grimly clinging to the swaying boxcar, blackened with soot and cinders, and wondering just how much farther away Westminster could possibly be.[8]

Gettysburg, Pennsylvania

"Towards morning came on a terrible storm, one of those instances which seem to establish a connection between battles and rainfall. In this instance, at any rate, the downpour was in proportion to the violence of the cannonade." The official historian of the Second Corps was awed by the severity of the thundering downpour: "The soldiers were drenched in an instant; and sudden torrents swept over the hills, as if to wash out the stains of the great battle. One of the Second Corps hospitals, around which had been collected hundreds of the Confederate wounded, was flooded; and some of the helpless prisoners were actually in danger of drowning where they lay, but were with great haste dragged or carried to higher ground."[9]

"The field hospital, which had been so directly in range of the enemy's guns in the afternoon was now threatened with a new peril," wrote another victim of that miserable drenching. "In the lower levels of the valley the ground quickly flooded and it required prompt action to save some of the helpless patients from drowning." The quiet meandering banks of Rock Creek, level on one side to facilitate the unloading of ambulances, that so appealed to Captain Livermore during the daylight now took on the sinister appearance of a floodplain in the early morning scramble to pull the helpless, wounded men back from the rising waters.[10]

Lt. Charles A. Fuller awoke from his drug induced sleep to the sound of rain still drumming on the canvas of one of the very few tents at the hospital, feeling for the first time the empty spot in bed where his left leg should have been. Isolated in this amputee ward from the events outside, he could only rely on the bits and pieces of information carried in by the doctors to know what was transpiring outside. "The

---

8. Haupt, *Reminiscences of General Herman Haupt*, pp. 213-15, 236; Cross, *The War and the Christian Commission*, p. 11.
9. Walker, *History of the Second Army Corps*, pp. 306-7.
10. Stewart, *History of the One Hundred and Fortieth Pennsylvania*, p. 127.

day of July 4 we had a drenching rain. Some men out lying in the low places and who could not move were, it was said, drowned. On the whole, I presume the rain was a benefit to the wounded."[11]

The injured men still out on the field, lying where they had fallen, were not all nearly so optimistic about the "benefit" of the rain. For many, the downpour had added just one more misery to a night of painful agony and burning thirst. "It had been a fearful night for our poor wounded men who had been lying out in the storm all night long. It was reported that some of the wounded were found lying in the water from two to four inches deep."[12]

Dawn did eventually arrive on the battlefield, the rain replaced temporarily by fair weather and cooler temperatures, but with it came no signs of rations or commissary wagons. For men who had fought for three days on unpalatable hard tack and scavenged coffee, or nothing at all, the need for food had become critical. Many took advantage of one untapped source of supply: "The famishing boys had discovered plenty of fresh, unsalted meat and raised biscuits in the haversacks of the rebel dead, and, yielding to the necessity that rises above all law, they had speedily foraged enough to give us all a hearty meal."[13]

The men of the 14th Connecticut Volunteers had already reached the same conclusion in the late night hours of July 3: "We crawled out on the battlefield after dark, where the enemy's [dead and] wounded lay, and took the haversacks from those who had been killed in the fight that day; these haversacks were nearly full of nice hoe-cakes. Some that we found were stained with blood where it had run into their haversacks from their wounds. But we were so hungry that we didn't stop for that. This may seem a tough story," confided Cpl. Edward H. Wade, "but it is true."[14]

For some, however, the sudden change in diet had some distinctly unpleasant side effects. "Like the rest, I ate heartily and was not on friendly terms with my digestive organs for twenty four hours

11. Fuller, *Personal Recollections*, p. 102.
12. Aldrich, *The History of Battery A*, p. 223.
13. Thompson, *Personal Narrative*, p. 47.
14. *Ibid.*; Coco, *On the Bloodstained Field*, p. 33. There were few, if any, facilities for washing on the battlefield. Beside the bloodstained food, many men had hands and uniforms sticky with the blood from their own injuries, and of the wounded whom they had assisted.

afterwards," ruefully commented Capt. Benjamin W. Thompson of the 111th New York.[15]

"On awakening on the morning of July 4th, it was found that the Confederates had advanced their skirmish line and a vigorous picket firing was kept up through the day. At times there was shot from long range guns and shells, necessitating some one of the regiment to be on the alert and warn the men of danger. The rain was very severe through the day which must have been trying to the great number of Confederate wounded who lay directly in front of the regiment, but too far out toward their skirmish line to enable the men to give them any relief."[16]

In spite of the deadly fire laid down by the Confederate pickets, volunteers from the various regiments accompanied the stretcher-bearers as they crept cautiously out to help as many of the enemy as could be reached. "That day our men went out into the fields in front, though savagely fired [on] by the hostile pickets, to bring in the suffering rebel wounded lying there in hundreds, moaning and shrieking in their pain—as indeed we have heard them all through the night previous." Although some were brought in and carried back to the hospitals, a great many of the injured Confederates from the action of July 2 and 3 were still beyond reach, kept from medical care by the fire of their own men.[17]

Assistant Surgeon Francis M. Wafer, the punctilious Canadian still serving the aid station at the Peter Frey Farm on the Taneytown Road, was incensed by this malicious activity of the Confederate pickets toward those trying to render medical assistance. "The enemy kept up a strong skirmishing line in our front which was very active in firing at every living object within possible range. Our stretcher bearers had removed most of their wounded from our front during the night, but some unfortunates had escaped observation, or were, in the hurry of the occasion, considered too hopelessly injured to remove. On our men attempting to remove these during the day they were deliberately

15. Thompson, *Personal Narrative*, p. 47.

16. Page, *History of the Fourteenth Connecticut*, p. 167.

17. Stevens, *Souvenir of Excursion to Battlefields*, p. 36. The enemy skirmishers were apparently under orders to keep the Union forces pinned down, at all cost, while the Confederate forces began their withdrawal.

fired at by the enemy's sharpshooters. Consequently they were doomed to lie there another day by the recklessness or barbarity of their comrades, as I cannot well apply milder terms to such conduct, because the stretcher bearers' vocation is always known by the mode of carrying the stretcher on the field, that is carried open when empty, looking when far away like a long and narrow white flag, if clean."[18]

Down by the extreme left of the Second Corps line, the Southerners had reformed their skirmish line in such a way as to allow Union rescuers more freedom in reaching the wounded. "During the night, the enemy had drawn back his pickets to the other side of the Emmittsburg [*sic*] Road, and left us free to assist the wounded. The appearance of the litters and ambulance wagons strengthened them, by giving them hope," wrote one observer of the evacuation of these marooned men. "They related their engagements of the evening before, and their sufferings during the night. One of them, pointing out the dead lying around him, said: 'This one lived only till sundown;—that one last[ed] until about midnight.—There is one who was still groaning but an hour ago.'"[19]

"The whole ground around us is a great hospital," wrote Thomas Galwey of the 8th Ohio. Members of each command, still in line of battle along Cemetery Ridge, were moving through the vast number of dead and dying in their vicinity, engaged in the heartbreaking job of looking for their missing comrades. "We have been attending to our wounded and have been picking up such of our dead as we could recognize. Each regiment selects a suitable place for its dead and puts a headboard on each individual grave. The unrecognized dead are left to the last, to be buried in long trenches."[20]

"Our regimental dead were buried on the ridge, near our position," wrote Chaplain Henry S. Stevens of the 14th Connecticut Regiment. "The graves of five corporals stand in a row, all neatly marked with the

---

18. Francis Wafer, diary. "The first removal of helpless wounded from the battlefield was usually effected by hand-litters, of which the number issued during the war exceeded fifty thousand. There were a number of patterns used, of which the best weighed twenty-four pounds, was quickly collapsible when not required, and possessed legs, which made its temporary use as a cot readily possible." [Edward L. Munson, "Transportation of Federal Sick and Wounded," in Francis T. Miller, ed., *The Photographic History of the Civil War*, 10 vols. (New York: The Review of Reviews Co., 1911), 7:302.]
19. Trobriand, *Four Years with the Army of the Potomac*, pp. 513-14.
20. Galwey, *The Valiant Hours*, p. 121. Most headboards were nothing more than a shingle, or a box lid, with the name, company, and regiment scrawled in pencil. Nothing more permanent or dignified was yet possible.

name, date, and regiment," recorded Maj. W. B. Hincks of that morning's sad and gruesome exertions.[21]

Even the simple act of digging in the rocky soil of Cemetery Ridge was a discouraging and frustrating challenge. "With one of my sergeants I dug a grave in a place I could designate and buried my Lieutenant," remembered Captain Thompson in later years. "We could get no tools but bayonets and tin plates, and, do the best we could, we were not satisfied."[22]

For many of the Pioneer troops of the Second Corps, July 4 would rank as one of the most hideous days of their lives. Sgt. T. P. Meyer picks up the narrative:

> On the morning of July 4th, according to orders, I reassembled my pioneers and took them out on the field of Pickett's charge and fight to bury the dead. The field presented a dreadful sight; the dead were already in a terrible state of putrefaction. Faces black as charcoal and bloated out of all human semblance; eyes, cheeks, forehead and nose all one general level of putrid swelling, twice the normal size with here and there great blisters of putrid water, some the size of a man's fist on face, neck and wrists; while the bodies were bloated to the full capacity of the uniform that enclosed them.
>
> It was a rare occurrence to find one who had not been robbed by the battlefield bandit or robber of the dead. Generally the pockets were cut open and rifled through the incision. The battlefield robbers were well known by the large amounts of money they had, and the watches, pocketbooks, pocket knives and other valuable trinkets they had for sale after the battle. All regiments had them.
>
> First we collected the dead men into rows, as usual, laying one against another, heads all one way, Union and Confederate in separate rows. Then some would collect and

21. Stevens, *Souvenir of Excursion to Battlefields*, p. 36.
22. Thompson, *Personal Narrative*, p. 47. "I informed his family as to his burial place," continued Thompson, "and [in] due time, they took his remains and buried him at his New York home."

arrange in rows while the majority of men buried them in trenches as heretofore described. These burial trenches were dug here, there and everywhere over the field and contained three or four or fifty as the number of dead near required. Few of these men had anything about them by which they could be identified, and were buried as 'unknown.'

The Confederates still had sharpshooters in the trees beyond the Emmittsburg [*sic*] road, and several times during the day they drove us off the field. The day was hot, sultry with frequent heavy showers. The stench on the battlefield was something indescribable, it would come up as if in waves and when at its worst the breath would stop in the throat; the lungs could not take it in, and a sense of suffocation would be experienced. We would cover our faces tightly with our hands and turn the back toward the breeze and retch and gasp for breath.

The dead were found in all manner of positions, lying, sitting, isolated, in groups, in heaps. Many there were without a visible wound or mark to cause death. Down beyond the 'Bloody Angle,' there remained standing a few panels of post fence, only the lower rails remaining. Against this a smooth faced soldier boy was sitting, his elbow resting on the second rail, his head resting on his right hand, his head upright the face turned toward us. Thinking he was sick or wounded I went out to offer assistance, and found he was dead. We examined him and found he had been shot through the left breast, in the hand to hand fight at the 'Bloody Angle' with Pickett's men the day before, then sat down just as we found him, and died without a struggle. Being perfectly poised he did not even roll over. There was nothing about him by which he could be identified. His accoutrements were all still in place, his cartridge box nearly empty.

...The field was thickly strewn with knapsacks containing the sundries of a soldier's outfit. Haversacks filled with biscuits and sweet cakes, the proceeds of forages among the people of Pennsylvania; blankets, tents, hats, coats, caps, belts, swords, letters, portfolios, books, bibles, testaments, playing cards, etc., etc., scattered everywhere. The day wore on. Our skirmishers were advanced; no enemy in force was found; our work at Gettysburg was finished.[23]

The artillerymen who had supported the Union center on July 3 were picking up their scattered tools and counting the losses of yesterday's action. The five batteries attached to the Second Corps had taken a severe hammering, losing 150 men and 250 horses in the process; of the five artillery commanders, three were dead and one mortally wounded. When finally relieved by fresh cannon, the gunners had moved their shattered ordnance to the artillery park on the Granite School House Road.[24]

Now members of each battery were heading back up the ridge to bury the lifeless bodies of comrades they were forced to leave behind when they fell back. "Three men from our battery rode back to the battle-ground to inter our dead, but found them already buried by Battery C, Rhode Island," wrote fellow Rhode Islander Theodore Reichardt of Battery A in his diary. "[Patrick J.] Lannegan was buried near our camp; also, Lieutenant Cushing, Battery A, Fourth Regulars."[25]

Thomas M. Aldrich, another member of Battery A, was also headed for the front. "As soon as I could get away from the battery, I went up to the hospital and saw the boys, and then went over to view the battlefield, and must say that on some portions of the field the sights were sickening, although they were gathering and burying the dead as quickly as possible. There was no firing of any kind, and our soldiers were well out on the field, some beyond the Emmitsburg road."[26]

"I went over the wall in front of our position and found the ground covered with muskets. Upon picking one up I found it loaded and cocked, which made it a dangerous weapon to be lying around. I called out to some soldiers near by and told them to be careful with the guns,

23. Muffly, *The Story of Our Regiment*, pp. 465-66, 467.

24. Hancock, *Reminiscences of Winfield Scott Hancock*, pp. 217-18.

25. Reichardt, *Diary of Battery A*, p. 97. The surgeons at the aid station had refused to treat Lead Driver Lannegan when it was discovered that "his stomach refused whisky." [Aldrich, *The History of Battery A*, p. 220.]

26. Aldrich, *The History of Battery A*, p. 221. Apparently, the galling Confederate skirmish fire was confined to certain areas, and must have slacked off from time to time.

then stuck the one I had in the ground. I did the same to a number of other muskets, and when I left the locality it very much resembled a large field of bean poles, as every one who picked up a musket, after looking at it, stuck it in the ground."[27]

Inspector General Morgan, still strongly disliked by many of the Second Corps troops for his cavalier attitude when enforcing the fully-shod fording of a branch of Monacacy River during June 29th's hard march, was riding by and witnessed this unique spectacle. "The field of battle presented a curious sight. Parties were gathering up the arms abandoned by the enemy and sticking the bayonets in the ground, so that there were acres of muskets standing as thick as trees in a nursery."[28]

Out beyond the bristling forest of inverted muskets, among the bloating bodies and screaming wounded, Virginian John Dooley recovered consciousness after spending the night on the bloody, rain-soaked field. "July 4th, 1863," he jotted in his diary while laying on the field. "I have slept a little despite a steady but light fall of rain which has undoubtedly proved extremely refreshing and grateful to thousands of fevered brains and burning wounds."[29]

Young Dooley was severely wounded, shot through both thighs. "This morning I am unable to walk a step and have myself carried about ten yards off the road to where Col [Lewis B.] Williams lies mortally wounded. . . . In the charge yesterday, foolishly and insanely he rode cooly [*sic*] and deliberately in front of the regiment, mounted on his horse. . . . Poor Williams! His spinal bone is broken, the shot, I think, striking at the neck joint and running down the spinal column. He suffers continual and intense agony. No position in which he may be placed affords any relief and he constantly seeks some change in the disposition of his head. There is a Yankee Col close by who is doing all he can to alleviate the sufferings of those around him, and he most cheerfully offers to assist our Col whenever he appears to suffer most. But Williams shows a dislike to be thus waited on, and frequently asks *me* to give a more comfortable position to his head, which on account

27. *Ibid.*
28. Walker, *History of the Second Army Corps*, p. 307.
29. Dooley, *John Dooley*, p. 108. Dooley must have been unconscious during the torrential downpour in the night.

of the stiffness of my own wound, I am unable to do without giving him much additional pain."[30]

The Second Corps ambulance crews had now worked their way out as far as Dooley's location, picking up Northerners and the more severely wounded first, the Confederates and the less seriously wounded whenever possible. "I make several of the officials who have direction of the ambulances promise me to have [the] Col removed to the field hospital where medical attendance may be had; and toward the middle of the day I have the satisfaction of knowing he had been removed."[31]

For the Irish officer, however, transportation would have to wait, as ambulance after ambulance rattled by without stopping. Dooley made himself as comfortable as possible, and continued scribbling in his diary.

Chaplain J. H. W. Stuckenberg, 145th Pennsylvania, had been up all night at the division hospital, helping to physically care for the soldiers of his regiment, and offering spiritual comfort and guidance whenever possible. Beside his duties at the hospital, so many of the officers of the 145th were struck down that the young German immigrant was forced to assume some of the regimental administrative functions. Finally, with all the paperwork finished, and the men as comfortable as possible, "I mounted my horse and proceeded to the front of our regiment. They occupied the same position as [the] previous day. A squad being sent to carry together the bodies of our wounded, I accompanied them."[32]

The detachment sent out to retrieve casualties still on the field scoured the same area that the 145th had battled over on July 2. "Beyond the wheatfield was a meadow, beyond that some woods. There were many rocks and bushes behind which the rebels had hid.

30. *Ibid.* Dooley apparently fell in the Emmitsburg Road, or some farm lane leading off the Emmitsburg Road. Colonel Williams was ill before the charge, and had pleaded with one of General Pickett's aides to be allowed to advance while mounted, in violation of the general's explicit orders. Finally swayed by the colonel's adamant appeals, the aide replied: "Mount your mare, I will make an excuse for you." [R. A. Bright, "Pickett's Charge," *Southern Historical Society Papers*, 31:228-30.]

31. *Ibid.* Dooley somberly added: "I never saw him afterwards. He died after 4 or 5 days' intense suffering."

32. Stuckenberg, *I'm Surrounded by Methodists*, p. 81.

But so suddenly did our men charge on them, that they threw down their arms and surrender. . . . Guns, bayonets, and bayonet and scabbards, cartridge boxes, and cartridges, haversacks and canteens were thrown and scattered in all directions."[33]

It wasn't long before they picked up the path of the attack; a trail of Union dead led up to where men from the two opposing sides had collided. Northerners and Southerners now lay intermingled, quiet and still in sudden death. "Among the dead we soon recognized those of our own regiment—[Pvt. H. L.] Tallmadge, Co I; [First Sgt. James D.] Cochran, Co C; [Cpl. J. Milton] Taylor and [Pvt. Joseph] Marsh, Co B; and [Pvt. Ira] Corbin, Co D. They were carried to an apple tree, under whose shadow they had fought. I offered a prayer and left the bodies there to be buried."[34]

"Immediately to the right of the ledge of rocks were our sharpshooters, some of them behind trees, firing constantly. I saw the tree, behind which some were posted, a few days later, its barks cut on its sides by rebel bullets aimed at our sharpshooters." The detail from the 145th had now reached the extreme front of the Union army; although there were still wounded visible from their position, they were effectively unreachable due to the heavy skirmish fire. Enemy pickets soon zeroed in on the small party. "Whilst looking for our dead a bullet, perhaps aimed at some one of us whistled past us, warning us that we were exposed to rebel sharpshooters."[35]

Having gone as far forward as possible to retrieve the wounded, the small party reluctantly turned back, followed by a chorus of pitiful cries—for help, for water, for medical attention, for an ambulance—from the wounded of both sides, stranded in the murderous no-man's-land between the two hostile forces. Many would not live to see the arrival of the next rescue detail.

Troops all along the Union line were feeling the effects of the heavy picket fire. "This day, Saturday, July 4th, the enemy kept us pinned to the ground by a most active and vigorous skirmishing. We could not show our heads above the hill without drawing the fire of their sharpshooters. Occasionally they varied the program by shelling from a few guns and throwing Whitworth bolts with uncomfortable

33. *Ibid.*
34. *Ibid.*
35. *Ibid.*, p. 83.

frequency and precision. All the forenoon we expected another attack and General Meade did all he could to draw them on."[36]

Beside gathering the wounded and burying the dead, July 4th was spent in respectful and reverent observance of Independence Day. As they had done in civilian life, many regiments commemorated the day by attending worship services with their regiment. Some regiments did not have a chaplain, and J. H. W. Stuckenberg's skills were much in demand this July morning. "I was requested by the Major of the 64th NY to hold services in his regt. I did so immediately after leaving our dead. The men were behind their breastworks, I stood in front of them. Brisk skirmishing was going on all the time, rebels and our men, and rebels as well as our men could be seen running and firing. A rebel flag was also seen at the edge of the woods. Worship at such a place, at such a time, with fearful scenes just enacted and being enacted, was very solemn. I thanked God that we had been spared, prayed for the many wounded, and remembered the relatives and friends of the killed. The soldiers felt deeply and many were moved to tears."[37]

When the somber time of prayer and remembrance was over, Stuckenberg moved down the line to his own men. "I passed on to our regt and was going to hold services there. But just then I saw a regt of our troops marching forward where the skirmishing was going on. A rebel battery concealed in the woods opened on them, enfilading the regiment. The regt faced about and retired—one shell passed over them, then came grape[shot] and canister, which struck directly in front of us. I was advised to retire. Whilst doing so a shell passed directly over my head and unpleasantly near and struck by a barn in which my horse was tied."[38]

With the possibility of holding Fourth of July services in his own regiment out of the question for the time being, Stuckenberg mounted up and headed for Rock Creek by way of several neighboring hospitals. "I returned to the 2nd corps hospital, visiting several others

---

36. Thompson, *Personal Narrative*, p. 47. The Confederate artillery had a few British Whitworth guns, which fired a "bolt" rather than a standard shell. In flight, it produced an unearthly howl; although no more accurate than any other artillery, the psychological effect of the Whitworth guns was immense.

37. Stuckenberg, *I'm Surrounded by Methodists*, p. 83. Maj. L. W. Bradley was now the senior officer in the 64th New York. In his official report, he wrote: "On the 4th we buried our dead and held short religious services conducted by Chaplain John H. W. Stuckenberg, of the one hundred and forty-fifth Pennsylvania Volunteers." [*OR*, vol. 27, pt. 1, p. 407.]

38. *Ibid.*, p. 83.

to look for wounded of our regt. I found Lt G. H. Finch, Co E, since dead. He was wounded through [the] l[eft] thigh and r[ight] ankle—and suffered greatly. He was faithful and brave—peace to his ashes." Tying up his horse at the Second Corps Hospitals, Stuckenberg immediately went back to work, comforting and encouraging the ever increasing multitude of wounded men.[39]

While the army was still in the vicinity, a steady trickle of men, authorized and otherwise, wandered through the hospitals, intent on finding fallen friends and family, living and dead. While the hospital was a terminal for the wounded, the medical facilities also served as a temporary morgue for officers carried to the rear and awaiting transportation home for interment. Laid off to the side away from the bustle and traffic of the hospital, bodies were arranged with all the dignity and care possible, deadly wounds cleaned and disheveled clothing straightened by personal servants, orderlies, and fellow staff officers attending their fallen commander and friend. Meanwhile, others were busy at headquarters and in town, picking up a coffin, visiting an embalmer, getting passes and leaves of absence signed for those that would travel with the deceased, and securing transportation for the body and the little group of mourners.[40]

Lt. Charles A. Fuller was delighted to see a regimental comrade walk through the doorway of the amputee tent.

> The morning of the 4th of July Capt [Willard] Keech came to see me and said he was to have a short leave of absence

39. *Ibid.* Lt. George H. Finch, Company E, died of his wounds on July 6, 1863. [National Archives and Records Administration, Service Records of George H. Finch.]

40. M. H. Bassett, *From Bull Run to Bristow Station* (St. Paul: North Central Publishing Company, 1962), pp. 32-33. Army life and death had spawned a traveling industry that moved with or in close proximity to the gargantuan army. Coffins of differing quality and price were available to suit the taste and pocketbook of the buyer. Hermetically-sealed models were quite popular when there was a delay before the body could be sent home, or during spells of pervasive summer heat. Embalmers shadowed the advances of the Army of the Potomac, even advertising their services in broadsides and newspapers.

on account of the wound he received in the neck, which came near effectually cutting it. He wanted to know what word he should convey to my people. I said tell them that I am doing as well as one can under the circumstances.

He replied, 'Don't you want them to come down here?'

I said, 'No! They can do no good here, and will be in the way.'[41]

Reluctantly, the two parted company, and Keech headed off for the railroad station. Both were painfully aware of the fact that they might very well never see each other again.

New York, New York

The telegram was short and ambiguous: "If you are going to Gettysburg, let me know." Young George Anna Woolsey received the message, addressed to her, at her family's posh Fifth Avenue townhouse, and the family gathered to intently pore over the scrap of paper. "If you are going to Gettysburg, let me know." It was signed by Frederick Law Olmstead, executive secretary of the United States Sanitary Commission.[42]

By July of 1863, George Anna, cousin of Yale College president Theodore Dwight Woolsey, was already a skilled volunteer nurse. Her experience had begun early in the war, when she cared for the wounded in Washington from the Battle of Bull Run, working side by side with fellow-volunteer Frederick Law Olmstead. Desiring to hone her abilities, she took a special course offered by Dr. Elizabeth Blackwell at New York Hospital in war nursing. (Although not yet the minimum thirty years of age at the time, she used her family's name and influence to gain admittance). As the United States Sanitary Commission began gaining momentum in its war relief efforts, Olmstead, now its executive secretary, tapped George Anna as one of only four women to work in the headquarter staff of the organization.[43]

---

41. Fuller, *Personal Recollections*, p. 103. Both men knew that an amputation as close to the body as was Fuller's was often fatal.
42. George Anna Woolsey Bacon and Eliza Newton Woolsey Howland, *Letters of a Family During the Civil War, 1861-1865*, 2 vols. (New: Privately printed, 1899), 2:526.
43. Anne L. Austin, *The Woolsey Sisters of New York* (Philadelphia: American Philosophical Society, 1971), pp. 38-40. The U.S. Sanitary Commission was a volunteer organization, roughly equivalent to the modern Red Cross.

This last year had been a grueling one for George Anna. The year 1862 saw her working with her sister Eliza Howland in the Transport Service, evacuating sick and wounded soldiers from the Virginia Peninsula by steamers. When this service was turned over to the military, she was off to Portsmouth Grove, Rhode Island, serving as assistant superintendent of a new military hospital. By May 1863, she was on the move again, this time to Virginia to care for the wounded at Falmouth following the disastrous Battle of Chancellorsville.[44]

Back home in New York for a few days to rest, George Anna now mulled over the cryptic telegram from her boss. Did Olmstead know some ominous news of twenty-three-year-old Charles Woolsey, George Anna's only brother, and staff aide to Brig. Gen. Seth Williams, adjutant general of the Army of the Potomac? Was he trying to break the news of young Woolsey's wounding or death as gently as possible? Unable to reach Olmstead for further clarification, the family "jumped at the conclusion *he* knew of bad news from Charley." George Anna and her sixty-three-year-old widowed mother immediately packed their bags, and "started at once to go to him,—Uncle Edward taking us as far as Baltimore."[45]

Westminster, Maryland

The slow freight from Baltimore finally hissed its way to a halt, couplings clanking heavily as it came to rest. Covered from head to toe with railroad dirt, the Christian Commission representatives climbed stiffly down from their boxcar roost and looked at the scenes of frantic

---

While initially considered by the Army's Medical Department to be a group of busybodies sticking their noses in where they did not belong, the Commission's dedication to sanitary conditions in all hospitals, commitment to swift and monitored transportation of the wounded, and attention to suitable diet and care in medical facilities were instrumental in raising Civil War medicine to a new level in cleanliness and effective treatment.

44. Brockett and Vaughn, *Woman's Work in the Civil War*, pp. 299-315, 324, 327-28; Frederick Law Olmsted, *Hospital Transports* (Boston: 1863); Olmsted (edited by Jane Turner Censer), *The Papers of Frederick Law Olmsted*, p. 324.

45. Bacon and Howland, *Letters of a Family During the Civil War*, pp. 525-26. Thirty years later, Olmsted commented on George Anna Woolsey's abilities in administration and crisis. The Sanitary Commission secretary avowed that he felt she "would, upon orders, take command of the channel fleet; arm, equip, man, provision, sail and engross the enemy, better than any other landsman I know." High commendation indeed. [Olmsted, *The Papers of Frederick Law Olmsted*, p. 324.]

activity going on all around. "We arrived at Westminster at noon Saturday. Just as we landed there was a report that [Brig.] General [John] Buford's cavalry were ordered off, as some supposed, to head [off] Lee's army, or to bring some aid to General Meade."[46]

"At Westminster everything was in the utmost confusion," observed Andrew Cross as the commissioners set about getting their freight unloaded. "Dozens of men were loading hard crackers, others meat and sugar, &c., from cars into army wagons, which, as soon as loaded, were hurried away for the army, which was not supplied. A little farther along the track, under guard, stood about 1,000 Confederate prisoners, waiting to enter the cars for Baltimore."[47]

More and more wounded men were beginning to arrive from the battlefield, but the crowd waiting by the tracks was still primarily composed of officers, some of the wounded from the first day's action, and those with significant political or military connections. "Several hundred of our wounded had reached here, and were attended to by our delegates. General Hancock, of the 2d Army Corps, who was wounded on the 2d day [*sic*], was here, and had his wound dressed and the smoke and dust of battle washed from him by one of our Commission, (Mr. Stillson). From him we learned positively that our army was victorious."[48]

There was obviously much to be done on the battlefield, and the men of the Christian Commission quickly set about to get out of the milling throngs along the railroad and on the road to Pennsylvania. "General Buford had ordered an army wagon to take our supplies, which we immediately had removed from the car to the wagon. While in this work, and just as we had nearly finished, one or two cavalrymen rode up to us, inquiring which was the road to some stone church? In a few moments there was a new commotion. Wagons, horses and footmen were hurrying along. We sought to know what this meant, and were informed that General Buford's cavalry was in motion."[49]

"Feeling that we were shut up to the duty of reaching the wounded, we pursued the steps to accomplish it. A proposition was made to hire a carriage. Knowing what difficulty we had in getting our stores that far, we concluded to stick by the wagon, while others went in a

---

46. Cross, *The War and the Christian Commission*, p. 11.
47. *Ibid.*, pp. 11-12.
48. *Ibid.*, p. 12.
49. *Ibid.*

carriage, and as we knew from General Hancock how great was the need in the army, we resolved to go with it at once."[50]

One last difficulty arose before the weary and grimy commissioners could pull out of the railhead community. "Just as we were about starting a cloud suddenly arose, which, with great rapidity, gave evidence of a severe storm. In a few moments it was upon us in torrents. Umbrellas and wagon covers were of but little use. We fled to a house, and after waiting until the first furious shower had slackened a little, we started."[51]

Ellen Orbison Harris, the secretary and field representative of the Philadelphia Ladies Aid Society, had been moving about through the wounded men all morning and into the afternoon, cleaning and dressing wounds, feeding the famished men, and encouraging them as best she could with her limited supplies. The cargo was finally unloaded from the Baltimore train, and the human load of wounded soldiers was placed on board for the return trip. Prisoners under guard climbed up sullenly, and the wounded were gently laid in the now-empty freight cars. "Late in the afternoon I was placed in a box car on a train with many other wounded," remembered General Gibbon. Lieutenant Haskell was still with his commander, "seeing him transferred from an ambulance to the cars for Baltimore, on the 4th." Hancock was also put on board; in a final act of gallantry, he provided transportation to the field for Ellen Harris. "General Hancock has ordered the ambulance which brought him here to carry me back."[52]

As the train slowly steamed out of the station, the Philadelphia volunteer nurse gathered together her depleted supplies, and climbed into the donated ambulance for the trip across the state line into Pennsylvania. "It rains heavily; the streets are blocked with wagons; may find trouble," she wrote tersely as she sat waiting to get under way. "Some of the Christian Commission will go with me. My heart fails me; know I go to mourn and lament." With the rain sluicing down from leaden skies, Andrew Cross' wagon and carriage, and Ellen Orbison

50. *Ibid.*

51. *Ibid.*

52. *Report of the Ladies Aid Society*, p. 12; Gibbon, *Personal Recollections*, p. 170; Byrne and Weaver, *Haskell of Gettysburg*, p. 193.

Harris' ambulance, all headed out of town, intent on reaching an obscure crossroads village named Gettysburg.[53]

York, Pennsylvania

The news of the Union victory was moving across the state as fast as newspapermen, cut off from the normal conveniences of telegraph and railroads, could get word out of Gettysburg. "On the morning of Saturday, July 4, 1863, came the glorious news of our victorious arms and of the retreat of the enemy toward the border. We learned that by afternoon supplies could be forwarded to our army."[54]

The civic-minded citizens of nearby towns were quick to respond. "The public square in York rapidly filled with wagons packed with provisions, clothing, blankets and hospital stores waiting the arrival of the banished horses which had been sent across the river before the occupation of the town by General Gordon's command [on June 27]."[55]

Many civilian volunteers, male and female alike, were making preparations to travel to the site of the battle to assist in whatever way possible. One of them, Mrs. Mary Cadwell Fisher, wrote: "About 3 P.M. I started with two ladies and my oldest son in a two-horse wagon loaded with necessaries of every kind." A number of the folks in York seemed to view "necessaries" as being spirituous in nature and in distilled form. "A former Cabinet minister presented me with several dozen bottles of the purest imported liquors, with the request that we

---

53. *Report of the Ladies Aid Society*, p. 12. For the men on the train, the trip was going to be a long one. General Gibbon related that the train "ran out only a mile or two to a side-track where we remained all night in a pouring rain, arriving the next day (the 5th) at Baltimore, where my family had already received news of my death." [Gibbon, *Personal Recollections*, p. 170.] There were "no adequate sidings" on the Western Maryland Railroad. There must have been some serious delay that kept this one train from leaving on schedule with the rest of the military convoy. Either the train was small enough to squeeze onto a tiny siding to the east of Westminster, or the trainload of wounded men steamed *west* out of Westminster, laying over just far enough outside town to let the next convoy of trains arrive on schedule. When that next convoy headed back for Baltimore in the early morning hours of July 5, the stranded train carrying Generals Hancock and Gibbon traveled back with it.

54. Mrs. Mary Cadwell Fisher, "A Week on Gettysburg Field," *The Philadelphia Times*, December 23, 1882.

55. *Ibid.*

would distribute it ourselves, to which I added a quantity of fine old whiskey from one of our celebrated county distilleries."[56]

With the return of the horses, the wagons quickly hitched up and headed south out of town in the pouring rain, anxious to avoid any remaining Confederates and reach Gettysburg before dark.

Gettysburg, Pennsylvania

"In the afternoon it rained very hard," remembered Chaplain J. H. W. Stuckenberg of that afternoon's work. "There was not a hospital tent at our hospital. Some of the wounded were in shelter tents which sheltered them poorly, others lay in the rain and mud, covered with a woolen or rubber blanket—or nothing at all. I labored to shelter them till I was wet through, and returned to my tent very weary and sick."[57]

Pausing in his labors at the division hospital, what Stuckenberg saw as he looked about him was not at all encouraging.

> It was a sad sight to look at the hospital at any time, but especially when those severely and mortally wounded were thus exposed. And nothing could be done for them. After the rain I with [Pvt. Lewis] Stallman, Co I, got some hay and placed [it] under the wounded. I gave my rubber blanket to one of our men, my woolen one to [Sgt.] Wm Brown [also of Company I], and tore another woolen one belonging to Lt Col [David Berkley] McCreary and divided it between E[rastus] Allen and [Cpl.] H[orace] Mann[,] Co I.[58]
>
> What a hospital on or near the field of battle is can only be known by those that have seen one. There were between 2000 and 3000 wounded in our 2nd corps hospital. In 1st Division there were two operating stands, where the Surgeons were constantly consulting about operations and were performing amputations. Heaps of amputated feet and hands, arms and legs were seen lying under the tables and by their sides.
>
> Go round among the wounded and you witness the most saddening and sickening sights. Some are writhing in pain,

56. *Ibid.*
57. Stuckenberg, *I'm Surrounded by Methodists*, p. 83.
58. Cpl. Horace Mann of Company I was wounded in the thigh, and recovered from his injuries. [*Erie Weekly Gazette*, July 18, 1863; *Erie Observer*, July 11, 1863; Service Records of Horace Mann, National Archives and Records.]

> and deeply moaning and groaning and calling for relief which cannot be afforded them. The finest forms are horribly disfigured and mutilated. Wounds are found in all parts of the body. Here lies one with his leg shattered, the flesh torn by a shell, nothing but shreds being left. There lies one shot through the abdomen, the intestines protruding—his life cannot be saved, perhaps even opium gives him but little temporary relief. He is but waiting to die. Here lies one with his arm almost severed from his body—waiting for amputation. There lies one once young and handsome shot through the face and head—his eyes swollen shut and covered with a yellow, putrid matter, his hair clotted with blood, his jaws torn, a bullet hole through each cheek. Some of the wounds are dressed, some are not. From some the blood still oozes, in others maggots are perhaps found. Perhaps they are poorly waited on, there not being nurses enough. No physician may have examined their wounds and dressed them. Their physical needs may not have been attended to. They long for home and their friends, but they cannot get to one, the other cannot come to them. Through neglect, perhaps, they die. They are buried in their clothes, without shroud, without coffin, perhaps without religious services and a board to mark their resting place.
>
> The hospital soon becomes foul, especially in summer—the stench sometimes becoming almost intolerable. Medicines may be scarce, the food unpalatable—perhaps scarce.[59]

Yet in spite of the horror and suffering assailing all the senses, the Union and Confederate wounded were fortunate to be at the Second Corps Hospitals in the marshy bottomland of Rock Creek. "Near the battle field of Gettysburg many barns for miles around were filled with wounded, many of whom had neither surgeons, nor nurses, nor food." Staggered by the enormity of the task facing him, Stuckenberg went back to work, ministering to the men of his regiment and those lying closeby in his section of the hospital in the only way he knew how—one at a time.[60]

---

59. Stuckenberg, *I'm Surrounded by Methodists*, pp. 83-84.
60. *Ibid.*, p. 84.

The chaplains of all the regiments had already mapped out the division hospitals, dividing the workload as equally as possible between them. "We districted the ground, and each chaplain gave his especial attention to the wounded of his own regiment, and to those of other regiments having no chaplain lying nearest to his own." In that way, every man, Southerner or Northerner, had access to spiritual comfort and encouragement as they came face to face with their own mortality while enduring the long wait for medical care.[61]

Out on the field, ambulance crews continued the herculean job of removing the wounded, gradually working their way further and further from the Union lines along Cemetery Ridge. For Virginian John Dooley, shot through both thighs out by the Emmitsburg Road, transportation arrived some time after he had succeeded in getting his mortally wounded colonel carried off to the hospital. "A few hours after, I am also removed and placed in an ambulance along side a wounded Yankee. Poor fellow, he is wounded in many places and appears to suffer very much. He is a coarse bloated looking Irishman and is whining and groaning continually except when the vehicle jolts over a stone or gully, and then he gives a loose to horrid oaths and imprecations. I long to get rid of my loathsome companion and hail with delight the approach of the field hospital."[62]

The weather had again taken a turn for the worse, with heavy storm fronts moving over the area of the battlefield. "The rain is pouring down as we reach the field hospital, which differs from the battle field only in this respect, that we have some kind of medical attendance and rations of crackers and substitute-coffee. But the accommodations are the same, viz., the wet muddy hillside, sans tents, sans blankets, sans fires, sans water, sans every thing relating to exterior comfort."[63]

After being unloaded from the ambulances, many of the Confederates were carried over Rock Creek onto the opposite hillside, and there laid tightly together to make room for the continuing arrival of still more wounded. "The whole ground for miles around is covered with the wounded, the dying and the dead. Confederate and Yankee are often promiscuously thrown together, although the officials

---

61. Murphey, *Four Years in the War*, p. 124.
62. Dooley, *John Dooley*, pp. 109-10.
63. *Ibid.*, p. 110.

separate us generally as much as is convenient. The Yankees are nearly all comfortably quartered, having tents and blankets and many little comforts which they have of course received of their comrades. This is only natural and none of our boys expect to receive attentions in preference to the enemy's wounded."[64]

"The little grove, containing some two or three acres, was literally filled with the victims of the demons—treason—rebellion—war," wrote Rev. Thomas G. Murphey, chaplain of the 1st Delaware Volunteer Infantry, of the hospital by the creek. "Most of the Federal soldiers were, in a measure, protected from the rain by shelter tents, which they had brought with them, or had been picked up by their comrades and friends for that purpose. But the Confederates were unsheltered. Men and officers were laid on the wet ground with nothing under or over them. They lay so close that in passing from one to another to try to do something for them, great care was necessary not to step on them, and their imploring calls for relief or shelter was distressing, for our supplies were limited."[65]

Dooley at once found other members of his regiment on the soggy floodplain of Rock Creek. "The first man who attracted my attention upon being assigned to my position on this dreary hillside was one of the members of my company, John Scammel. Poor Scammel! He is standing up in his usually inert way, and wringing water from a blanket which he had been fortunate enough to preserve. There appears nothing very grievous in his condition, but he opens his shirt and quietly points to a piece of shell which is half buried in the hollow between his breasts. He tells me in a low complaining voice that he feels his time has come and that no one will by proper care give him a chance, if there be any chance, to recover from his wound. I bade him lie down and keep as quiet as possible and if I should meet with a surgeon that I would get him some attention."[66]

Surgeons were at a premium at the hospital, each doing as much as physically possible with what limited supplies they had to meet the

64. *Ibid.*, p. 111. Conditions were so bad that Dooley felt the Union troops "comfortably quartered" if they had a scrap of shelter tent or one blanket. Subsequent visitors to the hospital were appalled by the lack of adequate shelter, cots, blankets, food, etc.

65. Murphey, *Four Years in the War*, pp. 121-22.

66. Dooley, *John Dooley*, pp. 110-11.

needs of the still-growing number of wounded being unloaded from ambulances and arriving on foot. Capt. Jack Adams of the 19th Massachusetts had a front row view of the doctors as they struggled to keep up with the influx of bleeding men. "Directly in front of us were two amputating tables which were always busy. We saw several men whom we knew placed on them and removed, minus a leg or an arm. The groans of the wounded were constant, and the dead were being carried past us nearly all the time."[67]

Surgeon Albert Vander Veer of the 66th New York, first assistant to Chief Operator Charles Squire Woods on the First Division surgical team, outlined the system used to determine who would be treated first. "It seems hardly proper to repeat that in our work at the time of such battles cases of hemorrhage were to be looked at first as promptly as possible. Serious fractures of the bone of the limbs requiring amputations were also attended to as promptly as possible. But among the wounded were many cases that were too serious to be moved but needed immediate attention: abdominal cases were almost immediately fatal." In spite of the many shortfalls that the Second Corps Hospitals were experiencing, Vander Veer could happily report that "we had plenty of surgical dressings, of anaesthetics, etc."[68]

To open up as much space as possible along the crowded creek banks, the surgeons were transferring those with lesser wounds to the railroad for evacuation from the battlefield. "We lay side by side until the morning of July 4, when the ambulances came to take us to the station," wrote Jack Adams, anxious to be on his way, via the depot, to a general hospital somewhere—anywhere away from the sounds of death and dying, and the perpetual macabre cartloads of severed limbs being trundled past him from the operating tables. "One after another was loaded in. I said, 'Save a good place for me,' but was informed that the orders of the surgeon were not to take me. I sent for the surgeon, who came and said that I must not be moved for two weeks." The news was devastating to the New York captain; suddenly all the shock, exhaustion, hunger, excitement, and anguish of the last four days

---

67. Adams, *Reminiscences of the Nineteenth Massachusetts*, p. 71.
68. Albert Vander Veer, Vander Veer Papers, DB 560, Albany Institute of History and Art, Albany, New York; transcribed copy in the 66th New York Infantry Vertical File, Gettysburg National Military Park Library. Surgeon Vander Veer continues: "In fact during my more than three years of service there was never a time but [that] we had sufficient chloroform and ether so that our patients were relieved from pain and suffering as much as possible."

rushed in like an overwhelming flood. "I saw the ambulance drive away, then buried my face in the ground and cried like a baby."[69]

Unknown to the doctors of the Second Corps, there would be no trains running out of Gettysburg this Independence Day. The Confederates had done quite a thorough job on the little single track running east out of town, effectively sabotaging every railroad bridges, from the one spanning Rock Creek north of the hospital, and on southeasterly toward Hanover Junction. Until those trestles and the quantity of torn-up track could be repaired, the wounded in those ambulances were on a short trip to nowhere.[70]

The harried ambulancemen quickly unloaded their charges by the railroad, then jumped back in their vehicles—there were still thousands more casualties to pickup and transport to the hospitals. Whipping up their horses, the Second Corps ambulances rattled away, leaving the stranded wounded by the side of the tracks with no food, no shelter tents, no doctors to dress their wounds and attend to their needs, and nowhere to go.

The Christian Commission "Eating Saloon," trackside east of Gettysburg

Fortunately, members of the Christian Commission had seen the transportation snag developing at track's end, and were moving rapidly to meet the need. "After the battle a stream of Federal soldiers, weary, weak from loss of blood, hungry and disheartened, could be seen coming in from the various field hospitals which had been suddenly extemporized three or four miles from town, hoping to find cars to take them to Baltimore or Philadelphia. To feed these men, to wash their wounds, to give them clean clothing, to encourage them to continue their journey till they should reach the place, a mile beyond town, where the trains were at first obliged to stop, was a part of our work."[71]

With the Army of the Potomac Commissary Department critically overtaxed following the battle, and hobbled by devastated roads and railroads, rushing food and water to these stranded soldiers was of critical importance. "An eating saloon was, therefore, imperatively

---

69. Adams, *Reminiscences of the Nineteenth Massachusetts*, pp. 70-71.
70. *OR*, vol. 27, pt. 1, p. 23.
71. *The United States Christian Commission for the Army and Navy. For the Year 1863. Second Annual Report.* (Philadelphia: April, 1864), p. 69.

called for, and immediately established, by the Christian Commission, at which, in the words of Dr. Bellows, 'some thousands of tired and hungry soldiers were fed.' The superintendence of this saloon was undertaken by Mr. Louis Muller, of Baltimore, a work in which he was assisted by Mr. Woodward, of the same city, both delegates, who cooked the food eaten, and personally attended to its distribution. In this work Mr. Woodward furnished an example of the most untiring industry and devotion, laboring till near midnight, rising with the first dawn of day, and deserves to be held in lasting remembrance for his faith and zeal and labors of love."[72]

Beside touring the battlefield, Second Corps Inspector General Morgan also visited the hospital facilities, monitoring the workings of the vast medical facility. "Our men . . . as always, according to my observation, were full of kindness for the wounded, and I saw them sharing with the prisoners at the hospital their coffee and crackers."[73]

While moving through the crowded creek bottom, Morgan came across an old acquaintance. "Lying on the ground here, in the rain, smoking a little old pipe, with an expression of satisfaction and content quite observable, I saw Colonel Fry, of the Thirteenth Alabama, formerly an officer of our army." Birkett Davenport Fry, born in 1822 in Kanawha County, [West] Virginia, had led something of a checkered military career: he resigned from the Virginia Military Institute, was released from West Point, had been a first lieutenant in the Mexican War, and then had gone on to take part in William Walker's abortive invasion of Nicaragua. Finally giving up on the military, he tried law for a while, before finally settling as an Alabama cotton mill manager when war finally overtook him once again.[74]

"On inquiring whether he was wounded, the colonel showed me a compound fracture of the thigh-bone." [In addition to the leg wound, Fry had taken a nasty blow to the shoulder from a shell fragment while approaching the Union lines during the Confederate assault of July 3.] "I went away, pretty certain that a man who could, with such a

72. *The United States Christian Commission for the Army and Navy. For the Year 1863*, p. 69. For more on the concept of the "Eating" or "Refreshment Saloon," see "Mary W. Lee, 72nd Pennsylvania Volunteer Nurse" in Appendix 3.

73. Walker, *History of the Second Army Corps*, p. 307.

74. *Ibid.*

desperate wound, lie all night in a rain so heavy as to cover the ground where he lay some inches with water, and then smoke his pipe with apparently so serene a satisfaction in the morning, was not going to give up the ghost yet, and was not surprised afterward to hear of the colonel's recovery."[75]

In the midst of all the amputations, the wounded being carried in, the dead being carried out, and the ululating background of thousands of voices in pain, prayer, and conversation, some men were trying to carry on a semblance of normal life. George Washington Beidelman of the 71st Pennsylvania propped himself up as best he could along the low ground by Rock Creek, pulled out writing utensils and paper, and dashed off a quick letter to his father about his wounding at the Angle on July 3:

> Hospital
> Battlefield of Gettysburg
>
> July 4, 1863
> My Dear Father,
>
> We have just fought, in old Pennsylvania, the greatest battle of the war. The 2d Corps has covered itself with glory. I am slightly wounded. A 'Minie' ball cut across both legs above the knees, just bruising the left, and cutting a gash in the right about the depth of my little finger. Otherwise I am very well and in the best of spirits.[76]

---

75. *Ibid.* Fry did indeed recover. After losing his leg on a Union operating table, and spending six days at the Second Corps hospital, Colonel Fry was shipped off to Fort McHenry as a prisoner of war. Moved from prison to prison, Fry was slow in recovering his strength; however, he was finally returned to the South by special prisoner exchange in March of 1864. [Service Records of Birkett D. Fry, National Archives and Records Administration.] Fry not only survived, but was promoted to brigadier general in active service. He would return to cotton production after the war until his death January 21, 1891. ["VMI Civil War Generals, Biographical sketches of VMI alumni who became general officers, 1861-1865." http://www.vmi.edu/~archtml/cwgen.html.]
76. Vanderslice, *The Civil War Letters of George Washington Beidelman*, pp. 178-79. Beidelman further described his wound in a letter dated July 14 and mailed from Chestnut Hill, a U.S. General Hospital in Philadelphia. He was wounded "in the battle of the 3rd. by a Minie ball, going through my pants

> Our losses are very heavy—in our whole corps they will probably average one-half of each regiment. The enemy's loss is equal to ours in killed and wounded, and they are all in our hands. We took more prisoners than we had men. Gen Longstreet and other generals are prisoners. We fought Lee's whole army and whipped him worse than at Antietam. I doubt if he will ever recross the Potomac.
>
> This is a glorious fourth of July for us. To God be all the glory!
>
> Your Affectionate Son
> George
>
> P.S.-Do note [*sic*] write till you hear from me again, which will be in a few days.
>
> N.B.-Please publish this note in the first Bloom[sburg, Pennsylvania] newspaper issued.[77]

At general headquarters, grave decisions had been facing General Meade on this Independence Day. One of the most pressing needs lay in rounding up the troops, scattered by the three days of fighting, and getting them reassembled into some approximation of companies, regiments, and brigades. Initial calculations showed that the Union army had suffered 23,049 casualties; those regiments most severely engaged had lost very heavily, with regiments reduced to the size of companies, and some companies having only a few individual soldiers remaining, and those often having no officers of any rank left uninjured.[78]

This problem was compounded for the army and the Second Corps Hospitals by the number of healthy men, well-meaning and otherwise,

---

and merely scratching my left leg, while it cut a piece out of my right leg, leaving a furrow about the length, breadth, and half the depth of my thumb; and that isn't very large. My knee, however, made a very narrow escape, the wound being on top, or in front, and only about two inches above the knee-cap." Beidelman was one of the very lucky ones. [*Ibid.*, pp. 179-80.]

77. *Ibid.* The wounding and capture of General Armistead led to the widespread, and erroneous, rumor that General Longstreet had been captured. Mail service was invariably disrupted after a major battle; it was far easier to get letters out than to get mail in to the men scattered throughout camps and hospitals, or even separated from their commands.

78. Coddington, *The Gettysburg Campaign*, pp. 540-41.

who found their way to the medical facilities. Surgeon Justin Dwinelle, overseeing the operation of the Second Division Hospital, was deeply troubled by this situation. "According to an order there were to have [been] fifty extra nurses & attendants left at corps Hospital. I took such men as I required and sent all others not on duty to the Provost Martial [*sic*] at Gettysburg as fast as I could find them. I had occasion at one time to send two Hundred and a number of times afterward from five to twenty. I think one thousand a low estimate of the number of able-bodied men who found their way to the Second Corps Hospital by the night of the fourth of July Who had no business there and ought to have been with their regiments."[79]

Beside the confusion and disruption caused by so many unauthorized people at the hospital, the situation was proving to be a tremendous drain on the limited resources of the Medical Corps. "This should be prevented in the future," continued Doctor Dwinelle in his report, "as these skulkers are mostly useless as help and often consume the food and occupy the shelter provided for the wounded. The usual excuse of these men is that they have been detailed by some Lieut, Captain or Chaplain."[80]

Meade was also facing the overwhelming challenge of getting adequate supplies to the famished Army of the Potomac. Thanks to the determination and foresight of General Haupt, the supervising genius of Union railroad transportation, there were sufficient provisions on hand at Westminster, Maryland. The weak link in the supply chain lay in moving the badly-needed food by creaky wagon trains over the intervening twenty-five miles of country roads to Gettysburg. In spite of the best efforts at the railhead in Westminster, the first caravan of supply wagons had not taken to the road until early on July 4.[81]

The Second Corps Hospitals had been making do with what could be begged, borrowed, or confiscated in order to feed the swelling number of wounded laying by Rock Creek. "Up to the Morning of the fourth[,] the Divisions of the corps being seperated[,] the Surgeons in charge of each division had provided rations for their own wounded," wrote Justin Dwinelle to his medical director, Dr. Alexander N. Dougherty. "But now that the divisions had got together[,] You will recollect that you made it a part of my duty to provide rations for all."[82]

79. Dwinelle, *Medical Report.*

80. *Ibid.*

81. Coddington, *The Gettysburg Campaign*, p. 541.

82. Dwinelle, *Medical Report.*

It had to have been a great relief to Surgeon Dwinelle when a portion of one supply train pulled to a halt on the level bank of Rock Creek and started to unload. "I received this day [July 4] delivered at the Hospital (6,000) Six thousand rations of Tea Coffee Sugar crackers Soap Salt Candles Salt Pork and three thousand six hundred pounds of Beef on the hoof." For now, at least, the hospitals would be able to give the men something to eat as they arrived, and have candlelight to push back the shadows as evening approached.[83]

Unfortunately, so much of the hospital staff was apparently detailed to the immediate care of the wounded that insufficient manpower was left to carry out an orderly distribution of the food and supplies. Even though there were crackers, salt pork, and fresh beef in the camp, many of the waiting wounded continued to suffer hunger pangs and growling stomachs.

Somewhere South of Gettysburg, Pennsylvania

The miniature supply train of the Christian Commission was still on the road northward, and the going was not getting any easier. The ambulance carrying Ellen Orbison Harris and her parcels of anaesthetics and stimulants had long since outdistanced the heavily loaded wagon, disappearing over the horizon toward Gettysburg. "It continued raining until about 5 o'clock. We pressed on through mud and rain and over the rough, stony and hilly roads to Taneytown."[84]

At Taneytown, it was necessary to give the weary horses a breather, so the commissioners took advantage of the stop to pay a brief call on a local acquaintance. "While our horses were eating, we called at the house of our friend, Rev. Mr. Scarborough, the Presbyterian preacher in that place, whose good wife insisted on giving us some supper, adding to our stores some loaves of bread. Soon as our horses were done eating we urged our driver to start."[85]

---

83. *Ibid.* "By the exertions of Colonel [Henry F.] Clarke, chief commissary, 30,000 rations were brought up on July 4 and distributed to the hospitals," wrote Surgeon Jonathan Letterman, medical director of the Army of the Potomac, in his official report. "Some of the hospitals were supplied by the commissaries of the corps to which they belonged. Arrangements were made by him to have supplies in abundance brought to Gettysburg for the wounded; he ordered them, and if the railroad could have transported them they would have been on hand." [*OR*, vol. 27, pt. 1, p. 197.]
84. Cross, *The War and the Christian Commission*, p. 12.
85. *Ibid.*

Now a new difficulty arose—the recalcitrant wagon driver felt that he had traveled quite far enough for one day. "He soon began to falter and make excuses to stop for the night. Presently a sound of horses' feet, which proved to be cavalry guarding the beef cattle of General Meade's army, aroused him sufficiently to journey on as long as they were in hearing. Very soon after he turned into a field where were three ambulances spending the night." No threats, promises, or pleading could move the obstinate teamster one step further, so "here we waited until daylight."[86]

Baltimore, Maryland

George Anna Woolsey and her mother, exhausted by the unexpected trip and anxious for news of brother and son, undoubtedly checked in at the Sanitary Commission headquarters upon their arrival in the city, intent on getting any update from the battlefield. "There the news reached us that Charley was safe, and the rebels, repulsed at every point, were, at that date, July 4, in rapid retreat toward the Potomac. . . . They left all their dead and dying in our hands at Gettysburg. 7,000 of the dead of both armies were buried at once; and all the buildings on the hillsides and in the little town, both private houses and shops, were full of wounded men. That July 4th saw also Pembroke's [*sic*] entire army of 31,000 surrender to Grant at Vicksburg; and Charley was safe! So it was a day always to remember with wonder and solemn thankfulness, though with horror at the suffering and distress all around us."[87]

Considering the fact that they had come so far already, and that there was such desperate need for help at Gettysburg, the two women decided to press on for Gettysburg without delay. A load of Sanitary supplies was scheduled to leave on the next train, and they would be on board to accompany it.

Hanover, Pennsylvania

It was becoming clear to Mary Cadwell Fisher and her companions that they were not going to reach Gettysburg before darkness set in.

---

86. *Ibid.*

87. Bacon and Howland, *Letters of a Family During the Civil War*, pp. 526-27. Although George Anna does not specifically relate that they stopped at the local Sanitary commission headquarters, it was the logical place for a message to reach them.

The persistent rains, combined with the severe damage done to the roads by heavy Union and Confederate traffic, had significantly slowed their progress. The need was so great, however, that they doggedly pressed on through the dim twilight. "The urgent call for help from Gettysburg decided us to go through without stopping. We took a circuitous route, avoiding the turnpike, and traveling with great caution, as we were in danger of meeting squads of desperate fugitives from the defeated army."[88]

"Before nightfall a pouring rain came on, and fearing to continue our journey in the darkness, as the swollen streams might render the bad roads impassable, we stopped at Hanover until the storm subsided."[89]

Gettysburg, Pennsylvania

Capt. Benjamin Thompson had done as much for his shrunken company of the 111th New York as was possible under the circumstances. The burials from his command were finished, corpses just barely covered in the stubborn rocky soil of Pennsylvania, the dead and wounded noted down for the muster rolls, any possible provisions sought out, and it was shaping up to be another night of sleeping on their arms. The little company was still in line with the rest of the regiment, along the littered slopes of Cemetery Ridge, waiting.

With the adrenaline-charged hours of hectic battle behind him, the exertions of the last week were beginning to catch up with the young captain. Although he was healing nicely from the nasty lacerations suffered when a shell sprayed rock chips into his face during yesterday's bombardment, it was the varicose veins in his legs that were now causing him the most discomfort. "My limbs and feet were so swollen and sore[,] and I was so exhausted, that the Colonel sent a man with me to the rear to find a place where I could be sheltered and get some rest. We found an abandoned shack where I was protected from the showers and I rested undisturbed."[90]

---

88. *The Philadelphia Times*, December 23, 1882.
89. *Ibid.*
90. Thompson, *Personal Narrative*, pp. 47-48. The "abandoned shack" was probably a primary aid station that had been cleared of wounded as the Ambulance Corps continued to evacuate casualties back to division hospitals along Rock Creek.

Far out across the Emmitsburg Road, behind the enemy skirmish line, Jacob Cole of the 57th New York still lay on the battlefield as rain sluiced down around him. It had been two days now since he had been wounded, once in the arm by a bullet, once in the leg by a shell fragment, in the bloody back-and-forth fighting in the Wheatfield. Two days without shelter of any kind; two days without any food or water except what he was carrying when he went into battle; two days without any pain killers as his two wounds began to swell and throb.

It was hard to get any rest with the procession of stealthy footsteps passing by—Southern skirmishers were silently falling back. "By midnight of the 4th there was not a living rebel left on the battlefield of Gettysburg, as early in the evening their picket line was withdrawn and I was left all alone among the dead." The New York soldier made himself as comfortable as possible, preparing to spend a third night alone in what had become one vast charnelhouse all around him.[91]

It was certainly not going to be a restful night in the teeming Second Corps Hospitals along Rock Creek, as wounded continued to be unloaded from a never-ending train of ambulances. Captain Thomas Livermore, after getting all the wounded that could be reached on the field into regimental aid stations, had turned his attention to evacuating these front line primary stations as quickly as possible to the division hospitals in the rear. Granite School House Road was clogged with ambulances heading east, turning south to the Bushman farm lane, then bumping and jouncing cross country to Rock Creek. Once unloaded, they turned their jaded horses around and headed back immediately for another load. What seemed like an inexhaustible flow of bleeding and torn soldiers was rapidly overwhelming the exhausted Second Corps surgeons.

Virginian John Dooley had finally managed to attract the attention of one of the overworked doctors. "A young surgeon is near me now, and after examining my wounds and asking a great many foolish and ignorant questions, I urge him to look at my man's (Scammel's) breast. He assures me positively that he will do so as soon as he has taken a

91. Cole, *Under Five Commanders*, p. 209.

bite of something to eat. Oh humanity!" exploded the young Confederate. "A human life or a cup of coffee!"[92]

With their portion of the burials in front of the Union lines finally completed, a weary and nauseous Sgt. T. P. Meyer and the 148th Pennsylvania Pioneers moved on to their next assignment. "In the fore part of the night I head the pioneers over to this hospital to bury some dead. The wounded all lying on the bare ground were generally quiet; the majority seemed to be sleeping. The head surgeon told me that they had discovered, in kerosene, a specific remedy for the extirpation of maggots from the wounds of the men, and triumphantly stated that there was no longer a maggoty wound in the place. Up to this time soldiers were frequently seen in the field hospitals, flipping maggots from their wounds with a stick whittled sharp for the purpose."[93]

As if to prove the "head surgeon" wrong, "one young soldier wounded under the arm asked a surgeon to dress his wound; he could not raise his arm. The surgeon took hold of his hand and jerked it violently up and a handful of big maggots fell out." So much for "the extirpation of maggots!"[94]

Captain Nickerson of the 8th Ohio found a familiar and welcome person at the hospital. "By a strange piece of luck, one of the hospital attendants had picked up my servant, whom he brought to me. 'Jerry' was a mite of a fellow[,] . . . very young, too, and about as broad as he was tall. His duties had heretofore been confined to blacking my shoes when in camp, and carrying my haversack and rubber coat when on the march. To these latter-mentioned articles he had still clung, so that when it commenced to rain the little rubber coat was used to partially cover me. It would only cover a small portion of my person, but, inadequate as it was, it was more than many of my comrades had."[95]

---

92. Dooley, *John Dooley*, p. 111.
93. Muffly, *The Story of Our Regiment*, p. 467.
94. *Ibid.*, pp. 467-68. One can only imagine the fiery agony of having an open wound washed out with kerosene.
95. Nickerson, "Personal Recollections of Two Visits to Gettysburg," p. 21.

The weather continued rainy and miserable, with drizzles interspersed with heavy cloudbursts. "The rain poured down in torrents, saturating the exposed portions of my clothing until, with the aid of a shallow pool that formed where I lay, it permeated the whole and I was thoroughly drenched," continued the Ohio officer. "At times I became unconscious, but recovered enough to miss the little cover which the rubber coat had afforded. Although it was very dark, I felt all around for it and could not imagine where it had gone, but gone it certainly had."[96]

"To add to this uninterrupted round of pleasure, toward morning I was seized with an awful thirst. Though the rain was pouring down my face and over my now totally unprotected body, I wanted water as I never before wanted it. I called, and called again and again, but no one came. Those who were not disabled were sleeping too soundly for one feeble voice to awaken them. Finally a sergeant of my regiment, who was lying near, answered, and said that he would try and get some water for me. I heard him get up and the rattling of his canteen, as he started down to the creek for the coveted drink, but he did not return."[97]

As it became evident that the sergeant was not going to return with a container of water, even the sound of the Rock Creek in the background took on it's own form of taunting torment. "The hope that had been raised and disappointed seemed to make me more thirsty than ever. A stream of water was boiling, bubbling, and running within my hearing; my face and body were drenched; and yet it seemed as though I should die of thirst. At last a blessing, though terribly disguised, came to my relief; I became delirious, unconscious."[98]

---

96. *Ibid.*, pp. 21-22. "The next day the mystery was explained. Little Jerry had visited me during one of the unconscious spells and, believing that I was dead, had constituted himself my executor and sole administrator, and as such had taken charge of my effects, consisting of the haversack and the aforesaid rubber coat." [*Ibid.*, p. 22.]
97. *Ibid.*, p. 22. "He had been badly wounded himself, and daylight showed that in his effort to succor his fellow-soldier, he had fallen near the banks of the stream and there bled to death. 'Greater love hath no man,' than was here shown by poor Sergeant Tracy." [*Ibid.*]
98. *Ibid.*

Confederate John Dooley, laying back from Rock Creek on the level banks used for ambulance unloading, was enduring a man-made suffering as the long night hours slowly passed.

> This is a horrid night, cold and wet and rainy. Groans and shrieks and maniacal ravings; bitter sobs, and heavy sighs, piteous cries; horrid oaths; despair; the death rattle; darkness; death. The Yankees near me ([male] nurses, they are called) instead of alleviating to some degree the fearful sufferings around us, are indulging in curses, the most ignorant curiosity, and obscene tales.
>
> All night long I lie awake shivering with cold save when my wearied eye lids droop for a moment, again to be opened by a convulsive start as the wheels of the ambulance all but run over my feet. And the infuriated drivers curse and whip their refractory horses, or some yell or shriek louder than the rest tells how near the horses' hoofs have approached some helpless wounded wretch. All night long these ambulances move among us, still bringing more and more from that field of blood.[99]

99. Dooley, *John Dooley*, pp. 111-12.

Chapter 9

SUNDAY, JULY 5: PRE-DAWN—SUNDAY, JULY 5: 11:00 P.M.

"Two boxes of soda crackers in a hospital of over 3000 wounded men."
Christian Commissioner Andrew Cross

Hanover, Pennsylvania

The storm front that had stranded Mary Cadwell Fisher and her traveling companions in Hanover had finally moved out of the area, leaving behind a cloudless, though muggy, night. The small band of relief workers from York, intent on reaching Gettysburg as soon as possible, hitched up their team and headed northwest toward the battlefield.

> After a few hours rest we again started in the clear starlight. A hushed calm brooded over the whole earth, as if nature herself had participated in the fearful combat and had lain down to rest.
>
> Day gradually broke with a strange, solemn light. Slowly the Sabbath sun came up over the distant hill-tops as if reluctant to look upon the scenes of horror on the battle ground, only yesterday filled with fierce combatants, and the incessant roar of artillery drowning the groans of thousands of poor wounded fellows; to-day covered with the unburied dead and the wrecks of the bloody strife.
>
> As we neared Gettysburg, still cautiously proceeding, we heard firing at regular intervals, while an occasional report told that the artillery was still doing its fatal work. We were

> repeatedly stopped by sentinels who refused to allow us to pass the lines, representing the danger of meeting with skirmishing parties, or of being struck with a chance shell, but a note from our Chief Burgess stating our errand prevailed and we were allowed to pass.[1]

Delayed for another hour by an Army of the Potomac corps marching out after the retreating Confederates, Mrs. Fisher and her comrades finally arrived at their destination, and were busily at work in a hospital in town by 7:00 a.m.[2]

Gettysburg, Pennsylvania

"July 5th," jotted wounded Confederate prisoner John Dooley in his diary by the weak light of early daybreak. "Morning dawns at last. Though raining still the chill of the small hours before day break no longer make me shiver, and soon the carriers come around with their vessels of coffee, and this does much towards comforting the inner part of man."[3]

"An officer (Yankee) is inquiring if any one here is acquainted with John Scammel. I tell him he belongs to my company. 'Here then,' he said, 'are some little things I took from his pocket; he died a few minutes ago a few yards off.' These little effects consist of a five dollar Confederate bill stained with his blood, and a paper showing the date, etc. of his enrollment. Poor fellow, he might have lived if proper care had been shown him." But there just were not enough surgeons to go around; even working as fast as possible, there were still thousands to be treated, and always someone with a worse wound than the previous patient's. "Our poor fellows are dying all around us and but little surgical attention might save them," grieved Dooley.[4]

General Meade also was up bright and early this July morning, overseeing the departure of a heavy reconnaissance, led by Brig. Gen.

---

1. Mrs. Mary Cadwell Fisher, "A Week on Gettysburg Field," *The Philadelphia Times*, December 23, 1882.
2. *Ibid.*
3. Dooley, *John Dooley*, p. 112.
4. *Ibid.*

Gouvenour K. Warren, to determine what the Confederates were up to. Plans were also being put in place for the entire Army of the Potomac to pull out of Gettysburg in pursuit of the defeated Southern army—the severely-used Second Corps would travel with the Twelfth Corps under the overall supervision of Maj. Gen. Henry W. Slocum.[5]

While all these arrangements were being put in place, Brig. Gen. Herman Haupt clattered up to army headquarters in a buggy, pausing long enough to bring Meade up to date on the efforts of his railroad maintenance teams. Working westward toward Gettysburg, the repair crews were laboring round the clock to reestablish rail service. Nineteen bridges had been totally wrecked by the Confederates on the right-of-way leading to the battlefield, and numerous culverts and tracks sections were severely damaged or weakened. The railroader confirmed the worst—it was still going to be a few more days before any trains steamed into the isolated village.[6]

The skirmishers, out in the lonely fence rows and pasturelands to the west of the Union position, were the first to notice the total lack of movement around the Confederate picket lines. "I think my regiment [5th New Hampshire] was in the skirmish line when the rebels retreated in the night," wrote Captain Livermore of the Ambulance Corps, "and the men were among the first to discover the retreat."[7]

With the battlefield now abandoned by the enemy, the Army of the Potomac could finally get on with the work of tidying up what had once been peaceful countryside, but now more closely resembled an immense refuse heap of bent, bloody, and battered military equipment, interspersed randomly with the bodies of mutilated men and animals. "Details were sent out to collect abandoned arms, and others to bury the masses of the rebel dead—a sad, sad job," wrote Chaplain Henry S. Stevens, 14th Connecticut Volunteers, of that gruesome task. "They found the dead in some places so numerous that the ground appeared covered with them, and one could walk for distances stepping only on bodies of the slain. The Emmettsburg [*sic*] road directly in our front

5. Coddington, *The Gettysburg Campaign: A Study in Command*, pp. 544-45.
6. Haupt, *Reminiscences of Herman Haupt*, pp. 216, 223-24.
7. Livermore, *Days and Events*, p. 269.

seemed packed with them—a vast hecatombs to the insatiate Moloch of the cruel and causeless slaveholders' rebellion."[8]

As the Union men moved further from their own lines, they encountered still more corpses, both Northern and Southern, stretching as far as the eye could see, which had lain for three days in the sultry summer heat. "The sight of some of the dead was moving to the sternest hearts. Some were in the attitudes indicating that life went out in agony, and others holding likenesses of home loved ones they had spent their last moments in gazing upon, or staring with glazed eyes upon the blessed scriptures that had solaced the dark hours when 'all *men* had forsaken them.'" Scattered in and among the twisted heaps of dead men and horses, discarded equipment, and bloody firearms were the wounded, moving about painfully, feebly calling out to their Northern rescuers. "One not yet dead, a mere lad, lying on the wet muddy ground, [was] groaning and writhing in his physical torture." When asked if he were in much pain, the boy replied: "Dreadfully! dreadfully! O that my mother were here!"[9]

Assistant Surgeon Francis Moses Wafer, wrapping up aid station operations at the Peter Frey Farm on the Taneytown Road, kept track of the activities out on the field. It was "a drizzly & foggy morning," he scribbled in his diary, and "much of the forenoon was spent in burying their dead & removing their abandoned wounded."[10]

The Second Corps, which had taken much of the brunt of the Confederate onslaught on July 2 and 3, was given the mixed blessing of being the last to leave Gettysburg in pursuit of the retreating Southerners. Their place in the marching order certainly gave them more time to rest after their strenuous fighting, but it also left General Hancock's men with the odious task of mopping up operations on the battlefield and interring the festering dead.

The burials, begun in earnest on July 4, were a long way from being complete. Even in death, the army regimen of "forming ranks" and "counting off" prevailed. "On Sunday morning, July 5, large details of our corps are made up to bury the dead," recalled one Ohio soldier.

---

8. Stevens, *Souvenir of Excursion to Battlefields*, p. 36. Moloch (or Molech) was an idol worshipped by the ancient Ammonites in the Middle East. The hollow metal deity was heated red hot, then first-born children were sacrificed by laying them in his outstretched, scorching hands.
9. *Ibid.*, pp. 36-37.
10. Wafer diary.

"The corpses are brought into rows and counted, the Confederate and Federals being separated into different rows."[11]

"A detail was soon made from each regiment, with pickaxes and shovels to perform the last sad rites. Our own dead were buried in groups, the name and regiment of each placed at the head of the little mounds. . . . The bodies of Union soldiers were buried in separate graves and each grave marked with the name and organization to which the soldier belodged [*sic*]. When that information could not be obtained, the grave was marked with that distressing word, 'Unknown.'"[12]

The Confederate dead were not afforded the luxury of separate graves, nor was time taken to determine individual identities. "At the feet of each row of fifty or a hundred dead, a trench is dug about seven or eight feet wide and about three feet deep—for there is not time for normal grave depth. Then the bodies, which are as black as ink and bloated from exposure to the sun, are placed in the shallow ditch and quickly covered with dirt."[13]

"Some of the bodies having lain upon the ground since the 2nd of the month, exposed to the hot rays of a July sun, were badly decomposed, and the stench from the battlefield was something fearful," remembered a former Maine infantryman, the memory still vivid and distasteful after forty-six years.[14]

No monuments, not even a cracker box lid with each man's name hastily scrawled, preserved the distinctive uniqueness of these Southern men. Most, in fact, were already rendered unidentified or unidentifiable by the fatal work of exploding and slashing shells, or by the marauding hands of scavengers from both armies which had removed all possible tokens of recognition. Across a landscape dotted with groves, copses, and orchards, scattered trees were pressed into service as makeshift memorial markers. "On an adjacent oak the burial parties would hew off the bark from one side and place in lead pencil the number buried in the trench," wrote J. Howard Wert, a local resident, who witnessed the ghastly work; "thus: '73 rebs buried to the right': '45 rebs, in this trench,' etc." For these veteran troops of the

---

11. Galwey, *The Valiant Hours*, p. 121.
12. Smith, *History of the Nineteenth Maine*, pp. 100, 93.
13. Galwey, *The Valiant Hours*, p. 121.
14. Smith, *History of the Nineteenth Maine*, p. 93.

South, the glorious Pennsylvania campaign came to a bitter end here, under the very ground that they had come to invade.[15]

As Northern details combed the field, picking up the litter of discarded military issue, a veritable arsenal of weaponry, running the gamut from state-of-the-art rifled muskets to archaic flintlocks, began accumulating out in the fields between Cemetery Ridge and the Emmitsburg Road. Union troops saw in this vast stockpile of abandoned equipment a golden opportunity to refit—many updated their old, lost, or damaged firearms from the flotsam of battle, replacing any equipment that had been discarded during the hot and dusty marches of June.

After a restful night in the shelter of an empty shack to the rear of the Union line, Capt. Benjamin Thompson of the 111th New York hobbled back to his regiment. Neither the lacerations to his face from flying stone chips during the July 3 bombardment, nor his painfully swollen feet and legs could keep him from reequipping his command. "I reached the field early in the morning of the Fifth and completed the equipment of my little company with the best the field afforded."[16]

As the first feelers of armed pursuit moved out after the retreating Confederates, Captain Livermore was busy dispatching long trains of ambulances across the battlefield. Where skirmisher and sharpshooter fire had swept the field with deadly accuracy the day before, the ambulancemen now were able to move about with complete freedom, picking up those wounded still desperately clinging to life, some after being left unattended for three days. Jacob H. Cole, nursing the two wounds he had received in Farmer Rose's wheatfield on July 2, was picked up by one of the Second Corps ambulance crews, and happily reported that "soon I was again among friends."[17]

---

15. J. Howard Wert, *A Complete Hand-Book of the Monuments and Indications and Guide to the Positions on the Gettysburg Battle-field* (Harrisburg, Pennsylvania: R. M. Sturgeon & Company, 1886), p. 201.
16. Thompson, *Personal Narrative*, p. 48.
17. Cole, *Under Five Commanders*, p. 209.

As inconceivable as it may seem, with so many soldiers still laying where they had fallen on the field, often with little or no food or water for days, groups of tourists wandered about the battlefield, totally oblivious to the needs of these gravely injured men. "Already the civilian souvenir hunters are scattered over the field, picking up relics of the battle. . . . The relic hunters, with satchels slung across their shoulders, provide us a good deal of amusement. Most of them have come from a good distance at the news of the battle, and have gained permission to journey to the field by representing themselves as volunteer nurses for the wounded. Some of them are medical men, some clergymen, and what not. But their innate curiosity is their main motive in visiting the places where anything remarkable occurred during the battle, and to gaze with ludicrous horror at the black and mutilated dead who are strewn everywhere. Cannon balls are especially sought by these people."[18]

"These people," as Thomas Galwey of the 8th Ohio described them, were scorned and derided by the troops, and frequently the butt of jokes and malicious pranks. "A practical joker of a soldier, seeing a middle-aged man thrusting his cane into the bloody grass, in search of relics, picked up an unexploded percussion shell and offered it to him. The civilian, who ought to have known better, took it thankfully and put it in his satchel, when another soldier, less jocosely inclined, warned the civilian of the dangerous character of his relic. Fearful lest the terrified greenhorn might throw the treacherous thing on the ground and bring havoc and ruin upon all around, the soldier took it from the satchel and laid it upon the ground as delicately as though it were a child."[19]

Spectators were also out and about on the fields which, only two days previous, had seen some of the most desperate fighting. Composed primarily of citizens from neighboring towns, as well as children and youths from Gettysburg, these locals wandered about the area goggle-eyed, witnessing the aftermath of the most exciting thing that had ever transpired in this bucolic part of Pennsylvania. Tillie Pierce, recovered from the horrors she had witnessed at the Jacob Weikert aid station on Friday night, was out sight-seeing along the Union battle lines with some of her friends. "While we were climbing up

---

18. Galwey, *The Valiant Hours*, pp. 121-22.
19. *Ibid.*, p. 122.

Little Round Top, we met one of the Pennsylvania 'Buck Tails,' who walked with us and pointed out the different places where the bodies lay among the rocks. . . . The view there spread out before us was terrible to contemplate! It was an awful spectacle! Dead soldiers, bloated horses, shattered cannon and caissons, thousands of small arms. In fact everything belonging to army equipments, was there in one confused and indescribable mass."[20]

While the scavengers and predators scoured the field for mementoes, and tourists took in the gruesome sights, genuine help was finally arriving on the ripped and gouged fields of Gettysburg. Ellen Orbison Harris and her borrowed ambulance had finally reached the Second Corps Hospital; she immediately started doling out what remained of her meager supply of chloroform and stimulants. Fortunately, the delegates of the Christian Commission were not far behind.

South of Gettysburg, Pennsylvania

For Andrew Cross and the men of the Christian Commission, anxious to reach the site of the recent battle, it had been a disgusting night spent in a lonely field with a recalcitrant teamster and a groaning wagonload of desperately-needed supplies. "Here we waited until daylight, when we had to put our wits to work to get him off without waiting for his breakfast. As he had two days allowed him in which to make his trip, we told him if he would get us to the hospital of the 2d Army corps, he might do what he pleased with the rest of the time, by which, and urging the condition of the wounded men, we induced him to start."[21]

"The heavy rain of the preceding day continued through the night and morning." The Christian Commissioners were traveling the same road over which the Army of the Potomac was rushing provisions from the Westminster railhead to the troops at Gettysburg, and the passage of the massive supply trains over this rural thoroughfare soon became readily apparent. "The immense wagoning which had been upon this clay road made it difficult to get along, even by going through the fields, and would have been utterly impossible in the night."[22]

---

20. Alleman, *At Gettysburg*, pp. 80-81.
21. Cross, *The War and the Christian Commission*, p. 12.
22. *Ibid*.

It soon became evident that the commissioners were drawing up on the edges of the Union army. "Very soon we came to squads of soldiers who had wandered off six to eight miles to see what they could obtain at the farm houses along the road; then along the road and in the field we could see dead horses, who, after being wounded, had probably fled as far as they could, and there had dropped down and died. From daylight we had noticed companies of cavalry turning in all the roads leading west from the Taneytown road. Since we [have] learned they were searching for the whereabouts of Lee's army, which that morning had moved in retreat."[23]

"As we advanced toward the round top, General Meade's extreme left, we came upon a portion of the 5th and 6th corps of [Maj. Gen. George] Sykes and [Maj. Gen. John] Sedgwick. These were scattered in every direction, in houses, barns, &c. Here were wagons, tents, stacks of guns, here a little fire, there a few men trying to keep on a place where they would not be in water or mud."[24]

The men at this far southern end of the field seemed to be as ignorant of the condition of the army as were the Christian Commission representatives. "One would inquire of us how many of the militia were out? Another, whether General McClellan was not in command of them? This part of the army did not know that the battle was over. With a knowledge of the severity of the preceding day's fight, it was very natural to be anxious for reinforcements. Many were waiting for orders to renew the fight."[25]

These isolated troops, marooned on the far left of the Union army, provided poor assistance in giving directions to the Second Corps medical facilities. "We inquired for the 2d corps hospital, but no one could tell. One said, in this barn, another in that, but none knew." Frustrated, the commissioners urged the wagoneer to drive on. "Seeing at a distance a train of about 30 to 40 ambulances coming from the battle-field, we made our way to them, and learned that they were going to the 2d corps. Beckoning to our driver, we followed them. . . ."[26]

Southwest of Harrisburg, Pennsylvania

Other Christian Commissioners were also making their way to the field. Bushrod Washington James, a prominent Philadelphia physician,

23. *Ibid.*, pp. 12-13.
24. *Ibid.*, p. 13.
25. *Ibid.*
26. *Ibid.*

had worked with the Commission the previous year following the Battle of Antietam. Now here was another opportunity to be of service, this time virtually at his doorstep. "When the terrible battle was in progress the news of it filled me with an enthusiastic desire to be again at the front, and in the midst of the surgical work which my experience at Antietam had shown me was a very necessary adjunct to the success of our cause of right."[27]

Unfortunately, there was some delay in getting started. "On account of a death in the family it was impossible for me to leave immediately on hearing of the battle." As soon as the funeral was over, Dr. James wasted no time in getting ready to depart for Gettysburg. "Just as rapidly as the work could be accomplished I gathered together a quantity of hospital stores, and in company with several others who were likewise provided, and all acting under the Christian commission, we shipped the stores to a point on the Pennsylvania Railroad a few miles south of Harrisburg, at Middletown, where large wagons were secured and the goods packed."[28]

With the railroad to Gettysburg demolished, and the bridges over the river at Harrisburg destroyed or sufficiently damaged to hinder the Confederate invaders, the only way to reach the battlefield from there was to be ferried across the river.

> A heavy storm had been raging all night, but in the early morning undauntedly we started to cross the Susquehanna River. Its waters were so swollen that we encountered the possibility of being swept down the angry stream or of being wrecked upon some of the rocks along the opposite shore. One who has only seen the river in time of quiet and sunshine would scarcely realize how turbulent and dangerous it becomes when the weather is stormy.
>
> Notwithstanding, our flatboat carried us over safely, and Providence favored our project in gaining a safe landing on the southern shore, from which we took the main road, known as the Harrisburg turnpike on the present map, southward to the now historic battle-field. The wagons were so laden with the goods that there was scarcely a foothold for the commissioners, so we, together with the drivers,

27. Bushrod Washington James, *Echoes of Battle* (Philadelphia: Henry T. Coates & Company, 1895), p. 98.
28. *Ibid.*, pp. 98-99.

walked nearly the whole distance to Gettysburg from our landing place.[29]

Hancock Bridge, New Jersey

For a number of months now, blonde, blue-eyed Cornelia Hancock had been casting about for some way in which she could assist in the war effort.

> After my only brother and every male relative and friend that we possessed had gone to the War, I deliberately came to the conclusion that I, too, would go and serve my country. I confided this resolution to my sister's husband, Dr. Henry T. Child, who lived in Philadelphia where he was well known in philanthropic and antislavery circles. He promised to let me know of the first available opportunity to be of use.
>
> The summons came on the morning of July fifth, 1863, when his horse and carriage was sent for me on a Fourth of July excursion boat that was returning to Salem [New Jersey] by the Delaware River. It arrived in the early morning and was driven the five miles beyond the town to where I lived. When it was driven up in front of our house, my mother threw up both of her hands and exclaimed to father: "Oh, Tom, what has happened?" I had not risen, but hearing Mothers exclamation, and surmising, I said: "Oh, nothing, Mother. Doctor has sent for me to go to war!" So it proved. . . .[30]

"In an hour's time I was off for Philadelphia." Cornelia, in her early twenties and a devout Quaker, was gravely concerned about decorum and appearances, especially on a Sunday morning. "I well remember when driving through Salem my friends were going to church, so I hid myself down in the carriage lest I should be stopped to be bidden good-bye or saluted by any of the formalities they might wish to

---

29. *Ibid.*, p. 99.
30. Cornelia Hancock, *South After Gettysburg: Letters of Cornelia Hancock from the Army of the Potomac, 1863-1865*, ed. Henrietta Stratton Jaquette (New York: Thomas Y. Crowell Company, 1937), pp. 4-5. Like the late night phone call or the out-of-town telegram, a decked-out carriage in backwater Hancock Bridge could only be the sign of bad news (or so Mrs. Hancock surmised).

indulge in. Much less did I want to hear them say: 'Why, Cornelia, thee is too young to go.'"[31]

So Cornelia Hancock rolled out of rural Salem, New Jersey, toward an unknown assignment, armed with only the vague promise of a brother-in-law in a distant city. One thing was certain, however. Her first stop would be Philadelphia.

Ascension Church, Philadelphia, Pennsylvania

"A suggestive scene was presented at Ascension Church, in Philadelphia, on the morning of the 5th of July, 1863. Two days before the great Battle of Gettysburg had been fought. The nation knew already that victory crowned our arms; but it stood yet on the tiptoe of expectation. As to the consequences of the rebel reverse suspense still prevailed. Hourly bulletins from the field announced the most terrible suffering among the wounded, and appeals for help—for nurses, surgeons, and stores—rung with painful pathos in the North. Thirty thousand men were lying on the field, helpless, dying, just as they fell. Ascension Church had acted upon this information."[32]

For the worshippers of this Philadelphia congregation, Sunday, July 5, 1863 would be like no other Sunday ever experienced before. "The hearts of its Christian men and women had been stirred by the sad appeal; and here, on this Sabbath morning, with the bells beating their morning psalms around them, two hundred or more, nimble-handed women chiefly, were assembled, busily at work preparing supplies for the field. In place of a sermon the clergyman had brought a sewing machine; instead of Sabbath-day finery each woman wore the more royal ornament of plain working-apparel. In every available niche a sewing-machine was shrined; even the pulpit-desk was removed, and a brood, noisy as so many canaries, clustered and chattered on the platform. Here were some preparing lint; there were others cutting shirts, drawers, bandages; while in another place others were sizing rags—of all things on a battlefield most necessary and useful."[33]

---

31. *Ibid.*, p. 5.
32. Foster, "Four Days at Gettysburg," p. 381.
33. *Ibid.* The sewing machine was one of the first mass-produced consumer goods which could be purchased on "time" payments. By 1863, many families, especially in the North, were paying $5.00 a month toward their new sewing machines. Some ladies were so proud of this new addition to their household that they even had their photograph taken with it. [Juanita Leisch, *An Introduction to Civil War Civilians* (Gettysburg, Pennsylvania: Thomas Publications, 1994), p. 11.]

Unknown to these conscientious volunteers, the shirts, drawers, bandages, and rags they were so assiduously laboring over would in a few days find their way to the Second Corps Hospitals at Gettysburg. But for now, however, these faithful civilians labored solely because they saw the need and desperately wanted to be of help. "Now and then young men staggered in under great burdens of material contributed at the houses in the vicinity, or poured into the treasury the gifts of friends and neighbors. The scene was a picture of wartime. Christian love and sympathy shone through it and over it like a benediction. There was a heart-beat in every click of the needle."[34]

Gettysburg, Pennsylvania

Falling in with the Second Corps ambulance train, Andrew Cross and his men walked ahead of their wagon, while the driver carefully navigated his team through the rocky terrain. "In a short time [we] reached the hospital of the 3rd Division of this corps. . . . This hospital was about 2 to 2 1/2 miles from the lines on our right, in a woods and along Rock Creek. The ground was very unfavorable, being flat, muddy and wet."[35]

Even these trained professionals, visitors to numerous battle-grounds and field hospitals, were totally unprepared for the sheer size and state of this medical facility. "Some little idea of the condition of this hospital and the destruction of the battle may be inferred from the fact that there were over 3,200 wounded in all, living, beside many dead lying around it, 2,308 Union and 952 Rebels. We came into the midst of these wounded and dying and dead, as they were lying on the ground, and being lifted from ambulances, and laid beside others who were on the ground, without anything under or over them. Many had lost nearly all their clothes in the fight; others when wounded had to have their clothes torn off to stop the blood and attend to their wounds."[36]

Reporting in to Dr. Isaac Scott, medical director of the Third Division, Cross and his men immediately volunteered to head back out on the field to assist the ambulance corps. "We proposed to go to the

---

34. *Ibid.*

35. Cross, *The War and the Christian Commission*, p. 13.

36. *Ibid.* Cross' count of "2,308 Union and 952 Rebels" wounded was the final total of patients cared for at all three of the Second Corps Hospitals. When the commissioners arrived at the hospital, the facility was still growing as wounded continued streaming in from the field.

battle-field to help gather up the wounded, dying and dead, but were informed that it would not be allowed, as the Rebel sharpshooters were still hidden about, and would fire upon any person that would come beyond a certain line, or unless connected with the ambulances; that the day before a Confederate officer had offered $500 to an ambulance driver if he would get him off the field. The Rebel commander kept these sharpshooters to annoy our ambulance drivers, and keep our army from the knowledge of his defeat and retreat. Some men in places had thus lay on the ground a day and a half longer than there was any necessity."[37]

Since they would not be allowed to go to the front to collect wounded, the commissioners walked through the hospital, getting a feel for their new surroundings. "The rain not only made the ground at this division hospital muddy, but at times so overflowed, that some of the wounded were drowned for want of help to move them from the low and flat places: at times it was with difficulty we could walk through the hospital. There were a few tents, some little shelter coverings, some gum cloths spread on two rails, with any cloth or covering they could get, but the great mass had no cover or shelter. Some with a pair of pants and no shirt, some a pair of drawers; the scarcity of everything was exceedingly great, no army provisions of any kind having yet come, and the men having been without food in many cases for three days."[38]

Jacob H. Cole was finally back inside his own lines again, arriving at the swampy "Second Corps hospital, where my wounds were dressed. There was such a number of wounded men brought to the hospital that we were obliged to take our turn in being attended to."[39]

As he bided his time awaiting treatment, Cole discovered that being in the hospital had its own forms of horror and despair. "While I was waiting for my turn to come I became an eye witness to a sight which I shall never forget while I live and one I hope never to witness again. I

---

37. *Ibid.* While the Southern army had fallen back the previous night, there may still have been scattered incidents of sharpshooters on the field as late as July 5.
38. *Ibid.*, pp. 13-14. For more on drownings at the Second Corps Hospitals, see the following chapter and Appendix 7.
39. Cole, *Under Five Commanders*, p. 209.

saw the physicians cutting off an arm from some, legs from another, and piling them in heaps outside the hospital to be afterwards buried."[40] The young New Yorker was most fortunate indeed that neither his wounded arm or leg were added to the horrible heaps of severed limbs.

"We were gratified on Sunday morning, the 5th, to find friends with stores for the wounded," remembered Chaplain Thomas G. Murphey of the 1st Delaware. "Commissioners from the Christian Commission, and volunteer aid societies, and individuals, some of whom had harnessed their teams and driven thirty or forty miles, were there with food and clothing."[41]

The news spread like wildfire throughout the Second Corps Hospitals that representatives of the Christian Commission had arrived in camp with supplies. "When the wagon came up the surgeons and men received us with the greatest gladness. Each would ask,—'Have you any bandages, lint, sheets, blankets, &c? we are in want of everything.' So of wines, breads, &c. We said to them, we have some of all these, and they are at your service at once. But what were they among such a multitude?"[42]

The supplies were going to disappear almost instantaneously unless the Commissioners set up some type of monitored distribution system. Fortunately, these men were well-schooled in emergency procedures. They immediately established a Christian Commission supply "station" at the Second Corps Hospital, with one senior delegate serving as "captain" of the "station." All other commissioners would work under his supervision in doling out the desperately needed supplies throughout the hospital, subject only to the orders of the surgeon-in-charge. "To make everything go as far as possible, we resolved to let nothing out but through one of our agents, and then only to extreme cases, as where a man had a leg or arm amputated, or was exhausted by his wounds and exposure. Painful as it was, the necessity was upon us, and we must do the best we could."[43]

40. *Ibid.*
41. Murphey, *Four Years in the War*, p. 123.
42. Cross, *The War and the Christian Commission*, p. 14.
43. *The United States Christian Commission for the Army and Navy. For the Year 1863. Second Annual Report*, pp. 69-70; Cross, *The War and the Christian Commission*, p. 14.

The Christian Commission had not come to provide supplies solely to the Second Corps; they had an interest in all the wounded men scattered around the battlefield. "Borrowing a horse of Dr. [Isaac] Scott, of the 7th [West] Virginia, and putting one of our Commission in charge of our goods, and procuring a guard, we hastened to the 3d and 5th corps hospitals. On inquiry of the Surgeons, the question was immediate,—'Have you any lint, bandages, sponges, stimulants, &c.?' We directed each of them to send over, and we would do for them what we could."[44]

Their visit to the Third and Fifth Corps Hospitals completed, the commissioners hurried back to their supplies at the Second Corps Hospital. A new realization was beginning to dawn of just how vast the need was in all of the field hospitals. "Coming back, the necessity for economy became so terrible, that when a poor fellow, who had periled his life for his country, and had a wounded arm or leg, begged for bread, we were often compelled to break a soda cracker in two, give him half, and the remainder to another wounded in his foot or leg."[45]

Having put their surgical supplies at the disposal of the doctors, the men from the Christian Commission set out through the masses of wounded men, personally passing out their meager dole of rations and delicacies. "A full description of the condition of the wounded would require the attention of one who was not so much occupied in getting the things needed to them and those of other corps," wrote Commissioner Andrew Cross in his report. "We can say, however, that in every direction lay men of all classes, the rich man and the poor man, the commander and the private. At one place, near a fence, lay privates, corporals, lieutenants, majors, and colonels, from New York, North Carolina, Indiana, Mississippi, Connecticut, Georgia, New Hampshire, Alabama, Maine and Delaware, side by side, on the bare ground, or on a little wet straw; no distinction. Men were gathered around trees, with their heads toward the body of the tree; occasionally, when able, one sat up and leaned against it. They were in every condition, from the slightest wound to the man dying in agony, from the terrible mangling of a piece of shell."[46]

The men were literally jammed together in the crowded creek bottom as they were unloaded from the ambulances, or carried in by

---

44. Cross, *The War and the Christian Commission*, p. 14.
45. *Ibid.*
46. *Ibid.*, p. 15.

stretcher crews to the hillside opposite, with absolutely no semblance of order by regiment, rank, or even army. "The first two men we supplied were of the 125th and 111th New York, the next two of the 21st North Carolina, then the 11th U.S. Infantry, an ambulance officer, then a Chaplain [Henry S. Stevens] of the 14th Connecticut, and Rev. Messrs. [J. E.] Adams [from New Sharon, Maine and] Chapin [also from New Sharon], &c. of [the] Christian Committee, for distribution."[47]

It did not take long for the surgeons from the other corps just visited by the commissioners to send men over to pick up the promised supplies. "While we were distributing from man to man, the men came from the 3rd and 5th corps, when we had to divide our goods into three parts, giving one to each of them. Think of two boxes of soda crackers in a hospital of over 3,000 wounded men, who had not anything to eat for three days! But what when divided among hospitals of three corps? It was all we had, and no appearance of supply from any other quarter."[48]

Andrew Cross and his men finally pulled out the loaf of bread that their kind hosts, the Presbyterian minister of Taneytown and his wife, had donated to their provisions the day before. Fresh bread was always a special treat to the troops, since the hardtack and other military staples were virtually inedible at the best of times, and now more so than ever to men weakened by serious wounds. "As we cut up a loaf of bread, which we had gotten at Mr. Scarborough's, to give it to those who had been wounded about the mouth and face, who could not chew a cracker, a man standing by begged us to sell him a slice. He would pay any price. How like Job's account: 'All that a man hath will he give for his life.'—[Job] 2, 4."

"But to him we could only say, 'We can't sell it to you at any price. We would gladly give it to you, but look at those men around you; say whether we ought to let you have it?'"

After a moment of awkward silence, the wounded soldier replied: "'It's all right; give it to them.' These men felt their gnawing hunger and wounds, but when they saw the condition of their companions they readily yielded."[49]

---

47. *Ibid.*, p. 14.
48. *Ibid.*
49. *Ibid.*

Pressed by the demands of the day and the size of the hospital, people lost all track of the date; even old friends sometimes failed to recognize each other.

> While giving out to the men, we noticed at the [distribution] table a man whom we had been supplying to give to others, who looked like a chaplain. . . . We were old acquaintances, and knew each other well, but during the day, meeting time and again at the same boxes, had never recognized each other. As we turned up to straighten our back, after getting things out, we recognized him.
>
> "Well, Murphy [*sic*], where in the world did you come from? I have been here all day; never noticed you before."
>
> "I am chaplain of the 1st Delaware," replied Rev. Murphey; "and am here attending to the wounded of my regiment."
>
> We said this was new work for two such old-fashioned Presbyterians, to be hard at work in boxes and bread, &c., on the Sabbath day.
>
> "What," said he, "it is the Sabbath day? Indeed, I had not the least idea what day it was. I can't tell anything about where I am, or what time has passed for three or four days."[50]

The Christian Commission men, many of them ministers, had also experienced the same unusual lack of consciousness of place and time. "We said that when day broke we recognized the Sabbath, but from that until the present we had not thought of anything but these goods, and to get them to the men that needed them, nor had it ever entered into our minds where we were. This was the first Sabbath we ever recollected spending in bodily labor or secular; but when the exception of necessity and mercy takes place, the exception becomes a duty."[51]

---

50. *Ibid.*, pp. 15-16.
51. *Ibid.*, p. 16. We tend to forget that, at that time, people simply did not work on Sunday, especially ministers of the gospel. The first day of the week was strictly set aside for worship and church attendance.

As the Christian Commissioners maneuvered through the cramped spaces between men, and as more wounded were continually being carried in, one member of the 108th New York took up his pen to scribble a quick note to a friend:

> July 5th/63
>
> God has given us the victory. The rebels are beat back and sides and fled for their lives. We took all their trains, and 6 miles long, but it is a dear victory if human life be taken into account. The Loss in killed and wounded is frightful on both sides. The 108 [New York] is only a name now. The regiment is gone. We had to support Rickett's [*sic*] regular battery close up to the guns and shot and shell did its work for the 108th. It numbers about 50 men for duty.[52]
>
> I hope all at home are well and happy. We will be sent to some hospital in a few days. We at present are lying in a marsh where there is some three inches [of] water under us, but it is no person's fault. It could not be helped. . . . I suppose Flanagan will be uneasy to hear of my death. I am living still thank God. Will write again in a few days.
>
> Yours most respectfully,
>
> James Moore[53]

Westminster, Maryland

After seeing his wounded commander, General Gibbon, safely off at the railway station on July 4, Frank Haskell had found a place to stay the night at Westminster. Rising refreshed in the morning, he sat down to compose a quick letter to his brother:

---

52. The 108th New York was in support of Battery I, 1st United States Artillery, commanded by Lt. George A. Woodruff, not the battery of Capt. R. Bruce Ricketts' 1st Pennsylvania Light Artillery. Because of their inappropriate placement between the limbers and the pieces, the New Yorkers suffered a fifty percent casualty rate without ever having fired a shot in its own defense. [*New York at Gettysburg*, 2:780; *OR*, vol. 27, pt. 1, pp. 465-66; Haskin, *The History of the First Regiment of Artillery*, p. 170.]
53. Letter, James Moore, July 5, 1863, copy in the 108th New York Vertical File, Gettysburg National Military Park Library, copied by permission of the USAMHI, Carlisle, Pennsylvania, original at the University of Rochester. All underlinings and parenthetic emphases are those of James Moore.

Westminster, Md.

July 5, 1863

I can write you but a hasty note now -- but must say to you that I am unharmed, after the terrific battles of the 2nd and 3d of July, at Gettysburg.

I cannot go into particulars,—the battle has been desperate,—you need not fear the result, but thank God for it.

On the 2nd I had a horse I rode, shot with three bullets,—on the 3d, another horse I then rode was shot with three bullets and a piece of shell.

But now more than ever before I think that I am not to be harmed in the battles, for on the 3d a bullet struck my saddle, and glanced going through my pants, drawers, but stopped at the skin above my right knee, and gave me but a *bruise*.

This place is 24 miles from the field, whither I came with the Genl after the fight of the 3d, and shall return there today. I shall be able to be in the saddle again in a day or two.

Genl Gibbon is severely wounded in the left shoulder with a bullet,—and will be off duty for some months,—but his wound is not at all dangerous.

He has consented that I may go back to the field, and back I shall go where duty and inclination call me.

Congratulate me upon my part in the great battle of Gettysburg.

I will give you a full description of it in a few days. Direct your letters as usual.

Much love to you all.
Frank A. Haskell[54]

Sealing up the envelope, Haskell gathering his few possessions together, and, heading north through town, paused only long enough to post his letter. Painfully favoring his bruised leg, the staff aide rode out of town, slowly covering the twenty-odd miles back "to the field, to his [Gibbon's] Division, since his wounding in the command of Gnl Harrow."[55]

---

54. Byrne and Weaver, *Haskell of Gettysburg*, pp. 88-89, 193.
55. *Ibid.*, p. 193.

As morning turned to afternoon, things had not improved for the harried surgeons at the Second Corps Hospitals along Rock Creek. If anything, it had gotten worse—ambulances still continued to disgorge their gory passengers along the soggy floodplain of Rock Creek. All the ground around the medical facilities and along the vehicle approaches was churned into a thick gooey muck by the passage of countless wheels and the ceaseless tramp of heavy boots.

"To say in such a field that the surgeons were busy, is needless. What else could they do but work; unless appalled at the mass of ragged, naked, torn and mangled mortality! There was not more than one for ten that were needed. Every man that could tie a bandage, or give a drink of water, or pour it upon a wound, was at work."[56]

With the distribution center set up by the Christian Commission busy passing out supplies to the surgeons of three different corps hospitals, the other representatives had rolled up their sleeves and fanned out through the hospital. "As we pass through them, in every direction we turned, men would call us. 'Doctor, oh, doctor, won't you attend to my case? Won't you fix my arm, or leg, or shoulder, or head?' As we stopped at their earnest cries, we could only say, we are not physicians or surgeons, but acting for the Christian Commission, and will do for you what we can. Until the Dr can attend to your case, we will furnish you with some wine, biscuit, crackers, bandages, lint, shirts, &c. They would then beg us to send the Dr; but to whom could we go?"[57]

Overwhelmed by the incessant flood of wounded, surgeons worked to the point of exhaustion, some collapsing from fatigue, others breaking down and weeping at their inability to do more for the long-suffering troops. The hands of the surgeons at the tables were becoming increasingly bruised and swollen from long hours of grasping scalpels and bearing down on saws. "The labor performed by these officers was immense," wrote Army of the Potomac Medical Director Jonathan Letterman. "Some of them fainted from exhaustion, induced by over-exertion, and others became ill from the same cause.

56. Cross, *The War and the Christian Commission*, p. 15.
57. *Ibid.*

The skill and devotion shown by the medical officers of this army were worthy of all commendation; they could not be surpassed."[58]

The operating tables were gruesome spectacles; around the clock, without pausing except to rotate one exhausted doctor for another, the amputations continued. The tables were soaked with the blood of the patients, the surgeons spattered and gory from their work. It became necessary to dig small drainage ditches wherever possible to carry away the runoff of blood from the tables, lest the ground around them become a gooey morass that would actually hinder the surgeons in their work. "On the amputation table one case succeeded another as fast as they could be operated on and removed," wrote one of the Christian Commissioners. "We little thought we could become so familiar with the sight of feet, legs, arms, just taken from our fellow-men, and look upon the operations without a thought except the inclination to take hold of the man and try and help him."[59]

As the Christian Commission representatives continued to slowly work their way between the bleeding soldiers, their carefully regulated stock of supplies was running dangerously low. Even an entire wagonload of medicines and foodstuffs could only stretch so far among the injured men of three corps hospitals. Often kind words, a tract, and a word of prayer was all that the representatives could share with the suffering men. Moving carefully to avoid stepping on the wounded, the commissioners stopped to talk, to comfort and listen to the men, no matter what color uniform they wore, providing the personal attention and individual care that the surgeons simply could not give.

"During all this time, Mr. Stillson and myself had never thought of eating, having forgotten breakfast, when a man told us Dr. Scott had some dinner prepared for us. His name was Lewis Morgan, Delaware, Delaware county, Ohio, Co I, 4th Ohio. His kind, pleasant and attentive manners left an impression on us not soon to be forgotten. Dr. Scott detailed him to attend us."[60]

Promising the wounded that they would return as soon as possible, Andrew Cross and J. B. Stillson followed the Ohioan, sidestepping and

---

58. *OR*, vol. 27, pt. 1, p. 197. It is probably not surprising that a higher than expected number of these men were later committed to insane asylums. [Record Group 94. Adjutant General's Office, Personal Papers of Medical Officers and Physicians, National Archives and Records Administration.]
59. Cross, *The War and the Christian Commission*, p. 15.
60. *Ibid.*

zigzagging their way through the wounded, back to the Third Division Medical Director's office to grab a quick bite to eat.

As the afternoon wore on, none of the members of the ambulance crews apparently thought it necessary to inform the medical directors or surgical staff at the Second Corps Hospitals that the wounded they were blithely transporting to the railroad station were not actually going anywhere. Ambulances continued to roll to a stop by the ominously empty tracks and disgorge their battered riders. Meanwhile, Baltimore Christian Commissioners Muller and Woodward, manning a makeshift "Eating Saloon" at track's end, worked round the clock to feed the incoming soldiers.

It is clear from Surgeon Justin Dwinelle's report that the doctors were totally unaware of the problem with the rail transportation. "It was adviseable [*sic*] at first that as soon as possible all the slightly wounded[,] those that could walk to Gettysburg[,] should be sent there to take the cars for Baltimore and Harrisburg[,] where they could be cared for in old established General Hospitals[.] As soon as this class were forwarded all those that could sit up in an ambulance and ride with safety were permitted to go[,] and subsequently those that could lie down and ride[.] This arrangement made it better for those that went away and those that remained[.]"[61]

So a growing number of wounded, happily anticipating evacuation from the festering atmosphere and frantic activity of Gettysburg, effectively fell through the cracks of the army transportation system, as more and more of the corps hospitals sent their walking wounded, then those with more serious injuries, off to the Gettysburg depot. Some of the wounded, noticing the lack of normal railroading activity around the station, began to suspect that the line might be broken further down the track toward Hanover Junction. Those capable of walking started to painfully shuffle along the roadbed; for them, there was only one way to go—the railroad ended at Gettysburg.

---

61. Justin Dwinelle, *Medical Report*.

Preparations were already under way for the Army of the Potomac to get under way in pursuit of the retreating Confederate army. Second Corps Medical Director Alexander Dougherty sat reading orders he had just received for the disposition of his Second Corps Hospitals from army headquarters:

> Head Quarters 2nd C[orps] Army of the Potomac
> Med Director's Office, July 5th 1863
>
> The Army may be ordered to move at any moment, and the following arrangements for the care of the wounded on the battlefield will at once be carried into effect. All the hospital tents will be left, and such medical and hospital supplies only as will be required for four or five days. There are twenty five wagon loads of medical supplies at the White House Church on the Baltimore Turnpike—more are ordered there including a sufficient number of bed sacks & will be on hand promptly.
>
> Surgeons in Chief of Divisions will accompany their Commands. One third of the operating staff, & sufficient number of Med[ical] Officers, attendants, &c will be left. Their places will be supplied by other officers at Frederick in a few days. Apply to your Corps Commander for a sufficient guard for the Hospital.
>
> The Quartermaster Dept has detailed 4 wagons for each of the Corps Hospitals.
>
> The Ambulances will also be left.[62] Commissary supplies will be at Westminster where they must be sent for. Cattle will be in this vicinity.

---

62. Contrary to what the order *seems* to say, not all of the ambulances were left behind. "Before the army left Gettysburg, and knowing that the wounded had been brought in from the field, six ambulances and four wagons were ordered to be left behind from each corps, to convey the wounded from their hospitals to the railroad depot, for transportation to the other hospitals." Unfortunately, the railroad into Gettysburg was not up and running when the army pulled out of town; the six ambulances for each corps were woefully inadequate to transport the huge backlog of wounded troops. Letterman continues: "I was informed by [Brig.] General [Rufus] Ingalls that the railroad to Gettysburg would be in operation on the 6th, and upon this based my action. Had this been the case, this number would have been sufficient. As it proved that this was not in good running order for some time after that date, it would have been better to have left more ambulances." The medical director of the Army of the Potomac ruefully added: "I acted on the best

Surgeon Henry Janes, US Vols is assigned to duty in general charge of all the Hospitals.

Very respectfully,
Your Obdt Servt
By command of
Maj. Gen'l Meade
Jona Letterman[63]

Putting down the order, Dougherty sent one of his aides to summon his senior staff members. There was a lot of work still to be done before this day was over.

Over lunch at the Third Division Medical Director's office, the men of the Christian Commission compared notes on their morning activities. It was painfully obvious that their carefully transported supplies were all but exhausted, the entire wagonload distributed within the space of only a few hours. But as more and more terribly wounded men were carried in from the ambulance trains, there was an ever-increasing demand for more of those same supplies, as well as more surgeons, assistant surgeons, and nurses. It was clear that they needed to act immediately to get more supplies sent from the nearest Christian Commission warehouse.

"As soon as we had eaten, we started to try some plan to get more surgeons, but were stopped by a report that any private surgeons were forbidden on the field. Just then Dr. Scott said he and all the surgeons that could in any way be spared were ordered forward with the army, which would be or was in motion. What! take away surgeons here where a hundred are wanted, and where, if the men have not immediate help, hundreds must die for want of attention. But so it is, and we can do no better."[64]

---

information that could be obtained." [*OR*, vol. 27, pt. 1, p. 198.] Capt. Louis C. Duncan, writing of the conditions in the hospitals after the battle, states that "it appears that but thirty [ambulances] were left" when the army marched away on July 6. [Duncan, *The Medical Department of the United States Army*, p. 263.]

63. Jonathan Letterman, Order to Medical Director's Office, July 5, 1863, copy in the Union Field Hospital Vertical File, Gettysburg National Military Park Library.

64. Cross, *The War and the Christian Commission*, p. 16.

Of the more than 650 medical officers present at the battle, all except 106 were moving out with the Army of the Potomac; "no more could be left, as it was expected that another battle would within three or four days take place, and in all probability as many wounded thrown upon our hands as at the battle of the 2d and 3d, which had just occurred." Jonathan Letterman, medical director of the Army of the Potomac, further felt that "the greater portion of the surgical labor was performed before the army left. The time for primary operations had passed, and what remained to be done was to attend to making the men comfortable, dress their wounds, and perform such secondary operations as from time to time might be necessary." Letterman did note, however, that the surgeons were still performing surgery "day and night, with little rest, . . . in the Second Corps, until July 7."[65]

To make matters worse, only one out of every three "medical officers" being left behind were actual cutters; the other two-thirds were merely "dressing surgeons," capable only in assisting the surgical teams, giving medication, and bandaging wounds. This meant that only about thirty-five operating surgeons were to be left at Gettysburg to deal with some 20,000 wounded men.

Incredibly, in the light of these facts, the surgeon general's office in Washington, D.C., was graciously declining numerous offers of medical assistance from the private sector. On July 4, Pennsylvania governor Andrew Curtin sent a dispatch to Surgeon General Hammond, inquiring "how many volunteer surgeons I may send." Hammond responded: "The Medical Director of the Army of the Potomac has plenty of surgical aid."[66]

An offer of surgical assistance by the "medical men in the hospitals of Philadelphia," on the very day that the Army of the Potomac was pulling out of Gettysburg with eighty-five percent of its medical staff, was refused, saying that "if their services would be needed they will be thankfully called upon. It is believed that at present there is sufficient hospital accommodations and that tents are not needed." As late as July 8, the *Pittsburgh Gazette* published a private dispatch: "The only way of getting to Gettysburg is by horse and carriages. Do not send any more surgeons."[67]

---

65. *OR*, vol. 27, pt. 1, pp. 197-98.
66. Hammond to Curtin, July 5, 1863, Office of the Surgeon General, Letters and Endorsements Sent 1818-1889, General Correspondence, volume 35, Record Group 112, National Archives and Records Administration.
67. *Ibid.*; J. R. Smith to John M. Cuyler, July 6, 1863; *Pittsburgh Gazette*, July 8, 1863.

(While this may be seen as an astounding and horrifying decision in hindsight, it must be remembered that civilian practitioners and medical men from the private sector were widely considered, at best, as a doubtful source of assistance by Medical Director Jonathan Letterman, Second Corps Surgeon-in-Charge Justin Dwinelle, and many other reputable military surgical personnel within the Medical Department of the United States Army. Volunteers like Dr. Bushrod Washington James—men who pulled their weight without complaint, worked as diligently as did their military counterparts, did what they were told to do when they were told to do it, and worked smoothly within the sometimes harsh regimen of an army hospital—were seen as the exception, certainly not the rule.)

While most of the Second Corps surgeons packed up their tools and personal effects, preparatory to moving out with their regiments, Andrew Cross hurriedly made arrangements to go into Gettysburg to seek assistance for the Second Corps Hospitals. "As Dr. Scott was ordered off, we had to try and get another horse. After searching, we found a wounded officer—Major Richard E. Cross, of the 5th New Hampshire, (brother of Col Edward E. Cross, who was killed on the 3d day), both formerly of Baltimore. He loaned it to us to go into Gettysburg and see if we could not make some arrangement for surgeons and supplies, but wanted it in the morning, as he was going to try and keep up with the army."[68]

The number one priority was to find a way of getting more medicines, clothing, and foodstuffs into Gettysburg. When Cross and his men had finally arrived at Westminster the day before following a thirty-hour trip, they had dashed off a quick note "to Mr. Griffin, chairman of [the] Commission, not to send any more supplies by that way. Knowing the communication by Northern Central Railroad, Hanover and Gettysburg, we started [off] to see the President of Gettysburg Road, hoping to be able to do something in the way of facilitating supplies." Mounted up double on Major Cross' long-suffering horse, Andrew Cross and one of his men clambered up out of the creek bottom, riding carefully to avoid the speeding ambulances still rattling in from the battlefield along the narrow farm lane.[69]

---

68. Cross, *The War and the Christian Commission*, p. 16.
69. *Ibid.*

After notifying his staff of the impending move of the army, Medical Director Dougherty dictated an order to one of his aides detailing the contingent of surgeons to be left behind at Gettysburg:

Headquarters 2d Corps
Med Directors Office

July 5th 1863

Capt

I am directed by Dr. Letterman to organize the hospitals of this Corps, Substantially on the following basis.

One-third of the operating staff will be left, and fifty nurses, attendants etc. etc. to each Corps. The three Division Hospitals will constitute a Corps hospital under Dr. Dwinelle, Surgeon 106th Penn Vols.

The operating staff and med attendants will be as follows.
1st Division
Surg. [Charles Squire] Wood 66th NY V
Chief Operator
Asst. Surg C[harles] T. Kelsey 64th NYV
" " [Uriah Q.] Davis 148th Penn Vols
" " [Charles] Smart 63d NY "
" " [W. P.] Bush 61st " " "
Assistants

2d Div
Surgeon N[athan] Hayward 20th Mass Vols
Chief Operator

Asst. Surg. [Henry C.] Levenseller [*sic*] 19th Maine "
" " [Frederick F.] Burmister [*sic*] 69th Penn "
" " [Theodore O.] Cornish 15th Mass "
" " [A. Stokes] Jones 72nd Pa "
Assistants

3d Div
Surgeon [Harry M.] M[c]Abee 4th Ohio "
Chief Operator

Surg. Fred[eric]k Wolfe [sic] 39th NYV
Asst. " Jno. [James] D. Benton 111th " " "
" " [J. W.] McCullough 1st Del "
Assistants

I respectfully request that the above details be made from Hd Quarters. Also, that a guard of a sergeant and thirty men be detailed to attend at the hospital reporting to Dr. Dwinelle.

And that the Chief Quartermaster be directed to leave four baggage wagons for each Corps Hospital.

Respectfully
A. N. Dougherty
Surg. USV & Med Director
2d Corps[70]

Fourteen surgeons and an administrator were to be left behind to treat a combined corps hospital of over 3200 wounded men. Even with fifty nurses and attendants to assist, there was still a huge backlog of patients awaiting primary amputations, and others would soon need secondary surgical attention. "The Surgeon of the 2d corps hospital gave me a list of his supplies when the army commensed its pursuit of the rebels," wrote Rev. Isaac W. Monfort, Military Agent of the State

70. Dr. A. N. Dougherty, order dated July 5, 1863, courtesy of Scott Michael Dwinelle. In his *Medical Report*, Surgeon Justin Dwinelle's list of surgical staff remaining in Gettysburg differs somewhat from the medical director's dispatch. In the First Division, Dwinelle does not list Assistant Surgeon Charles T. Kelsey of the 64th New York, but names Assistant Surgeon W. W. Sharp of the 140th Pennsylvania instead. Dwinelle adds Surgeons William J. Burr of the 42nd New York and John Aiken of the 71st Pennsylvania to Dougherty's list for the Second Division, and mentions Assistant Surgeon Ebenezer Day of the 39th New York with the remaining medical staff of the Third Division. However, a testimonial to the efforts of the Christian Commission was issued from the Second Corps Hospital staff on July 24, and included Assistant Surgeon Kelsey's signature, as well as those of Burr and Day, among other surgical staff from Dougherty's original order. [*United States Christian Commission for the Army and Navy. For the Year 1863. Second Annual Report*, p. 88] Apparently, Sharp, Burr, Aiken, and Day were left in addition to the fourteen men that Dougherty had originally detailed when it became clear that the wounded were still continuing to pour into the hospitals. So, at the very maximum, 18 surgeons and assistant surgeons were detailed to care for over 3200 gravely injured men.

of Indiana, in his official report to Governor Oliver O. Morton. "A few stretchers, eight pounds of chloroform, one box of bandages, sixteen rolls of plaster and three pounds of lint; and sixteen hundred wounded." But it was going to have to do—everyone else was ordered forward with the army, and another clash, possibly even bloodier than Gettysburg, was expected whenever the rebel forces were finally brought to bay.[71]

With the sounds of thousands of men and their activities—medical wagons being loaded with the surgical equipment and personal belongings, the moans of the wounded, and the singing of the bone saws from the amputating tables—coming in from outside the tent, Dougherty signed and blotted the order, then dispatched it with an orderly to Dr. Letterman's staff. The paperwork finally finished, the medical director started his own packing for the upcoming march.

The feverish delirium of the long night hours finally passed for Capt. Azor Nickerson in the afternoon heat of July 5. "The first thing I afterward recalled, except the wild phantasmagoria that always accompanies hours like these, was when, on the day following, an old friend, a captain in my regiment, lifted me out from among the dead, who had died during the night, and the muddy pool in which I had been lying."[72]

Nickerson's servant, although he had absconded with the captain's rubber coat, probably saved the Ohioan's life by mistakenly thinking that he was dead. "Little Jerry had returned to camp that morning and reported that 'De captain done gone died last night.' So my friend, with several others officers of the regiment, had come to try and find my body. Poor Jerry! he little knew how nearly the carrying away of the rubber coat came to finishing me, and thus confirming his story."[73]

"Our visitors remained with us for a very short time, as the regiment with the remainder of the army was already on the march following Lee. Every available man was ordered forward, and the fate of the immense

71. *Indianapolis Daily Journal*, July 23, 1863. It was still unclear exactly how many patients were at the Second Corps Hospitals, since ambulances still rumbled in with patients from aid stations and the remote corners of the field.
72. Nickerson, "Personal Recollections of Two Visits to Gettysburg," p. 22.
73. *Ibid.*

number of wounded was left to the care of the citizen-nurses who were expected to soon be there to assist the few soldier-attendants left with us." As yet, however, only Ellen Orbison Harris and a handful of Christian Commission and Sanitary Commission representatives comprised the hoped-for corps of "citizen-nurses," left alone with a handful of overworked doctors and over 3000 desperately wounded men.[74]

The vast Union army was indeed finally bestirring itself, and, piece by piece, corps by corps, was setting out in ponderous pursuit of the already-departed enemy, traveling three separate roads in an attempt to converge on the retreating Confederates. The Second Corps, last in the marching order, had to wait until all the other corps were safely on their way before setting out. The surgeons managed to delay their going as long as possible, working up to the very last minute, but the men in the ranks were ready, anxious in fact, to leave; as one man put it, anything was better than "laying around and doing nothing but see[ing] the sickening sights and smelling the miserable smells."[75]

"I do not know when Lee's retreat was discovered, but at this time [July 5] most of the troops had left and our Corps was left to bring up the rear. The battle field was put under guard, for, beside a number of captured cannon, there were from twenty five thousand to thirty thousand stand of small arms and an immense amount of other property."[76]

"After all the dispositions had been made our Corps marched to a little village called Quakertown. The Quartermasters were sent out with wagons and a guard to impress or buy food for the march." For Capt. Benjamin Thompson, shepherding his much-reduced company of the 111th New York along the short road to Two Taverns, it was a trip filled with pain and great discomfort. "My limbs and feet were so swollen that I could not get my shoes on, and I kept with my company by riding bareback on a broken down horse that we picked up."[77]

---

74. *Ibid.*
75. Walker, *History of the Second Army Corps*, p. 134. "All the surgeons of the corps remained with me untill [*sic*] the [morning of] the seventh when a part of them left with army," wrote Surgeon Justin Dwinelle in his Medical Report.
76. Thompson, *Personal Narrative*, p. 48.
77. *Ibid.*

Capt. Thomas Galwey of the 8th Ohio kept the ranks of his company closed up as they marched away in search of another battle. "About 3 p.m. we took the Baltimore pike and at nightfall halted two miles from Two Taverns for bivouac." The plucky Irishman from Ohio was well on the mend from his three wounds suffered out by the Emmitsburg Road, contrary to the doomsayer in his outfit who predicted that the third blow would be fatal. In fact, Galwey would survive the war and go on to live a highly successful life.[78]

---

78. Galwey, *The Valiant Hours*, p. 123. The 8th Ohio took a severe pounding at Gettysburg, suffering 102 casualties in the three day clash (with an effective strength of only 209 men going into combat, this was a 48.8 percent casualty rate).

Thomas Galwey, the staunch Irishman from the 8th Ohio who never fell out of a march except on the grueling move to Gettysburg, survived his three Pennsylvania wounds. Marching with Grant in the 1864 Overland Campaign against Richmond, Galwey even came to enjoy his remaining time in the military. "Perhaps soldiering in a splendid regiment is not so bad," he mused after the regiment was pulled out of the Petersburg trenches and mustering out of service on July 13, 1864. "Where could we find civilian friends to compare with soldier comrades?"

After the war, Galwey went on to distinguish himself in journalistic, religious, academic, and political arenas. With a discipline honed by his service with the 8th, he earned his B.A., M.A., and Ph.D. in rapid succession. Possessed of a natural linguistic aptitude, he learned and mastered ten languages (including Latin and Greek). His name frequently appeared in the editorial credits of prominent American journals and magazines. He served as editor-in-chief of a major Cincinnati newspaper, and was appointed associate editor of the *Catholic World Magazine* in 1880.

Settling for a time in Harlem, New York, he met and married Mrs. Mary V. Mitchell, daughter of a distinguished Cincinnati judge, in 1882. Their union produced four children—David, Frances, Geoffrey and Thomas, Jr.

The old Emmitsburg Road wounds gradually began to take their toll on Galwey's health. Spurred by his war-related disability, the old soldier uprooted his family and moved them off to the warmer weather of Galveston, where Thomas again became an editor, this time of a local Texas newspaper. But the call of the North was strong, and the family soon relocated again to New York. Upon his return, he assumed a professorship in French and Logic at Manhattan College. But the ever-restless Galwey soon turned to civil service, serving for twenty years as an attorney for one of New York City's departments.

Prominent in The Military Order of the Loyal Legion of the United States, as well as in several other veteran organizations, Galwey never lost his keen interest in the greatest adventure of his life—marching away to war with the men of the 8th Ohio. He died on February 20, 1913, just a few months short of the fiftieth anniversary reunion in the small town of Gettysburg. Mercifully, he never knew of the death of his namesake, Thomas Galwey, Jr., in another battle in another war on a distant continent just a few short years later. [Galwey, *The Valiant Hours*, p. 236-38].

Capt. Thomas Livermore was bringing up the rear, marshaling most of his contingent of Second Corps ambulances. By orders from above, only a handful of ambulances were left behind to transport the many thousand wounded at the Second Corps Hospitals. When he would later hear stories of the lowland flooding of Rock Creek, his only reply was that "they ought not to have been there." He would never admit to any culpability in the choice of the Rock Creek site.[79]

---

79. Livermore, *Days and Events*, pp. 258-59. Captain Livermore never evidenced any signs that he lost sleep over his disastrous choice of the Rock Creek bottoms as a fallback site for the Second Corps Hospitals. But then, his had already been a full life by the time the nineteen-year-old captain chose floodplains as hospital grounds.

Livermore had been born February 7, 1844, in the river town of Galena, Illinois. Galena was frontier country in those days, and his parents soon succumbed to the siren call of the west. When he was just seven, his family emigrated to California, spending three months on the trail. The young boy rode the entire way on horseback.

The west coast held few educational opportunities, so Livermore, now in his teens, returned to a now-more-settled Illinois to enroll at Lombard University in Galesburg. It was there that he first learned of the outbreak of war. In youthful impetuousity, he immediately left school and traveled to Washington, D.C. to be as near as possible to the action. At Poolesville, Maryland, he stumbled across the encamped 1st New Hampshire Volunteers, and promptly enlisted. He later moved to the 5th New Hampshire.

Colonel Cross, even in death, proved to be annoyingly right in the end—Captain Livermore was eventually replaced as head of the Second Corps Ambulance Corps. But Livermore thrived, and by war's end, mustered out with the rank of colonel. He became a lawyer, but the civilized grind of east coast life wore at him. He toyed with the idea of becoming a rancher in South America.

Jaded with his humdrum life in front of the bench, he became manager of the Amoskeag Mills in Manchester, and seemed to flourish there for a time. After seven years away, he again resumed his practice in Boston, but soon felt unfulfilled and cramped in his narrow metropolitan office. The offer of the vice-presidency of the Calumet & Hecla Mining Company came as a welcome relief, and he abandoned law for the next twenty-one years to pursue mining.

By now, the years were starting to creep up on the former ambulance commander. He left the mining company, and eventually retired to Boston, where he died on January 9, 1918. One Beacon Street associate wrote of his last years: "Never was he richer in service than when he passed to the beyond; never was he held in higher honor; never more beloved."

There is no record that he ever expressed any desire to return to Gettysburg, where in the heat of battle, as a young and inexperienced man, he was sent to make a critical choice, and instead made a horribly wrong decision that cost the lives of a number of helpless men. [Henry M. Rogers, in the Introduction to Livermore, *Days and Events*, pp. vii-x.]

"On Sunday July 5th, the enemy having retreated, our regt left the field of battle at 5 P.M. [and] went to a place called Two Taverns where they remained till Tuesday morning the 7th," wrote Chaplain J. H. W. Stuckenberg of the 145th Pennsylvania. "I was sick on the morning of the 5th and concluded to go somewhere in the country to rest and recuperate."[80]

There were, however, a few very personal details to attend to before the young German minister would leave Gettysburg. "I first buried E[rastus] Allen, who had died at 8 the evening previous." Allen had been cut down, along with nearly eighty of his friends, near the Rose Wheatfield, on July 2.[81]

The chaplain also "took the names of all our wounded and did all I could for them. I then went to Littletown about 10 miles distant[,] arrived there about 2 P.M." Settling in comfortably at a local farm, where he was referred by the local Lutheran minister, Stuckenberg did some visiting and slowly began to recover from the overwork, lack of sleep, and sickness of the past week.[82]

Philadelphia, Pennsylvania

It had been a flying trip for Cornelia Hancock as Dr. Henry T. Child's carriage tore along the road from Hancock's Bridge to Philadelphia. "It was late afternoon when we reached Philadelphia. The City was wild with excitement over news of a terrible battle which had just been fought on Pennsylvania soil—no one knew exactly where—but it finally became known as having occurred at a little town called Gettysburg. The Rebel army was at first supposed by many to be on its way to Philadelphia. Every hour was bringing tidings of the awful loss of life on both sides."[83]

The carriage bore Cornelia directly to her brother-in-law's residence, where she found a swirl of activity as preparations were being finalized for his impending trip to the battlefield. "Dr. Child, with a number of other physicians, had determined to leave that night by the eleven o'clock train for Gettysburg. I was to accompany him. He and

---

80. Stuckenberg, *I'm Surrounded by Methodists*, p. 84.
81. *Ibid.*
82. *Ibid.*
83. Hancock, *South After Gettysburg*, p. 5.

the Hon. Judge Kelly had aided Miss Eliza Farnham, a well-known public-spirited woman, with a number of others of 'suitable age' to get passes as volunteer nurses. The ladies in the party were many years older than myself, and I was under the especial care of Miss Farnham."[84]

Everyone seemed to have something to do, or somewhere to go, rushing here for supplies or there to confer with someone, except Cornelia. Trying to stay out from underfoot, she took the opportunity to visit with her sister, and waited impatiently for eleven o'clock to arrive.

Gettysburg, Pennsylvania

Christian Commissioner Andrew Cross and his companion, riding double on their borrowed horse, were still trying to reach Gettysburg to arrange for supplies to be brought in on the Northern Central, Hanover and Gettysburg railroad. Having to deal with army regulations was not making it any easier. "On our arrival at the cross road, on the [Baltimore] turnpike, a mile south of Gettysburg, we were stopped by a guard. We went down the turnpike a mile further, where Gen Meade then had his headquarters, to state our case and get passed."[85]

Col. G. H. Sharpe, deputy provost marshal general in charge of the Bureau of Information at Meade's headquarters, was not about to take the responsibility for passing these two unknown men through the lines, especially at this late hour. Being a good military man, the intelligence officer promptly delegated the responsibility. "Col Sharp [*sic*] said we would have to go to [Brig.] Gen [Marsina R.] Patrick's headquarters, which was nearly two miles further."[86]

"It was now after 9 o'clock, damp and dark at that. To comfort us, he said he would go along, and let us share his bed, which was on the barn floor, near the 3d corps hospital, as far from the town as where we had started."[87]

Frustrated with the waste of time and the snarl of military red tape, Cross and his companions cautiously rode on in the darkness toward the headquarters of the Provost Marshal General, located in a "barn

---

84. *Ibid.*
85. Cross, *The War and the Christian Commission*, p. 16.
86. *Ibid.*
87. *Ibid.*

near White Church" on the "Baltimore Road."[88] The Baltimore Pike still served as the Army of the Potomac's chief supply conduit, and army wagons and ambulance convoys rumbled past in wet darkness. So far, all this frustrating night had seen accomplished by Cross and his friend was a ride toward Gettysburg and then back out again, all without achieving a single thing.

Fortunately, a warm welcome awaited them at provost headquarters. Making their way past groups of Confederate prisoners, looking sullen and downcast at the Union troops standing guard over them, Sharpe and the two exhausted commissioners dismounted and went in. "The General ordered the pass, preferred we should go in town, but on our remonstrating as we were from Baltimore, had brought supplies for the wounded, had been all day on our feet in water and mud distributing them, he said we might lodge in the barn with him; that these people around here he could not trust."[89]

The past four days had been grueling ones for Cross and his companion. The night of July 2 had been spent pacing the station platform, waiting for the military supply train to pull out of Baltimore; the night of July 3 had seemed like it would never end, clinging to the roof of a swaying train as it steamed through the darkness; last night had been a miserable campout with a surly wagon driver in a muddy field south of Gettysburg. The big Pennsylvania barn, redolent with the warm aroma of straw and farm animals, looked mighty inviting to the weary and bedraggled Christian Commissioners. "Col Sharp [*sic*] having ordered some one to tie up our horse, we laid down on the barn floor, where we slept more soundly than we have often done in the most comfortable bed."[90]

There was at least one hopeful sign along the boggy banks of Rock Creek this miserable Sunday night. Another supply train had arrived,

---

88. Marsena R. Patrick, *Inside Lincoln's Army: The Diary of Marsena Rudolph Patrick, Provost Marshal General, Army of the Potomac*, ed. David S. Sparks (New York: Thomas Yoseloff, 1964), p. 266. This was at the Aaron Sheely Farm. Farmer Sheely wrote that Provost Marshall General Patrick "came up to the barn with his retinue. I invited him to the house. He refused, saying he preferred to stay in the barn." [Aaron Sheely, memiors, Adams County Historical Society.]
89. Cross, *The War and the Christian Commission*, p. 16.
90. *Ibid.*, pp. 16-17.

leaving behind almost a duplicate of yesterday's delivery—6,000 rations of tea, coffee, sugar, crackers, soap, salt, candles, and salt pork. These army issued foods, largely inedible by the severely wounded, were augmented from the supplies of the various volunteer organizations as they gradually arrived at the hospitals. "In the earliest days of the Hospital," wrote Surgeon Justin Dwinelle to Medical Director Dougherty, "I received large supplies of soft Bread Wines & Cordials Oranges and Lemons various articles of light diet and needful articles of clothing from the Sanitary and Christian commissions[,] Adams Ex[press] Co[mpany,] Fireman's Associations of Baltimore and from various other associations and individuals[.]"[91]

Unfortunately, with every able-bodied person pressed into the care of those still arriving in ambulances and by litter, there just didn't seem to be enough hands to distribute the foods. Thousands of wounded were arrayed haphazardly along both banks of Rock Creek, demanding immediate attention, and the number-one priority was saving the lives of these men. The food was parcelled out, but it was a slow and uneven process, and many were passed over.

As if the continuing flood of incoming wounded, lack of proper shelter, inadequate staff, shortage of food, and marshy location were not enough of a challenge to the harried surgeons, they were also forced to carry on a running battle with the weather. Periodic showers continued to sweep through the Gettysburg area, some sudden and very forceful.[92]

"I was the first assistant to Surgeon Charles S. Wood, Surgeon of our regiment, who was a most competent operator and we were a busy lot of medical men," remembered Surgeon Albert Vander Veer of the 66th New York. The First Division Hospital operating theater on July 5 "consisted of just a frame-work constructed of wooden posts and cross pieces with a fly, and a tent was used as a covering from the heat of the sun and we performed a number of operations at night."[93]

91. Dwinelle, *Medical Report.*

92. Weather records of Dr. Michael Jacobs of the Pennsylvania College at Gettysburg, Gettysburg National Military Park Library.

93. Albert Vander Veer, Vander Veer Papers, DB 560, Albany Institute of History and Art, Albany, New York, transcribed copy in the 66th New York Infantry Vertical File, Gettysburg National Military Park Library.

Surgeon Vander Veer had vivid memories of one particular unexpected downpour. "Late in one afternoon Doctor Wood was performing an amputation of the thigh and I was controlling the artery with my thumb and finger when such a pronounced thunder storm came up that our lights were extinguished and Doctor Wood said to the physician in charge, watch your anaesthetic carefully and Doctor Vander Veer be sure that you do not lose control of the artery."[94]

"When the storm had past and Doctor Wood was able to continue the operation he said in a most comforting manner, 'I do not think that the poor fellow has lost much blood.' This proved to be the case for he rallied nicely and was able to be taken back the next day to the base hospital, the nearest of which I think was Baltimore where a number of our wounded were sent."[95]

Pvt. Elbert Corbin of Battery B, First New York Light Artillery, looked around for a unoccupied piece of ground, than sank down exhausted on the boggy creekbank. Left behind to care for Lt. Albert S. Sheldon, who had been shot down during the furious infighting at the peak of Pickett's attack, Corbin had finally gotten Sheldon settled for the night. Pulling out pen and paper, Corbin hurriedly scribbled a few lines home in the dim light from a nearby lantern:

> SUNDAY, July 5—9 P.M.
>
> I was kept very busy in the rain all day yesterday, taking care of the wounded. It was a hard storm, and thousands of the wounded were exposed, without cover.—At 12, midnight, I lay down wet through and through, after getting Sheldon and the boys a partial shelter. I had but six hours sleep in the last seventy hours, and been in battle two days. I have twelve wounded men to cook for, and have to take care of their wounds. The groans of the wounded have been in my ears for two days and nights, and the screech of shot, roar of cannon, explosion of shells, whistle of bullets for two days previous. I have seen eighteen amputating tables at work from daylight to dark, for *our Corps alone*, and others

94. *Ibid.* Surgeon Charles Squire Wood was acting in a supervisory capacity at this surgery. This was one of the roles of the surgeon in charge of each division.

95. *Ibid.*

> have suffered as severely. But the enemy are retreating and our forces are following them up. They have left all their wounded.—Seventy ambulance loads came in here last night.[96]

Virginian John Dooley had spent long hours surveying his surroundings, trying desperately to distract himself from the painful thrumming of his thighs. Now he lay awkwardly propped up, writing in his pocket diary in the cool dampness of the fading light, recording with dispassionate clarity the plight of the wounded prisoners surrounding him.

One in particular kept passing him again and again throughout the long day; shifting once again to ease the agony, he carefully started to describe him: "Here is a poor wounded Confederate who is walking up and down, wandering anywhere his cracked brain directs him. Just on top of his head and penetrating to his brain is a large opening made by a shell in which I might insert my hand. He walks about as if nothing was the matter with him, and pays no attention to any advice given him."[97]

As both Union and Confederate wounded struggled to get comfortable in their pain and hunger, and the bone-tired surgeons continued their thankless work around the operating tables, Rock Creek rushed and foamed its way between the two halves of the hospital. The water level had risen dangerously last night, and, although it had dropped some, it continued to boil through the tortuous s-curve channel south of town.

Now an ominous sound was faintly rolling in from the distant horizon. It was thundering again; another summer storm was bearing down on the waterlogged countryside around Gettysburg. The drenched ground would absorb no more rainfall; any precipitation would simply run off into the surrounding streams and creeks. If it started to rain again, Rock Creek was quickly going to reach flood stage.

---

96. Letter of Pvt. Elbert Corbin, July 5, 1863, courtesy of Mr. Stephen J. Dreher.
97. Dooley, *John Dooley*, p. 112.

CHAPTER 10

SUNDAY, JULY 5: 11:00 P.M.—TUESDAY, JULY 7: PREDAWN

". . . the waters cover them, extinguishing the little spark of life. . . ."

John M. Scoville
First New York Light Artillery, Battery B

Philadelphia, Pennsylvania

"At eleven P.M. we were wending our way out Washington Avenue to Broad and Prime streets, then the depot." The caravan of carriages made their way quickly through the deserted streets of Philadelphia, sending ghostly echoes bouncing off the shadowed buildings.[1]

Dr. Child and his medical friends, accompanied by Miss Eliza Farnham, a group of middle-aged volunteer nurses, and a wide-eyed young Quakeress named Cornelia Hancock sat back as the train for Baltimore rolled out of the station. "The darkness, the uncertainty of everything, was appalling, and when we reached Havre de Grace, we heard the cars creaking weirdly on the pontoon bridges over the Susquehanna River." Once on the other shore, the train picked up speed and soon disappeared into the darkness.[2]

Gettysburg, Pennsylvania

John M. Scoville of Captain Rorty's First New York Light Artillery, Battery B had been spending a very uncomfortable night at the Second

1. Hancock, *South After Gettysburg*, p. 5.
2. *Ibid.*, pp. 5-6.

Corps Hospital. Scoville's participation in the fighting had been very brief—"all I saw of the battle was about one-half hour of the second day," he told a reporter in later years. "I was carrying ammunition from a caisson to the piece—the ammunition was an armful of shells—and about to lay them near the muzzle of the gun. As I turned a minnie ball struck me a few inches below the shoulder blade, passed through my body and entered my arm midway between the elbow and shoulder. I found all this out afterward, and later on it was cut from the wrist." In shock and pain, Scoville turned and stumbled over the crest of the ridge in search of the nearest aid station.[3]

"When the time came to be removed, the wounded, I among the rest, were carried to a piece of woods and a camp hospital was established," remembered the miller-turned-artilleryman; "and for five days my wounds were uncared for, and it was pretty tough living. The wounded and dying were on every side; very many were worse off than I."[4]

The only bright spots in the past three days of pain, hunger, and drenched clothing had been the continued visits of Scoville's friend and fellow batteryman, Charles Minard. Minard had been on detached duty at Second Corps headquarters since February; on receiving word of his friend's condition, the New Yorker immediately sought and was granted leave to go find his injured messmate.[5] "As soon as I learned of Scoville's being wounded, I went to the hospital and hunted him out. I found him in a wood lying near the bank of a creek. He had been marked for the amputating table, but, hunting up an old friend of his, Dr. [Nelson] Neeley of the Fifty-seventh New York volunteers, we begged like dogs for the 'fin.'" Assistant Surgeon Neeley, surrounded by thousands of wounded men clamoring for his attention, was pressed for time and less than optimistic. "The doctor shook his head, but said he would do all he could to save it."[6]

Not at all encouraged by Neeley's tepid assurances, Minard talked in turn with each of the division surgical staff—all proved even less hopeful than Neeley. "The surgeons insisted that the arm must come off, and, as a last resort, I appealed to the medical director of the corps, Doctor Dougherty." Moved by the dogged determination of Scoville and his faithful friend, the medical director threaded his way carefully through the crowded creek bottom to Scoville's side. "He made an

---

3. "Wounded at Gettysburgh. The War Experiences of Commander Scoville, of Moses Summers Post," *The Syracuse Sunday Herald*, March 8, 1885, p. 5.
4. *Ibid.*
5. Stephen J. Dreher, Letter to author, April 17, 1995.
6. "Wounded at Gettysburgh," p. 5. "Fin" was Civil War slang for arm.

examination of the wounds, and said it would be a miracle if he lived with the arm on, but he gave directions for dressing the wounds, and especial direction for his future care."[7]

The first order of business was to get the wounded gunner moved to a quieter location. "Scoville lay within sight of the amputating table near which arms and legs were piled up like cord wood. It was thought advisable to move him into some other ward out of sight of the 'butchering block.' It was done in a hurry, as a heavy rain had been falling and the creek had risen very rapidly, flooding the whole space where Scoville and his comrades were."[8]

The persistent rains ever since the battle had finally brought Rock Creek to flood stage. "Of course no one foresaw that the little stream which ran around us would soon overflow its banks, or doubtless more men would have been left, at least for this emergency," wrote one stunned survivor. "As it was, the stream, swollen to an unusual height, did soon overflow its banks, and sweeping through our dismal ranks, drowned many helpless fellows before the few attendants there could get them out of the way."[9]

With the Army of the Potomac pulling out of Gettysburg in pursuit of the retreating Confederates, only the smallest skeleton crew remained with the divisional surgical staff of each hospital to care for the injured. Even with the aid of individuals such as Pvt. Elbert Corbin and Charles Minard, left behind by their commanding officers to assist in the care of the wounded from their own units, a hospital guard detail of thirty soldiers, fifty male nurses and attendants assigned by the medical director, a few volunteer commission agents, a handful of Confederate surgeons and assitants, and various hospital stewards and musicians, there could scarcely have been more than 225 able-bodied men left scattered throughout the three Second Corps divisional hospitals, left to care for nearly 3000 desperately wounded men, spread over several acres of bottomland, in the inky dark of night.

Now the waters of Rock Creek were moving silently, inexorably into the tangled ranks of pallets, blankets, and stretchers laying along the low banks of the stream. Except for the sperm oil lamps dimly

7. *Ibid.*
8. *Ibid.*
9. Nickerson, "Personal Recollections of Two Visits to Gettysburg," p. 22.

illuminating the gory scenes at the operating tables, and the solitary lanterns carried by the attendants as they moved through the camp, the hospital facility was in total darkness. Alerted to the danger by the changing pitch of the rushing stream and the feel of water creeping along their bodies, some of the wounded feebly cried out, raising the alarm.

"It was terrible!" remembered John M. Scoville. "Men who were lying on the banks of the stream and were unable to move, remained in their helplessness and drowned. We who were equally helpless were lying where we could see the waters cover them, extinguishing the little spark of life left from the wounds."[10]

"The mean little creek got mad and rose over seven feet," wrote 8th Ohio hospital steward Charles H. Merrick to his sister. "It flooded our Camp so quick we had to wade in the water to remove the wounded. It was an awful thing to hurry out several hundred wounded and dying men, the rain falling in torrents all the time. How I did work, and how the poor fellows did suffer."[11]

Anyone that was able to walk or painfully limp snatched up all available lanterns and hurriedly sloshed out into the churning water to rescue as many of the wounded as possible. The surgical staff of each table made sure that their equipment, upon which literally rested the lives of so many men, was above the rising waters; then they waded out into the widening stream to carry, to assist, even to drag their patients to safety.

Charles Minard made sure that his friend Scoville was out of danger, then rushed back to the water's edge to assist in getting the helpless away from the danger. The water was rising faster now. "I pulled two of the wounded up the hill at one time; I had one by the arm and the other by the hair; I had no time to get a better hold, for if I had let go of either he would have gone under the water."[12]

---

10. "Wounded at Gettysburgh," p. 5.
11. Charles H. Merrick, Letter to his sister Min Merrick, July 10, 1863, William P. Palmer Collection, Container 1, Folder 3, MSS 3088, Western Reserve Historical Society, Cleveland, Ohio [underlining is by Merrick]. Merrick mistakenly dated the flooding as taking place July 9, rather than early morning July 6. By July 9, all the Second Corps Hospitals were high and dry on the farmland of Jacob Schwartz.
12. "Wounded at Gettysburgh," p. 5.

Some rescuers went to elaborate lengths to save endangered men too injured to transport. "The man who was looking after me, finding that he could not, alone, carry me to higher ground, cut some stakes, drove them into the ground, placed poles on them, and then breaking up an old barrel, took the staves and laid them across the poles, thus making quite a comfortable bunk, several feet above the water," wrote gravely wounded Captain Nickerson of the 8th Ohio. "Upon this, after great labor on his part, and no little anguish on my own, this faithful man succeeded in placing me out of reach of the angry waters that swept through our camp and under my cot."[13]

"The overflow was probably not over two feet in depth, but to men who could not raise their heads, this, like Mercutio's wound, was enough—it sufficed. The few attendants there worked like Trojans, but it was impossible to save all, and quite a number of the more helpless ones were drowned within the range of my limited vision."[14]

"Many of the wounded on the bank of a brook were in danger of drowning from the rapid rise of the water. There were no stretchers, and some of the badly wounded could not be carried in the arms of the men without great pain." A pair of Christian Commissioners looked around desperately, searching for something, anything, that would allow them to move the critically injured. "'Lay them on my back,' said a Delegate, going into the water on his hands and knees, and thus, bent with his face to the ground, he conveyed them tenderly out of the reach of danger."[15]

Surgeons, stewards, commission representatives, and hangers-on alike waded out into the chilly waters, grabbing the wounded men and physically dragging them to higher ground. It was obvious that the entire western bank was in danger of being engulfed, so the injured were manhandled up the steep opposite bank, often crying out from the pain of the jostling, then laid out unceremoniously on the top as their rescuers hurried back for more. Many of the wounded lost what few remaining possessions they still had in the process, seeing blankets, shelter tents, letters, Bibles, and clothing carried downstream by the rising water. Now the survivors lay gasping and bleeding from reopened wounds, unsheltered on the bare rocky ground—dazed and drenched, but alive.

---

13. Nickerson, "Personal Recollections of Two Visits to Gettysburg," p. 22.
14. *Ibid.*, pp. 22-23. The question of just how many wounded actually drowned at the Second Corps Hospitals is addressed in depth in Appendix 7.
15. Rev. Edward P. Smith, *Incidents of the United States Christian Commission.* (Philadelphia: J. B. Lippincott & Co., 1869), p. 173.

Baltimore, Maryland

The train from Philadelphia rattled to a stop in the early morning darkness at the Baltimore depot, and disgorged a steady stream of passengers, all intent on stretching their cramped legs or making the connection with other trains. Cornelia Hancock took in the crowded platform, the bustling passengers, and the vast expanse of the depot with wide eyes; she had never been this far from rural New Jersey before. "The morning [July 6] found us in Baltimore where there was stir and some knowledge of events."[16]

"Here Dorothea Dix appeared on the scene." Standing like a sentinel in the center of the platform, Dix—famed social reformer, founder of insane asylums, and now superintendent of female nurses—carefully scrutinized the passengers stepping down from the coaches. She was a deceptively unimpressive, quiet woman of sixty-one years with a chronic respiratory ailment. But what she lacked in physical presence she more than made up in experience. Being acquainted with the landmark work of the British Sanitary Commission during the Crimean War, and having personally visited and toured the Black Sea hospitals of Florence Nightingale, Dix brought the highest possible credentials to her government nursing position.[17]

She also brought extremely stringent standards for "her" nurses. All candidates were expected to be over thirty, healthy, "plain almost to repulsion in dress, and devoid of personal attractions." Important skills included the knowledge of "how to cook all kinds of low diet," "look neat themselves, and keep their boys and wards the same. Must write and read for their boys, but not from [just] any book or newspaper." Personal habits were very strictly limited—"they must be in their own rooms at taps, or nine o'clock unless obliged to be with the sick; must not go to any place of amusement in the evening; must not walk out with any patient or officer in their own room except on business; must be willing to take the forty cents per day that is allowed by the government, to assist them in supplying what the rations . . . will not furnish in food," as well as use the remainder to succor their patients. Her strict moral standards also forbad frippery such as "colored dresses, hoops, curls, jewelry, and flowers on their bonnets." And only devout Protestants need apply. The ratio of these new

---

16. Hancock, *South After Gettysburg*, p. 6.
17. *Ibid.*; Adams, *Doctors in Blue*, p. 176.

female nurses to their existing male counterparts was generally about one to every four or five, varying from hospital to hospital.[18]

Alerted to the battle in central Pennsylvania, and the public outcry for more citizen assistance for the wounded, she immediately left Washington, setting up her temporary headquarters in Baltimore, the rail terminus from which any connecting trains to Gettysburg would leave. Intent on intercepting and carefully inspecting any female citizens heading for the battlefield, she had become a fixture at the depot since her arrival in town.

Now she turned her eagle eye on the group of volunteer nurses disembarking from the Philadelphia train. "She looked the nurses over and pronounced them all suitable except me," wrote young Miss Hancock. "She immediately objected to my going farther on the score of my youth and rosy cheeks. I was then just twenty-three years of age. In those days it was considered indecorous for angels of mercy to appear otherwise than gray-haired and spectacled. Such a thing as a hospital corps of comely young maiden nurses, possessing grace and good looks, was then unknown." Her personal sponsor, Eliza Farnham, quickly spoke up in her defense. "Miss Farnham explained that she was under obligation to my friends who had helped her get proper credentials."[19]

At this point, Cornelia took things into her own hands. Frustrated by the abundance of talk and lack of any positive action, Cornelia sought out the train for Gettysburg. "The discussion waxed warm and I had no idea what conclusion they came to, for I settled the question myself by getting on the car and staying in my seat until the train pulled out of the city of Baltimore. They had not forcibly taken me from the train, so I got into Gettysburg the night of July sixth—where the need was so great that there was no further cavil about age."[20]

---

18. Adams, *Doctors in Blue*, pp. 177-78.
19. Hancock, *South After Gettysburg*, p. 6.
20. *Ibid.* Cornelia Hancock was not the only volunteer nurse to run afoul of Dorothea Dix's stringent standards. When seeking to go to Gettysburg to help the "mangled victims" of the battle, young Sophronia Bucklin had also been refused by Dix's curt: "No, you are too young for field duty." When tapped by a member of the Sanitary Commission to go help distribute stores, with the assurance that the Sanitary Commission representative would stand between Sophronia and Dix, she jumped at the opportunity. A confrontation scene (much like what Cornelia Hancock recorded) ensued in the lobby of a Baltimore hotel, with similar intercession by a sponsor. Unlike Cornelia Hancock's situation, this one ended amicably enough: "The kind superintendent [Dix], with no chiding, forgave me, and said, 'Report to the

Gettysburg, Pennsylvania

Christian Commission representative Andrew Cross and his companion were up early at the headquarters of the provost marshal, reluctantly leaving the warmth and comfort of the straw-filled barn in which they had passed the night in order to saddle their borrowed horse. With a military pass signed by Provost General Marsena R. Patrick in their pocket, the two were intent on getting into town as soon as possible to arrange transportation of additional Christian Commission supplies on the Gettysburg Railroad. Mounting up double on their borrowed horse, the pair cantered off towards town along the Baltimore Pike in the early light of dawn.

"At daylight we were off to Gettysburg, where we saw Mr. McCurdy, the President of the railroad, and learned that the Government had the road in hand; that cars would be up as soon as they could have the road ready." Having done all that was possible at this end to arrange for shipment of supplies, Cross and his associate took the opportunity to visit other hospitals in town and assess their need for additional supplies. "We went to the Seminary and College hospitals, and around the town, in court house, churches, &c., where we found a continued specimen of what we had down the country [at the Second Corps Hospitals], only that they were sheltered and dry, and had some attendants."[21]

As they were passing through town, the two stumbled across something literally worth its weight in gold in this war-ravaged town. "When we left the [Second] corps hospital, the cry began to be heard, 'Bread! bread!' We did not know where to turn to get it. After we came to town, as we came down from one of the hospitals in the town, we espied a wagon with bread, &c. We hailed the man to lay violent hands on it, to send it down to the hospital, when he told us that it was in charge of Mr. Latimer Small, of York, who had passed us but a moment before, in a carriage with some other persons. We hurried up to him, learned that there was more coming, and urged him to send it to the 3d division of the 2d corps. He gave direction, and afterwards we heard of the joy which it gave many wounded men."[22]

Sanitary Hospital for duty.'" [Sylvia G. L. Dannett, ed. and comp., *Noble Women of the North* (New York: Thomas Yoseloff, 1959), pp. 253-54.]

21. Cross, *The War and the Christian Commission*, p. 17.

22. *Ibid.*

With the coming of morning it was finally possible to look around and see the condition and new location of the Second Corps Hospitals. The rising waters in the black of night had driven the medical facilities up the steep eastern bank of the creek and onto the property of local farmer Jacob Schwartz. The tract of land, consisting of several hundred acres, had been purchased by Jacob Schwartz, Sr. and his wife around 1812. After raising twelve children and working the farm for more than three and a half decades, Jacob, Sr. sold the property to one of his children, Moses, in 1849. Moses moved to Cashtown a few years after buying the family estate, selling it in turn to his brother, Jacob, Jr. Even as late as 1863, however, it was still known locally as the "Moses Schwartz place." During Jacob, Jr.'s ownership, the farm had grown to some three hundred acres, and had become the site of several other large corps hospitals in addition to the three divisional hospitals of the Second Corps.[23]

The hospitals were now set up on something of a peninsula, with the flooded Rock Creek rushing directly behind and below them, and the neighboring White Run winding around to both the east and south where it linked with Rock Creek. The First and Second Division replanted themselves directly up the slope from their location in the lowlands along Rock Creek. The Third Division, however, decided to distance themselves from the other two divisions—probably motivated by the problem of too many men crammed together and too little fresh water and food to go around. Medical Director Isaac Scott notified Chief Operator Harry M. McAbee of his plans, and together they moved the division hospital away from the other divisions, ". . . going to an open hill half a mile further south."[24]

The first order of business in each division hospital, after getting everyone up the steep bank and spread out haphazardly on the ridge above, was to reestablish the amputating tables. Men with shattered arms and legs, with no hope whatsoever of saving their mutilated and ravaged extremities, were rapidly dying in the summer heat as infection,

---

23. J. Howard Wert, "In the Hospitals of Gettysburg, July, 1863," No. I, *Harrisburg Telegraph*, July 2, 1907, p. 7; Coco, *A Vast Sea of Misery*, p. 91.
24. Dwinelle, *Medical Report*; Coco, *A Vast Sea of Misery*, p. 91; Theodore Dimon, *Report of the General Agent of the State of New York for the Relief of Sick, Wounded, and Discharged Soldiers* (Printon, New York: Comstock and Cassidy, 1864), p. 53.

septic shock, and fever set in. The hurried evacuation of the hospitals the previous night, with the accompanying manhandling of the patients to safety, had reopened a number of battle wounds. Hemorrhage was always a persistent danger, and last night's rough handling could suddenly and fatally undo all the careful work of both doctors and patients.

As harsh as the reality was, the lives of many men were dependent on the surgical removal of one or more of their limbs. With the surgeons once again laboring around the bloody operating tables, the soaked survivors of last night's flooding, many with little clothing and no shelter at all, pragmatically set about trying to make themselves as comfortable as possible under their new circumstances.

Quakertown, Pennsylvania

Capt. Benjamin W. Thompson of the 111th New York was still suffering terribly from the thirty-three mile forced march of June 29. His varicose veins and the terrible misuse of his feet over the last week had left his extremities so badly swollen that he was not even able to get his shoes on. Fortunately, the previous day's march had been only a few miles long, but even that had necessitated his riding the short distance on a broken-down horse someone had scrounged up.

"At Quakertown I spent the night in a home where the good woman baked bread all night and sold it to the soldiers at fifty cents a loaf. Her man had to go out after midnight and buy more flour as trade continued brisk. And there were plenty of other generous, patriotic families doing the same. Some few even sold as low as twenty five cents, but not many."[25]

But even a good night's rest, sheltered from the intermittent rains in the home of these loyal townsfolk, had not helped reduce the swelling in his legs. "The next morning my regimental Surgeon refused to allow me to go with my company, and the ambulance corps had positive orders to allow no one to ride, so I was left at Quakertown." Unable to march forward with his men, forbidden to go in an ambulance, even if he continued on the sway-backed nag he had been riding, there seemed but only one place left to go. As his regiment marched off into the distance, Captain Thompson reluctantly turned his mount's head, and slowly headed back to Gettysburg.[26]

---

25. Thompson, *Personal Narrative*, p. 48.
26. *Ibid.*

Gettysburg, Pennsylvania

Frank Haskell was also making his way back to Gettysburg from the army bivouac. "On the 6th of July, while my bullet bruise was yet too inflamed and sensitive for me to be good for much in the way of duty,—the Division was then halted for the day some four miles from the field on the Baltimore turnpike,—I could not repress the desire or omit the opportunity to see again where the battle had been. With the right stirrup-strap shortened in a manner to favor the bruised leg, I could ride my horse at a walk, without serious discomfort."[27]

Riding leisurely along in the company of an old acquaintance from Wisconsin, Haskell took in all the sights along the way. Riding toward town, "it seemed very strange upon approaching the horse-shoe crest again, not to see it covered with the thousands of troops, and the horses and guns, but they were all gone,—the armies, to my seeming, had vanished,—and on that lovely summer morning the stillness and silence of death pervaded the localities where so recently the shouts and the cannon had thundered."[28]

Few soldiers may have been in evidence, but sight-seers were out in force on the field. "Numbers of civilians and boys, and some girls even, were curiously loitering about the field, and their faces showed not sadness or horror, but only staring wonder or smirking curiosity. They looked for mementoes of the battle to keep, they said; but their furtive attempts to conceal an uninjured musket, or an untorn blanket,—they had been told that all property left here, belonged to the government,—showed that the love of gain was an ingredient at least of their motive for coming here. Of course there was not the slightest objection to their taking any thing that they could find, now; but their manner of doing it was the objectionable thing."[29]

After riding along the Confederate lines and touring through the town itself, Haskell and his companion turned their horses' heads toward Cemetery Ridge. "I rode through the Cemetery on 'Cemetery Hill.' How those quiet sleepers must have been astounded in their graves when the twenty-pound Parrott guns, thundered above them, and the solid shot crushed their grave stones! The flowers, roses and creeping vines, that pious hands had planted to bloom and shed their

27. Byrne and Weaver, *Haskell of Gettysburg*, p. 193.

28. *Ibid.*

29. Byrne and Weaver, *Haskell of Gettysburg*, p. 194. In all fairness, some of the civilians may have been hoping to recoup some of their losses sustained during the battle.

odors over the ashes of the dear ones gone, were trampled upon the ground, and black with the cannon's soot. A dead horse lay by the marble shaft, and over it the marble finger pointed to the sky. The marble lamb that had slept its white sleep on the grave of a child, now lies blackened upon a broken gun-carriage. Such are the incongruities and jumblings of battle."[30]

The ambling tour of the battlefield ultimately led to the scene of the height of the battle for the men of the Union Second Corps. "I look away to *the group of trees*,—the Rebel gunners know what ones I mean, and so do the survivors of Pickett's Division,—and a strange facination [*sic*] led me thither. How thick are the marks of battle as I approach,—the graves of the men of the 3d Division of the 2nd Corps,—the splintered oaks,—the scattered horses,—seventy-one dead horses were on a spot some fifty yards square, near the position of Woodruff's Battery, and where he fell."[31]

"I stood solitary upon the crest by *'the trees'* where less than three days ago I had stood before; but now how changed is all the eye beholds. Do these thick mounds cover the fiery hearts, that in the battle rage, swept the crest and stormed the wall? I read their names—them alas, I do not know,—but I see the regiments marked on their frail monuments,—'20th Mass Vols'—'69 PV'—'1st Minn Vols'—and the rest,—they are all represented, and as they fought, commingled here."[32]

Awed and humbled by the tour, Haskell and his friend stood silent in the shade of the battle-scarred trees, looking out at the scenes of devastation and desolation spread out on all sides.

Ambulances continued to clatter into the Second Corps Hospital, but with a longer drive to reach the newly relocated medical facility, and at an ever slower rate. The departure of the army had severely curtailed the number of ambulances available to the hospital, and the few that could be secured were forced to divide their efforts.[33] One portion continued to transport the wounded capable of evacuation to the depot in Gettysburg, still suspiciously empty of any railroad trains

30. *Ibid.*, pp. 198-99.
31. *Ibid.*, p. 199.
32. *Ibid.*
33. Of the more than one thousand ambulances at Gettysburg during the battle, medical director of the Army of the Potomac Jonathan Letterman left only *thirty-two* behind when the Army pulled out. [*OR*, vol. 27, pt. 1, p. 197.]

or personnel, and increasingly more crowded with weak, bandaged, and damaged men huddled around the limited shelter of the Christian Commission "Eating Saloon."

The remaining ambulancemen kept scouring the battlefield, searching for the last few isolated casualties not yet recovered, hidden by the rocky terrain or laying incapacitated in tangled overgrowth. Now, fully three days after the close of the fighting, virtually all of the Union wounded had been retrieved from where they had fallen. The ones now being recovered were largely Confederates from the more remote areas of the battlefield, and a bone-jarring ambulance ride over fields and rugged terrain was often necessary to even reach roads leading to the hospital.

Unfortunately, reaching the Second Corps medical facilities was no guarantee of having their injuries cleansed and bandaged. Many awaited examination by a doctor—in fact, by anyone at all—until long after their arrival. Those with wounds not considered life-threatening had to remain untreated until such a time as the overworked surgeons could finally attend to their cases. Even those needing immediate amputations were often forced to wait for those that had arrived ahead of them, with wounds just as serious, if not worse.

Although the hospital was now out of the lowland quagmire along the eastern bank of Rock Creek, conditions were still deplorable for the wounded. Representatives from various volunteer organizations continued arriving in Gettysburg by foot or on horseback; one, a Reverend Williams from the Sanitary Commission, was absolutely shocked at what he found at the Second Corp Hospitals. "There were at least 2,500 wounded men in this hospital, which was located in a grove about a mile south of the Baltimore Pike, and between two and three miles from town. The men were in a terrible condition. They were upon the damp ground, many of them with nothing under them. In this hospital there was an unusually large number of amputations, the amputated stumps lying directly upon the ground, except when now and then elevated upon a handful of straw, or a bunch of old rags."[34]

"Many of the men, perhaps most of them, were in want of clothing. Suitable food was not to be had. The surgeons were overworked, there was an insufficient number of attendants—every able-bodied man that

---

34. *United States Sanitary Commission Report for the Army and Navy—[Its] Work and Incidents, First Annual Report, Philadelphia, 1863.* Quote of either Rev. E. F. Williams or Rev. J. W. M. Williams—no first name is given.

could possibly be spared having accompanied the army in pursuit of Lee."[35]

The condition of the Confederate wounded was, if possible, even worse than that of their Union counterparts. "There were nearly or quite a thousand Rebels, most of them severely wounded, lying on the outskirts of the hospital, shrieking and continually crying for assistance. The appearance of those connected with the Third Division of this corps beggars description. Destitute of clothing, many of them nearly naked, lying in the mud—for the sudden rise of the little stream by which they had been placed rendered it impossible to avoid this—cursing, praying, begging their visitors to put an end to their sufferings; here one and there another laid out by himself to die, these wretched men made the strongest appeal to Christian sympathy and benevolence."[36]

In spite of the horrible conditions and the severity of their wounds, the Confederates continued to be intensely interested in the safety and whereabouts of General Lee and their army. "Two or three days pass by and we can hear nothing reliable about the movements of the army. The Yankees tell us the most ridiculous stories of the hasty and disastrous retreat of our army, how large detachments are daily captured and how the whole will be destroyed before they reach the Potomac." John Dooley, however, was highly skeptical of all such bluecoat rumors. "But we know too much to believe anything the Yankees say, and know too well how glad these same gallant blue coats will be when Genl Lee is agitating them no more and is again in Va."[37]

"Ah, these days go slowly by," continued his entry, "and yet new scenes are daily being enacted around us and serve to excite, tho' far from pleasing."[38]

With the constant influx of bleeding and mutilated men also came a procession of the lame, the sick, the handicapped, and diseased. Cpl. David Stoup of Company E, 63rd Pennsylvania, from the decimated Third Corps, was there, crippled so severely by rheumatism

35. *Ibid.*
36. *Ibid.*
37. Dooley, *John Dooley*, p. 114.
38. *Ibid.*

aggravated by the damp weather and wet ground that the slightest movement of his gnarled limbs brought excruciating pain.[39] Twenty-one-year-old Pvt. Charles F. Buzzell, Company E, 12th New Hampshire (also from the Third Corps) had also come in for treatment, but he was kept apart (as much as possible) from the other wounded. It was clear that he was suffering from typhoid fever.[40]

With the excitement of battle now past, more and more men began showing the effects of the mammoth march of June 29, hobbling painfully to the hospital complaining of boils, blisters, and lesions of their feet. In the rush to save the lives of those with dreadful wounds, such routine cases were often forced to shift for themselves. With thousands in need of immediate attention, the overworked surgeons simply had no time to spare to attend to the routine complaints of camp life, and only the barest minimum of time and attention could be given them by the limited number of dressing surgeons, hospital stewards, and others at the Second Corps medical facilities.

Nor had the fighting halted the onset of the mundane ills of camp life and personal ailments—diarrhea and camp fevers, the effects of venereal diseases, digestive ailments, hernias, and men needing teeth pulled. One such case was that of Pvt. Austin A. Carr of the 82nd New York Infantry, who had been developing a serious case of hemorrhoids, aggravated by the largely indigestible nature of army cuisine. "On the march to Gettysburg, the piles did not bother [me] much, except to feel a little sore at times. At the close of the fight at Gettysburg on the 3rd of July, volunteers were called for to go for rations; as the men were weary after two days of hard fighting. I volunteered to go, but when called upon was unable to respond. The tumors had come down."[41]

---

39. Stoup died on July 24, and was buried on the Jacob Schwartz farm lane. He was ultimately reinterred in Plot A-72 in the Pennsylvania Plot of Gettysburg National Cemetery. The official cause of death was listed as rheumatism.

40. Buzzell died July 14 of the effects of the fever, and was buried in the Schwartz cornfield on Rock Creek. He, too, was reinterred in the National Cemetery, in Plot A-5 of the New Hampshire section.

41. Austin A. Carr, *A Casualty at Gettysburg and Andersonville: Selections from the Civil War Diary of Private Austin A. Carr of the 82nd N. Y. Infantry*, ed. David G. Martin (Hightstown, New Jersey: Longstreet House, 1990), p. 10.

After spending a miserable night stretched out on the bare ground, trying to find some relief from the pain, Carr was ordered to report to the nearest aid station. "Shortly after reaching the Hospital Building, firing began at the front, and I then returned, the officer in command again ordering me to the rear, but I told him that I was in so much pain that I would lay down awhile. I then lay down, covering myself with my rubber blanket, as a heavy rain had commenced falling. I lay there untill [*sic*] the storm ceased, about 4 P.M., when I was again ordered to the rear. By that time I was in a fearful condition, the lumps having swollen, and I was rapidly getting so that I could not walk."[42]

With great difficulty, the ailing private made his way back to the aid station. "I managed to get to the building used as a hospital, but that being filled with the wounded, I went to a field below and laid down, and laid there from the afternoon of the 4th untill [*sic*] the morning of the 6th. On Sunday the 5th, a couple of Minnesota boys passing bye [*sic*], seeing that I was helpless brought me a fresh canteen of water, and with that I kept the tumors moistened, as I did not know what else to do, except as I heard it spoken of. On the morning of the 6th the tumors bursted, issuing a considerable amount of matter and blood, affording me almost instant relief."[43]

Once again, the New Yorker headed back to the aid station. "As soon as I could, I got to my feet, and walked to the building used as a hospital, and explained my case to the physician there in charge. He dressed my wound, for I was struck in the collar bone with a piece of shell, making a slight wound, the missile glancing off. I did not pay much attention to the wound, as my attention was attracted to something more serious. I was still very sore, and could walk only in pain. The doctor sent me to a hospital farther down the road."[44] Carr was, undoubtedly, dispatched off to the Second Corps Hospitals at the Schwartz Farm.

After seeing his regiment break camp and march off in pursuit of the retreating Confederates, Capt. Benjamin W. Thompson reluctantly turned and headed back to Gettysburg. Following the short ride back

42. *Ibid.*
43. *Ibid.*
44. *Ibid.*

from Quakertown, he had finally managed to track down the location of the Second Corps Hospital. After picking his way over the unfamiliar terrain to the Schwartz farm, he was directed still further south to the detached Third Division Hospital, where the wounded of the 111th New York Regiment were being treated.

Slowing his horse to a walk when he reached the site, he gazed in wonder at the "hospital." There were no buildings, no tents, and almost no blankets. The collection of bleeding and shattered men, some with no shirts, some with no pants, some almost stark naked, were scattered randomly around Farmer Schwartz's south meadow and the hills along Rock Creek. The captain slid stiffly down off his broken-down nag, wincing at the pain from his swollen feet and legs, and limped off in search of his wounded comrades. "I found my way back to the Second Corps hospital and there had plenty of work caring for men much worse than myself."[45]

"Our hospital was on the bank of a stream and led up into a clover field. We managed to get straw enough from the neighborhood to put on the ground for our wounded men and we had such blankets as we could get hold of—and this was all there was to the hospital except the operating tables. During the time we were there it rained terribly and the men were wet to the skin a number of times, so that it was evident to anyone that they should be gotten away from such a place and sent where they could be reasonably cared for. We had not only the severely wounded of the Corps, but a large number of wounded rebels."[46]

As for the medical staff of the Third Division, Thompson had nothing but the highest commendation for their skills. "The work of the surgeons and their helpers, most of whom were, like myself, unable to be with the army, was very arduous. They all worked like heroes and did everything in their power for the good of the men. There were no shirkers there."[47]

Unfortunately, Captain Thompson did not lavish the same praises on the civilians living nearby. "The patriotism of the neighboring farmers did not shine very brightly. A well to do farmer near us refused us straw for our men. I took a squad and read him a warm army lecture

---

45. Thompson, *Personal Narrative*, p. 48.
46. *Ibid.*, pp. 48-49.
47. *Ibid.*, p. 49.

and then took all the straw we needed. Not a man or woman in the vicinity offered a hand to help or a drop of milk for the poor sufferers."[48]

Philadelphia, Pennsylvania

There was no shortage of patriotism in Philadelphia on July 6, however. After a day of strenuous activity, the members of the Ascension Church in downtown Philadelphia were ready to send off their handmade supply of shirts, drawers, bandages, and lint. Members of the congregation, as well as friends and relatives from around town, had delved into their own larders and canning cupboards, contributing jams, jellies, pickles, relishes, and other homegrown goods. "By the following noon [July 6], through the efforts of the women and young men, several tons of stores, including garments, delicacies, and medicines, with a large money collection, had been accumulated." Many of those that had a hand in producing, packaging, and loading the relief stores were turned out to see off the wagons and their staff of relief workers.[49]

"With these a delegation of active workers was immediately dispatched to the field," wrote John Y. Foster, a member of the congregation. "It was my fortune to accompany these young men." With high hopes of getting to the battlefield as quickly as possible, the teams were whipped up and the caravan lurched into motion. Within the hour, the supply train had headed west out of Philadelphia on the road to Gettysburg.[50]

The members of the Ladies Aid Society of Philadelphia were also hard at work on this hot July day. Normally meeting only on Fridays to

48. *Ibid.* Despite the harsh words of Thompson and many others, there were some of the local residents that took an active hand in helping the casualties. At the Second Corps Hospital, a neighbor from down the road, Catherine Houghtelin Wert, mother of J. Howard Wert, was affectionately known as "Aunt Katy." She assisted many of the wounded, and became a particular favorite of the Confederates. [Coco, *A Vast Sea of Misery*, p. 79.]
49. Mrs. Edmund A. [Emily Bliss] Souder, *Leaves from the Battle-Field of Gettysburg. A Series of Letters from a Field Hospital. And National Poems.* (Philadelphia: Caxton Press of C. Sherman, Son & Co., 1864), pp. 6-7.
50. Foster, "Four Days at Gettysburg," *Harper's New Monthly Magazine*, vol. 28 (December, 1863, to May, 1864): 381.

read the reports of the their Field Secretary, Ellen Orbison Harris, and to manufacture and process relief goods, news of the battle brought them hurrying back to their meeting rooms, rented from the 10th Presbyterian Church, early on Monday morning. "Attendance was very large, strangers who never met with us before came in, and one of the pleasantest features of the work was the voluntary offerings of different denominations, and their gathering in with us to labor,—as our Association has no respect to sect,—but previously, with less success than desirable. Divine favor seemed to rest upon us, in the union of feeling, the very liberal contributions of the public, and the prompt and efficient aid we were enabled to furnish."[51]

The Society had worked hard to build up a backlog of emergency supplies, storing them in rooms rented from the managers of the Philadelphia Bible Society. These were immediately dispatched to Secretary Harris at Gettysburg, and arrangements were made to ship relief goods directly to the battlefield from outlying areas without having to first funnel them through the Philadelphia office.

Meanwhile, as the business was being conducted, the rank and file members of the Society were hard at work in other parts of the building, cutting and stitching clothing and bandages. Many of the poor and indigent residents of the city, paid by private charities, assisted in the work. Other Aid Society ladies were out gathering donations of money and food from local citizens, as well as soliciting assistance from out-of-town benefactors.

As each shipment was finished, it was picked up by the Railroad and Express companies and immediately shipped off to Gettysburg.[52]

Somewhere Northeast of Gettysburg, Pennsylvania

Dr. Bushrod Washington James and his friends were also pushing on toward Gettysburg. Now a full day after crossing the Susquehanna River by ferry boats, the heavily loaded wagons cut deep ruts into the sodden roads. The doctors, forced by the overloading of the wagons to walk alongside the convoy, were well beyond footsore by now, and rest stops were becoming more frequent. At this rate, it did not look as though they were going to reach the battlefield before nightfall.

---

51. *Report of the Ladies Aid Society*, pp. 2-3.
52. *Ibid.*, pp. 4-5.

Somewhere East of Gettysburg, on the Railroad

The last leg of the rail trip was turning out to be anything but rapid for Cornelia Hancock and her party. The Rebel invasion had thrown northern rail transportation into a major upheaval—non-military freight shipments had been totally suspended, and passenger business was severely curtailed. In the meantime, military trains had priority as supplies and equipment were rushed to the Army of the Potomac.[53]

The train had steamed north out of Baltimore on the Northern Central, a stretch of tracks heavily damaged by the Southerners during the Gettysburg campaign. Repairs were just being completed on the stretch between Baltimore and York, Pennsylvania, and rolling stock crept tentatively up the grades over rebuilt culverts and new trestles.

South of York, the train had taken the switchoff onto the Hanover and Gettysburg branch of the North Central. A little single-track line, just twenty-five miles long, it had taken a tremendous beating from the Confederate invaders. They had effectively destroyed every bridge between Harrisburg and Hanover Junction, including three key bridges on the Hanover and Gettysburg line.

Now, the right-of-way swarmed with a detachment of Herman Haupt's 400 man army repair corps; teams of oxen, piles of tools, timbers, and prefabricated bridge trestles all added to the impression of a bustling commercial jobsite. Progress of the train slowed to a glacial crawl. Any other time, the passengers would have been in Gettysburg long ago—now those on board could only look out in helpless frustration as the train inched its way past piles of twisted iron rails, splintered and charred ties, blackened bridge supports, and squads of toiling gandy dancers and foremen, all sweltering in the July heat.[54]

In addition to Doctor Child's contingent of doctors and volunteer nurses, two other notable passengers were on board this train. George Anna Woolsey and her mother, Jane Eliza Newton Woolsey, had managed to secure tickets to Gettysburg, no doubt because of George

---

53. Thomas Weber, *The Northern Railroads in the Civil War, 1861-1865* (New York: King's Crown Press, 1952), p. 64.
54. Samuel Richey Kamm, *The Civil War Career of Thomas A. Scott* (Philadelphia: 1940), pp. 161-162; George Anna Woolsey, *Three Weeks at Gettysburg* (New York: Privately Published, 1863).

Anna's association with Frederick Law Olmsted and the United States Sanitary Commission. Now the unlikely pair, one a vivacious New York socialite in her twenties, the other a sixty-three-year-old widow from a Virginia slave-owning background, accompanied two rail cars stuffed with medicines, tents, clothing, and food for the wounded. Watching the landscape passing by the coach windows with agonizing slowness, mother and daughter sat side by side and anxiously willed the locomotive to pick up speed.[55]

Gettysburg, Pennsylvania

After touring a number of hospitals in and about the city limits of Gettysburg, it was becoming evident to Andrew Cross and his fellow relief agent that they were going to have to move the Christian Commission operations closer to the center of hospital activity. "We had been directed to make headquarters at the 2d Army corps, but we at once saw that it was not the place, as reference to the map will show. The town was full of hospitals, and east, north and west of the town Rebel hospitals, among which were many of our own wounded."[56]

First, the two needed to return Major Cross' long-suffering horse and let the other commissioners know of the change in plans. "We rode back to the 2d corps, left the horse, and came back to the town. Here we met with other members of the Commission, and united in securing Mr. Schick's store for reception of goods."[57]

The need for a larger, centralized facility was readily apparent to everyone present. The influx of relief supplies was increasing exponentially, "coming to the Commission from citizens around [the area], York, Hanover, Carlisle, Harrisburg, Lancaster, Baltimore, Philadelphia, &c., and indeed from almost every direction. But a few days before they were in dread of the invading army; now, with grateful hearts and willing hands, they were bringing of what had been saved, and offering it to supply food and clothing for the wounded, who had borne the burden of their defence [*sic*]."[58]

---

55. *The Sanitary Commission of the United States Army. A Succinct Narrative of Its Works and Purposes*, p. 151.
56. Cross, *The War and the Christian Commission*, p. 17.
57. *Ibid.*
58. *Ibid.*

Cross and his team busied themselves with sweeping out any debris left in Schick's store during the Confederate occupation of the town. Others cobbled together a makeshift sign advertising the presence of the Christian Commission, while the remainder began receiving the first trickles of what promised to soon be an avalanche of emergency relief supplies.

As things began to quiet for the night, 8th Ohio hospital steward Charles H. Merrick paused long enough in his duties to finish a letter he had been writing to his sister:

> 2nd Corps hospital at
> Gettysburg, Pa. July 6th, 1863
>
> My Dear Min,
>
> It pleased me much to get a letter from you yesterday and I was glad to lie down away from the sounds and sight of misery to read it. Such a time as we have had and are having still. There are from our Reg alone ninety six wounded men, many of them seriously wounded. Since the battle four have died, making our killed sixteen. Two more will die tonight. Lieut [Stephen] Strange is here near me as I write. He is not hurt badly. Capt [Azor] Nickerson continues very low and I doubt very much his recovery. We have several hundred rebels here to feed and take care of which adds much to the horror of the scene. Dr. [Joseph L.] Brenton was ordered to the Reg this morning, and he left me to take care of our wounded. I have about fifteen to help me, but for all that, the work is very great, and I can scarcely get a moment's rest during the day or night. Loads of rebel wounded still come in and they say the field is just covered with dead. Lieut Miller, Co G, (a big dutchman) is quite a hero now. He rushed forward and killed the colorbearer of the rebel regiment in our front and took his flag away. Our boys say the whole rebel Brigade fired at him, and it seems astonishing that he was not cut into strings.
>
> We are shut out from all news. But I suppose the papers are full of rejoicing. The[y] ought to be, for I believe the "army of the Potomac" has gained <u>one</u> victory, and a great one too. I hope I shall not be here many days. My health [is]

not good, But I only need rest and good living to cure me. Direct as usual. Love to all. . . .

As ever, Charles[59]

"Twenty-four hours we were in making the journey between Baltimore and Gettysburg, places only four hours apart in ordinary running time," wrote an exasperated George Anna Woolsey, "and this will give you some idea of the difficulty there was in bringing up supplies when the fighting was over, and the delays in transporting wounded."[60]

As the first train to reach the outskirts of Gettysburg approached the scene of the fighting, everyone anxiously peered out the windows in the fading light, trying to catch a glimpse of the recent battle. "Coming toward the town at this crawling rate, we passed some fields where the fences were down and the ground slightly tossed up: 'That's where Kilpatrick's cavalry men fought the rebels,' someone said, 'and close by that barn a rebel soldier was found day before yesterday, sitting dead;' no one was found to help, poor soul, 'near the whole city full.'"[61]

The locomotive slowed from its snail-like pace as it neared the battered little town of Gettysburg and rattled to a final stop. Ahead was what had once been the railroad bridge spanning Rock Creek, now a twisted ruin after the departure of the Confederates. Union repair crews, illumined by blazing fires and lantern light, were swarming over the scene of destruction, hard at work installing new trestles, ties, and track. This was the second effort to rebuilt the span; initial attempts were now somewhere downstream, washed away by the flooded Rock Creek. For now, this was the end of the line.

"The railroad bridge broken up by the enemy, [the] Government had not rebuilt as yet, and we stopped two miles from the town, to find that, as usual, just where the Government had left off the [Sanitary] Commission had come in." Just off to the side of the tracks, on this side of Rock Creek, several large Sanitary Commission tents had just been

---

59. Charles H. Merrick, Letter to his sister Min Merrick, July 6, 1863, William P. Palmer Collection, Container 1, Folder 3, MSS 3088, Western Reserve Historical Society, Cleveland, Ohio [underlining is by Merrick].

60. Woolsey, *Three Weeks at Gettysburg.*

61. *Ibid.*

pitched, preparing to receive the wounded as they arrived from the field hospitals.[62]

During the past several days, the Commission had been frantically rushing emergency supplies to the battlefield from storehouses in Maryland. While waiting for rail transportation to be restored on the Gettysburg Railroad, eight loads had been forwarded overland from Westminster. In addition, four more wagon loads were moved out of warehouses in Frederick. A schoolhouse, about three miles southeast of town on the Baltimore Pike, had been pressed into service due to its proximity to the various corps hospitals. Shoving school desks and educational paraphernalia into one corner, the small building was soon stuffed to the rafters with medicines, hospital supplies, foodstuffs, and clothing. From that central field depot, eleven wagon-loads of badly-needed supplies were rushed to the corps hospitals and to individual groups of wounded still stranded in various remote parts of the battlefield. Preparations were already under way to move the facility to larger quarters in Gettysburg.[63]

Knowing that the railroad would be up and running in a few days, Sanitary representatives from Baltimore busied themselves setting up a transit hospital; the work was just being completed when the train carrying the Woolseys rolled to a stop at Rock Creek. "The temporary terminus of the railway was then over a mile from the town, and to this terminus crowds of slightly wounded men came, limping, dragging themselves along, silent, weary, worn. The moment the cars stopped, the crowd of weary and wounded soldiers accumulated there, indicated that point as a place for a Relief Lodge."[64]

Dr. John Hancock Douglas, the associate secretary of the Commission, was there to personally oversee the establishment of the new Sanitary Lodge. "I immediately had two of our largest tents, together capable of sheltering seventy-five men, pitched, stoves erected, and a lodge established. The wise foresight of Mr. [Frederick Newman] Knapp [supervisor of the division of special relief of the Sanitary Commission] had included these articles among the first

---

62. *Ibid.*

63. J. H. Douglas, Sanitary Commission Pamphlet No. 71, *Report on the Operations of the Sanitary Commission During and After the Battles at Gettysburg, July 1st, 2d, and 3d, 1863* (Washington, D.C.: Privately Published, 1863), pp. 12-13; *The Sanitary Commission of the United States Army. A Succinct Narrative of Its Works and Purposes*, pp. 151, 154.

64. *The Sanitary Commission of the United States Army. A Succinct Narrative of Its Works and Purposes*, pp. 152.

invoice. The two Germans, whose names I have unfortunately lost, volunteered as cooks." For the wounded and exhausted men hobbling painfully out from town along the deserted tracks, the sight of the oversized canvas tents, awnings, and cookhouse of the Sanitary Commission in the distance must have been a tremendous relief. "That night our tents were full, and we had the great satisfaction of not only affording shelter and attention to the wounded, but also supplying good nutritious food to those within our tents, and those who had taken refuge on the cars."[65]

"There stood the temporary lodge and kitchen," wrote George Anna of the first sight to meet their eyes as they clambered down from the railroad carriage, "and here hobbling out of their tents came the wounded men who had made their way down from the Corps hospital expecting to leave at once in the return cars." The train, however, was not going to depart until morning, so the passenger and freight cars were quickly transformed into rolling hospital wards as soon as everyone had disembarked and all the freight had been offloaded.[66]

When the doors of the Sanitary Commission boxcars were opened, George Anna and her mother pitched in with the other relief agents to get the desperately needed supplies over to the hospital tents; then, rolling up their sleeves, the two started ministering to the wounded making their painful way from Gettysburg.

While the Woolseys were busy getting the Sanitary Commission Lodge up and running, Cornelia Hancock, Doctor Child, Eliza Farnham, and the others from Philadelphia tramped the two miles into town in a muggy, drizzling rain. "We were met by Dr. [Robert] Horner, at whose house [on Chambersburg Street] we stayed. Every barn, church, and building of any size in Gettysburg had been converted into a temporary hospital."[67]

There certainly was a tremendous need for volunteer nurses, skilled or otherwise, and Doctor Horner was quick to find them a place to be of service. "We went the same evening to one of the churches," wrote Cornelia, "where I saw for the first time what war meant. Hundreds of desperately wounded men were stretched out on boards laid across

65. *Ibid.*, pp. 154-55.
66. Woolsey, *Three Weeks at Gettysburg*.
67. Hancock, *South After Gettysburg*, p. 6.

the high-backed pews as closely as they could be packed together. Thus elevated, these poor sufferers' faces, white and drawn with pain, were almost on a level with my own. I seemed to stand breast-high in a sea of anguish. The townspeople of Gettysburg were in devoted attendance, and there were many from other villages and towns. The wounds of all had been dressed at least once, and some systematic care was already established."[68]

While those volunteer nurses with some skill in the care of the injured efficiently set to work among the wounded and battered men, Cornelia cast about for some way that she could be of use in the crowded church. "Too inexperienced to nurse, I went from one pallet to another with pencil, paper, and stamps in hand, and spent the rest of that night in writing letters from the soldiers to their families and friends. To many mothers, sisters, and wives I penned the last message of those who were soon to become the 'beloved dead.'"[69]

When the Sanitary Commission representatives finally had the last of the wounded fed and settled in for the night at the Lodge (all to the accompaniment of shouts, hammering, and the bellowing of the ox teams of the military rail crews rebuilding the Rock Creek bridge), mother and daughter Woolsey headed into town in search of supper for themselves. "The first day Mrs. and I reached the place we literally begged our bread from door to door—but the kind woman who at last gave us dinner would take no pay for it. 'No, ma'am, I shouldn't wish to have that sin on my soul when the war is over.' She, as well as others, had fed the strangers flocking into town daily, sometimes over fifty of them for each meal, and all for love and nothing for reward."[70]

The same selfless woman generously put them up for the night, and for the nights following. "One night we forced a reluctant confession from our hostess that she was meaning to sleep on the floor that we might have her bed, her whole house being full. Of course we couldn't allow this self-sacrifice and we hunted up some other place to stay in. We did her no good, however, for we afterwards found that the bed was given up that night to some other stranger who arrived late and

68. *Ibid.*
69. *Ibid.*, pp. 6-7.
70. Woolsey, *Three Weeks at Gettysburg.*

tired—'An old lady, you know, and I couldn't let an old lady sleep on the floor.'"[71]

Such open-handedness was not common in and around Gettysburg, however. Almost universal vilification was expressed by doctors, nurses, volunteers, and the wounded toward the "Dutch farmers" that lived in the rural areas surrounding the outskirts of town. Even the male residents of town were not much praised by those visiting the crossroads town. "Such acts of kindness and self-denial were almost entirely confined to the women," noted George Anna Woolsey acerbically.[72]

Out on the property of Farmer Schwartz, the Second Corps divisional hospitals were also settling down for another long dark night. The surgeons, still laboring by guttering lamplight at the amputating tables, cast weird flickering shadows over the crowded hospitals wards, now pitch-black under overcast skies. Men knew of the life or death of their neighbors only by sound and touch. Groans, sighs, sharp exclamations of pain, prayers, muttered conversations, and maniacal ravings punctuated the night, making it difficult for the exhausted men to find the longed-for release of sleep.

Many of the Confederate wounded still remained untreated, and were wracked by extreme pain. "There is one poor youth near by whose agonies are frightful, especially at night. Both his thigh bones have been broken by a ball, and really his anguish is enough to move a heart of stone. The worst is that he lingers in this terrible agony for three days, and it was a real satisfaction to learn that the unfortunate boy had expired."[73]

"Another victim and a member of my regiment is deliriously moaning and shouting all the night," continued diarist John Dooley. "He begins in a low tone of voice and shouts louder and louder, using only one phrase all the time, until he becomes exhausted. Thus he repeats frantically a hundred times at least the words, 'I'm proud I belong to the 1st Va Regiment!' Then he stops and begins another sentence, shouting and singing until he is exhausted."[74]

---

71. *Ibid.*
72. *Ibid.*
73. Dooley, *John Dooley*, p. 114.
74. *Ibid.*

Some injuries were simply beyond the abilities of even the most skilled medical corps surgeons to repair, leading to strange and slow deaths. "Another of the 19th Va has a jaw fractured and throat lacerated and is actually dying of pain and hunger."[75]

There were few comforts anywhere in the hospital, and Union men still suffered almost as much as the Southern wounded. "The groans of the wounded were constant, and the dead were being carried past us nearly all the time. On my left lay a young boy. He suffered much, but did not complain. One night, when it was time to go to sleep, he whispered, 'Good night, lieutenant, I think that I shall go up before morning.'"[76]

Capt. Jack Adams moved painfully in the dark, turning toward the boy as he favored his three untreated wounds. "I urged him to keep up his courage, but he said it was no use, he should die." Sometimes it just seemed easier to stop fighting and let go of life in the long dark privacy of the night.[77]

As the hours of blackness passed painfully and slowly from midnight to the early hours of morning, the camp settled into as near a semblance of quiet as it was going to achieve. Surgeons, numbed with fatigue and appalled by long hours of bloody amputations, collapsed for a few hours of troubled sleep as weary counterparts relieved them. Men, wracked with pain and anxiety, finally passed out from sheer exhaustion. All found at least some release in the murkiness of unconsciousness, or the haunted dreamings of sleep, or in the confidential arrival of death, in the inky July darkness.

75. *Ibid.*
76. Adams, *Reminiscences of the Nineteenth Massachusetts*, p. 71.
77. *Ibid.*

CHAPTER 11

TUESDAY, JULY 7: DAWN—TUESDAY, JULY 7: MIDNIGHT

"... for five miles around, there is an awful smell...."

Cornelia Hancock
Volunteer Nurse

Gettysburg, Pennsylvania

The stiffness and pain of his untreated wounds awakened Capt. Jack Adams in the feeble light of dawn. Remembering the conversation of the night before, he awkwardly rolled over on his side to face the young lad laying beside him. "In the morning I looked and saw that the poor boy had answered the last roll-call. He lay by my side until afternoon, before they could find time to take him away. I had forgotten to ask his name, and no one knew him. His grave no doubt bears the mark 'unknown,' and the records of his regiment say, 'missing in action.'" The battle at Gettysburg had claimed still another victim.[1]

Cornelia Hancock was up bright and early on July 7, and anxious to attend to the needs of any troops from back home. "Learning that the wounded of the Third Division of the Second Corps, including the 12th Regiment of New Jersey, were in a Field Hospital about five miles outside of Gettysburg, we determined to go there early the next

1. Adams, *Reminiscences of the Nineteenth Massachusetts*, p. 71.

morning, expecting to find some familiar faces from among the regiments of my native state."[2]

There were ambulances rolling through town, returning empty from the depot on their way back to the corps hospitals. Cornelia and her companions flagged down one with "Second Corps" emblazoned on it's side, and were soon clattering along through town and out into the ravaged countryside. "I being interested in the 2nd, because Will [her brother] had been in it, got into one of its ambulances, and went out at eight this morning and came back at six this evening."[3]

"As we drew near our destination we began to realize that war has other horrors than the sufferings of the wounded or the desolation of the bereft. A sickening, overpowering, awful stench announced the presence of the unburied dead, on which the July sun was mercilessly shining, and at every step the air grew heavier and fouler, until it seemed to possess a palpable horrible density that could be seen and felt and cut with a knife. Not the presence of the dead bodies themselves, swollen and disfigured as they were, and lying in heaps on every side, was as awful to the spectator as that deadly, nauseating atmosphere which robbed the battlefield of its glory, the survivors of their victory, and the wounded of what little chance of life was left to them."[4]

The ambulance lurched off the Baltimore Pike and onto a narrow rutted farm lane. Finally forced to leave even this small thoroughfare, the vehicle bucked and jounced overland toward the Third Division Hospital, a half-mile south of the other two division facilities. "As we made our way to a little woods in which we were told was the Field Hospital we were seeking, the first sight that met our eyes was a collection of semi-conscious but still living forms, all of whom had been shot through the head, and were considered hopeless." With not enough attendants to go around for the still-living wounded, no one could be spared to minister to the soon-to-be dead. There they lay alone, dying one by one—not through lack of care or kindness, but through lack of manpower. "They were laid there to die and I hoped that they were indeed too near death to have consciousness. Yet many a groan came from them, and their limbs tossed and twitched."[5]

---

2. Hancock, *South After Gettysburg*, p. 7.
3. *Ibid.*, p. 10.
4. *Ibid.*, p. 7.
5. *Ibid.*

The medical teams had been quite busy since setting up in the Schwartz woodlot, systematically working through the wounded where they had been deposited after the flooding. Under the supervision of dressing surgeons and cutters not on duty at the tables, male nurses and attendants had grouped the men according to their injuries, setting up a primitive system of triage. "The few surgeons who were left in charge of the battlefield after the Union army had started in pursuit of Lee had begun their paralyzing task by sorting the dead from the dying, and the dying from those whose lives might be saved; hence the groups of prostrate, bleeding men laid together according to their wounds."[6]

What Cornelia Hancock saw as she looked around the Third Division hospital absolutely appalled her. "There are no words in the English language to express the sufferings I witnessed today. . . . There was hardly a tent to be seen. Earth was the only available bed during those first hours after battle. . . . The men lie on the ground; their clothes have been cut off them to dress their wounds; they are half naked, have nothing but hard-tack to eat only as the Sanitary Commissions, Christian Associations, and so forth give them."[7]

The hospital was still struggling to get organized after the forced withdrawal from the banks of Rock Creek. While the wounded, many of them still untreated, lay without shelter and inadequately clothed, the surgical teams were continuing their seemingly endless work of surgery in the trees. "A long table stood in this woods and around it gathered a number of surgeons and attendants. This was the operating table, and for seven days it literally ran blood. A wagon stood near rapidly filling with amputated legs and arms; when wholly filled, this gruesome spectacle withdrew from sight and returned as soon as possible for another load."[8]

"There was a tiny brook running down from where the surgeons were working, and the blood of the soldiers mingled with the water of the brook until it was all red, and was a veritable river of blood," remembered Cornelia in later years. "Oh! if we had only known about carbolic acid in those days! We knew nothing about antiseptics, and the gangrene and rotting came so quickly. I spent hours with a spoon scooping out from wounds."[9]

---

6. *Ibid.*, pp. 7-8.
7. *Ibid.*, pp. 8, 10.
8. *Ibid.*, p. 8.
9. *The National Tribune*, August 16, 1934.

"I was the first woman who reached the 2nd Corps after the three days fight at Gettysburg," wrote Cornelia Hancock to her cousin that night. I was in that Corps all days, not another woman within half a mile. Mrs. [Ellen Orbison] Harris was in the first division of the 2nd Corps. I was introduced to the surgeon of the post [Dr. Harry M. McAbee], went anywhere through the Corps, and received nothing but the greatest politeness from even the lowest private."[10]

"So appalling was the number of the wounded as yet unsuccored, so helpless seemed the few who were battling against tremendous odds to save life, and so overwhelming was the demand for any kind of aid that could be given quickly, that one's senses were benumbed by the awful responsibility that fell to the living. Action of a kind hitherto unknown and unheard of was needed here and existed here only."[11]

The immediate pressing question was: what could be done right now, this very minute, with the materials at hand, that was not already being done by the surgeons and hospital stewards? "From the pallid countenance of the sufferers, their inarticulate cries, and the many evidences of physical exhaustion which were common to all of them, it was swiftly borne upon us that nourishment was one of the pressing needs of the moment and that here we might be of service. Our party separated quickly, each intent on carrying out her own scheme of usefulness." Cornelia's internship of last night was over—from now on, she was on her own.[12]

Charlotte Elizabeth Johnson McKay was in Washington, D.C., when the July 4, 1863, newspapers announced the three days of fighting that had taken place at Gettysburg. Mrs. McKay (who early in the war had lost her husband and only child, not to battlefield wounds,

10. Hancock, *South After Gettysburg*, p. 10. Although Cornelia Hancock was indeed part of the first group of women to reach the Third Division hospital of the Second Corps on Tuesday morning, Ellen Orbison Harris had actually arrived Sunday, July 5. In fact, she had spent part of the previous night at the Eleventh Corps Hospital with "one of the delegates of the [Christian] Commission . . . in giving to some hundreds of wounded soldiers the first soft bread they had tasted since the fight." [*The United States Christian Commission for the Army and Navy. For the Year 1863. Second Annual Report*, p. 77.]

11. *Ibid.*, p. 8.

12. *Ibid.* While Cornelia Hancock boldly claimed to be the first one to reach this hospital, here she admits that other women were with her.

but to sickness at home) had been tireless ever since in her work as an independent nurse in the field hospitals of the Army of the Potomac. When the Union army marched north in pursuit of Lee in June, 1863,

> the field hospitals in Virginia were all broken up, and the wounded sent to Washington. Thither I followed, to remain in Washington until we should see where the next blow should fall.
> . . . I immediately went to Baltimore, and thence to Hanover Junction, the point nearest Gettysburg that could be reached by rail. From this point, about thirty miles distant, the railroad had been torn up, and there was no conveyance, either public or private, to be obtained. The horses had all been sent into places of concealment, in case of a rebel raid, which was hourly expected. Heavy rains had made the roads so muddy that it was impossible for pedestrians to cross the street at the station where I had stopped.[13]

With no way to go forward, Charlotte McKay faced the prospect of being stranded in Hanover Junction indefinitely. She therefore must have been delighted to see a large government wagon train, loaded down with a shipment of grain, creaking its way over the horizon, headed in the general direction of Gettysburg. On board was Rev. Isaac W. Monfort, military agent of the State of Indiana, stationed in Washington, D.C. He and his five assistants had left Westminster, Maryland, on July 6, hitchhiking a ride on the only vehicles they could find heading toward the battlefield. It had been slow going as the supply train felt its way cautiously ahead through regions rumored to be infested with Confederate raiders. Monfort and his associates were on their way to the battlefield to supervise the care of wounded Hoosiers, and they graciously invited Mrs. McKay to ride along.[14]

> I would probably have been obliged to return to Washington, but for the kind and persevering efforts of Mr. Montford [*sic*], military agent of the State of Indiana, who,

---

13. Mrs. C. E. McKay, *Stories of Hospital and Camp* (Philadelphia: Claxton, Remsen, & Haffelfinger, 1876; reprint, Freeport, New York: Books for Library Press, 1971), p. 50.
14. *Indianapolis Daily Journal*, July 23, 1863, p. 2; Frank M. Keaton, Letter to O. P. Morton, July 10, 1863, Correspondence of the Indiana Military Agencies, Archives Division, Indiana State Library, Indianapolis.

> seeing my dilemma, invited me to join a party for whom he was seeking transportation to Gettysburg. I gladly availed myself of his offer, and, after having waited nearly a day, we found ourselves seated, or rather reclining, on bags of forage, very near the canvas covering of a huge Government wagon, one of a train going to the front—a conveyance which we thought ourselves fortunate to obtain.[15]

It was a hot and dusty way to reach Gettysburg, stifling under the heavy canvas canopy of a forage wagon, but it was still better than walking. "When the train halted for the night, we found lodgings at a farm-house." In the morning, Monfort and his party hopped out when the wagons reached Littletown, staying on there to check on the care of any Indiana wounded. Charlotte rode on into Gettysburg, where "I found my division hospital near the battle-field, five miles from Gettysburg. There, lying along a little stream, and spread out over the adjacent fields and hills, were our wounded men, their sufferings increased by want of food and clothing. Agents of the Sanitary and Christian Commissions, men and women who had come for the emergency, medical officers and soldiers detailed for hospital duty, were all hard at work." After checking in with the divisional staff, Charlotte pitched right in, busied herself preparing and distributing food to the needy sufferers.[16]

Others volunteers were also making their way out to the Schwartz Farm. Mrs. Mary Cadwell Fisher, who had set out from York, Pennsylvania, with her oldest son and two other ladies in a two-horse wagon loaded with "necessaries of all kinds" for the wounded at Gettysburg, had been hearing rumors of the deplorable conditions out at the Second Corps in the town hospitals where she and her team had been working. She immediately determined to see if she could get her party transferred from the Fifth Corps to the Second Corps. "On Monday I was, by request, assigned to the Second Army Corps' Hospital, temporarily located on the ground along Rock creek, about

15. McKay, *Stories of Hospital and Camp*, pp. 50-51.
16. *Indianapolis Daily Journal*, July 23, 1863, p. 2; McKay, *Stories of Hospital and Camp*, p. 51.

two and a half miles south of Gettysburg. I began work there on Tuesday morning [July 7]."[17]

Looking back in retrospect over almost thirty years, she was still horrified by the memories of what she saw when the Schwartz Farm came into sight on that bright July morning. "More than two thousand wounded men lying on three hill sides, which gently sloped down to a ravine. At their base two of the hills were crowded with our own brave boys in blue, and the third with the no less brave boys in gray."[18]

The handful of volunteers quickly encountered the same problem that was confronting Cornelia Hancock and her party. "What a tiny band of workers we seemed to clothe the naked, feed the hungry and shelter the dying from the fierce rays of the sun. On our arrival it seemed hopeless to attempt to do anything with such an array of destitute, starving men before us, and with so few hands to perform the work; but a system of divided labor was adopted, assigning to each assistant a certain field and certain duties." Mary Cadwell Fisher and the folks from York got busy in the only way possible—focusing on one wounded soldier at a time.[19]

Littlestown, Pennsylvania

Chaplain J. H. W. Stuckenberg was up bright and early, getting ready for his return to the battlefield. The German-born minister, rested up from his exhaustion in the peaceful rural setting of nearby Littletown, was anxious to be back with his men of the 145th Pennsylvania, and had persuaded his host, the Lutheran pastor in town, to accompany him. "On the morning of the 7th I started back to our Hospital with Rev [Samuel] Henry, he having his saddle bags [packed] with bread and cakes, and I having eggs, butter and bread for our wounded." Laden with their precious foodstuffs and supplies, the pair set off for the battlefield.[20]

---

17. Fisher, "A Week on Gettysburg Field."
18. *Ibid.*
19. *Ibid.*
20. Stuckenberg, *I'm Surrounded by Methodists*, p. 84.

Climbing down, stiff and dusty, from a lumbering government wagon, Indiana Military Agent Rev. Isaac W. Monfort and his five associates immediately discovered the flotsam and jetsam of the distant battle, washed up in the appropriately-named village of Littlestown. "On Tuesday, the 7th, we reached Littlestown, where we parted with our trains. At this point, though eight miles from Gettysburg, there was sad and abundant evidence of the fierceness of the late conflict. Hundreds of wounded were there in church and school house—in barns and shops."[21]

Monfort and his men had carried supplies of "lint, bandages, shirts, drawers and wine for the relief of our soldiers wounded in the late engagement." Each man, loaded down with relief items, spread out through the makeshift hospitals, intent on finding, relieving, and recording the names of injured Hoosiers. "Wounded men came around us asking for lint and bandages and were supplied." The presence of government officials, even from far-off Indiana, forced one recalcitrant proprietor to open his large brick building for additional hospital space.[22]

Within hours, all the hospitals in the hamlet had been canvassed, and Monfort and his team were ready to proceed to Gettysburg. "At this point, three wagons were pressed into our service, and dividing our company into pairs, we started for the different Corps Hospitals."[23]

Washington, D.C.

United States Army Medical Inspector Edward P. Vollum carefully reread the orders from the Surgeon General of the United States, then folded them and slipped them into his pocket. The dispatch was certainly clear enough—he was to leave immediately for Gettysburg, scene of the recent battle, and oversee the rail evacuation of the wounded from the town. While there, he was to report directly to Medical Inspector John M. Cuyler, Army of the Potomac Medical Director Letterman's representative and overall coordinator of the entire medical effort at Gettysburg.[24]

After packing his few belongings, Vollum was on the first train to Baltimore. Lieutenant Colonel Vollum had a fairly good idea of how to

---

21. *Indianapolis Daily Journal*, July 23, 1863, p. 2.
22. *Ibid.*
23. *Ibid.*
24. *OR*, vol. 27, pt. 1, pp. 25-26.

handle the rail movement, but he was going to have to see just how bad things were in Gettysburg before coming up with any final plan. There was nothing to do now but sit back, relax, and wait until he could assess the situation first-hand.

Gettysburg, Pennsylvania

Dr. Bushrod Washington James and his companions had been doggedly pushing on after crossing the Susquehanna River, pausing only long enough to rest and water the horses. Now the tiny wagon train, flanked by the weary and footsore commissioners, was coming into the outskirts of Gettysburg from the north.

"Nearing the camps and hospitals, we proceeded with our needed freight on through the scene of the first day's fight, then through the town, passing over Cemetery Hill and through the scene of the second and third day's battle, then down along the Baltimore pike over Rock Creek and a small run until we reached White Creek, the point at which three large hospitals were located, filled with thousands of the wounded and dying, who were suffering still more from the need of the very goods and hospital stores with which we had been willingly supplied by the self-sacrificing and liberal-hearted citizens of Philadelphia."[25]

The representatives had stumbled across the three division hospitals of the Second Corps, scattered along the bare ridge known locally as Red Hill. "On the right-hand side of the road, looking southward, we found in a long line of woods, on a hillside, at the foot of which a fine stream flowed, three thousand untented soldiers, including men of both armies, wounded, suffering and dying for the need of the surgical aid and provisions of the kind which we had brought. Here we halted and distributed as much of the goods as were necessary."[26]

These commissioners immediately faced the same supply challenge that had confronted Andrew Cross and his men. "[We] straightway sent some to another hospital contiguous to this on the same road, about one-eighth of a mile northward, where there were estimated to be twenty-five hundred more wounded men, and the remainder of the

---

25. James, *Echoes of Battle*, pp. 99-100.
26. *Ibid.*, p. 100. The hospital tents arrived during the day of July 7 [Dwinelle, *Medical Report*], so the latest Doctor James and his group arrived at the Second Corps hospital was early morning of the seventh.

supplies were sent a quarter of a mile to the south, to an old barn hospital with about fifteen hundred, on the east side of the road; the one I labored at was on the west. They required these stores equally as sadly [*sic*] as ours. Every house, barn and available building throughout this part of the country was filled with the wounded."[27]

Stunned by the magnitude of the task, but intent on getting their medicines, foodstuffs, and clothing delivered, the men split up into distribution teams. After divvying up the supplies between them, they methodically spread out through the hospitals sprawled around Rock Creek and the Farmer Schwartz's adjoining countryside, offering their goods to wounded and surgeon alike, Union, Confederate, no distinction, no difference.

Reverend Monfort and his team, in their three appropriated wagons, were coming into the outskirts of Gettysburg from the east. "Along the line of travel before reaching the hospitals we met hundreds of the wounded, who, being able to walk, but bearing in many cases dangerous hurts, had been permitted to make their way as best they could to the nearest depot, which was some 27 miles from Gettysburg."[28]

The crass and blatant gouging of the wounded men's pocketbooks astonished Monfort. "The road from Littlestown was thronged with the wounded, hungry, faint and weary. We met a benevolent gentleman selling them bread at fifty cents a loaf. He was a native of the State. Others were heard of who had *cultivated* the grace of benevolence, and could readily ask one dollar a loaf! The loaves may have been large—I did not see them."[29]

As the Hoosier contingent came into sight of the massive hospital complex east of Gettysburg, it became apparent that surveying this group of wounded would take days, not just a few hours, as had the Littlestown's hospitals. "During this day (the 7th) visits were made to the 1st, 2d and 3d Corps Hospitals, and the next day to the 12th Corps, and the names of the [Indiana] wounded obtained, reports of which were forwarded to you [Gov. Oliver O. Morton] last week. The stores we carried were the first to reach the battle-field." It was going to be a

27. *Ibid.*
28. *Indianapolis Daily Journal*, July 23, 1863, p. 2.
29. *Ibid.*

long, long week for Monfort and his men, working their way through thousands of patients in search of the few men from Indiana.[30]

It had taken less than two days for the Sanitary Commission to outgrow their headquarters at the little Baltimore Pike schoolhouse. Even though Commission supplies were being distributed as expeditiously as possible to the surrounding corps hospitals, the tiny building was now insufficient to house the barrels, crates, boxes, and bundles of relief supplies being disgorged from Sanitary Commission transports. While the school was "near the different corps hospitals, and about three miles out from Gettysburgh," construction was finally nearing completion on the Rock Creek bridge, and trains (along with the boxcars of Sanitary Commission supplies they carried) would soon be rolling into downtown Gettysburg. New quarters were needed, and soon.[31]

Representatives had been combing the town of Gettysburg, looking for a building large enough to hold the ever-increasing flood of emergency supplies now beginning to flow into the region by road and rail. The best that could be secured under the circumstances was the small dry-goods store of Robert F. McIlhenny, located in the corner room of the David Wills building on the diamond in downtown Gettysburg. Just a city block away from the Gettysburg depot, supplies could be easily transferred from the trains to the new location. Even though the new room was not substantially larger than the old facility, "on Tuesday morning, July seventh, a store-house was taken in town, and the school-house closed."[32]

---

30. *Ibid.* Actually, Doctor James and his group from Philadelphia, Mary Cadwell Fisher and her delegation from York, the Sanitary Commission, and the Christian Commission had all arrived with supplies before or during the 7th, as well as Reverend Monfort and his group. Most Indiana troops served in the Western Theater. There were only five Hoosier regiments with the Army of the Potomac—the 7th and 19th in the First Corps, the 14th in the Second Corps, the 20th in the Third Corps, and the 27th in the Twelfth Corps. In addition, Companies I and K of the 1st Indiana Cavalry served as Eleventh Corps General Headquarters guard, while six companies of the 3rd Indiana helped make up Brig. Gen. John Buford's First Division of the Cavalry Corps.
31. Frank Moore, ed., *The Rebellion Record: A Diary of American Events*, 11 vols. (New York: D. Van Nostrand, 1864-68), 7:125.
32. Frassanito, *Early Photography at Gettysburg*, p. 98; Moore, The Rebellion Record, 7:125.

The Christian Commission had managed to sneak a march on the larger, better funded Sanitary Commission—they already had a centralized headquarters facility, up and fully operational, a full thirty-six hours earlier than the Sanitary Commission. "On Monday, [July 6], F. E. Shearer, Esq., agent of the Commission at Washington, D.C., reached the town of Gettysburg, where he found a number of the delegates already occupied in the hospitals, with the centre of their operations at the office of R. G. Harper, Esq., editor of the 'Adams Sentinel.'"[33]

Shearer immediately saw the necessity of expanding the warehouse and distribution operation beyond the cramped confines of the newspaper office. "Through the aid of Mr. J. Bevan, Mr. Schick's store was soon obtained as a depot for supplies, the only such depot in town till another was opened by Adams' Express Company, twenty-four hours afterwards, and a third twelve hours later still by the Sanitary Commission."[34]

Schick's Store on the Diamond (the center of town) was literally a stone's throw away from the Sanitary Commission's facility in the McIlhenny Dry Goods store. The two neighboring volunteer Commissions, while outwardly so similar in their desire to aid the wounded, could scarcely have been more unlike internally.

The Christian Commission had sprung from the Young Mens' Christian Association, with the goal of attending to the spiritual good of the soldiers of the army, and incidentally, their intellectual improvement and social and physical comfort. Christian Commission "delegates" passed out Bibles, tracts, and other reading and writing

---

33. *The United States Christian Commission for the Army and Navy. Work and Incidents. First Annual Report* (Philadelphia: United States Christian Commission, 1863), p. 68. There was also a Christian Commission station, complete with tent, supplies, and delegates in every corps hospital except the Sixth Corps. With only a few hundred wounded, the surgeon-in-charge there told Commission delegates that he needed no supplies. Consequently, the Fifth Corps delegates visited the Sixth Corps Hospital from time to time to share the Gospel with the patients and to conduct funerals. The captain of the Christian Commission station at the Second Corps Hospital was Rev. J. E. Adams of New Sharon, Maine, who was ably assisted by J. B. Stillson of Rochester, New York, and twelve other delegates. [*The United States Christian Commission for the Army and Navy. For the Year 1863. Second Annual Report*, pp. 70, 76.]

34. *Ibid.*

material along with relief supplies. The Christian Commission was quietly guided by a committee of pastors, missionaries and Christian workers.

The Sanitary Commission, one the other hand, was founded by a consortium of highly influential Northern business professionals. Sanitary "commissioners" concerned themselves solely with providing relief supplies and improving the care of the wounded. The Sanitary Commission was steered by an Executive Committee, chaired by Secretary Frederick Law Olmsted, fresh from his triumph as the master designer of Central Park in New York.

The Christian Commission had quickly become the arch-rival of the Sanitary Commission for private support and legislative recognition. Donations regularly flowed from church congregations nationwide, and the ladies aid societies that they supported. With so many pastors, missionaries, and church leaders involved in the Christian Commission, the Sanitary Commission discovered that its charitable support base was being seriously undercut by the rival Commission. To further add insult to injury, the Christian Commission had been readily accepted and encouraged by the government; meanwhile, highly placed officials still viewed the Sanitary Commission, with undisguised distrust, as a threat to the Medical Department.

By mid-1863, matters had reached the point of heckling and name-calling from key members of the Sanitary Commission. George Templeton Strong, high-powered New York lawyer and Sanitary Commission treasurer, was harshly outspoken of the upstart Christian Commission. He characterized their chairman, Rev. George H. Stuart, as "that evangelical mountebank and philanthrope." Their officials were "an ugly-looking set. . . . Some were unctuous to behold, and others vinegary; a bad lot." The Christian Commission, in his opinion, was "no more a commission than it is a corporation, or a hose company, or a chess club" that seemed "to me one of many forms in which the shallowness, fussiness, and humbug of our popular religionism are constantly embodying themselves."[35]

But now, with the Sanitary Commission moving in their operations just across the Diamond, the Christian Commission facility was forced to again expand their facility. The upstairs rooms of the Apollo Hall, a building across the Diamond from Schick's Store, were secured as additional storage space. "The rooms thus provided were soon filled

35. George Templeton Strong, *Diary of the Civil War 1860-1865*, ed. Allan Nevins (New York: MacMillan, 1962; reprint, 1982), pp. 589, 311.

with goods, which were kept in almost constant motion by receipt and distribution. Fifteen hands were employed, and were occupied day and night in the labors of the warehouse. Every visitor was drafted for service, and it was a rare sight presented in the mixed corps of laborers, consisting of ladies, clergymen, teachers, lawyers, merchants, mechanics, and colored laborers. The boxes and barrels upon the pavement at times reached more than half way to the second story, and drays and carts were before the door, loading and unloading, during nearly the whole day. The clerks and laborers of the warehouse were so completely worn down, that service was imposed upon every one that came in."[36]

In addition, the Christian Commission was running its own Commissary Department. On July 8, Louis Muller, the delegate in charge of the facility, would write: "We have fed at least two thousand wounded men in this town today, and about the same number of rations have been sent by our delegates to those in the field, beside wagon loads of all kinds of supplies. No man can estimate the amount of suffering we are relieving. . . . The rebels have swept this country of everything eatable." The Christian Commission even placed ads in the area papers, headlined "Help the Wounded Soldier," in an effort to procure items that were needed but not currently available to the wounded.[37]

The headquarters and distribution facility was a beehive of activity and enterprise. "Cars were to be unloaded, boxes to be unpacked and repacked, transportation to be obtained, telegraphing to be done, invoices to be verified, the books of the Commission to be kept, letters of acknowledgment to be written, those of inquiry from friends of the wounded to be answered—a work which engaged the services of one man all the time—delegates to be assigned on their arrival to the different corps hospitals or sent to our stations among the rebels, Sabbath and weekday services to be arranged, strangers seeking tidings of relatives or friends to be aided—in short, all the work of a great establishment was here planned and done."[38]

Now the supplies began arriving in ever larger shipments. "On Tuesday (July 7) two large loads of the choicest hospital supplies from

---

36. *The United States Christian Commission. Second Report of the Committee of Maryland, September 1863.* (Baltimore: Sherwood & Co., 1863).
37. *Ibid.*
38. *The United States Christian Commission for the Army and Navy. For the Year 1863. Second Annual Report*, p. 80.

Philadelphia, comprising something like eighty boxes, and accompanied by nearly thirty delegates, came round the mountain from Carlisle. . . . About this time other loads of stores arrived from Columbia, Harrisburg, York, and the 'Patriot Daughters,' of Lancaster."[39]

Even Dr. Henry W. Bellows, president of the Sanitary Commission, was forced by the circumstances to swallow any rancorous opinions he held when he commented favorably on "the enterprise, zeal and blessedness of the labors of this sister institution."[40]

Even as massive amounts of supplies began arriving at the McIlhenny and Schick Stores in downtown Gettysburg, the First and Second Divisions hospitals were struggling to get the wounded under some kind of shelter. The buildings of the Jacob Schwartz Farm were visible from the top of the ridge, where the hospital had fled after being flooded out of the Rock Creek bottomland, and Dr. Justin Dwinelle was quick to appropriate them for the use of this portion of the hospital. The injured men were picked up as gently as possible and borne by stretcher, cot, or blanket across the rugged pastureland to the farmstead; with even the most gentle handling, however, these longsuffering veterans were again subjected to yet another painful jostling of their wounds.

The new shelter included a two-story house, the brick and wood barn, and a scattering of outbuildings including a wagon shed, corn crib, carriage house, and smoke-house. "The old farmhouse [was] occupied by the men of Hancock's corps," wrote one Christian Commission agent who attended to the wounded in the Schwartz barn. "Its every room was a chamber of death and the boards of the shambling porch . . . were stained with the blood of the men for whom there was no room inside."[41]

"West of the farmhouse . . . stood the old barn," continued the Christian Commission agent. "This was devoted exclusively to the wounded of the Confederate army. The smaller of the barn doors had

39. *Ibid.*, p. 68.
40. *New York Times*, July 16, 1863.
41. H. S. Peltz, "Two Brass Buttons," *Gettysburg Compiler*, March 15, 1887. This source is somewhat doubtful in its authenticity, and contains numerous errors or inconsistencies. Additional critical notes on this source by Kathleen Georg Harrison (January 1981) are available at the Gettysburg National Military Park Library.

been unhinged to serve as surgeon's tables. . . . Every available inch of space was occupied [eighty men were in the barn]. The men lay close to each other, side by side in long rows. . . . The cattle pens, too, still reeking with the litter of the barnyard, were densely packed with victims as [was] the threshing floor above, and I noticed with horror, as I assisted the dressing of a bleeding wound, that the blood of the patient [above] filtered through the cracks . . . and dripped upon the sufferers below."[42]

Twenty-five-year-old Maj. William Watson, surgeon of the 105th Pennsylvania Volunteer regiment, was hard at work at the Third Corps Hospital, up and running just a pasture's length away from the big rambling Schwartz barn. "Day before yesterday I performed fourteen amputations without leaving the table," he wrote on July 7 in a hurried letter home; "I do not exaggerate when I say I have performed at least calculation fifty amputations." In two days, as soon as a few final operations were performed at his own division hospital, "I will turn my attention to wounded Rebels. There are about one hundred of them in a Barn near us in a most distressing condition. Many of them require operating. Old Army Surgeons say that the wounds are more serious and amputations more numerous in this than any previous battle."[43]

J. Howard Wert, from the neighboring Wert Farm, got a crash course in amputations when he wandered over to check out the excitement at the Schwartz place. Years later, he vividly recalled the scenes around the swarming farmyard that day. "By the barn of Mr. Schwartz out in Mt. Joy Township . . . stood the amputation tables, and the work on them was incessant—sickening, and gruesome—until the legs and the arms were piled by cords and hauled off by wagonloads to be dumped in trenches where a century hence the plowman will upearth the moldering bones of those who fought at Gettysburg."[44]

---

42. *Ibid.* Apparently this same barn was used by portions of the Third Corps hospital for shelter and care of their Confederate wounded as well. Mentioned in several different sources, it is always referred to as being "filled with rebel wounded," and all descriptions are consistent with the building on the Schwartz property. [*United States Sanitary Commission Report for the Army and Navy—[Its] Work and Incidents, First Annual Report.*]

43. William Watson, *Letters of a Civil War Surgeon*, ed. Paul Fatout (West Lafayette, Indiana: Purdue University Press, 1961; reprint 1996), pp. 108, 109-10.

44. J. Howard Wert, "In the Hospitals of Gettysburg, July, 1863," No. I, *Harrisburg Telegraph*, July 2, 1907, p. 7.

If possible, the move gave Surgeon Justin Dwinelle and his dead-tired doctors even more to do than before. Now the dressing surgeons and the Second Corps surgical staff found themselves spreading out their efforts even further, dividing their attention between the house and barn to attend to the injured, listening to the incessant murmur of thousands of voices echo and reecho off the sides of the barn and farm house. Edging cautiously along as they sidestepped through the crowded yard and driveway packed with sufferers, the medical attendants moved through the cramped confines of the smokehouse and corn crib to dress wounds, then made their rounds out to the surrounding pasturelands to check on the thousands of wounded not able to take advantage of the limited amount of shelter. The few chaplains who had remained behind with the wounded had long ago given up any hope of ministering to only the men from their own regiments; now they gave spiritual comfort and encouragement to any and every soldier, enemy and friend alike, as they worked their way through the maze of stretchers and blankets, slipping in congealed pools of blood, carefully plotting each step to avoid treading on someone's wounded arm or shattered leg.

To further complicate the situation, other Union corps hospitals had fallen back to this general vicinity behind the battlelines when setting up their facilities, and the Second Corps found themselves sharing their new-found shelter with other hospitals whose needs were nearly as great. With the Third Corps now also using a portion of the Schwartz property, each hospital continued to swell with newly-arriving wounded; the two medical departments inexorably expanded toward each other, then began overlapping around the two wells in the center of the farmer's lot. So tightly did the hospitals become compacted that the Second Corps hospitals occupied the farmyard, commingling with Third Corps wounded; some of Sickles' Third Corps wounded were moved into the farm house and outbuildings and quickly became interspersed with Hancock's men. The barn seems to have been shared equally between the two corps as a Confederate ward.

The First and Second Divisions of the Second Corps Hospital in their entirety were now on the Schwartz property, with the Third Division still a half mile off to the south. Sufficient water supply and adequate shelter were further threatened by the fact that the Second Corps hospitals, and the symbiotic Third Corps hospitals, were bordered and partially hemmed in by portions of the Fifth Corps hospitals; closely adjoining them were the First, Sixth, and Twelfth

Corps hospitals. Only the Eleventh Corps had their facilities at any distance from this swelling medical complex of Gettysburg.[45]

Death and dying in the 145th Pennsylvania Volunteers had continued unabated in Chaplain Stuckenberg's absence. "Lt [George H.] Finch, was dead," noted the chaplain in his diary upon reaching the hospital. The severe wounds in his left thigh and right ankle were too much for the young officer of Company E, and he had died the day before.[46]

First Lt. Horatio F. Lewis of Company D was gone too, and his death staggered the chaplain. Stuckenberg could vividly remember letting the officer, totally exhausted and ready to straggle, climb wearily on to his horse during that horrible never-ending march of June 29, now seemingly an eternity in the past. "Lt Lewis had his leg amputated. He looked feeble and sallow, suffered a great deal (had been lying on the field till a rebel for 25 doll[ar]s brought him into our lines to a house to their rear, but they stole his canteen, his money ab[out] 80 dollars, haversack et cet.) and could not sleep. He has since then died. He was a noble young man, knew a good deal about military affairs and made a good officer. He was brave, ambitious and hopeful. There was an innocence and simplicity about him, which were well calculated to gain one's affection. His loss is felt severely by us all. We loved him, we admired him. He is one of the many truly noble sacrifices given to our country. He was calm and resigned when I saw him, and frequently, I was told, was found praying. The thought of his death greatly saddens me, for I loved him and had great hopes for him."[47]

But by far the majority of the wounded were on the road to recovery, or appeared to be, although many would be permanently maimed for the rest of their life. "Lt [Jeremiah] Birtcil Co F was wounded in the arm,

45. Dwinelle, *Medical Report*; Coco, *A Vast Sea of Misery*, p. 91; Dimon, *State of New York Report*, p. 53.

46. Stuckenberg, *I'm Surrounded by Methodists*, pp. 84, 82, 86; Service Records of George H. Finch, National Archives and Records Administration.

47. Stuckenberg, *I'm Surrounded by Methodists*, pp. 84-85, 76, 86; Samuel P. Bates, *History of the Pennsylvania Volunteers 1861-5*, 5 vols. (Harrisburg, Pennsylvania: B. Singerly, 1869-71), 4:532; *Erie Weekly Gazette*, July 16, 1863; Service Records of Horatio F. Lewis, National Archives and Records Administration.

but will recover." The injury to the right arm was slight, and the second lieutenant was looking forward to soon rejoining the regiment.[48]

Other members of the regiment seemed to be able to boast of wounds in almost every part of their collective anatomy. "Lt Hamlin Co I was wounded in the heel," noted Stuckenberg. The first lieutenant was fortunate indeed to avoid the amputating tables—at least this time around.[49]

Some losses came long after the firing had ceased. "Capt Geo[rge G.] Griswold Co I was wounded in the hand. It was regarded as a slight wound. He went to Philadelphia. Erysipelas set in and he has since died. He was universally beloved. There was a peculiar amiability and gentleness about him which were very winning. The news that he would probably die surprised and saddened us, and when the news came that his spirit had gone 'Home,' our hearts were filled with grief."[50]

When he checked in with Surgeon Charles Squire Wood, chief operator of the First Division hospital, Chaplain Stuckenberg learned that the regiment had bivouacked a few miles east of town, and were expecting orders to move out at a moment's notice. "I was desirous of reminding [*sic*] with our wounded; but another battle was soon expected, and as our troops were moving, all the surgeons of our Division, except 6, and chaplains, except one, were ordered to join their regiments. I bid the boys farewell and started with Rev Henry for the battle field."[51]

After showing his companion quickly around the scene of the recent battle, the chaplain was soon spurring his mount southeast along the Baltimore Pike toward his regiment, taking one last look around at the effects of the army's unkind visit to this rural setting. "Near Gettysburg every road and field, farm and house and barn

---

48. Stuckenberg, *I'm Surrounded by Methodists*, p. 85; Bates, *History of Pennsylvania Volunteers*, 4:537; *Erie Weekly Gazette*, July 16, 1863; *Erie Observer*, July 11, 1863; Service Records of Jeremiah Birtcil, National Archives and Records Administration.
49. Stuckenberg, *I'm Surrounded by Methodists*, p. 85; Service Records of James H. Hamlin, National Archives and Records Administration.
50. Stuckenberg, *I'm Surrounded by Methodists*, p. 85; Bates, *History of Pennsylvania Volunteers*, 4:545; *Erie Observer*, July 16, 18, 23, 1863; Service records of George G. Griswold, National Archives and Records Administration.
51. Stuckenberg, *I'm Surrounded by Methodists*, p. 86.

indicated that troops had been there and that a great battle had been fought. With what feelings I left that field!"[52]

Fortunately, not everyone associated with the military was inching away from Gettysburg in pursuit of the retreating Confederates. Some of the Second Corps hospital stewards, volunteer aides, and musicians had been left behind, to serve as hospital staff. While not qualified to perform surgery, these men helped with the myriad of details involved in the care of over three thousand men.

Among this group were Principal Musician Robert A. Cassidy and Acting Hospital Steward William H. Mayes, both of the 148th Pennsylvania Volunteers. Surgeon Uriah Q. Davis of the 148th had specifically directed them to remain behind to "care for the wounded of the Regiment."[53]

Robert and "Billy" first made sure that all of their comrades had been collected from the battlefield. Once they had successfully gathered them all at "the First Division Hospital on the east bank of Rock Creek, a short distance south of the town of Gettysburg," they set about to follow Dr. Davis' daunting orders: "Our instructions were to make the men as comfortable as wholly inadequate shelter and food supplies would permit."[54]

In this, the two men proved themselves far more resourceful than most of the other Second Corps caregivers. "An 'Autenreith,' in charge of Billy Berry, brigade hospital steward detailed from Company

52. *Ibid.*, p. 87. Stuckenberg left the 145th in October, 1863, to return to the three congregations he served in Erie, Pennsylvania. He had arrived for the chaplaincy of the 3rd Regiment, raised from northwest Pennsylvania on September 10, 1862.

Following graduate study in Germany in 1865, he served parishes in Indianapolis and Pittsburgh. From 1873 to 1880, Stuckenberg taught at Wittenberg College before returning to Europe for fifteen years. He wrote extensively, publishing books in the fields of sociology, theology, and biography. He died quite unexpectedly on May 28, 1903. Even though separated from his military comrades in 1863, Stuckenberg never stopped being concerned for their spiritual well-being. For the remainder of the war, he frequently donated money to the American Tract Society with the proviso that the purchased materials be sent to his former regiment. [Stuckenberg, *I'm Surrounded by Methodists*, pp. 1, 3, 8.]

53. Muffly, *The Story of Our Regiment*, p. 312.

54. *Ibid.*

G of our Regiment, afforded us excellent advantages in the matter of hospital supplies. By collecting abandoned shelter tents wherever obtainable and appropriating uncut wheat from an adjacent field for bedding, we were enabled to protect and render our wounded more comfortable than those of any other command in the Division." Their careful attention in providing shelter and dry bedding for their messmates had a significant affect on the recovery rate of their friends and neighbors. "Mortality among our wounded was much lighter than among those of other commands less fortunately provided for."[55]

When the volunteer nurses from Philadelphia split up at the Third Division hospital, Cornelia Hancock looked around to see where she could be of the most use. "No one paid the slightest attention to us, unusual as was the presence of half a dozen women on such a field; nor did anyone have time to give us orders or to answer questions." Cornelia was just going to have to shift for herself, without help from anyone else.[56]

Looking around, she spotted an unattended wagon of supplies, probably part of the shipment from York that Christian Commissioner Cross and his associate had directed to the hospital. "Wagons of bread and provisions were arriving and I helped myself to their stores. I sat down with a loaf in one hand and a jar of jelly in the other; it was not hospital diet but it was food, and a dozen poor fellows lying near me turned their eyes in piteous entreaty, anxiously watching my efforts to arrange a meal."[57]

Even the simple act of making jelly sandwiches became a grueling test of ingenuity, fraught with monstrous difficulties in this abnormal setting. "There was not a spoon, knife, fork, or plate to be had that day, and it seemed as if there were no more serious problem under Heaven than the task of dividing that too well-baked loaf into portions that could be swallowed by weak and dying men. I succeeded, however, in breaking it into small pieces, and spreading jelly over each with a stick. A shingle board made an excellent tray, and it was handed from one to another. I had the joy of seeing every morsel swallowed greedily by

55. *Ibid.* Autenreith was a medical supply house, offering a full line of medical wagons and surgical instruments.
56. Hancock, *South After Gettysburg*, p. 8.
57. *Ibid.*

those whom I had prayed day and night that I might be permitted to serve."[58]

Encouraged by her initial success, Cornelia rummaged around in some of the other wagons, intent on finding different ways to meet the physical needs of the vast number of wounded sprawled all around her. "An hour or so later, in another wagon, I found boxes of condensed milk and bottles of whiskey and brandy. It was an easy task to mix milk punches and to serve them from bottles and tin cans emptied of their former contents."[59]

Within a matter of a few hours, all the relief items brought by Dr. Bushrod Washington James and his Philadelphia volunteers had been distributed; there was nothing left to offer now except Doctor James' skills as a physician and surgeon. "Having distributed the stores in as diplomatic a manner as possible, I returned to the first hospital [Second Corps] to offer my services where they would be most available. Here I found a corps of ladies, several of whom were of my clientele in Philadelphia, who had come down to the battle-field to do what good they could for the poor afflicted soldiers. Samaritan-like, they had given up their own comfort for a time in order to help the wounded and dying."[60]

The volunteer nurses immediately made Doctor James' presence known in the camp, and the news quickly reaching the ears of Justin Dwinelle. "They announced my arrival to the surgeon in charge, telling him that I was a surgeon, and he immediately placed me in charge of a row of hospital tents, the occupants of which had all undergone the severe operation of amputation at the hip-joint or along the femur. I made a careful examination of the general condition of the cases, instructed the nurses and the hospital stewards what should be done in case of hemorrhage occurring, which in the large vessels in that region of the body would cause rapid death in the event of the ligature giving way, and instructed them as to other emergencies."[61]

58. *Ibid.*, pp. 8-9.
59. *Ibid.*, p. 9.
60. James, *Echoes of Battle*, pp. 100-1. This "corps of ladies" were probably part of Cornelia Hancock's group.
61. *Ibid.*, p. 101. Note that between his first visit to the hospital ["three thousand untented soldiers"] and his return later in the day ["a row of hospital tents"], the medical tents had arrived and were already being pitched and occupied.

Satisfied that everything was under control in the amputee ward, "I proceeded to the chief surgeon and asked if there were any additional duties that I could perform. My services were gladly accepted, and for several days, in conjunction with these responsible cases in the tents, which were my special care, I spent my available time at the operating tables, which were situated in the woods on the crest of the slope which receded to White Creek; the hospital tents were run in rows along avenues on the level area to the north."[62]

At the amputating tables, the surgeries continued unabated, and the presence of a fresh surgeon was gladly welcomed. Dazed doctors, worked far beyond the point of exhaustion, stood swaying precariously at the tables, held upright by assistants. Cutting hands were painfully swollen and bleeding from the constant exertion, and scalpels fell from numbed and nerveless fingers. Some doctors fainted from exhaustion. Now a full four days after the end of the battle, men continued appearing, as if by magic, on the operating tables, in a continuing parade of oozing and infected wounds.[63]

In the torrid heat of July, "green-bottle" flies were a noisome scourge, swollen to massive proportions on the blood of the wounded and dead. The proximity of the hospitals to the Jacob Schwartz Farm, with its barnyard litter and manure pile, brought insects in biblical swarms to the medical facility. Fence posts, tent poles, canvas, prostrate bodies—any surface, especially where blood had splashed or splattered—were literally black with the buzzing hordes. Many of the injured now appearing at the tables had wounds crawling white and alive with maggot infestation.[64]

"To give you some idea of the extent and numbers of the wounds, four surgeons, none of whom were idle fifteen minutes at a time, were busy all day amputating legs and arms," wrote Cornelia Hancock to her cousin that night concerning the activity at the Third Division hospital. "I gave to every man that had a leg or arm off a gill of wine, to every wounded in the Third Division, one glass of lemonade, some

---

62. *Ibid.*

63. *The Sanitary Commission of the United States Army, A Succinct Narrative of its Works and Purposes* (New York, 1864), p. 159.

64. Coco, *A Vast Sea of Misery*, p. 190.

bread and preserves and tobacco—as much as I am opposed to the latter, for they need it very much, they are so exhausted."[65]

As morning passed into afternoon, and then early evening, the young Quakeress continued moving through the troops, feeding them, giving drinks, comforting, encouraging, writing letters, and being a mother, sister, or friend as each situation dictated. "The first volunteer attendant I saw on the field at Gettysburg was a woman," wrote gravely wounded Captain Nickerson of the 8th Ohio. "I find that she wrote her name in my diary, on July 7, 1863, 'Miss Cornelia Hancock, New Salem, N. J.' She carried writing materials, envelopes, and postage stamps, and wrote letters to the friends of those who were too desperately wounded to do so themselves. She took down just what each wanted to say, without abridgment, and in this manner many a mother, sister, and sweetheart received their first, last, and only message from their loved ones, whose lives ebbed out on this fatal field. It was a thoughtful, sensitive, and delicate service, faithfully performed."[66]

It had also been a long and busy day for Mary Cadwell Fisher and her delegation of York citizens after they had divided up the duties to be performed and went their individual ways. "Some were able to materially aid the surgeons in their herculean task, and with firm hands and steady nerves assisted in dressing wounds; others devoted themselves to feeding and clothing the men. The good work was forwarded with marvelous rapidity, and before nightfall the ground was dotted with tents and the store and kitchen tents were in order."[67]

"Our first work was to satisfy the hunger of the men, taking them row by row as they came in regular order. We made no difference between the Union soldiers and the prisoners in the distribution of food, clothing and medicines which the nurses could administer. Many were not so badly wounded but that they could help themselves somewhat, and after being revived and strengthened by food, clean clothing and needed stimulants could, in turn, assist in the care of their helpless comrades."[68]

65. Hancock, *South After Gettysburg*, p. 11.
66. Nickerson, "Personal Recollections of Two Visits to Gettysburg," p. 23.
67. Fisher, "A Week on Gettysburg Field."
68. *Ibid.*

Mrs. Fisher took it upon herself to distribute the "needed stimulants"; in fact, the generous upper-class residents of York had so liberally supplied her with "the purest imported liquors" and "a quantity of fine old whiskey from one of our celebrated county distilleries" that she basically became a mobile tavern to the wounded, many of whom had not tasted a drop of alcohol in well over a week. "Fortunately my private stores enabled me to give prompt aid in many cases where stimulants were required. Nothing was more needed and nothing more difficult to obtain than good liquors. My stock, like the 'widow's cruse of oil,' held out in marvelous manner, and the surgeons often told me that Judge Black's brandy bottle saved more lives than their instruments and medicine combined."[69]

The volunteers from York found the hospital staff, and especially Doctor Dwinelle, to be most supportive of their work to aid the men. "The head surgeon of the Second Army Corps was most curteous to the volunteer nurses, and untiring in his efforts to render more tolerable the situation of his command. Naturally a broad humanitarian, he looked upon those in his care as men, and not mere 'food for powder.' He placed at my disposal an ambulance and two boys in blue to assist me, thus enabling me to send to town at any time for delicacies which could not be prepared or obtained on the ground."[70]

"It was an important circumstance that our Hospital wagons containing tents, blankets, cooking utensils, provisions, shovels, axes, and Medical Stores could not follow the army as usual," wrote Surgeon Dwinelle in his official report of the Second Corps Hospital. "They did not arrive so as to be available untill [*sic*] the seventh. As soon as we got the tents up we were able to put every wounded man under shelter."[71]

Even with the arrival of the hospital tents, it was still going to be some time before the thousands of wounded were all moved under shelter. "It took a number of days for the large hospital tents to be put up," remembered Lt. Charles A. Fuller of what he could see through the flaps of the amputee tent. "All the sound part of the army that could be spared followed up the enemy. Of course, it took a large number of

69. *Ibid.*
70. *Ibid.*
71. Dwinelle, *Medical Report.*

soldiers detailed for the purpose, to partially care for the thousands of wounded from each army."[72]

The operating tables continued full of patients, and no surgeons could be spared, even for the crucial task of getting patients under cover. Saving lives was still more important than sheltering bodies. The doctors were forced to let others, some displaying recent wounds, pitch the big white medical tents while they doggedly pressed on with their medical duties at the tables, protected from the elements by makeshift lean-tos and pieced together sun shades.

After being treated by the surgical staff, the wounded were left largely to shift for themselves; occasionally a dressing surgeon would look in on them, but that was rare with thousands needing attention, and only dozens of attendants. "The surgeons were continually engaged upon new cases that had received no attention. Those of us that had been treated knew this, and we found no fault at what otherwise would have been terrible neglect."[73]

Slowly, the hospital was getting back to some semblance of a normal routine. As medical attendants, the hospital guard, and any volunteers got tents pitched, the wounded, treated and untreated alike, were moved inside for the first time since the battle. "Soon after the men were got under shelter they were put on to Stretchers and temporary bunks."[74]

With the shelter needs of the men cared for, attention was then turned to clearing and policing the hospital grounds. "From necessity the tents were arranged in the woods as close to the wounded as we could get them. The trees were cut down for several rods around the tents and the grounds were thoroughly policed." Shovels were broken out and drainage trenches dug around the tents and amputating tables.[75]

The commissary department, which had been operating ever since arriving at Gettysburg with borrowed pots and scavenged provender, was up and running again with government-issue gear. Regular army chow of hardtack, beans, and salt pork, as well as fresh beef briskets,

---

72. Fuller, *Personal Recollections*, p. 102.
73. *Ibid.*
74. Dwinelle, *Medical Report.*
75. *Ibid.*

were once more available to the men. Sadly, few of the seriously wounded could stomach the coarse provisions, and many passed still another hungry day at Gettysburg.

Throughout the pitching of tents, carrying of blankets and cots, the sounds of axes and shovels, the amputations had continued constant. "All the surgeons of the corps remained with me," wrote Surgeon Dwinelle, "untill [*sic*] the [morning of the] seventh when a part of them left with army."[76]

But now, as all but a skeleton crew of exhausted surgeons packed up their belongings and prepared to link up with the Army of the Potomac, there was the first encouraging news in many days—the end of the first round of operations was in sight. "At that time three fourths or more of the necessary amputations had been performed. Most of those remaining to be done were not in a favorable condition to be operated on."[77]

"An operating staff was left with me for each division," continued Dwinelle in his report, "and also Surgeons with their Hospital attendants and stewards to act as dressers and perform other duties.... These Surgeons were relieved from time to time as their services could be dispensed with. There also reported to me for duty on the seventh Eight or nine contract Surgeons; [Army] Surgeons Walker, Norris, & Morris; Asst Surgeon Barry of the eleventh corps; several Confederates; and about Thirty volunteer Surgeons." The end was in sight, but there was still a very long and painful way to go, for surgeons and patients alike.[78]

Whenever there were momentary lulls in the cries of the wounded, 8th Ohio Hospital Steward Charles Merrick dutifully pulled out paper and pen to finish the letter he was scribbling home to his sister:

> Tuesday, July 7th, 1863
> Gettysburg, Pa.
> Dear Min,
>
> I wrote to you yesterday and have but little to say to day. I know you will be glad to hear almost daily from me and the

76. *Ibid.*
77. *Ibid.*
78. *Ibid.* For the probable identity of "Surgeons Walker, Norris, & Morris," see Appendix 2.

poor boys, so I write again. We have not so many to care for now—some have died and the slightly wounded have been sent away. I have 40 now who need constant care. When I wrote day before yesterday we had about 1,200 lying around here. I think we have about 800 now. This includes about 300 rebels. In our Reg. 18 have been killed or died since the battle. James Kelly, whose mother lives in Cleveland, cannot live long. I thought sure he would die last night. I wish you would see her, or see Capt Renny's folks, and tell them to see her.

She lives at 148 Crolon St. They are Irish. I told him there was no hope of his living. He said: "All right; I am willing and reconciled to what ever be my fate." His leg is badly shattered, and has never rallied from the shock sufficient to receive an opperation [*sic*]. He speaks of his Mother often, and says she is all he has to care for.

I feel almost alone here with the boys. No one to boss me, or no one to run to for advice. Many times I have wished you could be here, But I know it would be more than you could endure. It is pleasant though to see now and then a woman flitting around among the sufferers. The Christian and Sanitary Commission are here with a small amount of supplies and are doing all the good they can.

But our Brigade Surgeon, Dr. [Harry McKindree] McAbee, [4th Ohio Volunteers]. Oh, how I hate that man, and long to slop [*sic*] his face for him. But we are in the military rules now and he can insult and domineer, I must tamely submit to his insolence.

I have one awful case. [Pvt. William] Welsh [Welch] , Co I, was shot in the cheek, the ball went diagonally down, lodged in the lower Jaw, or below the Jaw in the throat. This morning some of the arteries broke and fresh blood run in streams from his mouth and nose. I ran to him and placed my thumb on the carotid [artery]; when the blood stopped, We fixed a tourniquet so as to hold the artery for the time. But what can be done but tie the carotid and that you know seldom if ever succeeds in saving life. To cut out the ball is equivalent to cutting his throat and sure death. But it is hard to see a healthy man lie and bleed to death.

Capt [Azor] Nickerson, I fear, is sinking.

I hear our Reg moved this morning towards Baltimore. I fear it will be several weeks before I can Join the Regiment.

> Not because I tire of taking care of the boys, but I cannot expect any letters from you. They will all follow the Regiment.
>
> Since I wrote that last word "Regiment," we have buried Kelly—Our boys get better burial than some—we bury them within ten minutes after they die. I counted 19 in one row who have been lying three days above ground. I have wished some of the Chaplains, instead of preaching and praying around here nights when men want to sleep, would take a shovel and bury our dead. Perhaps I am uncharitable towards army Chaplains, but my conviction is strong that they are, as a whole, all a humbug, and a burning shame to their profession.
>
> I have written you a <u>horrible</u> letter this time in many senses. I will try next time and be more cheerful and not speak of the horrors of war so much.
>
> Love to all at home.
>
> Charles
>
> I shall be anxious to hear whether you got the last 30 dollars I sent. I hear the rebels captured a mail about that time.[79]

No doubt feeling better after venting his spleen, Merrick sealed up the letter and walked it over to be posted.

Capt. Azor Nickerson was not doing well at all, having been shot through one arm and through the lungs. Wounds that penetrated the chest cavity were notoriously fatal in this pre-antiseptic era. News of his critical condition had immediately been forwarded to his family in Ohio.

> My father had been summoned from a neighboring State, and soon after he came an incident occurred that aptly illustrates the peculiar phases of this war. He became very much interested in the Confederate soldier who was lying in my tent, and was careful to divide any luxury he got for me

79. Charles H. Merrick, Letter to his wife, July 7, 1863, William P. Palmer Collection, Container 1, Folder 3, MSS 3088, Western Reserve Historical Society, Cleveland, Ohio. All underlinings are by Merrick.

with him. The man, though apparently grateful, said little, and I think half suspected that my father was not aware that he belonged to the Confederate army. One day, however, the old gentleman had prepared a couple of milk-punches, and, while "Johnnie" was partaking of his, he suddenly asked him to what regiment he belonged. The patient hesitated for a moment, and then answered: "The ----th Mississippi."

"The ----th Mississippi!" echoed the good Samaritan, as he staggered and nearly fell to the ground. "Why," said he, "you may be the very man who shot my boy!" and the tears sprang to his eyes at the thought. In a moment more he recovered his equanimity, and taking the wounded Confederate by the hand, said: "Never mind, my boy, pardon me for having such an unwelcome thought. I am sure you believed you were doing your duty, whatever you did."

I was quite proud that, from this time on until all the Confederates were removed from among the Union troops and placed in a camp by themselves, my father showed the man even more attention than he did me, so anxious was he to demonstrate that he made no difference because he might have "shot his boy."[80]

The Second Corp ambulance dropped Cornelia Hancock off at the door of Doctor Horner, then clattered away into the growing darkness. After trimming the lamp in her room, Cornelia sat down to write a hurried note:

Gettysburg, Pa. July 7th, 1863.
My Dear cousin,

I am very tired tonight; have been on the field all day—went to the 3rd Division 2nd Army Corps. I suppose there are about five hundred wounded belonging to it. They have one patch of woods devoted to each army corps for a hospital. . . . You can tell Aunt that there is every opportunity for 'secesh' sympathizers to do a good work among the butternuts; we have lots of them here suffering fearfully. . . .

80. Nickerson, "Personal Recollections of Two Visits to Gettysburg," pp. 24-25.

. . . I feel very thankful that this was a successful battle; the spirit of the men is so high that many of the poor fellows said today: "What is an arm or leg to whipping Lee out of Penn." I would get on first rate if they would not ask me to write to their wives; *that* I cannot do without crying, which is not pleasant to either party. I do not mind the sight of blood, have seen limbs taken off and was not sick at all.

It is very beautiful, rolling country here; under favorable circumstances I should think healthy, but now for five miles around, there is an awful smell of putrefaction. Women are needed here very badly, anyone who is willing to go to field hospitals, but nothing short of an order from Secretary Stanton or General Halleck will let you through the lines. Major General Schenk's order for us was not regarded as anything; if we had not met Miss Dix at Baltimore Depot, we should not have gotten through. It seems a strange taste but I am glad we did. We stay at Doctor Horner's house at night—direct letters care of Dr. Horner, Gettysburg, Pa. If you could mail me a newspaper, it would be a great satisfaction, as we do not get the news here and the soldiers are so anxious to hear; things will be different in a short time. Cornelia[81]

As Surgeon Justin Dwinelle sat wearily down at his field desk, the light of his lantern cast ghostly illumination over an order just arrived from Medical Headquarters:

Gettysburgh, July 7th
Doctor,

The trains will start tomorrow, at 8 A.M., 12 noon, and 3 or 4 P.M.

You may send those able to walk, and who are decently clothed. About 300 can be sent in each train.

Let them take one days ration with them.

Henry Janes
Surg. in Charge of
Hospitals about Gettysburgh

81. Hancock, *South After Gettysburg*, pp. 7, 8.

Surg. Dwinell [*sic*]
In Charge of 2nd Corps
Hospital[82]

Dwinelle sat staring at the order. Numbed by emotional and physical exhaustion, it took a moment for the full impact of the words to strike home. "The trains will start tomorrow. . . ." That could only mean that all the wounded that they had been so carefully sending off to the railroad station ever since the battle had been sitting, most likely unattended, beside empty railroad tracks, waiting for trains that never came.

But now, the trains really were up and running. Finally, the wounded would be leaving this festering, diseased mausoleum called Gettysburg. At long, long last.

82. Henry Janes to Justin Dwinelle, Order dated July 7, 1863, Copy in the Union Field Hospital Vertical File, Gettysburg National Military Park Library.

Chapter 12

WEDNESDAY, JULY 8: DAWN—THURSDAY, JULY 9: MIDNIGHT

"Soon there was no lack of attendents."

Lt. Azor Nickerson
8th Ohio Volunteer Infantry

Hanover, Pennsylvania

Medical Inspector Edward P. Vollum, U.S. Army, stepped down from the railroad coach at Hanover on this rainy Wednesday, chafing at the unexpected delay in reaching Gettysburg. He was supposed to make his way as quickly as possible to the site of the recent battle to oversee the railroad transportation of the wounded. Now some unnamed problem down the track had stranded the train here at Hanover. Undaunted, Vollum asked directions to the nearest hospital, then walked over to check on the care of the wounded.

"I was detained a few hours, on the 8th, at Hanover, Pa., where I found about 150 wounded, chiefly from [Brig. Gen. Judson] Kilpatrick's cavalry, under charge of Assistant Surgeon [Perin] Gardner, First [West] Virginia Cavalry. They were comfortably situated in a school-house and in dwellings."[1]

Vollum walked throughout the town during his layover, visiting homes and businesses where wounded soldiers were being housed and treated, asking about the welfare of the men and personally checking on the cleanliness and comfort of the facilities. After his brief inspection, he was pleased to report that "the inhabitants had

1. *OR*, vol. 27, pt. 1, pp. 25-26.

furnished them with bunks, bedding, dressings, utensils, and food in sufficient quantity, the people in each street in the town furnishing food delicacies, nurses, &c., two days at a time."[2]

Satisfied with the quality of care shown by the inhabitants of the small town, the medical inspector made his way back to the Hanover Station where the locomotive, with a full head of steam up, was sounding its whistle prior to departure. Vollum must have idly wondered how the care of the wounded still left at the battlefield compared with that given here in this rural stopover. Taking his seat, he watched the station and then Hanover itself disappear over the horizon as the engine and cars slowly picked up speed, heading northwest toward Gettysburg.

Gettysburg, Pennsylvania

With the railroad finally up and running (at least in a limited and tentative fashion), the trickle of visitors that had been reaching the battlefield on foot, by wagon, or on horseback quickly swelled to a steady influx. Foremost among them were average citizens of both sexes, moved with compassion for the suffering of the wounded left behind at Gettysburg. These hearty souls, representing a great variety of abilities and skills, were willing to come from the next town, the next county, or several states away to do what it took to make the injured men comfortable, and to assist the surgeons in getting these men on the road to recovery.

"Soon there was no lack of attendants," related one wounded Ohioan. "Every walk in life appeared to be represented. Some gentlemen brought their wives and daughters, and remained for weeks doing with their own hands the most disagreeable drudgery, sleeping on the ground, and enduring other privations with the heroism of veteran soldiers."[3]

In some ways, there had been more personal attention provided for the Confederate wounded in the early days after the battle than for many of their Union counterparts. "Genl Lee, like the Noble thoughtful General he is, has left behind (before retiring) many hundreds of nurses (from among our private soldiers) and many surgeons of his army to assist and to care for the thousands of the brave men whom he knew could not receive the attention they required from the hands of the

---

2. *Ibid.*
3. Nickerson, "Personal Recollections of Two Visits to Gettysburg," p. 23.

enemy. These nurses and surgeons are afterwards detained as regular prisoners of war."[4]

Now, however, with the news of the battle and the sufferings of the wounded in Gettysburg being spread by telegraph and newspapers, there was a wholesale response from people all over the North. "The whole country has learned tidings of the battle of Gettysburg," remembered the wounded Ohioan, "and the nearest towns and cities are sending out generously medical stores, provisions, money, *preachers*, and 'sanitary committees.' The Sisters of Charity and Mercy are in many parts but as yet I have not seen any."[5]

Pennsylvania in particular was lavish in its outpouring of generosity and support for the wounded stranded at Gettysburg. "The old Keystone state outdid herself; her quota being filled by some of the wealthiest and most accomplished men and women within her borders," recalled Capt. Azor Nickerson of the 8th Ohio. "One group from Chester County was composed entirely of Quakers, or members of the Society of Friends. They were of the best and most reputable of that exceedingly respectable county. I saw ladies of this delegation, with their own hands, cooking delicacies at an open fire, where the wind blew smoke and ashes in their faces with the persistence proverbial of all such out-of-doors cooking 'ranges.'"[6]

William and Anna Holstein from Upper Merion, in Montgomery County, Pennsylvania, were a husband and wife team that had come to be closely identified with the Second Corps hospitals. The couple was described by hometown acquaintances as "people of considerable wealth, and unexceptionable social position, beloved and honored by all who know them." William, at forty-six, started visiting battlefield hospitals in 1862, while Anna, nine years younger and fiercely domestic, had contented herself with staying at home, collecting and publishing her husband's hospital stories for use by aid societies. However, she found herself frequently moved as she heard the tales of suffering and courage brought home by her husband from the

4. Dooley, *John Dooley*, p. 115.
5. Nickerson, "Personal Recollections of Two Visits to Gettysburg," p. 23. There is no record of members of these two Catholic orders working at any of the Second Corps hospitals.
6. *Ibid.*

Maryland hospitals in September following Lee's Northern invasion. When William returned to the general hospitals around Antietam and Frederick, Maryland, after a brief visit home, Anna was by his side. The two also served together in hospitals near Falmouth, Virginia, following the Battle of Fredericksburg in December of 1862, and near Potomac Creek following the clash at Chancellorville in May of 1863.[7]

Anna's husband contracted a malarial fever in Washington, so the Holsteins traveled back to their home in Upper Merion in June, to rest and recuperate in the clear, country air of Pennsylvania. "We remained at home only long enough for Mr. H. to recuperate sufficiently to bear the fatigues of travel. While he was still unfit for the journey, the great battle of Gettysburg, July 1st, 2d, and 3d, 1863, was fought; within one week after it, we were on our way thither."[8]

Accommodations were still at a premium in the overcrowded crossroads village when they arrived, even with five small local hotels. The Holsteins, however, were old campaigners, and any kind of shelter would suffice for the night. "Reaching the town late in the evening, [we] spent the night upon the parlor floor of one of the hotels; with a satchel for a pillow, slept soundly. In the morning went to the Field Hospital, where we were warmly welcomed by our old friends of the second corps."[9]

"The wounded at that time, lay just where they had been placed when carried in from the battle—friend and foe resting together." William started working his way through the hospital, doing whatever was necessary to comfort and assist the wounded; Anna, a dietitian experienced in the preparation of specialized hospital foods, started unpacking her stove and other culinary utensils, apparently as the tents were being set up on or about July 8. "We soon found where and how to resume work, which we had so lately left off: a tent was promptly prepared for our use; it was not many hours until the 'diet kitchen' was in full operation; with the large and valuable supplies taken on with us, the 'institution' moved on in a wonderfully smooth, efficient manner."[10]

---

7. Brockett and Vaughn, *Woman's Work in the Civil War*, p. 251; Conklin, *Women at Gettysburg*, p. 255; Holstein, *Three Years in Field Hospitals*, pp. 37-38.
8. Holstein, *Three Years in Field Hospitals*, p. 38.
9. *Ibid.*
10. *Ibid.*, pp. 38-39.

Among these volunteer attendants who had come to Gettysburg with the specific goal of attending to the needs of the wounded were a group of determined, unmarried women, boldly venturing out on their own to accomplish this purpose in a time when feminine independence was frowned on, if not viewed with outright ridicule by most men. Seeing the needs and responding to the crisis, some of these stalwart women endured extreme hardship in reaching their destination.

One such was Miss Clarissa Fellows Jones, a Philadelphia school teacher. "The Christian Commission in Phila sent no females to the Battlefields, when I applied to Mr. Geo[rge] H. Stuart for a Pass as Nurse to go to Gettysburg, he directed me to Mr. G. S. Griffith [Chairman of the Christian Commission] in Baltimore." Undaunted by the buck-passing, Miss Jones set out for Baltimore, still intent on gaining access to the wounded. She was "a woman who had enough backbone to go to Baltimore after the Philadelphia commission had refused her a commission, saying the battlefield was no place for a woman," as one newspaper writer described her. At Baltimore, she so forcefully presented her case that she "succeed[ed] in convincing the Baltimore men that she was needed at Gettysburg. . . ."[11]

"So furnished with letters to that gentleman [George H. Stuart] I went with my baggage consisting of 8 barrels of the finest Drugs from the druggists of Phila, my trunk and a large basket. Arriving early in the morning I was cordially received and started for Gettysburg. . . . Mr. Griffith very promptly accepted my services and directly obtained transportation for me, sending me to the Second Army Corps Hospital with a letter to Mr. and Mrs. Moore of Baltimore who were already at work."[12]

Just as she was about to set out for Gettysburg, her goal now apparently within reach, events turned unexpectedly ugly for the young teacher, the result of a tragic case of mistaken identity. "My barrels arrived the next morning, were seized by the Court Martial and contents distributed.[13] The people had carelessly read Miss C. F. Jones [as] the name of a noted rebel woman *Mrs. C. F. Jones* instead of Miss C. F. Jones. I got across the Street quickly, sat down upon my trunk

11. Clarissa Fellows Jones, Pension file, submitted February 5, 1917, National Archives and Records Administration; Philadelphia *North American*, Sunday, June 29, 1913, special section, p. 4.
12. Clarissa Fellows Jones, Pension file, submitted February 5, 1917, National Archives and Records Administration; Philadelphia *North American*, Sunday, June 29, 1913, special section, p. 4.
13. Miss Jones meant provost marshal, not court martial.

which a black man was about to get into with a hatchet. I still sat there and he finally report[ed] me to the C[ourt] M[artial] [*sic*] who came down and I explained to him that this was my trunk. I told him those empty barrels were also mine. He examined and found the mistake apologized etc."[14]

All the apologies in the world could not restore the precious medicinal contents of those barrels, however, and there was no time or money to immediately replace the looted goods. Nothing was left but press on empty-handed to Gettysburg, bearing nothing but her trunk of personal possessions and her Christian Commission Pass. The trip was apparently uneventful, but identity trouble again awaited her at the battlefield, where she was "threatened with arrest as a Southern spy, one Mrs. C. F. Jones." Again, her explanations won the day, and, after receiving directions, she set off in search of the Union Second Corps hospital.[15]

Upon reaching the complex of hospital tents at the Schwartz Farm, Clarissa Fellows Jones, in spite of the loss of all her supplies and threats of arrest due to being confused with a Southern sympathizer and spy, "volunteer[ed] to nurse the rebel wounded, considered an unpleasant task indeed for a Yankee girl. . . ." In fact, no other Northern civilian seemed interested in caring for the Confederate wounded when the casualties of the two armies were moved into separate wards of the tent city going up in Farmer Schwartz's pasture, out behind the barn and outbuildings. "When the wheat field of 14 acres was garnered the Gov[ernment] with all speed rushed cots and tents and the men were carried across the creek (Rock) and the blues on the right and the greys on the left. There were plenty of nurses but when all the Blues were furnished with nurses the rest fled to Gettysburg and upon a call for volunteers I was the only one to offer myself. . . . Dr. Dwinell[e] Sur-in-chg asked me to take charge of the Rebel wounded whose tents were on one side of the fourteen acre field."[16]

---

14. Clarissa Fellows Jones, Pension file, submitted February 5, 1917, National Archives and Records Administration; Philadelphia *North American*, Sunday, June 29, 1913, special section, p. 4.
15. Clarissa Fellows Jones, Pension file, submitted February 5, 1917, National Archives and Records Administration; Philadelphia *North American*, Sunday, June 29, 1913, special section, p. 4.
16. Clarissa Fellows Jones, Pension file, submitted February 5, 1917, National Archives and Records Administration; Philadelphia *North American*, Sunday, June 29, 1913, special section, p. 4.

Her thoughtful care of the Southerners quickly raised some serious questions as to her loyalty, especially among the Northern patients.

> The Union men could not understand my devotion to the Confederates, and finally I noticed among them a coldness to me.
>
> I asked them what was the trouble, and one of them said: "Miss Jones, where are you from?" I told them I was from Philadelphia.
>
> "Are you a rebel sympathizer?" another asked. I answered most decidely no.
>
> And then I had a heart to heart talk with them, and told them of the sufferings of the rebels and how desperately they needed the affectionate care of a woman, just as much as they did. The boys soon saw the other side, and agreed with me. "That's right, Miss Jones, you do all you can for those Johnnies; they are not such a bad sort, after all."[17]

With the full approval of the Yankee patients, she spent long hours caring for the grieviously wounded Rebels. She fondly remembered those generous Northerners, even many years later: "We became better friends after that."[18]

In turn, the Confederate wounded idolized her and her selfless care. "The men were always courteous to her, ever anxious to do her a favor, and . . . they appreciated everything she did for them. 'I never heard one word out of the way. I was a woman alone, and I appealed to them.'"[19]

Some nurses, such as Mary Lee, followed the Second Corps for purely personal reasons. Mary had been a leading light in the Union Refreshment Saloon movement in Philadelphia, an organization sparked by the spontaneous generosity of the City of Brotherly Love's citizens to the regiments passing through town on their way to the front. Under Mrs. Lee's guidance, the effort rapidly outgrew its quarters in a dilapidated old boat house, annexing buildings on both

17. Philadelphia *North American*, Sunday, June 29, 1913, special section, p. 4.
18. *Ibid.*
19. *Ibid.*

sides, until soldiers could find dormitory rooms, bathing facilities, and hot food at all hours of the day and night. But when Mary's son William enlisted in Company B of the 72nd Pennsylvania, she decided to leave the refreshment saloons in the hands of others, choosing instead to follow her son's unit as a regimental nurse.[20]

A skillful and innovative cook due to her experience at the Refreshment Saloon, she proved to be an immediate favorite after the Battle of Antietam. At a field hospital where she was nursing, commissary supplies were limited to "a barrel of flour, a barrel of apples, and a keg of lard. To a practical housekeeper, as she is, this combination seemed to point to apple dumplings as the dish in which they could all be employed to the best advantage; and the good-natured astonishment of the poor fellows, who looked for nothing but black coffee and hard-tack, was merged in admiration for the accomplished cook who could there, almost on the battlefield, serve them with hot dumplings."[21]

Following the debacle at Fredericksburg in December, 1862, she returned to Philadelphia to nurse her sick son back to health, and worked as time allowed at the Refreshment Saloon. Making her way back to the Second Corps in March, 1863, she nursed their wounded following the trouncing at Chancellorsville, now accompanied by her daughter Amanda, who served as a personal aide to her busy mother.[22]

With the dissolution of the field hospitals along Potomac Creek prior to the march into Pennsylvania in June, 1863, she headed first to Alexandria, then home to Philadelphia. The news of the battle reached her there, and she made preparations at once to leave for the hospitals of the Second Corps. "Arriving several days after the battle, she went directly to the Second Corps Hospital, and labored there until it was broken up." No doubt her culinary wizardry was immediately put to good use upon her arrival.[23]

---

20. Brockett and Vaughn, *Woman's Work in the Civil War*, pp. 480-81; Marjorie Barstow Greenbie, *Lincoln's Daughters of Mercy* (New York: G. P. Putnam's Sons, 1944), pp. 134, 135. By the end of the war, between 800,000 and 900,000 troops had been served by this Philadelphia institution.
21. Frank Moore, *Women of the War; Their Heroism and Self-Sacrifice* (Hartford, Connecticut: S. S. Scranton & Co., 1866), p. 151.
22. Conklin, *Women at Gettysburg*, p. 201.
23. Brockett and Vaughn, *Woman's Work in the Civil War*, p. 486.

Clarissa Fellows Jones referred to receiving from the chairman of the Philadelphia Christian Commission "a letter to Mr. and Mrs. Moore of Baltimore who were already at work" in the Second Corps hospital at Gettysburg. While surviving records do not show a Mr. and Mrs. Moore, a *Miss* Jane Boswell Moore and Mrs. Moore, her mother, a team of independent nurses from Baltimore, were already there, busily caring for the wounded at the Schwartz Farm, when Miss Jones arrived.

Not being associated with any outside agency meant that the Moores paid all expenses out of their own pockets. "We drew liberal supplies from both Sanitary and Christian Commissions, as well as largely from individuals," wrote Jane Boswell Moore, "but have ourselves belonged to no association, and received no compensation from any quarter. None of our expenses were defrayed, except in the matter of government passes. As southern women who had no relatives to give to the cause, we endeavored to be behind none in our devotion."[24]

The Moores were very private citizens, and their work as nurses seems to be the only thing ever recorded about them for posterity. Beside working with Clarissa Fellows Jones at the hospital, jotting down some personal experiences, and a passing mention in a letter by an ambulance driver, the only mention of the Moores is in a book of reminiscences of Civil War nursing, quoting newspaper articles which have not survived. They truly served to unselfishly succor the wounded, then quietly returned to the anonymity of civilian life without notoriety or ado.

Some had not come to Gettysburg with any intentions of ever nursing at the Second Corps Hospital. One such lady was Mrs. Hanness.

Mrs. Hanness (no one ever seems to have asked her for her first name) came to Gettysburg from central New York State. There she had presided over a happy and prosperous household made up of her husband and their only child, a son of seventeen. When war came to America in 1861, both father and son, filled with patriotic enthusiasm, rushed out to join the same Empire State regiment. Both fell, severely wounded, in the fighting on July 1, 1863.

24. Moore, *Women of the War*, pp. 569-70.

Receiving news of their wounding in an obscure little Pennsylvania town, she left their New York home, intent on reaching the battlefield at any cost. Seeking permission to enter the battle zone, she was directed to Harrisburg.

> Amongst the earliest arrivals on that field of death was the stricken mother. With difficulty she obtained from the Harrisburg provo-marshal [*sic*] a permit to continue her journey. She walked ten miles through the mud from New Oxford to Gettysburg and found a home in the house of that noble man, David Warren, on Carlisle street, whose latch-string was ever out, through this whole period of calamity, to those who searched for their loved ones.
>
> Her husband mortally wounded had been carried into a private house and had already breathed his last. Her son could nowhere be found. She searched over miles and miles of hospitals, in fields and barns, in churches and warehouses. She enlisted hundreds in the quest.
>
> As the days past with no sign of her missing son, the practical Mrs. Hanness turned more and more of her sorrow and despair over her lost son and her dead husband into useful ministration to the wounded men that she found laying scattered everywhere.
>
> Then, with a lifelong grief in that gentle heart, she turned to the suffering crowd around her and went to the Second corps field hospital, where thousands moaned as they hovered between life and death. Daily as a volunteer nurse she passed from cot to cot, prayed with the dying, soothed the anguish of the living; yet all the time hoping against hope that, in some mysterious way, she would find that lost son.[25]

J. Howard Wert, a neighbor of the Schwartzs who became a historian in later life, remembered the sad-eyed Widow Hanness very well. "After a day of labor, she would seek my mother's humble home for a few hours of rest." Wert remembered her as "a woman of fine presence, with a pleasant face, a wealth of auburn hair and clear, blue

---

25. Wert, "In the Hospitals of Gettysburg, July, 1863," no. 11, *Harrisburg Telegraph*, July 25, 1907, p. 4.

eyes," a gracious woman who invariably ". . . had a cheerful word and a subdued smile for all."[26]

A new song was making the rounds, published in a series of popular hymnals—W. B. Bradbury's "Sweet Hour of Prayer." After each day of labor among the Second Corps wounded, with muted agony in her own heart and eyes no longer able to cry, Mrs. Hanness would give vent to her sorrow in the only way she knew. Many of the men in the hospital would remember Mrs. Hanness as the nurse who sang them to sleep at night.

> Each evening as fell the shades, with a voice of rich compass and tender pathos, that lone woman whom a single hour of battle had rendered a widow and childless, would sing:
>
> Sweet hour of prayer, sweet hour of prayer,
> That calls me from a world of care,
> And bids me at my Father's throne
> Make all my wants and wishes known;
> In seasons of distress and grief
> My soul has often found relief,
> And oft escaped the tempter's snare
> By thy return, sweet hour of prayer.[27]

To the desperately wounded, groaning in agony, reaching out with tenuous fingers to find arms and legs forever lost to the surgeon's knife, struggling to lay comfortably as maggots squirmed in festering wounds, begging for water that tasted of blood and death, the crystal-clear notes of the widow's voice brought soothing comfort and thoughts of far-off homes:

> Sweet hour of prayer, sweet hour of prayer,
> Thy wings shall my petition bear
> To Him whose truth and faithfulness
> Engage the waiting soul to bless;
> And since he bids me seek his face,
> Believe his word, and trust his grace,
> I'll cast on him my every care,
> And wait for thee, sweet hour of prayer.[28]

---

26. *Ibid.*
27. *Ibid.*
28. *Ibid.*

To the dying men of the Second Corps hospital, writhing in anguish with pain that no anesthesia could dull, with brain tissue exposed to the fetid air, or jawbones shot clean away, men with perforated bowels, or air hissing harshly out of chest wounds with each agonized breath, to men consumed with racking fevers from unchecked infection, the music floating on the night air brought strength to face the final hurdle of one's own mortality:

> Sweet hour of prayer, sweet hour of prayer,
> May I thy consolation share;
> Till, from Mount Pisgah's lofty height,
> I view my home and take my flight;
> This robe of flesh I'll drop, and rise
> To seize the everlasting prize;
> And shout while passing through the air,
> Farewell, farewell, sweet hour of prayer.[29]

Beside the large turnout of mostly untrained volunteer nurses, several groups of skilled (or at least semi-skilled) medical personnel were making their way to the battlefield. One group, called "contract surgeons," were doctors allowed to wear uniforms and be addressed as "acting assistant surgeons"; however, none of these men held a current military commission. Some had been in the army and left (for a variety of reasons); some had no military experience whatsoever. Each served under his own individual contract with the army.

While ideally employing only medical school graduates that had passed examinations before Army Medical Department boards, many underqualified or nonqualified "practitioners" managed to find their way into these contract positions. Botanics, Thompsonians, vegetarianists, hydropaths, chromothermalists, even self-taught native "doctors" all ended up serving side by side with the skilled surgeons of the Army Medical Corps in times of extreme crisis.[30] Those

---

29. *Ibid.*

30. Botanics, also called homeopaths, used vegetable and herbal mixtures to treat sick and injured men. They were especially fond of preparations based on cayenne pepper. Thompsonians were a small group of quacks who followed the "medical" teachings of their founder, Samuel Thompson. Vegeterianists were a group, founded by Sylvester Graham, that advocated the use of a vegetarian diet, and vegetable-based treatments, to cure a wide

with training were frequently the least skilled in their profession, often men who had failed in private practice through incompetence, drunkenness, or just sheer laziness. Even undergraduate medical students managed to find their way to the scenes of recent fighting as "contract surgeons," each one eager to try out their unused medical knowledge, and seeing this as an exciting opportunity to gain important "practical experience" toward their degrees.[31]

The Second Corps hospital employed some of these contract surgeons to deal with the overwhelming rush of patients, especially to fill the gaps when most of the regimental surgeons were ordered to pack up and march with their units in pursuit of the retreating Southern army. "There also reported to me for duty on the seventh Eight or nine contract Surgeons," reported Justin Dwinelle, surgeon in charge.[32]

A second group of medical men arriving at Gettysburg and wandering out to the various corps hospitals were volunteer physicians, doctors in private practice from small towns as well as metropolitan areas, taking time away from their familiar but mundane practices to come to the scene of the recent battle. Whether inspired by a sense of compassion, or patriotism, or a desire to be involved with the movers and shakers of current medical technology, or sometimes just by plain boredom or curiosity, these private physicians showed up unexpectedly at Doctor Dwinelle's headquarters tent, fully expecting to be allowed the run of the Second Corps hospital.

Dwinelle had seen enough of these men to know what to expect. "Volunteer Surgeons as a class are not reliable. Of the large number who reported to me only four or five were realy [*sic*] of much benefit. A number reported for duty and I never saw them afterwards. They came & went at their own pleasure and in several instances after being assigned to duty they left without giving notice. Most of them did not choose to operate. Yet they would insist upon expending their time at the operating table. Not a few of them seemed to have a horror of dressing a stump."[33]

---

range of sicknesses and injuries. Hydropaths firmly held to the beneficial medical effects of certain waters, whether bathing in them, drinking them, or using them in preparations. General Thomas J. "Stonewall" Jackson was an avid believer in hydropathy.

31. Adams, *Doctors in Blue*, pp. 174-75; Harold Elk Straubing, *In Hospital and Camp: The Civil War through the Eyes of its Doctors and Nurses* (Harrisburg, Pennsylvania: Stackpole Books, 1993), pp. 3, 6.
32. Dwinelle, *Medical Report.*
33. *Ibid.*

Many of these volunteer practitioners, with no military experience whatsoever, seemed to view the corps hospital more as a vacation getaway or a tourist attraction than an medical institution filled with men fighting for life. "I have had them report to me at night stating that they would be ready to go to work in the morning and that they would remain as long as their services were required," continued Dwinelle. "They would then stroll about the hospital a couple of hours get their supper lodging & Breakfast and leave immediately after."[34]

In a time when most of the nation's doctors had never seen, let alone performed, an amputation, numerous country doctors and big city practitioners saw this as a golden opportunity to try their hand at this radical form of surgery. "At one time two Medical Gentlemen came to me and stated that they had been sent down by the Surgeon General to assist about the hospital but as they found the operations nearly all performed they came to report that they were going to leave on the next train. This was the first and last that I saw of those gentlemen. Like many others of this class they decline to do anything unless they can take off limbs. [I] Cannot myself understand why it is that professed Surgeons will come several hundreds of miles to assist after a battle and then refuse to go to dressing Stumps. I have never been able to get more than one sixth of the volunteer Surgeons who have reported to me for duty to go to work as dressers and remain over six hours."[35]

As a dedicated medical man and administrator bearing responsibility for the well being of thousands of patients, Dwinelle did not mince words when stating what he expected from any doctor who showed up unannounced and uninvited on his doorstep. "If good Surgeons of undoubted reputation can be sent to us in time[,] stay with us while their services are needed[,] conform to the same rules and regulations and put up with the same inconveniences without fault finding that the corps Surgeons have too [*sic*], Their services will be appreciated. But if men of whom we know nothing and are not willing to work except at the operating table We must decline to assign them to so responsible a position. It would be a manifest injustice to the Surgeons of the corps to make them of Secondary Importance to citizen Surgeons. The Medical department of the Second corps is mostly composed of men who are practical from large experience and observation."[36]

---

34. *Ibid.*
35. *Ibid.*
36. *Ibid.*

Still another class of professional volunteers—a large contingent of pastors, priests, and clergymen representing various denominations—were disembarking from the trains, and arriving daily by wagon and horseback, in Gettysburg. While most were indeed sincere in their concern to minister to the physical and spiritual needs, both to the wounded members of their own congregation as well as others, there were some that had come merely as sightseers and adventure seekers. Others seemed determined to harangue or bombast the lost of this captive audience into the Kingdom of God. The injured soldiers, having encountered a vast array of humanity during their military experience, were quick to differentiate between those who came to work and those who came only to talk. "Clergymen of all denominations were there," wrote wounded Ohioan Azor Nickerson.

> They may, however, be divided into two classes—those who depended upon prayer and works, and those who relied exclusively on prayer without works. The difference between the two will be better understood by a brief description of the course pursued by one of each class, who, during the early part of my stay, paid daily visits to me.
>
> One was a portly man, about fifty-five years of age. He carried with him a large bible and a hymn-book. I do not recall that he ever brought anything else, or even asked a patient to take a glass of water. When he came in he asked me how I felt, and if I was prepared to die. Then he adjusted his spectacles and read a chapter from his bible. That finished, he selected what seemed to be the longest hymn he could find, and in a wheezy voice sang it all through without skipping a stanza. These interesting exercises were then closed by a lengthy prayer in which advice to the Creator was the most prominent feature. He daily inflicted this programme upon me at a time when every breath I drew was like the thrust of a dozen daggers, until the surgeons finally found it out, and then they forbade his entering my tent at all.[37]

37. Nickerson, "Personal Recollections of Two Visits to Gettysburg," p. 23.

At least one instance of the callous nature of these spectator clergymen had occurred on July 7, before the hospital tents and cooking utensils had arrived at the Second Corps hospital. Pvt. Charles Muller of the 1st Minnesota Infantry noted the unusual instance of men carrying lumber into the hospital camp and erecting a handmade

> row of tables about 40 or 50 feet long. Then some other man came along with some baskets filled and covered with table cloth[s]. Then some ladies came and covered those tables [with] linen cloths and plates, saucers and cups, while other[s] were making coffee other[s] were cutting up some hams and roasted chickens and bread and I did see some nice cakes even dishes with candy and preserves, and from all appearances the man [*sic*] around the table were all preacher[s] and I did begin to figure out how long it will be before they will ask me over [and] begin to distribute but how much a man can be mistaken in his figurings. When everything was ready then the whole club of preachers their wives, sisters and daughters sat down around the table and had a good meal and they were telling stories as if they were on a picnic ground and not even a single one would look around to ask if we wanted something or not. Then towards 12 o'clock a girl of 19 or 20 came around and had [a] cup of coffee and ask[ed] me if [I] wanted a cup of coffee. I said yes and when she gave it to me she said now hurry up because I haven't much time to wait on you. I told her I did [not] call on her to wait on me at all. Then she wanted to take the cup away from me again but that was more than I could stand and told her to get away or else I would knock her down and then I took a dislike against all the preachers in the world and have not got over it yet.[38]

While there were isolated instances of clergymen coming to look or talk rather than to minister, the majority worked diligently and hard to meet the needs of the patients, whether spiritual or physical, no matter how demanding or difficult.

---

38. Charles Muller, unpublished memoirs at the Minnesota Historical Society, St. Paul, Minnesota.

In striking contrast with this [portly preacher with the big bible and hymnbook] was the course pursued by another wearer of the cloth—a stout, energetic man of about thirty-five years of age. As he never troubled me with any of the conundrums which others of his profession considered it their duty to propound to those of us loitering along on the brink of eternity, it was some time before I knew that he was a minister of the Gospel. He never came into my tent that he did not do something for my comfort. Without being told, he seemed to have an intuition of what was needed, and then off came his coat and the thing was done.

One of the many bad features in my case was the utter distaste I had for anything in the way of food. Such nourishment as I did take was taken like any other medicine, because the surgeons prescribed it. . . . I had conceived the idea that there was nothing in the world I wanted or could eat except a roasted potato: and as it was said that there was not a potato to be had within miles of our camp, of course I wanted one more than ever. I had long since ceased asking for them, but when food was mentioned that simple vegetable was the only thing that suggested itself to my mind. My clergyman friend was located in the Second Division hospital, some distance from ours, which was the Third Division, Second Corps [still camped south of the Schwartz farm]. But he always came to see me at least once a day, and I had my tent flaps turned back so that I could watch for his coming. One very hot Sunday morning I caught sight of him coming considerably earlier than was his usual custom. His coat was thrown across his arm, and the perspiration was rolling down his face, but when he looked up and saw me watching his approach he swung a little bundle he had tied in his handkerchief, and exclaimed, with all the enthusiasm of a boy: "I've got them, captain, I've got them!" Sure enough, he soon laid before me a dozen potatoes, two of which he immediately washed with his own hands, and roasted in the ashes. I saw Tiffany's collection of diamonds, at the Centennial of 1876, and also the most notable display of jewels ever made by one person in this country, . . . and yet I have never seen any diamonds, rubies, sapphires, or pearls that were at all comparable with the exquisite beauty of that cluster of Irish potatoes, brought to me at Gettysburg, on Sunday morning, by the Rev. J. E. Adams of New Sharon, Me. He had walked in the broiling sun over ten miles to gratify an invalid's whim.

Up to this time he had never held any religious services in my tent. So, while he was preparing another potato for one of my fellow-soldiers, I told the attendant that he might give my compliments to him and say that, as it was Sunday morning, I should be very glad, if he could spare the time, to have him offer a prayer. "Certainly," he replied, when they told him, and walking over to my tent he laid aside his hat and knelt by my rude bunk. He was still without his coat, his sleeves were rolled up, and his hands were grimy with the ashes from his potato roast. His throat was bare of necktie, the collar thrown open wide, and great beads of perspiration stood on his broad forehead; but what a prayer! Like his works it was fervid, earnest, and apropos. Nothing seemed to be forgotten, and yet it appeared to be such a short prayer. . . . When it was finished and the worthy man had gone, I felt as though I had really been with one who walked arm in arm with the Master, and knew when and how to work as well as when and how to pray.[39]

Another pastor was fondly remembered by Anna Holstein for his work at the hospital. "To aid in relieving the suffering among these wounded men was the 'Germantown Field Hospital Association' formed; I mention it here because this was the first point where it came prominently into notice. They sent as their representative the well-known rector of one of their churches, Rev. B. W. Morris; his services as chaplain are gratefully remembered by many in these eventful times."[40]

Beside ministering to the physical and spiritual needs of the wounded, the pastors and clergymen served as a great source of news to the bedridden men of the hospitals. Because of their mobility within the hospitals, their freedom to go into town to pick up supplies as the needs arose, and their frequent connection with outside organizations

39. Nickerson, "Personal Recollections of Two Visits to Gettysburg," pp. 23-24.
40. Holstein, *Three Years in Field Hospitals*, p. 39.

such as the Sanitary or Christian Commissions, these ministers were often up on the very latest news (or at least the most up-to-date army scuttlebutt). Unfortunately, the most recent information, after passing through the Army rumor mill, and the mouths of countless persons along the way, often bore little resemblance to reality, or was badly garbled and confused when it arrived at its destination.

Sometimes good news to one group of men was the worst possible tidings to another. One clergyman in particular, representing the Sanitary Commission, made an incredibly embarrassing gaff with one group of wounded. "This evening he came rushing into our tent, half frantic, and cried out, 'Glorious news, this evening, boys, glorious tidings of victory! Gen. Lee and his whole army have been intercepted before reaching the Potomac and have been destroyed or taken prisoners.'"[41]

The breathless messenger was greeted with deathly silence in the gloomy interior, and found himself transfixed by the baleful look of every man in the tent. Finally the quiet was broken by the ranking officer, Col. Birkett D. Fry of the 13th Alabama. "'Well, sir,' demanded our Col. Fry, 'supposing your news to be true, do you think that we can rejoice with you in the destruction of all that is dear to us?'"[42]

The Sanitary Commission representative stood gaping in the gathering twilight, furiously trying to come up with a graceful way out of this awkward predicament. "The preacher looked mortified for a single instant, then a sudden light flashing across his brain he exclaimed, 'Excuse me, boys, excuse me! Really I thought you were *our* boys, and rushed in without perceiving how you were dressed. Boys—,' he said with rising dignity, 'I am *too noble*, too magnanimous (those are his very words) to insult a fallen foe.' He then launched into a self glorifying account of what he and the Commission were doing hourly and daily for the wounded, without distinguishing rebel from truly loil [*sic*], and how the magnificent government of the Federal Union was going to fabylous [*sic*] expense in order to render us comfortable. 'Boys,' he said in conclusion, 'We love to heap burning coals upon the heads of our enemies, but we do not wish to insult them.'"[43]

Apparently feeling that he had sufficiently recovered his composure, and put in a good plug for the Sanitary Commission in the

41. Dooley, *John Dooley*, p. 120. Like so much army gossip, the story was totally false.
42. *Ibid.*
43. *Ibid.*

process, the befuddled clergyman hastened away, leaving a dour and unimpressed group of Southerners behind him. "We heard him crying his galorious [*sic*] tidings to more willing ears than ours," wrote an incredulous Lt. John Dooley.[44]

Most of the news, both factual and spurious, arrived at Gettysburg with each new gaggle of tourists and sightseers. As hard as it is to conceive, with its five mile stench, its black clouds of swarming flies, its gouged and mutilated landscape (complete with bloated horse carcasses and blackened human bodies), and its multiple thousands of damaged and bleeding men desperately fighting to hang on to life, Gettysburg was proving to be an immense tourist attraction. Driving in by horse-drawn vehicles from surrounding towns and counties, or else disembarking from the trains now arriving several times a day, the gawkers, the morbidly curious, and the thrill seekers streamed to the battlefield. Like moths to the flame, the battlefield, especially where congealed pools of blood still stood in the hollows, or where damaged equipment lay strewn about, or particularly where some bloody and bullet-riddled clothing lay abandoned on the field, irresistibly drew them to "ooh" and "ahh" in wonder. Some seemed totally callous or indifferent to the suffering around them; others, like John B. Linn, just did not seem to notice the needs of the wounded he encountered during his visit.

Linn, on leave from the 51st Pennsylvania Infantry, had caught the train into Harrisburg, then rode and walked into town on July 7, collecting interesting battle souvenirs along the way. He and his companion, a Doctor Harbaugh, called on local pastor T. P. Bucher, who provided them lodging. The two then leisurely toured some of the hospitals located in private homes in town, sociable to the wounded but unhelpful in their care. Munching on some doughnuts which he had been carrying in his pocket (but had failed to offer to any of the hungry wounded he encountered), Linn and his companion later accompanied Pastor Bucher, heading out of town to tour the Evergreen Cemetery and get an idea of the battle. "On the way [we met] Dr. Gerhart of Franklin and Marshall, who gave us an awful account of the suffering in the 2nd corps. Men lying with legs and arms amputated with nothing whatever to cover them, wounded crying for water, the air

44. *Ibid.*

itself burthened with distress. A young lady coming along in great excitement appealed to us for the sake of humanity to go out and assist in the 2nd corps." Unmoved by her impassioned entreaty or the state of the men hospitalized at the Schwartz Farm, Linn and company continued on with their sightseeing expedition.[45]

Many other visitors beside Linn were out combing the field on July 7. Jacob Hoke, a store owner from neighboring Chambersburg, picked up part of a pocket Bible laying near a severed leg, a grisly remnant of a once-whole and living man. Hoke seemed absolutely fascinated by the minutest details of his grisly find. "It had been cut nearly in two by some missile, the irregular edges and angles of which corresponded with both the marks upon the Bible and the soldier's leg. The soldier had evidently carried this Bible in the pocket of his blouse, and the same shell which had severed his leg had cut through his Bible. . . . The leaves of the Bible were stained with the blood of its owner. . . . We divided the leaves among us. . . ." Heading back to Chambersburg later the same day, Hoke took along a cache of souvenirs, "as did almost every one else who visited the field, some relic in the shape of bullets, bayonets, &c. Bullets could be gathered everywhere, and we saw persons engaged in collecting them by the bucketsfull [*sic*]."[46]

Sightseers seemed content to wander about the field, even if there were no genuine sights left to see. "The big show was gone, but they seemed content to look over the ground where it had been. A torn and bloody garment would attract a crowd, which would disperse only to concentrate again to look at a hat perforated with bullets." These people seemed "animated only by idle curiosity, seeming without thought or care for the hundreds of suffering men lying so near them without notice or sympathy."[47]

As for John B. Linn, he was back out on the field again on July 8. This time he went on an excursion with some newly-made friends, wandering through the area where the Second Corps had fought on

45. John B. Linn, "Journal of my trip to the battlefield at Gettysburg," Diary of John B. Linn, Centre County Library and Historical Museum, Bellefonte, Pennsylvania, typescript copy in the Hospitalization after Gettysburg Vertical File, Gettysburg National Military Park Library, pp. 1-6.

46. Jacob Hoke, *Historical Reminiscences of The War; or Incidents which Transpired In and About Chambersburg, during the War of the Rebellion* (Chambersburg, Pennsylvania: M. A. Foltz, Printer and Publisher, 1884), pp. 171-73.

47. Robert M. Powell, *Recollections of a Texas Colonel at Gettysburg*, ed. Gregory Coco (Gettysburg, Pennsylvania: Thomas Publications, 1990), p. 21.

July 2. There he was able to experience all the interesting and entertaining things to see and do and collect on a battlefield—stepping on a fresh grave and feeling the solid mass of the body under the soil, gawping in wonder at what was left of Farmer Sherfy's Peach Orchard and farm buildings, exchanging gossipy stories about the rumored misfortunes of local residents. "We returned picking up some letters, cards and cutting off some buttons for relics of the fight. On our way in Goodman picked up an Enfield rifle as a trophy. I found a testament with the name T. C. Horcraft, 34th Regt, N Y S V Excelsior eagle and shield, on the next page was written 'David Mitchell' 105 Virginia Regt. I picked up a letter from a boy to his father evidently stained with his father's blood[;] contents very interesting, it is among the relics I have from the field. Also one from a girl to her lover."[48]

As far as Provost Marshal Marsena Patrick was concerned, these tourists had come "in Swarms" for no other reason than "to Sweep & plunder." But even his order to impress looters into twenty-four hour shifts for burial detail work, seems to have barely slowed the gathering of mementoes by the macabre out-of-town visitors. Linn's party was stopped in Gettysburg and a companion's scavenged Enfield rifle confiscated, but Linn had his loot secreted about his person. Going back to where he was staying, he added his battlefield haul to the cartridge from a dead Confederate soldier and "a box marked '3 Second fuzes Richmond Arsenal'" which he had picked up on the way into town.[49]

The Second Corps hospitals were again a hot topic of discussion in Pastor Bucher's parlor tonight. "He told us of six rebels drowning today from the rising of the streams in which they were lying wounded. The suffering in the 2nd Corps [is] pitiful, men particularly rebels still lying there unattended." Once again, neither Linn nor any of his companions made any efforts to go to the Schwartz Farm and see if there was any way that they could be of assistance; instead, they sat and swapped stories of the battle with various visitors that dropped by the house until it was time for bed.[50]

Finally, on July 9, one of the party, Jim Duncan, decided to go back and actually visit the hospitals of the Second Corps. Linn, on the other hand, strolled over to the First Corps hospital, meeting "streams of wounded walking to town in order to get off in the cars." Along the

48. Linn, "Journal of my trip to the battlefield at Gettysburg," pp. 6-8.
49. Patrick, *Inside Lincoln's Army*, p. 268; Linn, "Journal of my trip to the battlefield at Gettysburg," pp. 3, 8-10.
50. Linn, "Journal of my trip to the battlefield at Gettysburg," p. 10.

way, he stopped to sightsee, pausing from time to time to greet old friends, and to pass the time with new acquaintances. For his part, Jim Duncan returned to town with three wounded friends in tow, all apparently from the Second Corps hospital and intent on reaching the railroad. He found overnight lodging for them at a private home and hired a "lady nurse" to care for them. Linn finally made himself useful by walking with Duncan over to the Sanitary Commission, where they were able to secure some clean shirts for Duncan's charges.[51]

"Sick of hospitals and tired of my dirty clothes," Linn finally caught a ride out of town on June 10 with some friends, heading for Carlisle and laden with souvenirs and "relics" of his interesting and informative visit to Gettysburg. It is extremely doubtful if any of the wounded in any of the Gettysburg hospitals, suffering in agony with infected wounds, groping for missing arms or legs, or shivering with fever as they lay dying, knew (or even cared) about his departure.[52]

Another kind of souvenir hunter had also arrived at Gettysburg. He was Dr. John H. Brinton, curator of the brand-new Army Medical Museum in Washington D.C. Brinton was a man on a mission; the trophies he sought were the stuff of nightmares—human remains. His assignment was to assist the field hospital surgeons, and to secure specimens of battlefield injuries that might be used as teaching tools in developing more effective medical treatments of traumatic battlefield wounds.

Dr. Brinton well understood the emotional and physical pressures of battlefield surgery. "It was hard enough to be worked day and night in those great surgical emergencies, accompanying fierce and protracted battles, and it really seemed unjust to expect the rough preparation, necessary to preserve for the Museum, the mutilated limbs."[53]

So his would have to be a hands-on type of work, carefully training surgeons what to look for, and taking the lead in finding suitable specimens. "To overcome all these difficulties and to set an example, I

51. *Ibid.*, pp. 11-12.
52. *Ibid.*, p. 13.
53. John H. Brinton, *Personal Memoirs of John H. Brinton, Major and Surgeon U. S. V., 1861-1865* (New York: Neale Publishing Co., 1914), reprinted as *Personal Memoirs of John H. Brinton, Civil War Surgeon, 1861-1865* (Carbondale: Southern Illinois University Press, 1996), p. 187.

visited frequently our battle-fields, as soon as the information was telegraphed to Washington. I then saw not only a great deal of active surgery, but I had the opportunity of showing practically to the operating surgeons, and to their assistant staffs, what it was that we really wanted, and how their part could be accomplished with the least amount of labor, and in the most satisfactory manner. Many and many a putrid heap have I had dug out of trenches where they were buried, in the supposition of an everlasting rest, and ghoul-like work have I done, amid surrounding gatherings of wondering surgeons, and scarcely less wondering doctors."[54]

After a bumpy ride in a boxcar from Hanover Junction with an acquaintance searching for the body of a friend, Brinton had "found quarters, I think, at the Medical Purveyor's, and busied myself for several days in visiting the hospitals in the town, in the churches and public buildings, and also the large field hospitals which had organized outside the town. These hospitals were generally in good condition, and accommodated large numbers of wounded."[55]

"My duty at this time was twofold, first to render what help I could surgically, and secondly, to collect specimens and histories for the Museum." During his rounds, Brinton stopped by to assist at the tables and in the wards of the Second Corps Hospital. At least one Second Corps patient joined Doctor Brinton's macabre museum as a specimen.[56]

"I was able to gather much for the Museum, and for the most part the medical officers were anxious to further me in my endeavors to carry out my Washington instructions. By the 16th or 17th of July, I had returned to Washington, and resumed my office duties."[57]

Another professional group of visitors that came to the battlefield, wherever there was death and dying to be found, were the itinerant embalmers and undertakers. Being astute businessmen, they set up their stands near the major field hospitals, where they would be seen by visiting relatives anxious to send the body of some loved one home.

---

54. *Ibid.*
55. *Ibid.*, pp. 241-42.
56. *Ibid.*, p. 246. See "Private Dawson W. Arnold, 5th Florida Infantry" in Chapter 15.
57. *Ibid.* The Museum still exists in Washington, D.C., and is a sobering look at actual skeletal remains of men who fought and died during the Civil War.

While many simply pitched a tent and set up two barrels with a plank lying across them as a work surface, others took great pains to appear as professional as possible with display items, attractive signs, and suitably somber apparel. One even took out advertisements in local papers, singing the praises of "metallic coffins for transportation of bodies to any part of the country"; deluxe features included a "warranted air-tight" design so that it "can be placed in the Parlor without fear of any odor escaping therefrom." Some even featured a recessed compartment in the lid that could be filled with ice to slow decomposition.[58]

One literally could not avoid coffins in Gettysburg. "Since the battle, Gettysburg has been an extensive coffin mart & embalmer's harvest field," wrote one Connecticut soldier. "The coffins were stacked on the streets blockading the side walks. These coffin speculators made an enormous profit." There was even a local source for hand-crafted coffins—carpenter Henry Garlach, with a workshop on Baltimore Street, was working day and night to keep up with the constant demand.[59]

"A great business is being done in disinterring bodies for embalming and shipment North," reported Sanitary Commission Secretary Frederick Law Olmstead during his visit to Gettysburg to monitor the Commission's relief efforts. "There are half a dozen fit embalmers competing for it. The Governor of Pennsylvania I believe pays for the removal of all Pennsylvania dead to their friends."[60]

Local residents often helped the bereaved with this last, ghastly detail, whether as a courtesy to guests lodging in their homes, or as a way of earning some type of income during the crisis. "A number of our citizens made quite a good thing out of this gruesome business of taking up the dead for those people and assisting them in preparing them for shipment to their homes." Not surprisingly, "men who were engaged in this work bought whiskies in large quantities" afterwards at the Globe Hotel.[61]

The provost marshal's office effectively depressed the market for the embalmers and their trade within a few weeks of the battle. It was

58. Advertisement formerly in the collection of the Kean Archives, Philadelphia.

59. Justus M. Silliman, Letters of Justus M. Silliman, New Canaan Historical Society, New Canaan, Connecticut.

60. Evelyn Page, "After Gettysburg—Frederick Law Olmstead on the Escape of Lee," *Pennsylvania Magazine*, 72, (October 1951): 442.

61. John C. Wills, Wills Papers, Adams County Historical Society, Gettysburg, Pennsylvania.

officially ordered that no further exhumations should be carried out until cooler weather arrived. The atmosphere was already nauseating enough without disinterring bodies that were already buried. The gravely disappointed undertakers would have to content themselves with providing services to the area hospitals. There was still plenty to keep them busy, especially at the Second Corps Hospital.

The Sanitary Commission was on the move again, but not by choice. The army was consolidating its various offices to downtown Gettysburg; officers had shown up at the door of the Robert F. McIlhenny dry-good establishment, carrying orders to evict the Commission from the facility which they had acquired not twenty-four hours earlier. "The next day [July 8]," wrote Dr. John Hancock Douglas, associate secretary of the Commission, and executive supervisor of the Gettysburg Sanitary Lodge, "our store-house was given up to the Provost-Marshal."[62]

Fortunately, continued Doctor Douglas, "another room on Baltimore Street was by his permission taken. The latter place, the store of Messrs. Fahnestock and Company [was] the largest in town." The new location, located at the corner of Baltimore and West Middle Street, was a clothing store owned by brothers James F., Henry J., and Edward G. Fahnestock. While Edward was off in Virginia serving with the 165th Pennsylvania, a local nine-month unit, the business was handled by his two older brothers.[63]

With its imposing three story brick construction and flat-roofed addition, the Fahnestock store was indeed the largest commercial structure in town. Union Maj. Gen. Oliver O. Howard had scrambled up on top of the building to make his initial observation of the battle unfolding west of town when he arrived in town on July 1. From this strategic vantage point, Howard quite probably finalized the critical decision as to where to rally the retreating Union forces.[64]

62. Moore, *The Rebellion Record*, 7:126.

63. *Ibid.*; Frassanito, *Early Photography at Gettysburg*, p. 99. Most of the Fahnestock merchandise had been moved out of town to safety before the battle even began. In fact, the paranoid Fahnestock brothers maintained their own railcar at the depot, for the express purpose of evacuating their inventory if Confederates were even suspected of being in the vicinity.

64. William A. Frassanito, *Gettysburg: A Journey in Time* (New York: Charles Scribner's Sons, 1975), p. 88; Frassanito, *Early Photography at Gettysburg*, pp. 98, 99.

The Fahnestock Brothers' emporium immediately "became the centre of the busiest scene which I have ever witnessed in connection with the Commission. Car load after car load were brought to this place," wrote Douglas, "till shelves and counter and floor up to the ceiling were filled, till there was barely a passage-way between the piles of boxes and barrels, till the sidewalk was monopolized, and even the street encroached on. These supplies were the outpourings of a grateful people."[65]

Many of the arriving parcels revealed handwritten messages as they were pre-sorted for distribution:

"These stockings were knit by a little girl five years old and she is going to knit some more, for mother says it will help some poor soldier."

"This blanket was used by a soldier in the war of 1812—may it keep some soldier warm in this war against traitors."

"This is a poor gift, but it is all I had," read a note stuffed in a small package of bandages, "I have given my husband and my boy, and only wish I have more to give, but I haven't."[66]

Just before leaving town after taking a number of photographs of battlefield dead and the aftermath of the struggle, Washington D.C. photographer Alexander Gardner and his crew stopped by to capture the bustling activity at the Fahnestock building on film.[67] An exposure made by Gardner, most likely in the morning sunlight of July 9, does indeed show boxes, crates, packing cartons, and trunks heaped up to the first floor windows, on the sidewalk, and out into the rutted street along the outside of the converted clothing emporium. There is even a confused swirl of people visible out front by the doorway, apparently Commission agents caught in the very act of manhandling supplies into the building through the main entrance. No less than three neatly-lettered signs, tacked up to a tree outside the front door and affixed to the building itself, announced the new home of the Sanitary Commission.[68]

---

65. Frassanito, *Gettysburg: A Journey in Time*, pp. 88-89; *The Sanitary Commission of the United States Army. A Succinct Narrative of Its Works and Purposes*, p. 155.
66. *Adams Sentinel*, March 22, 1864.
67. The Sanitary Commission was one of Gardner's favorite charities. So impressed was he with the relief work of the Commission that he personally produced an entire series of oversized album cards depicting the activities of the Commission during the Civil War, including the Gettysburg exposure of the Fahnestock building.
68. Frassanito, *Early Photography at Gettysburg*, pp. 98-99. Frassanito offers a detailed discussion of the date and time of the photograph.

Word of the move was rapidly dispatched to all the corps hospitals, and the new and greatly enlarged supply center threw open its doors for business at its third location in as many days. Little time was wasted before the growing mountains of supplies stacked inside, in front of, alongside of, and around the back of the big brick Sanitary Commission headquarters were on their way to the various corps hospitals. The Sanitary Commission also issued supplies to the twenty-four Confederate hospitals west of town, and the scene around the Fahnestock building—as Union blues intermingled with butternut and gray uniforms, as supply wagons manned by Confederates jostled for position with Union teamsters, and as Southern drawls were answered in Yankee twangs—must have astonished many visitors to Gettysburg.

In order to draw supplies, the Second Corps representatives had to deal with the ever-present paperwork incumbent upon any large organization. A clerk, under the watchful eyes of Mr. H. P. Dechert at the Sanitary Commission, and local lawyer R. G. McCreary at the Christian Commission, filled out the requisition form, securing the answer to a number of questions: What is your name? Where is your hospital? Who are the surgeons? How many wounded are currently at your hospital? Do you have any special needs today? "Each morning the supply wagons of the division and corps hospitals were before the door, and each day they went away laden with such articles as were desired to meet their wants."[69]

Even considering the huge inventory of the Sanitary Commission, there were bound to be some desperately needed items—supplies which had unexpectedly been exhausted, or equipment lost or broken—which were simply not immediately available. "If the articles needed one day were not in our possession at the time, they were immediately telegraphed for, and by the next train of cars thereafter they were ready to be delivered." If no one from the hospital was available to pick up the item(s), an agent from the Commission saw to it that the necessary goods were delivered promptly, and at any hour, to the proper medical facility.[70]

With the railroad up and running and once again carrying freight to Gettysburg, trainloads of refrigerated cars carrying perishable comestibles were arriving in staggering numbers. "Thus, tons of ice, mutton, poultry, fish, vegetables, soft bread, eggs, butter, and a variety

---

69. *The Sanitary Commission of the United States Army. A Succinct Narrative of Its Works and Purposes*, p. 155.
70. *Ibid.*

of other articles of substantial and delicate food, were provided for the wounded, with thousands of suits of clothing of all kinds, and hospital furniture in quantity to meet the emergency. It was a grand sight to see this exhibition of the tender care of the people for the people's braves. It was a bit of home feeling, of home bounty, brought to the tent, put into the hand of the wounded soldier."[71]

Another aspect of "home feeling" and "home bounty" were the visitors, families, and friends stepping off these trains at the Gettysburg depot. A fair share of these arrivals to the battlefield ended up in one of the corps hospitals, and the staff of the Second Corps were becoming well acquainted with some of these new arrivals. Noticeable among them were some very prominent men of the North, making their political presence felt even as they circulated among the casualties from their home states. "It is a very good place to meet celebrities; they come here from all parts of the United States to see their wounded. [Massachusetts] Senator [Henry] Wilson [chairman of the Senate Military Committee], [Illinois Representative] Mr. [Elihu B.] Washburn [*sic*], and one of the Minnesota Senators have been here."[72]

The Confederates were the focus of much attention from these visitors; the vast number of Northerners had never even seen anyone from south of the Mason-Dixon Line, and many now clustered about these unwilling guests of Pennsylvania to gawk and make sidelong comments. "We had no little fun (in all our misery, after this) and crowds of visitors were arriving every hour to inspect and examine in truly Yankee style, the wounded, and to see what kind of horns the rebels had upon their heads. Many came to assist in caring for the wounded, and brought clothes and blankets and cordials and medicines and what not."[73]

The Southerners managed to have a great deal of reciprocal fun at the expense of these Union sightseers, especially the ladies in the crowd. "Probably we enjoy the appearance of the inquisitive (female) portion of our visitors more than they did ours; and had no lack of fun at their expense. There is a celebrated Miss or Mrs. Farnsworth (I think that's the name); she views all around her with the eye of a

71. *Ibid.*
72. Hancock, *South After Gettysburg*, p. 15.
73. Dooley, *John Dooley*, pp. 118-19.

commanding general, and to hear the natives speak of her you might think that her sole coming was sufficient to heal all our wounds and save the dying from their menaced death.[74] Miss [Dorothea] Dix also is here, and condescends to converse with our party. This morning (July 10th) she spoke upon the harsh treatment of the Yankee prisoners in the South, and *we* spoke of the tyrannical rule of Yankee *rulers* in the South. She asked if we had ever heard of Gen. Dix; that he was a kind man; and that no one could accuse him of cruelty to any one under his command or control."[75]

A number of the male visitors voluntarily pitched in to help care for the flood of patients. "Scores of men, who at home had never been considered 'handy,' found themselves at once capable and willing nurses, washing and robing, as tenderly as a sister's hand could do, the poor, limp, grimy fellows, to whom a wash was as essential as powders and salves."[76]

For their part, the Southern wounded presented some disagreeable hygenic challenges for visitors and staff members alike. "The work was not in itself a pleasant one; many of those who fell into our hands were almost loathsomely dirty; one felt a desire often to get between them and the wind; and, probably, had we followed our inclinations, we should never have performed, in a single case, the process of ablution."[77]

Two other rather unique visitors stopped by the Second Corps hospitals during this time. Both were armed—not with musket and powder, or even with relief supplies, but rather with bulky camera apparatus, glass plates, and chemical solutions. Frederick Gutekunst had made the trip to Gettysburg within a few days of the end of the battle, accompanied by his assistant, Mr. J. Marshall. Gutekunst was

---

74. The "Miss or Mrs. Farnsworth" Dooley refers to is Eliza W. Farnham, Cornelia Hancock's sponsor.
75. Dooley, *John Dooley*, p. 119.
76. John Y. Foster, "Four Days at Gettysburg," *Harper's New Monthly Magazine*, vol. 38 (February 1864): 384-85.
77. *Ibid.*, p. 385.

born in 1831, but, by 1856, had already risen to prominence as one of the leading photographers in Philadelphia.[78]

Gutekunst's aim in coming to Gettysburg was philanthropic rather than merely photographic—he planned to donate all income from the sale of his battlefield photographs to aid the sick and wounded soldiers recuperating at Gettysburg. The August 1 *Philadelphia Inquirer* printed the following notice in the "City News" column:

> Views of the Battle-ground at Gettysburg, Pa.—F. Gutekunst, Nos. 704 and 706 Arch street, Philadelphia, respectfully announces that, aided personally by a prominent lawyer of Gettysburg, who was a useful guide to our forces during the battles there, he has succeeded in making several fine Photographic Views of prominent parts of the battle-ground at that eventful place.
>
> They are published in a series of seven 10 by 12 views, and will be sold by subscription only; the proceeds of sales to be used for the benefits of our sick and wounded soldiers.
>
> The subscription books and samples are now ready. The views are, viz:—
>
> 1. Major-General Meade's Head-quarters
> 2. The Field of Battle, July 1
> 3. Our Centre, looking east from Cemetery Hill
> 4. Gateway of the Cemetery
> 5. The Seminary
> 6. Residence of the "Old Patriot"[79]
> 7. Second Corps Hospital and Head-quarters United States Sanitary Commission [*sic*]
>
> The price of the set will be $10. Orders should be given at once to secure good prints and prompt delivery.—F. Gutekunst, Photographer, Nos. 704 and 706 Arch street, Philadelphia.[80]

Gutekunst's exposure of the Second Corps Hospital shows a grouping of tents pitched in the edge of a stand of trees, by the side of what was once a cornfield. To the right is a large hospital tent, with boxes, barrels, bales, carboys, jugs, and crates visible inside and out.

---

78. Frassanito, *Early Photography at Gettysburg*, p. 50.
79. A view of John Burns' home.
80. *Philadelphia Inquirer*, August 1, 1863, "City News" column.

On top of a barrel and a box, stacked precariously high, is a mounded heap of loaves of bread. Representatives of the Christian Commission, not the Sanitary Commission as Gutekunst mistakenly identified them, stand, sit, and lean against trees and boxes outside. In the background smaller hospital tents can be seen, standing in an orderly row.

Standing in the shadows, just to the right of the starkly-white tent on the left, are two women. The distance and the shadows make identification extremely difficult. However, on the other side of the tent, standing in plain view, is a folding amputation table. Cornelia Hancock mentions her tent's close proximity to the operating tables in her letters; at this early date, it is almost certain that one of these two women is Cornelia, pausing only long enough in her work to be photographed, and then back to work.

Off to the far left stand two men who appear to have been working in the July heat, since their sleeves are rolled up and they stand holding tools. These are most likely members of the crew pitching hospital tents, who just happened to wander by at the right moment. At least nineteen men can be seen in the photograph—one, an elderly gentleman seated in the foreground, incongrously attired in a top hat, another holding a straw boater, and the rest in an assortment of military and civilian headgear, or bareheaded. Clothing ranges from formal to casual.[81]

Central in the picture, leaning slightly against a tree, and standing dressed in black pants, vest, jacket, and hat, complete with gold watch chain, stands Justin Dwinelle himself, holding a book in one hand and a cigar in the other, and looking off into the distance. On the other side of the tree is another man—this one attired in a distinctive light patterned frock coat, with a Christian Commission ID badge on his waistcoat breast pocket, holding a paper in his right hand.[82]

---

81. Legend has it that the man in the top hat is the redoubtable John Burns, brought along specifically for the photo shoot.

82. Scott Michael Dwinelle, Letters to Roland R. Maust, January 16, 1999, and October 15, 1999; David Morris to Roland R. Maust, telephone call, April 19, 1999. This was most likely Mr. Andrew Cross, who headed the Second Corps Christian Commission depot. The badge, with its distinctive shape, was positively identified in an extreme enlargement of this photograph by Christian Commission reenactor Larry McGrane. See Gordon Dammann, *Pictorial Encyclopedia of Civil War Medical Instruments and Equipment, Volume III* (Missoula, Montana: Pictorial Histories Publishing Company, 1997), p. 115 for a picture of one of these ID badges. Made out of durable brass or German silver, they appear starkly white in black and white photography.

While Gutekunst records taking only one Second Corps hospital picture, a second photograph has surfaced that records another scene from the same hospital. This one transports the viewer to another view of Farmer Schwartz's fields, backed by a fringe of hardwoods and conifers, where a portion of the Second Corps Hospital is situated. If there was a crop growing in the field when the hospital arrived, it had long since been trampled into an unrecognizable mass of stalks and stubble by the time this picture was taken.

Seven tents are in evidence, three of which appear to be cobbled-together affairs of multi-colored and patterned blankets and tree branches. Each tent is rolled up from the bottom to encourage ventilation of the stale air inside. Behind one of the tents a medical supply wagon stands stationary, canvas sides drawn up to reveal the drawers and supplies within. Patients can be seen inside the canvas shelter tents, squinting out into the bright summer light at the photographer, laying supine on cots, each covered with blankets. An assortment of cups hang on the tentpost, ready when the call comes for a cool drink of water.

Staring back at the lens in solemn attention are staff and patients. To the right, members of the hospital guard are drawn up, some rigidly at attention, some slouching nonchalantly or leaning against a tent. Lined up in a segregated row to the left are the staff of surgeons, assistant surgeons, stewards, and one woman. Attired in a light dress, complete with jacket, bonnet, and wide hooped skirt, she stands partially blocking a man in a black silk top hat, this one bearded and far younger than the gentleman in the first photograph.

What visibly ties together these two scenes together is the presence of a man standing four persons to the right of the woman . . . dressed in a distinctive light patterned frock coat, with a Christian Commission ID Badge gleaming from his waistcoat breast pocket. The presence of the same man, dressed in exactly the same clothes, with the ID badge at the exact same spot on his coat, and appearing in both photos, in a hospital with over 3000 patients, plus staff, volunteers, commission agents, and visitors, strongly suggests that Gutekunst took *two* separate exposures on the same day, and chose to only use only one in his seven portrait series.[83]

---

83. Recently discovered evidence supports the suggestion that Gutekunst took two separate photographs of the Second Corps Hospital while in Gettysburg. A July 1863 *Philadelphia Press* clipping has been discovered included in a letter, dated July 20 in Philadelphia, and addressed to someone identified

Gutekunst returned to Philadelphia, developed his glass plates, and ran his advertisement in the July 23, 1863, *Philadelphia Inquirer*. He produced only a small number of sets; even at the price of ten dollars, the photographic essay of Gettysburg quickly sold out.[84]

Surrounded by a press of visitors anxious to reach the battlefield, United States Army Medical Inspector Edward P. Vollum stepped off the train as it reached the outskirts of town, and straight into the midst of railroad chaos. "I arrived at Gettysburg about 7 p.m. on the 8th, and, in consequence of some irregularity or delay in the railroad trains, there were about 2,000 slightly wounded men collected at a point a mile from town, where the trains stopped, without food, shelter, or attendance for the night. Fortunately, through the agents of the Sanitary Commission, these men were all fed, and some 300 sheltered that night."[85]

Obviously, something was going to have to be done, and done quickly, to get these men moved out of town before more seriously wounded soldiers started arriving. Fortunately, some preliminary efforts had already been begun at this end of the tracks. "No system had as yet been adopted for the transportation of the wounded, nor had this been possible in the deranged condition of the railroad, though Surg. J. D. Osborne, Fourth New Jersey, detailed for this purpose by Surg. H. Janes, U. S. Volunteers, in charge of the hospitals at Gettysburg, was using his best endeavors to work through the confusion and crowds of wounded with which he was surrounded, and I have to acknowledge the important services of this gentleman until the time of my departure."[86]

Surgeon Henry Janes, selected by Army of the Potomac Medical Director Jonathan Letterman to oversee the field hospitals at Gettysburg, must have been delighted to see Inspector Vollum walk

---

only as "S." The clipping refers to two separate exposures recorded by Gutekunst at the Second Corps field hospital in early July. "S" had arrived in Gettysburg sometime around July 8, and departed on July 17, 1863. [Frassanito, *Early Photography at Gettysburg,* p. 424, THE HOSPITALS, Second Corps hospitals, footnote 3].

84. *Philadelphia Inquirer*, July 23, 1863; Frassanito, *Early Photography at Gettysburg*, pp. 47-48.

85. *OR*, vol. 27, pt. 1, p. 26.

86. *Ibid.*

into his Gettysburg office. At thirty-one, Janes, a Waterbury, Vermont, native, had been practicing medicine for only eight years, including two years in the army. The bedlam and constant crises following the recent battle must have caused Janes to look back with longing eyes at his tranquil practice as house physician at New York's Bellevue Hospital.

Despite his youthful appearance, which even a bushy beard failed to disguise, Janes was widely regarded as something of an organizational whiz-kid. In fact, "his administrative abilities caused him to be selected more than once to establish and take charge of general hospitals for the Brigade and Division." But the arrival of another seasoned medical administrator from Washington was certainly a boon for both the overworked Janes and the accumulating backlog of battle casualties.[87]

Doctor Janes had already received a detailed description of the appalling conditions of the wounded from George K. Johnson, another medical inspector whom Surgeon General Hammond had sent to the battlefield. After touring the battlefield and hospital sites, he reported: "There were some in churches, some in barns, some in tents among the fruit trees, some in tents in the fields, some under such shelter as a farmer would be ashamed to show for his cows. Some were under blankets hung over cross-sticks, and some without even so much shelter as that. There were some scattered groups of men outside the hospitals. It sometimes appeared as if an experiment had been made to see how many wounded could be crowded into a given space in a house."[88]

As if the condition of Union hospitals was not grave enough, twenty-four Confederate hospitals had been discovered to the north and west of Gettysburg as the army set off in pursuit of Lee and his forces. Each was filled with horribly wounded men, with injuries too serious to risk the jouncing trip home to Confederate soil in springless wagons. Now these casualties, some 5,500 in number, were also thrown onto the mercy of Northern care. That was in addition to approximately 1,800 Confederate casualties already behind Union lines, plus the nearly 1,000 bleeding men gobbled up during the disastrous July 3

---

87. Gerard A. Patterson, "Gettysburg's Abandoned Wounded," *Civil War*, no. 54 (December 1995): 54, 56; Brig. Gen. W. T. H. Brooks, Commendation of Henry Janes, February 6, 1863, Medical Officers Files, Record Group 94, National Archives and Records Administration

88. Duncan, *The Medical Department of the United States Army*, p. 234.

offensive, plus an additional 800 or more Southern wounded packed into the buildings of Pennsylvania College. A supply shortage of catastrophic proportions was just a question of time.

It was going to be a massive job, but Vollum was determined to get the wounded evacuated as quickly and comfortably as possible. He immediately pitched into the job, working in close conjunction with Surgeons Osborne and Janes. The telegraph wires were soon humming, carrying messages from Vollum and Janes to the surgeon general's office and other authorities back in Washington.

The crisis hit with full force on July 9, the morning of Vollum's first full day in Gettysburg. Both medical and personal supplies were desperately needed by those wounded men still stranded back at the end of the line in Gettysburg, who did not benefit from the Sanitary Commission's efforts out by Rock Creek. There was no time to order the needed supplies through the quartermaster, fill out the proper requisition forms, and submit them through the standard channels. Surgeon Janes immediately handed the problem over to Medical Inspector Vollum, who proved himself up to the challenge. "On the day after my arrival, the demand for stationary, disinfectants, iodine, tincture of iron, and some other articles was so great and immediate, that I purchased them in Gettysburg, and sent the bills to the quartermaster there for payment."[89]

Even those measures were not sufficient to meet the shortfall, and Vollum had to go shopping again for still more supplies. "Before the arrival of Medical Inspector [Jonathan] Cuyler [Vollum's superior], as far as my time and opportunities admitted, I endeavored to make up the deficiencies in medical supplies at Gettysburg by telegraphing to Surgeon [Josiah] Simpson, U.S. Army, at Baltimore. In reply, he ordered liberal supplies of alcohol, solution chloride of soda, tincture of iron, creosote, nitric acid, permanganate of potassa, buckets, tin cups, stretchers, bed-sacks, and stationery of all kinds for 10,000 men in field hospitals."[90]

89. *OR*, vol. 27, pt. 1, p. 28.
90. *Ibid.*

Medical Director Jonathan Letterman sat in his headquarters with the Army of the Potomac on July 9, reading a plainly written wire from Surgeon Janes that must have given him pause to reconsider his decisions about the Gettysburg wounded: "The number of wounded here probably exceeded 20,000. We have been short of nurses, surgeons, and transportation, both ambulance and railroad."[91]

The very same day, the Surgeon General's office in Washington D.C. sent a telegram to one of its medical inspectors at Gettysburg. In four short sentences, the pencil-pushers in the capital demonstrated the unimaginable—their total lack of comprehension of the true situation in Gettysburg. "Unofficial reports are received that many supplies are needed at Gettysburg. Nothing official confirms these reports. Please answer at once. Do you need anything, ambulances or supplies?"[92]

---

91. *Ibid.*, vol. 27, pt. 3, p. 620.
92. Acting Surgeon General J. R. Smith, Letter to Medical Inspector Jonathan Cuyler, July 9, 1863, Office of the Surgeon General, Letters and Endorsements Sent to Medical Officers, Volume 4, Record Group 112, National Archives and Records Administration.

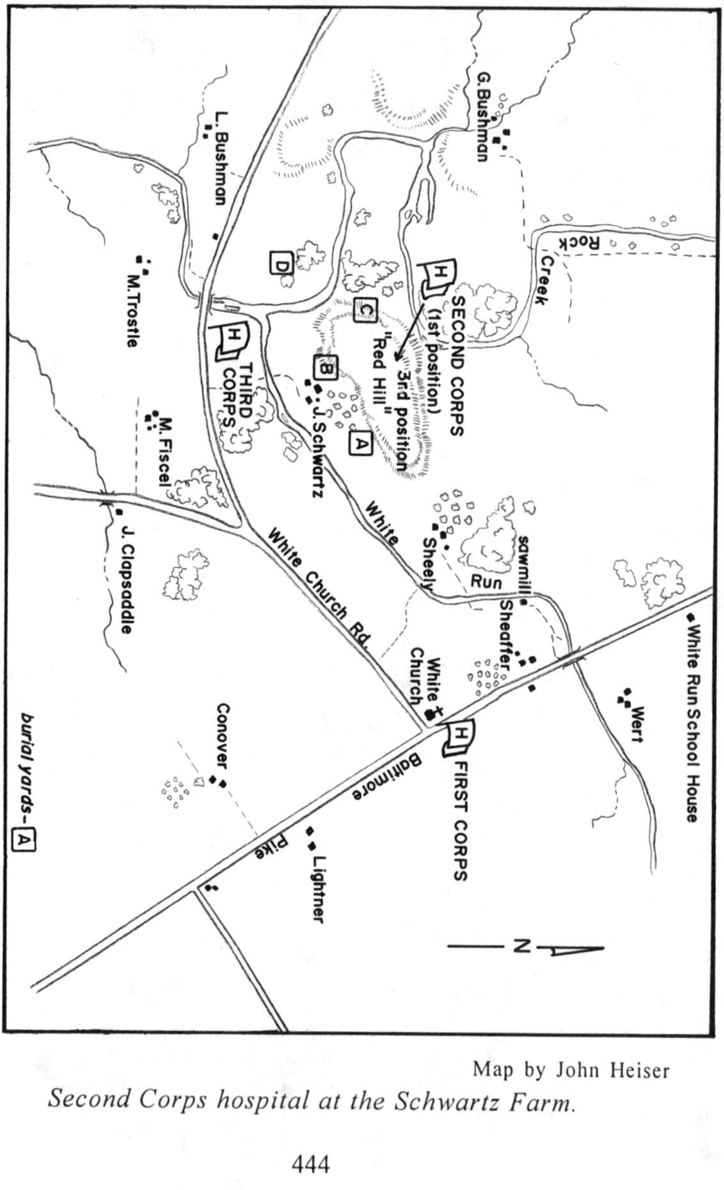

Map by John Heiser

Second Corps hospital at the Schwartz Farm.

CHAPTER 13

WEDNESDAY, JULY 8: DAWN—SUNDAY, JULY 12: MIDNIGHT

". . . am full of work and sorrow. . . ."

Ellen Orbison Harris
Ladies' Aid Society of Philadelphia

Gettysburg, Pennsylvania

As visitors continued to pour into Gettysburg, the volunteer nurses carried on their work faithfully and largely unnoticed—encouraging those that were improving, helping the men that were struggling, and comforting the wounded as they lay dying. Cornelia Hancock and the other volunteer nurses were out by the curbs of Gettysburg bright and early on the morning of Wednesday, July 8, waiting for their army transport to arrive. "We . . . go out about eight and come in about six—go in ambulances or army buggies. The surgeons of the Second Corps had one put at our disposal."[1]

Although yesterday's arrival of the medical supply wagons had brought sufficient army hospital tents to shelter all the wounded at the Second Corps, it was an ongoing process to get the great canvas monsters laid out and pitched for the thousands of men still lying in the open. There was a severe shortage of able-bodied men, or even wounded men with sufficient strength to render assistance, to erect the capacious walled tents, and the surgeons were still too busy to be of any assistance, especially with the departure of most of the surgeons and assistant surgeons to the Army of the Potomac on July 7. It was

1. Hancock, *South After Gettysburg*, p. 12.

still going to be a few more days before the job was finished, with everyone finally stretched out on regulation cots with army-issue blankets.

Even though it was beginning to look more and more like a normal army encampment, with the arrival of provisions putting everyone again in touch with standard army rations, the situation out at the Schwartz property when Cornelia Hancock and her associates arrived was still awfully grim. "I feel assured I shall never feel horrified at anything that may happen to me hereafter. There is a great want of surgeons here," wrote Cornelia to her sister; "there are hundreds of brave fellows, who have not had their wounds dressed since the battle. Brave is not the word; more Christian fortitude never was witnessed than they exhibit, always say[ing]—'Help my neighbor first he is worse.'"[2]

"For more than four weeks (beginning the first few days after the fight) we were engaged in the field hospitals of the Second Army Corps," wrote Jane Boswell Moore, who, with her mother at her side, cared for the needs of the Confederate wounded. "Words utterly fall short in describing the appearance of those woods in the morning we reached the hospital, after riding through swollen streams, amid the still unburied bodies of men and horses that lay putrefying on the field."[3]

Miss Moore describes in detail the state of things immediately following the flooding of Rock Creek. "The site of the hospital, which had been hurriedly chosen, was in a grove of trees on a piece of rising ground, surrounded nearly on all sides by a ravine, along which ran a creek near whose banks lay hundreds of wounded and dying Rebels, most of whom were exposed to the pitiless pelting of the storm. Such a thing as a cot, a bed, or a stretcher, was scarcely to be seen."[4]

Exposure was the common denominator to most of the Gettysburg wounded, Union and Confederate alike. "Scarcely had one man out of a thousand anything more than the ground, covered with an old

2. *Ibid.*
3. Jane Boswell Moore, "An Incident in Gettysburg," in *The United States Christian Commission. Second Report of the Committee of Maryland, September 1, 1863* (Baltimore: Sherwood & Co., 1863), p. 104.
4. *Ibid.*

blanket or oil cloth, to lay on, and hundreds had undergone amputation since the battle. Miserable little shelter-tents alone protected them from the rain, whilst numbers of the poor wretched Rebels had not even these, but were exposed through all the heavy rain of Tuesday night, with scarcely covering enough to keep warm in dry weather." She would be able to report with some satisfaction of the moving of the wounded, "ours mostly under the shelter of large tents."[5]

But as the tent city spread across the landscape, so, too, were the camp cemeteries expanding with each morning's burials. "But a few rods distant thirty or more interments were daily taking place. . . . Men were employed as grave diggers, and the dead lay at tent doors on the ground, as well as on the bloody stretchers, waiting burial."[6]

The five senses were constantly assaulted at the hospital with a barrage of sights, smells, and sounds. "Shrieks, cries and groans resounded on all sides, not only from those in the tents, but on the amputating tables, which were almost constantly occupied; and who could pass them without a dreadful shudder at those ghastly bleeding limbs heaped without, which the eye, however cautious, could not always avoid?"[7]

"All were clamorous for bread and butter; our own men were badly off; the Rebels begged piteously; the doctors were busily engaged in amputating; great piles of limbs being heaped up at the three different tents, and hundreds suffering to have their wounds washed and dressed. The air at times resounded with moans and shrieks of anguish."[8]

It was in this hellish maelstrom that Mrs. and Miss Moore turned their attentions to bringing about some semblance of order out of the discordant chaos. "We set to work immediately, buttering bread, making lemonade, changing bloody clothes for clean ones, giving out wines, brandy and towels. . . . We had many delegates on the ground, and yet how unequal to meet the wants of so vast a number!"[9]

---

5. *Ibid.*, pp. 106, 104.
6. *Ibid.*, pp. 104, 107.
7. *Ibid.*, pp. 104-5.
8. *Ibid.*, pp. 106-7.
9. *Ibid.*, p. 107.

Bushrod Washington James, as a medical representative of the Christian Commission, was working long, exhausting hours at one of those three operating tables, experiencing first-hand the critical shortage of skilled surgeons. "Every surgeon in the hospital was kept busy nearly a week amputating limbs, probing for and removing bullets, or sewing, bandaging and dressing the wounds of those who were too badly mangled and shattered to be aided in any more hopeful manner."[10]

Even with amputations going on nonstop, twenty-four hours a day, there were still not enough tables or surgeons to go around. "Every hour the improvised operating tables were full, and many of the poor fellows had to be operated upon while lying upon the damp ground. We could not help it," wrote a frustrated and anguished Doctor James. "Among the thousands, there were those who could not be allowed to wait until there was a vacant table."[11]

"Worse than that, my heart grew sick when I saw men, some officers among them, feverish and bleeding or weak almost to death because there were not then surgeons enough to operate upon the vast multitude in time to save them all ere gangrene set in, for the regimental surgeons had to join their commands on the march. With no bed but the earth, no comfort but a blanket, little food and drink, a knapsack pillow, and no possible surgical care, except the daily temporary dressings, they died, and we could not help it!"[12]

One volunteer nurse from Philadelphia published a gruesome report of the injuries that he saw in his rounds of the camp. His words are made all the more chilling by its matter-of-fact tone, more like a grocery list than a roll call of real, live, breathing and feeling men. "The wounds were of every imaginable description, and upon all parts of the person. There were wounds in the head, the breast, the abdomen, the legs, the feet, the hands; there were wounds of the flesh merely, and others affecting the vital organism; in some cases legs and arms were swept away so closely to the socket that it was impossible to gather up the

---

10. James, *Echoes of Battle*, p. 101.
11. *Ibid.*, pp. 101-2.
12. *Ibid.*, p. 102. Thirty-two years later, now a seasoned physician having seen all the challenges of a continuing medical practice, Doctor James still looked back aghast at the awful conditions at the Second Corps hospital at Gettysburg: "I have worked hard in my profession many a time, but the horror of that scene I can never forget! Nor the arduous labor of those days! It exceeded all that I have been called upon to perform before or since that fearful time." [*Ibid.*, p. 102.]

cords, and hurts were necessarily cauterized or left to fester and eat away the life; in others, the face would be partially shot away, leaving, perhaps, only a single eye or row of teeth; while in others still, simply an ear, or finger, or part of the nose would be missing."[13]

These were the kind of wounds that Doctor James was encountering at every turn, and the sheer immensity of human devastation was taking a horrible toll on the remaining Second Corps surgeons, and the few volunteer cutters. "We toiled nearly all day and night, snatching a few hours for rest only when we became too much exhausted to continue, began again as soon as nature would permit us to feel equal to the necessity. In fact, only the power of will kept some of us at our post. And we were such a pitiable few among so many wounded! The compulsory use of the knife was sadly trying, but, oh, it was far worse to see the wounded who were awaiting their turn, burning with fever or wasting with gangrene, which came quickly in the hot, sultry days of that weary season. It was July, and even those in health became almost exhausted in the sultry heat, but worse followed."[14]

The Confederates were also sweltering in the equatorial-like heat, and most were still not under any kind of shelter. Many whiled away the time by talking amongst themselves, even fraternizing with Union wounded and members of the hospital staff. Wounded Virginian John Dooley had struck up a conversation with another Irishman, an enemy soldier from Lowell, Massachusetts, as he sought to pass the long hours of tedium. The Northerner was seeking to learn news of some common friends from back home in Ireland.

After bringing the Bay Stater up to date with news of the mutual acquaintances, now fighting for the South, Dooley and another wounded Virginian berated the New Englander, who himself had experienced persecution in the Old Country, for now fighting on the side of the North. Dooley questioning how he could "consistently turn his back on his principles and for the pitiful hire of a few dollars do all in his power to crush a brave people asserting their right of self government; and now that he was engaged in the cause of tyranny,

13. Foster, "Four Days at Gettysburg," pp. 385-86.
14. James, *Echoes of Battle*, pp. 102-3.

fighting against honesty, Justice and right, and moreover against those very gallant young men he was seeking to hear of. . . ."[15]

The tongue-lashing worked a remarkable effect on the now-sheepish New Englander. "The poor fellow's eyes filled with tears. He said he didn't know how it was at all, but they got him to enlist and if he got back to Lowell he didn't think they'd 'get him again.'" The encounter had an unexpected outcome for Dooley and his comrades, laying exposed to the elements in the midday heat. "He then went off and returned with two good blankets and a fly-tent which he insisted on our taking from him; and then hastily bidding us good-bye was gone and we never saw him afterwards."[16]

Painfully working together, Dooley and his friends spread out the blankets under the meager shade of the fly tent, thinking all the while about the conversation with the Massachusetts man. "Perhaps we were too severe towards him," mused Dooley in his diary; "but when we see the Irishman supporting so foul a tyranny as ever blackened the pages of any history, our indignation cannot but be moved. . . ."[17]

Auburn, New York

For the overworked Second Corps surgeons, help was on the way in the person of Dr. Theodore Dimon. Dimon, like Dr. Bushrod James, had offered his professional services to the military in the past to care for the wounded; upon hearing of the need for medical help at the battlefield hospitals, he determined to volunteer his services again. On July 8, he sent off a telegram to the Surgeon General of the United States, offering to "report to any Army medical officer for duty, without expense to the Government if my services were needed, till the first of August." The following day, the return message came over the wire from Assistant Surgeon General Smith's office, "accepting [the] offer and directing me to report to Medical Inspector Cuyler U S A at Gettysburg."[18]

Dimon immediately gathered together his belongings, preparing to leave later in the evening of July 9. "Mr. James S. Seymour of Auburn

15. Dooley, *John Dooley*, p. 115.
16. *Ibid.*, pp. 115-16.
17. *Ibid.*, p. 116.
18. Theodore Dimon, *From Auburn to Antietam*, The Civil War journal of a battlefield surgeon who served with the Army of the Potomac 1861-1863, typescript copy in the Hospitalization after Gettysburg: Personal Accounts Vertical File, Gettysburg National Military Park, unnumbered pages.

with some other gentlemen advanced me one hundred dollars to defray my expenses while engaged in this service."[19]

Gettysburg, Pennsylvania

As if there were not already enough problems at the Second Corps hospital—shortage of surgical staff, lack of proper food, insufficient or inadequate shelter, and horribly unsanitary conditions—now a new problem was rearing its ugly head, and this one had the potential of being the most deadly of them all. "I begin now to suffer from thirst, for the only water they bring us is from a neighboring run which is warm and muddy and has the additional properties belonging to human blood and dead bodies." Being shot through both legs was bad enough for John Dooley, without having to drink contaminated water as well. "I have therefore determined to refrain from this nauseating and unhealthy draught as long as I possibly can."[20]

Dooley was absolutely right; the runoff from the almost daily thunderstorms, carrying the effluvia of decomposing and insufficiently buried soldiers, putrescent horse carcasses, and the hastily and carelessly located latrines of tens of thousands of men was tainting the water supply all around Gettysburg. In addition, the approximately 72,243 horses that came to town with both armies, from July 1 to 4, produced a staggering 433,458 gallons of urine, and over 1,950 *tons* of manure. All of this battlefield drainage had to go somewhere.[21]

Compounding the shortage of potable water was the fact that the water table of the entire region was being stressed far beyond its capacity. Most wells and cisterns had been drained dry within days by the mouths of thirsty soldiers, both friend and foe alike. Even with the extensive rainfall, it was simply going to take time to restore the depleted water table. In the meantime, all that remained for patients and staff of the Second Corps Hospital was the brackish and polluted drainings from the battlefield.

Dr. Bushrod Washington James remembered that noxious water and its effects very well. "There came a shower which washed the battle-field soil and drained it into the stream at the outskirts of the woods, it overflowed and infected the spring from which we obtained

19. *Ibid.* Seymour was the general agent of the State of New York for the relief of sick, wounded, and discharged soldiers, and reported directly to the governor. Dimon would serve as adjunct agent under Seymour.
20. Dooley, *John Dooley*, p. 113.
21. Magner, *Traveller and Company*, pp. 47-48.

water for drinking and cooking, and it was only a few hours until nearly every one in the camp was more or less affected with the dangerous poison."[22]

This was a problem with no apparent solution, because, in all the supplies being imported into Gettysburg, and then forwarded to the hospitals, from the very basic foodstuffs to the most exotic delicacies, there were no shipments of bottled water. "There appeared to be no help for it! We must use it or suffer with thirst. No one can tell how many more of those on that fearful field might have lived—maimed or crippled, perhaps—if it had not been for that infectious water, which must have involved almost every stream and spring near by the late field of carnage."[23]

Even the hospital staff were not immune to the effects of this fetid water; a number, including the indomitable Doctor James, suffered nausea and severe gastric problems from drinking the water, even after boiling it for protracted periods. James opted, like Dooley, to refrain from using the brown water, but the summer heat and exertion finally forced him to partake of it sparingly. "I refrained from drinking it until it was impossible to do without it longer, then I drank tea or coffee made with the water, and even after boiling, it had the power to sicken me; but it was the poor patients tossing with fever and begging for water who were most to be pitied. We knew that there was danger in the draught, and we gave it sparingly."[24]

With all the crises and difficulties at the hospitals, there was at least one bright spot on Wednesday, July 8—the primary operations, mostly amputations, were finally coming to an end. After the primary surgeries were completed on the Union wounded, the Confederates were then operated on and their wounds treated. Although it seems terribly harsh, it was a standard procedure in Civil War field hospitals, both Northern and Southern alike, that surgeons treated their own wounded first, then the wounded of the enemy. "Attending to our own first, which is our duty," as assistant Francis Wafer put it.[25]

---

22. James, *Echoes of Battle*, p. 103.
23. *Ibid.*
24. *Ibid.* "Even now, how vividly that row upon row of tents full of suffering humanity comes before my mind," added Doctor James, "and how powerless I felt to do even a modicum of good among so many!" [p. 103]
25. Wafer diary.

The remaining Second Corps surgeons had been putting in almost superhuman stints at the operating tables in order to process all the wounded men. At the First Division Hospital, Medical Director Richard C. Stiles stated in his after-action report that "Surg. [Charles Squire] Wood, who was left in charge of the division hospital, informs me that about 800 of our wounded & 200 of the enemy's were cared for in our division hospital—that he performed 120 capital operations, 150 operations in all—Surg. [William Warren] Potter performed 54 amputations & resections; and Surg. [J. W.] Wishart almost 30, making almost 230 operations in all."[26]

"It took nearly five days for some three hundred surgeons [in all seven of the Union Corps hospitals] to perform the amputations that occurred here [at Gettysburg], during which time the rebels lay in a dying condition without their wounds being dressed or scarce any food. If the rebels did not get severely punished for this battle, then I am no judge," added Cornelia Hancock sententiously.[27]

Since the Confederates had left only their most seriously injured men behind, there was an extremely high mortality rate among the Confederate wounded at the Second Corps hospitals. "We have but one rebel in our camp now [at the Third Division hospital south of the Schwartz farm]; he says he never fired his gun if he could help it, and, therefore, we treat him first rate. One man died this morning. I fixed him up as nicely as the place will allow; he will be buried this afternoon. We are becoming civilized here now and the men are cared for well."[28]

Their number now swelled by newcomers, the volunteer nurses continued to work their way through the growing city of hospital tents and its ever-increasing number of visitors, getting to know the wounded that they were treating. "The Second Corps did the heaviest fighting, and of course, all who were badly wounded, were in the thickest of the fight, and, therefore, we deal with the very best class of the men—that is the bravest. . . . The reason why they suffer more in this battle is because our army is victorious and marching *on* after Lee,

26. R. C. Stiles, Manuscript report of the First Division, Second Corps hospital operations during the Battle of Gettysburg, MSC 129, National Library of Medicine, Bethesda, Maryland, p. 5.
27. Hancock, *South After Gettysburg*, p. 13.
28. *Ibid.*

leaving the wounded for citizens and a very few surgeons. The citizens alone are stripped of everything they have so you must see the exhausting state of affairs. The Second Corps alone had two thousand men wounded, this I had from the Surgeon's head quarters."[29]

Cornelia Hancock was quickly discovering that she had a rather unique appeal to the seasoned veterans of Winfield Scott Hancock's corps. "My name is particularly grateful to them because it is Hancock. General Hancock is very popular with his men."[30]

As the condition of the men improved, their fighting spirit and political tendencies were beginning to return as well. Whenever a scrap of newspaper made its way onto the hospital grounds, the nurses would go from tent to tent, and then circulate throughout those still waiting to be taken to the tents as were pitched, reading and rereading the newsprint to each enthralled audience of listeners. "On reading the news of the copperhead performance, in a tent where eight men lay with nothing but stumps (they call a leg cut off above the knee a 'stump') they said if they hold on a little longer they would form a stump brigade and go and fight them."[31]

Along with a renewed interest in politics came a resurgence of partisan feelings between the Northerners and Confederates. Men who had magnanimously rendered aid to a fallen foe in the heat of battle were beginning to remember that this was the *enemy* that had put them in the hospital in the first place. Men in blue were put in tents with other Union men, while the Confederates were sequestered in their own tents or in Farmer Schwartz's barn.

Old campfire controversies and partisanships over favorite commanders were again popping up among the bored convalescents. "Most of the men are from New York here now; they are very intelligent and talk good politics. McClellan is their man mostly. Meade they think sympathizes with McClellan and therefore they like him. Hooker is at very low ebb except they think he fed them well—a circumstance that soldiers make great account of. Such feeders you never saw," enthused Miss Hancock.[32]

As for herself, the volunteer nurse from rural Hancock Bridge, New Jersey was taking to nursing as if she had been doing it all her life. After two challenging days spent at the Third Division Hospital of the

---

29. *Ibid.*, p. 12.
30. *Ibid.*
31. *Ibid.*, p. 13.
32. *Ibid.*, pp. 14-15.

Second Corps, she felt as if she was becoming quite the seasoned veteran of hospital care, and frequently looked down her nose at the new nursing arrivals and the other female visitors encroaching on her domain. "We have some plucky boys in the hospital, but they suffer awfully. One had his leg cut off yesterday, and some of the ladies, newcomers, were up to see him. I told them if they had seen as many as I had they would not go far to see the sight again. I could stand by and see a man's head taken off I believe—you get so used to it here. . . . I have torn almost all my clothes off of me, and Uncle Sam has given me a new suit. William says I am very popular here as I am such a contrast to some of the office-seeking women who swarm around hospitals. I am black as an Indian and dirty as a pig and as well as I ever was in my life—have a nice bunk and tent about twelve feet square. I have a bed that is made of four crotch sticks and some sticks laid on that with blankets on top. It is equal to any mattress ever made. The tent is open at night and sometimes I have laid in the damp all night long, and got up all right in the morning."[33]

"I have the cooking on my mind pretty much," she confided in one letter to her sister. Foodstuffs were now beginning to arrive regularly from both national and local relief associations, and kitchens cooking special diets for those unable to stomach standard army rations were up and running in each of the divisions. "The Christian Committee supports us and when they get tired the Sanitary is on hand. Uncle Sam is very rich, but very slow, and if it was not for the Sanitary, much suffering would ensue. We give the men toast and eggs for breakfast, beef tea at ten o'clock, ham and bread for dinner, and jelly and bread for supper. Dried rusk would be nice if they were only here."[34]

Unfortunately, fresh clothing and linens had not kept pace with the number of wounded coming into the hospitals. Every bit of water was needed for drinking and cleansing wounds; none could be spared for laundry purposes, and some things were desperately needed. "Bandages are plenty but sheets very scarce. We have plenty of woolen blankets now, in fact, the hospital is well supplied, but for about five days after the battle, the men had no blankets nor scarce any shelter. . . . Pads are terribly needed here. Bandages and lint are plenty. I would like to see seven barrels of dried rusk here."[35]

---

33. *Ibid.*, pp. 13-14. In this same letter, she writes that she was picked up in the morning and dropped off at night in Gettysburg. She apparently also had a tent at the hospital where she could stay over at night when the need arose.
34. *Ibid.*, p. 13.
35. *Ibid.*, pp. 13, 14.

With her shift coming to an end, a bone-tired Cornelia Hancock sat down to write a quick update to her sister as the sun set on another long day of ministering to the wounded:

> Gettysburg—July 8th, 1863
> My Dear Sister,
>
> . . . There is no mail that comes in, we send letters out: I believe the Government has possession of the road. I hope you will write. It would be very pleasant to have letters to read in the evening, for I am so tired I cannot write them. Get the Penn Relief to send clothing here; there are many men without anything but a shirt lying in poor shelter tents, calling on God to take them from this world of suffering; in fact the air is rent with petitions to deliver them from their sufferings.
>
> C. Hancock
>
> Direct boxes—E. W. Farnham, care of Dr. Horner, Gettysburg, Penna. for Second Corps Hospital. Do not neglect this; clothing is shockingly needed. We fare pretty well for delicacies sent up by men from Baltimore. If you direct your letters Miss Hancock, Second Corps, Third Division Hospital, do not scruple to put the Miss to it, and leave out Cornelia, as I am known only by that cognomen. I do not know when I shall go home—it will be according to how long this hospital stays here and whether another battle comes soon. . . .
>
> I do not know the day of the week or anything else. Business is slackening a little though -- order is beginning to reign in the hospital and soon things will be right. One poor fellow is hollowing fearfully now while his wounds are being dressed. . . .
>
> All is well with me; we do not know much war news, but I know I am doing all I can, so I do not concern further. Kill the copperheads. Write everything, however trifling, it is all interest here.
>
> From thy affectionate
> C. Hancock[36]

---

36. *Ibid.*, pp. 12-13, 15.

Volunteer nurse Charlotte McKay took upon herself the role of chief procurement officer for her divisional hospital. She made it her business to keep the larders stocked with whatever foodstuffs she could lay hands on, and set herself an arduous daily regimen to make it all happen.

> My programme for a day at Gettyburg was to rise as early as possible in the morning, and send out everything that was available in the way of food to the wounded. An item for one morning was a barrel of eggs, and as it was impossible to cook them all, they were distributed raw, the men who had the use of their hands making little fires in front of their tents, and boiling them in tincups, for themselves and their disabled comrades.
>
> Breakfast being over, I would ride to the town, and gather up everything in the way of sanitary supplies that I could get, from the Sanitary and Christian Commissions, the large and generously filled storehouse of Adams Express Co., or any quarter where they could be obtained I would take butter, eggs, and crackers by the barrel, dried fish by the half kentle [*sic*], and fresh meat in any quantity. . . .[37]

After making her early morning circuit of all the relief agencies, she returned to where she had left the army teamster and his vehicle, and told him where to go to pick up the requistioned supplies. "Having seen them loaded on an army wagon, [I] would return in my ambulance, which was well filled with lighter articles, in time to give some attention to dinner."[38]

With dinner cooked and served, there was still plenty of time before darkness closed on the camp to personally make the rounds through the camp. "The remainder of the day would be devoted to the distribution of such stimulants as egg nog and milk punch,—which would be prepared in large buckets, and served to the patients in little tin-cups,—or supplying there with clothing, pocket-handkerchiefs, cologne, bay rum, anything that could be had to alleviate their sufferings."[39]

---

37. McKay, *Stories of Hospital and Camp*, pp. 51-52.
38. *Ibid.*, p. 52.
39. *Ibid.*

When her visits were finally completed, she made the weary trip back to Gettysburg in an ambulance to catch a few brief hours of sleep, and then the demanding cycle of foraging resumed anew.

"Thus passed nearly six weeks at Gettysburg, with little variation in the daily routine, save that which came from urgent claims of special cases of suffering, which, indeed, were many. Men with both hands amputated or disabled, who would eat nothing unless I gave the food with my own hands; men discouraged and desponding from loss of limbs, and painfulness of wounds, to whom a few cheerful or playful words would do good like a medicine; men dying, to whom a few words of sympathy and encouragement as to the future were so precious."[40]

Charlotte's fellow hitchhiker on the government wagon train, Rev. Isaac W. Monfort, was also busy bringing supplies out to the hospital. The Indiana Military Agent, along with his five staff members, were delighted when the railroad reopened, and supplies were able to flow into town. "I had the pleasure of loading a six mule team several times with provisions for our wounded in the different corps hospitals," wrote Monfort. Gov. Oliver O. Morton had chosen his military agent well, and Hoosier troops scattered in and around Gettysburg benefitted from his compassion and wholehearted dedication to duty.[41]

With the primary operations now coming to an end, the surgeons, following their first real night of sleep in over a week, set to work on the morning of July 9 to dress the wounds of the men with serious, but non-fatal, wounds.

Men with wounds considered mortal were largely left alone to die, freeing up time to devote to those who had at least some hope of survival. Mary Cadwell Fisher, volunteer nurse from York, Pennsylvania, was one of the very few who paused to visit with these "fatalities." "Among the most harrowing in those days of horrible sights were those of sufferers who had been left to their inevitable death. There was no time or means on the first day or two after the

40. *Ibid.*, p. 53.

41. *Indianapolis Daily Journal*, July 23, 1863, p. 2.

battle to spend on the mortally wounded. Our strength and resources were taxed to the uttermost limit to even insufficiently help the men who had a chance of life, but those whose days were numbered and were pronounced beyond surgical aid had to depend upon their fellow-sufferers' care. Many a poor fellow died on the hard ground, with no shelter, and happy he who found a pitying comrade to close his eyes and fold his hands across his wounded breast. I could never pass the unfortunates without stopping a moment to say some word of sympathy or give the cup of cold water for which they thirsted."[42]

In this dumping ground of "mortally wounded" lay Capt. John G. B. Adams of the 19th Massachusetts Volunteers. With several serious wounds, his case had been pronounced hopeless almost a week earlier, but he had stubbornly clung to life, left to his own devices until now.

"I remained here [at the Second Corps hospital at the Schwartz Farm] six days, and my wounds received no attention only such as my comrades gave. They kept my canteen filled with water, which I used freely, to prevent inflammation. Do not think that I blame the surgeons. No nobler men ever lived than composed the medical staff of the Army of the Potomac; but there were twenty thousand wounded men, and the cases requiring amputation must receive attention first."[43]

Even though his wounds had still not been examined and cleaned by a surgeon, Adams was greatly encouraged by a visit from fellow officers of his regiment. "One day I was made happy. Lieutenant Shackley and Adjutant Hill came to see me. They had ridden back fifteen miles. Some of the boys had found a chicken, and they had made a broth and brought it to me in an old coffee pot. It was the first thing that had tasted good, and I shared it with [Duncan] Sherwood [Company A, 19th Massachusetts Volunteers]. Some think soldiers are hard-hearted. No hearts more tender can be found than in the breasts of brave men."[44]

After spending some time with their desperately wounded comrades, it was finally time for the visitors to ride back to their regiment. As far as they knew, this was the last time they would ever meet their "dying" friend Captain Adams, and it was terribly hard to say good-bye. "When those officers parted from me that day not one of us could speak, and tears ran down our cheeks as we pressed each other's hands."[45]

---

42. Fisher, "A Week on Gettysburg Field."
43. Adams, *Reminiscences of the Nineteenth Massachusetts*, p. 71.
44. *Ibid.*, p. 72.
45. *Ibid.*

Others of the wounded were being showered with gifts of food and "delicacies," foodstuffs thought to be desirable because of rarity or palatability—canned lobster and oysters, caviar, home canned pickles, preserves, fresh fruits, a vast range of domestic and imported wines, and alcoholic decoctions of every imaginable kind. "All of [the] home luxuries that *could* be carried, were lavished with an unsparing hand by a now deeply grateful people," noted Anna Morris Holstein.[46]

"Everyone who came to see me brought something that they thought might tempt the appetite," remembered one soldier wounded on July 3. "The Hon[orable] and Colonel [Levi] Maish, who was himself convalescing from wounds received at Antietam, made several journeys from his home at York, Pa., to Gettysburg, to bring me delicacies that would have been the delight of an epicure. One corner of the tent was literally packed with all sorts of canned provisions, baskets of champagne, native and foreign still wines and liquors of all kinds."[47]

Unfortunately, not all of the wounded were able to enjoy this windfall of goodies. Those with severe injuries to the mouth and throat often greatly desired these tempting items, but could not chew or swallow the foods. Others, with wounds about the chest and abdominal cavities, often did not desire to eat anything at all. Patients with life-threatening fevers and infections could not bear the rich fatty foods, and, for those that lay dying, thoughts were of friends and family in distant homes, and not of food, however epicurean it might be.

Even those with non-mortal injuries, such as amputations, were finding it hard to find someone to examine their wounds after surgery, and change their dressings. "The surgeons were continually engaged upon new cases that had received no attention. Those of us that had been treated knew this, and we found no fault at what otherwise would have been terrible neglect. I think it was six days after my amputation

46. Holstein, *Three Years in Field Hospitals*, p. 40.
47. Nickerson, "Personal Recollections of Two Visits to Gettysburg," pp. 23-24. Levi Maish was the colonel of the 130th Pennsylvania Infantry.

before a doctor could be found to look at my stump," remembered Lt. Charles Fuller of the 61st New York Volunteer Infantry.[48]

Fuller had been experiencing the full range of phantom pains and novel sensations from his missing leg. "The night before [the doctor's visit] I had been made very nervous by crawley [*sic*] feelings on that side of me, just where I could not tell. It is, I think, the rule with amputations, that the patient cannot from the feeling put his hand on the place of amputation. It takes a good while for the nerves to realize where 'the end' is. They were made to carry the news to the brain from the extremities, and, until the new arrangement has become somewhat acquainted with the change, these lines of communication are doing duty for parts of the body not there. My bad feelings were not at the end of the stump, but down in the foot and ankle, where there were constant beats, and pulls and cramps."[49]

By July 9, even the Confederate wounded were finally being moved under military shelter as the hospital tents continued to be put up. After spending the previous day beneath the meager shade of the fly tent provided by the conscience-stricken Massachusetts soldier, Dooley and his tentmates were upgraded to a full-size hospital tent. "My condition is somewhat ameliorated by the kindness of our Lowell Irishman, and today, Thursday [the] 9th, 5 or 6 of us are assigned to a larger tent and here for the first time my wounds are washed and some lint and bandage put over them. They give me no pain unless when I try to walk or stand. There are incipient maggots in them which further develop themselves in a few days."[50]

Maggots proved to be the bane of most of the Second Corps patients, regardless of uniform color or patriotic sympathies. "Great green flies in swarms of millians [*sic*] gathered in the camp, grown unnaturally large, fattened on human blood," remembered one Confederate casualty. "Fever-smitten, pain-racked, there came to us another terror: we were to be devoured while living by maggots—creeping, doubling, crawling in among the nerves and devouring the soldier while yet alive." Even the sound that the silent little creatures made, when present in sufficient number in an open wound, added to

48. Fuller, *Personal Recollections*, p. 102.
49. *Ibid.*, pp. 102-3.
50. Dooley, *John Dooley*, p. 117.

the feelings of loathing. "The noise they made as they doubled and twisted, crept and crawled, was that of hogs eating corn."[51]

After having finally been provided adequate shelter, and having his wounds cleaned and dressed for the first time, John Dooley lay back on his Army of the Potomac cot and waited to see what new experiences awaited him as a prisoner of war.

With the Second Corps hospitals now stepping down from emergency status and beginning to operate as a longterm convalescent facility, the primary focus changed from crisis surgery to the bedside care of thousands of wounded men. Secondary surgeries (for men who had not been strong enough earlier) and amputations (for limbs and members that developed gangrene or had not properly healed) were going on, but not at the frenzied pace of the past week.

Sadly, there were some injuries that could not be cured by all the surgery or medicine or care that could be provided at the hospitals. Sometimes, the effect of the minié balls or shrapnel were too devastating, ripping and puncturing what simply could not be fixed. Every day, the bodies of those that had died, furiously fighting for life to the very last instant in the heat of the bright daylight, or surrendering to quiet death in their feverish sleep, were laid outside tents doors or along the walkways of the hospitals, awaiting burial.

"The mortality, especially among the Confederates, was very great for several days after the battle," remembered Rev. Thomas G. Murphey, chaplain of the 1st Delaware Veteran Volunteers. "The surgeon [Harry M. McAbee] in charge of our [Third] Division Hospital assigned me to the duty of burying the dead. An idea of the scarcity of assistance and of the mortality may be inferred from the fact that, although every effort in our power was made to inter the dead, they accumulated, and lay for days unburied. At length we were obliged to call in assistance from another Division Hospital."[52]

---

51. W. C. Ward, "Incidents and Experiences on the Battlefield of Gettysburg," *Confederate Veteran*, vol. 8 (1900): 348-49. In actuality, the maggots were extremely helpful, eating only the necrotic flesh in the wound in a very efficient manner. However, to men feeling the frantic wriggling of the little white critters inside open wounds and sores, one might easily imagine being eaten alive from the inside out.
52. Murphey, *Four Years in the War*, pp. 123-24.

The shortage of able-bodied men was now acute at the hospitals. With the bulk of the army away pursuing the retreating Confederates, the only uninjured help in the medical facility were a now-drastically reduced contingent of eighteen Second Corps surgeons and assistant surgeons, a smattering of hospital stewards, a thirty-man hospital guard detail, fifty male nurses and attendants assigned by the medical director, a few volunteer commission agents, a handful of Confederate surgeons and assitants, and any soldiers specifically left behind by their commanders to care for the wounded of their regiment. Among these few were spread the necessity for medically caring for the wounded, moving the wounded as the need arose, pitching the tents, slaughtering and dressing the beef cattle, unloading incoming supply wagons, distributing clothing, medicines and food, and burial of the dead. Without the aid of the volunteers that continued arriving at the Second Corps, many of the jobs would simply not have been accomplished. As it was, the wounded still often found themselves laying side by side with the dead, waiting for someone to take the deceased away for burial. One soldier remembered a corpse "lay by my side [from early morning] until afternoon, before they could find time to take him away."[53]

The Second Corps wounded had left a trail of graveyards in their wake as they moved from the battlefield, on through the aid stations and divisional hospitals, finally to arrive at the corps hospital. The ground in the triangle between the Bryan Farm, the Peter Frey farmstead, and the Hummelbaugh place, even though sown with boulders and rocky scree, saw at least one hundred and sixty-three burials as the cemeteries of the two aid stations ran together and overflowed with the mortally wounded, and those dead on arrival from the battlelines. The First Brigade of the First Division buried at least three of their dead on the farm of the J. Bair family. Brig. Gen. Alexander S. Webb's "Philadelphia Brigade" of the Second Division seems to have had their own personal cemetery for their killed in action on July 3—the 69th, 71st, and 72nd Pennsylvania buried at least ten of their men in the fields of the G. Herling (or Herting) Farm. The Third Division aid station attendants at the Jacob Swisher house laid at least eight

53. Adams, *Reminiscences of the Nineteenth Massachusetts*, p. 71.

Second Corpsmen to rest out behind the farmhouse, including two troopers of the 6th New York Cavalry, which served as corps headquarter guard.

Back at the divisional hospitals clustered near the western end of Granite Schoolhouse Road, small cemeteries were created spontaneously around the back of this house, or on the other side of that barn, as patients in critical condition expired from the trauma of invasive wounds and massive shock. Six interments were made in various recognizable places on the William Patterson Farm (such as near a cedar tree, or near the fortifications, or near the Second Corps divisional hospital). Even Sarah Patterson had a few Second Corps burials on her property.

As the bodies of the dead began to accumulate at the Corps hospital out beyond Rock Creek, so, too, did the need for places to inter them. The Schwartz farmlands were soon dotted with four growing cemeteries, called "yards" in some records, near the three division hospitals. "Yard A" was a Union cemetery closely adjacent to the farm buildings, in a field to the northwest of the barn and house. "Yard B," holding both Union and Confederate bodies, was off to the southwest, between the Schwartz buildings and those of neighbor Lewis A. Bushman, whose farm sat on the western side of Rock Creek. "Yard C" lay on a hill along Rock Creek, in the woods on a ridge known as "Red Hill," and both Northerners and Southerners were interred there. "Yard D" lay along a lane through a cornfield, near a walnut tree, at an unspecified location, but probably south of the farmstead in the vicinity of the confluence of Rock Creek and White Run. It likewise saw burials of bodies clad in bloody blue uniforms, as well as those dressed in ripped and punctured butternut and gray.

Beyond the four official "Yards," there were also a series of other "unofficial" cemetery plots scattered about the expansive Second Corps facility. The Schwartz farm lane was flanked by the graves of at least nine casualties from the Third Corps, along with one lonely Confederate, interred under the cooling shade of a stand of walnut trees. The Third Division Hospital, a half-mile south of the other two division facilities, used Michael Trostle's "Walnut Row" as an extensive burial ground, with at least twenty-three interments from that division, as well as a few from other Second Corps divisions.[54]

54. This is the compilation of local Dr. J. W. C. O'Neal's physician's handbook, journal, and letters; local Dr. Rufus Weaver's letters, notes, and reports sent to various Southern women's organizations seeking reinterment of their

Death, even death on such a massive scale, was still a somber and humbling thing. Here, in the midst of mass pandemonium and medical chaos, some efforts were still made to observe the social mores of everyday life, and to honor the passing of those who did not survive.

The bodies were brought out to the nearest "yard" and laid out for burial. Nurses tenderly cleaned up each corpse after death, arranged the clothing as neatly as possible, and wrapped the remains in an army blanket. (Only those fortunate enough to have friends with ready cash were buried in coffins, and those in the price range of foot soldiers were often made of unadorned pine boards, hastily nailed together).

William and Anna Holstein from Upper Merion, Pennsylvania, had taken personal supervision of the burials at at least one of the cemeteries; they would walk out to the open graves when all was ready. After putting on his spectacles, William read a brief burial service and prayed over the deceased. When the ceremonies were completed, the burial detail (sometimes composed of friends and acquaintances of the soldier) would lower the corpse into the grave, then shovel the gaping hole shut in the hot July sunshine. Headboards, made of whatever flat boards were available, were erected by the hospital staff, and included name, rank, and regiment. Fitting remarks were sometimes added, written in pencil or crayon by friends or relatives. Frequently the nurses could be seen walking through the cemeteries in the evenings, reading the markers and silently grieving over the wounded men they had come to know and love, and had been unable to save.[55]

Nurses, and whatever other staff and friends were available, often came out to see the final disposition of favorite messmates or patients that they had befriended. With deadening regularity, the bearers

---

dead; S. G. Elliott's map of the disinterments; assorted recollections, memoirs, letters, diaries, and newspaper articles; and the detailed roster of known Confederate dead, compiled by Kathleen Georg Harrison from the handbook and burial lists of Dr. John W. C. O'Neal, J. G. Frey, the Weaver family and others, Gettysburg National Militray Park Library. In addition, the tracking and identification of the cemeteries reflect the statistical analysis by this author of the extant records of burials, disinterments, and reinterments which he compiled of the Second Corps hospitals.

55. Holstein, *Three Years in Field Hospitals*, pp. 41-42; Philadelphia *North American*, Sunday, June 29, 1913, special section, p. 4.

brought ravaged bodies out to the four cemeteries, and there they were buried. Swaddled in coarse army blankets, the corpses were laid out, the make-shift shrouds here and there stained red from seepage of death wounds; white faces, etched with pain, silent now, and still. No eulogies, no bands, and little pomp and glory attending these simple funerals; but then, dying at the Second Corps hospital was a very unglamorous end to the hopes and dreams of many young men.

As the sun went down on July 9, the situation at the hospitals was slowly improving, but the burial details were still running far behind. The sight of the dead, Union and Confederate, lying slack and cold awaiting burial grieved the nurses trying so desperately to save lives. Ellen Orbison Harris had been at the Second Corps hospitals since July 4, and the pressures of those five days were beginning to tell on the slender field secretary of the Philadelphia Ladies Aid Society. As she sat down to write to one of her constituents, fatigue and despair sounded heavily in each pen stroke:

> Gettysburg, July 9, 1863.
> My Dear Dr.:
> . . . Am full of work and sorrow. The condition of things here beggars all description. Our dead lie unburied, and our wounded neglected. . . . Our wounded in numbers have been drowned by the sudden rising of the waters around, and thousands of them are still naked and starving. God pity us! pity us![56]

Friday, July 10, found the hospital hunkering down to the long-term task of restoring the wounded men to some semblance of health, and getting them evacuated away from the pestilential atmosphere and poisonous water of Gettysburg to general hospitals back east as quickly as humanly possible. The time for frantic action was largely past now; what remained was the patient ministration to men doggedly fighting off infections and fevers; men struggling to recover from the

56. *Report of the Ladies' Aid Society*, p. 13.

trauma of losing an arm, a leg, or a combination of appendages; men mustering their strength to come back from the edge of death; men slowly dying, and knowing it.

"The events daily occurring in the hospitals were most painful," wrote Anna Ella Holstein; "they might be summed up, briefly, to be: fearfully wounded men; nurses watching for the hour when suffering would cease, and the soldier be at *rest*; parents and friends crowding to the hospital, hoping for the best, yet fearing the worst; strong men praying that they might live *just long enough* to see, but *once* more, wife, or child, or mother."[57]

"Not the least distressing sight, after a great battle, is that of friends in search of the wounded and fallen," wrote another nurse. "Ofttimes the claims of those suffering are so great that the dead can scarcely be thought of." In ever increasing numbers, these folks were now finding their way out to the clustered hospitals east of Rock Creek. From metropolitan neighborhoods and isolated farms they came—fathers and brothers, mothers, wives, and sisters, the wealthy and the impoverished—it made no difference now; all were on an equal footing as they made their way, with desperate hopes of who they would not find, and gnawing fears of who they *would* find, in the wards of the corps hospitals. These were mixed hopes and fears—hoping that their son, brother, or husband was really not there at all, but back at the regiment; then again, being wounded was far better than being shot dead on the field—or was it? For many, it was a desperate race against time and mortality to reach loved ones before it might be forever too late.[58]

Nurses and other hospital volunteers were now called upon to extend their care, not just to the thousands of wounded, but to frantic family members and friends as well. Sometimes this care involved going to incredible lengths to be of help, as illustrated by Baltimore nurse Jane Boswell Moore. "One evening a poor widow, with five little children at home dependent on her earnings as a seamstress, came from Philadelphia to look for her eldest boy on the field of Gettysburg. She had heard he was dead, but could not believe it. On reaching the hospital she was told he was in one of the tents. 'O,' she said, 'how my heart beat for joy! but when I went in, they told me he was dead.'"[59]

---

57. Holstein, *Three Years in Field Hospitals*, p. 40.
58. Moore, *Women of the War*, p. 562.
59. *Ibid.*

Those in the tent and other wounded related the story of his last fight. "He had written to her that nothing would induce him to miss this final battle, as on it depended the fate of Pennsylvania, and perhaps the whole country. During the last day's battle he had raised his head from behind a stone wall to fire, and being shot through the head, was instantly killed. 'O,' said the poor mother, 'if I could only know he was prepared!' She could be resigned to it all, she said, if her boy's body could go with her, and be buried where she could see his grave. And in perfect trust, she handed me fifteen dollars,—all she had—and begged me to tell her what to do."[60]

As a Second Corps nurse, Jane Boswell Moore's time was already consumed with the care of the wounded entrusted to her oversight. Still, she searched for a way to be of help to this distraught mother. "I had not a minute to spare, save early in the morning; but I made diligent inquiry, and found a comrade of her son, who described his grave. Then we went together to the man who removed and prepared bodies for transportation."[61]

The average price of embalming in Gettysburg was $20.00, with another $15.00 needed to cover the cost of the coffin and case. Transportation costs from the battlefield to the family cemetery or private plot back home were currently about $30.00. Payment of gravediggers on both ends of the trip, any food and lodging along the way, and other miscellaneous expenditures, could add still further to the overall expense.[62] It was painfully obvious to Miss Moore that the widow's fifteen dollars would barely begin to cover the costs of taking her son back to Philadelphia. "It was clear her money would amount to little. I said so while I was thinking what to do, and she fearfully caught at the words, assuring me she would sew at government tents and bags, any length of time after her return, to make it up. 'Such an idea never entered my mind,' I replied; 'I was only thinking of what was best to do. We will arrange it some way.'"[63]

After reassuring the grieving mother, the first necessity was to find her a place to stay while she waited for her son's body. "So I told her story to the grave-digger, whose wife at once gave her board in their humble house, while her husband reduced his charges. Then we walked to [the] Adams express office, passing a great pile of rusty

---

60. *Ibid.*
61. *Ibid.*, pp. 562-63.
62. Coco, *Wasted Valor*, p. 136.
63. Moore, *Women of the War*, p. 563.

muskets lately gathered from the battle-field. I could hardly get her away from these. 'I wonder if *my* boy's is there,' she said sadly; and then, as she entered the express office, where her feeling overcame her, 'It was through it,' she said, 'my boy used to send me his little bit of money!' Only the beginning, I thought, of sad memories to haunt her after-life."[64]

The Adams Express Company, a private cartage and rail freight carrier, had been instrumental in the transportation of much of the foods, relief supplies, and medicines for the various relief commissions, and Jane Boswell Moore felt confident she could look to them for help in shipping the boy's remains home. "Here I pleaded her case again, not doubting the result, as every facility possible had been afforded me during the war from the company. Transportation tickets to Baltimore were next procured, and I hurriedly wrote, in the office of the provost, a note to a friend who would pass her the rest of the way."[65]

With all the paperwork and transportation details cared for, the grim task of retrieving the body yet remained. "Then she rode in the ambulance as far as it went on her way to search for the grave, and I promised to see her again in the evening." With her shift at the hospital over, the young nurse from Baltimore made her way in the gathering darkness to the gravedigger's home to visit the widow. "The excitement was then over; she had found the grave, and though unable to see her boy, a lock of hair had been cut for her, and all was ready for her to leave on the morrow, a gentleman in Philadelphia having offered her burial-room in his lot. But words failed her when she tried to express gratitude; she could only pour out blessing."[66]

This same story, with minor variations, would be enacted again and again in the ensuing days and weeks, a mournful and unexpected Greek tragedy of epic proportions played out in the lives of unprepared relatives, in the shadow of departing armies following the end of battlefield fighting. But for these devastated family members and friends, however, the battle was only beginning as they made arrangements for funeral services in distant cities and remote villages, donning mourning bands on arms and hats, draping black crepe from their doorsills. For them, the war had forever ripped away a vital part of their very being that could never be replaced. For the widows, the

---

64. *Ibid.*
65. *Ibid.*
66. *Ibid.*, pp. 563-64.

orphans, for the grieving mothers, destitute fathers, and bereft fiancees of both North and South, the name "Gettysburg" would linger as a constant anathema, an ever-present malignant reminder of pain and irretrievable loss.

Relief in the form of volunteers and supplies continued arriving in Gettysburg. Dr. Cyrus Cort, pastor of the Reformed Church of Altoona, Pennsylvania, had walked most of the way from Carlisle to minister to the wounded. Arriving July 8, he noted in his diary the torrential rains that had swollen many of the neighboring creeks, and had caused much havoc at the Second Corps Hospital site along Rock Creek two days before. The pastor even had difficulty fording some of the streams, so much had they risen above their banks.

After working the battlefield area for two days, Cort and a companion found themselves in the fields south of the Schwartz Farm at the Third Division hospital.

> Friday July 10, 1863 I visited the 2nd Army Corps Hospital four miles from town where we saw sights never to be forgotten. The woods and creek bottoms were full of badly wounded rebels who piteously asked for water, medicine, attention to wounds, etc. Amputations were rapidly taking place by rebel and Union doctors. Most of the wounded were North Carolinians and Georgians who were hurled against the impregnable entrenchments of Round Top and swept down like chaff [probably referring to Pickett's Charge]. These men expressed abhorrence of the war and of their ambitious leaders who presipitated [*sic*] secession. We labored in behalf of the Christian Commission (Dr. Cort and friend were then young clergymen) until dark among these fallen foes.[67]

67. Ambrose Cort, Sr., Letter to R. L. Jones, October 25, 1933, photocopy in Hospitalization after Gettysburg: Personal Accounts Vertical File, Gettysburg National Military Park Library. While conditions were quite austere for all the Confederate wounded, they were especially so at the Third Division hospital. There, the Southern casualties were consistently mentioned by witnesses as laying on the slopes along Rock Creek. Even as late as July 11, these men were still waiting to be moved under some shelter. The Third Division hospital, separated as it was from those of the other two

Mary Cadwell Fisher and her companions from York had also found the Confederate wounded to be in poor shape.

> Much of my work lay among the Confederate troops, whom I found in a most deplorable condition. In some instances they were entirely destitute of clothing, being covered with a piece of old blanket. Others had nothing on but a ragged shirt or pair of drawers, those who were fortunate enough to have two garments sharing with those who had none. The long march had completely worn out the poor uniform, and the distance from the base of their supplies rendered it impossible to replace them. Providentially our ample stores enabled us to clothe them all decently.[68]

Working her way through the wounded Confederates, she struck up conversations with a number of them; for their part, they were glad to have someone with which to talk.

> How emaciated they were! Some of them told me they had subsisted almost entirely upon corn, gathered from the fields in their hurried march, which ravenous hunger often compelled them to devour green from the stalk. After the struggle was over and there was no longer need for exertion, nature seemed to have exhausted her resources, and they were for the most part indifferent, depressed and hopeless.[69]

With evening coming on, hospital steward Charles Merrick of the 8th Ohio, serving at the Third Division hospital, paused long enough to jot a quick note home to his wife, Dr. Myra Merrick, the first female physician to practice in Cleveland, Ohio:

---

divisions, and caring for the vast majority of the Confederates, was simply overwhelmed by the vast number of severely wounded men it was called upon to treat. Consequently, they lagged significantly behind the rest of the Second Corps in sheltering and clothing these wounded prisoners.

68. Fisher, "A Week on Gettysburg Field."

69. *Ibid.*

Gettysburg Hospital
July 10th, 1863
Dear Wife,
. . . Some of our slightly wounded are gone. I still have forty who need constant care. About six of them I have no hope of saving. Capt. [Azor] Nickerson is better to night. The various Sanitary Commissions are pouring in supplies and there are lots of women workers busy among the men.

I have not had time to criticize their work or their looks much. I notice one peculiarity. The[y] all seem to take awful long strides when walking. One abominable "Bloomer" is visible occasionally. Mrs. [Ellen Orbison] Harris is here. I like her quiet, lady-like Quakerish manner. She is prompt in business—quick in decision—pious in speach [*sic*]—uses no unnecessary words.

I have written to Dr. [Joseph L.] Brenton [regimental surgeon of the 8th Ohio] to day. I hope our boys will be removed soon to some City and I be sent to the Regiment, although I do not mean to be "weary in well doing."

I wish I could get a letter from you, but that I cannot hope at present. There is one case of Tetanus a few steps from where I now sit. But it is getting dark. Bless the dear ones at home.
Love as ever,
Charles[70]

That "quiet, lady-like Quakerish" Mrs. Harris was also sitting at the Third Division hospital, not far from Steward Merrick, penning a letter to Mrs. J. of the Philadelphia Ladies Aid Society, the woman responsible for the forwarding of all collected supplies to society representatives working in field hospitals. After working for a few days at the First Division hospital, Harris had moved her efforts down to the Third Division, most likely because of the primitive conditions still in existence there. Much had happened since yesterday, and much of the melancholy so evident in her last letter was now gone.

70. Charles H. Merrick, Letter to his wife, Dr. Myra H. Merrick, July 10, 1863, William P. Palmer Collection, Container 1, Folder 3, MSS 3088, Western Reserve Historical Society, Cleveland, Ohio.

Gettysburg, July 10, 1863.

My Dear Mrs. J.:

Since Saturday, the 4th, I have been on this "field of blood," seeing suffering of the most fearful character. Every hour brought to my view my own boys, maimed and mutilated, whose joyful greetings almost break my heart. The poor fellows, how bravely they bear the loss of members, and such extreme discomforts, which would be hard to bear by men in good health. Abijah, our Abijah is now dying; lost a leg; was taken off close to the body. But I cannot particularize.[71]

Thirty-eight boxes of stores from "Ladies Aid" have reached us. We are sending many to Frederick City. A battle is imminent there. . . .[72]

Have had opportunities of conversing with many rebel officers; they all admit the war to be "the slaveholders war." A chaplain from Florida, an intelligent and Christian man, justified the war, saying, "The preservation of slavery, one of God's wisest and most beneficial plans for Christianizing the African race, demanded and deserves all the blood and treasures given to its defence." Is it not wonderful?

Miss B. goes with me.[73] An ambulance has gone on with chloroform, sticking plaster, &c., to be ready at once, should a battle occur. The amount of stores here at this time is very large, more than adequate to meet present wants, indeed prospective ones, except in the matter of bread and butter.

---

71. Pvt. Abijah Crosby, Company C, 19th Maine had worked as an aide throughout the war with Ellen Orbison Harris and other members of the Philadelphia Ladies Aide Society. Crosby was wounded in the left leg on either July 2 or 3, and the leg was amputated at the middle third. He died July 12, and was buried at the temporary aid station at the Jacob Swisher Farm. In her letters, Harris sometimes referred to him as "Abijah the poet." [Conklin, *Women at Gettysburg*, p. 398, Harris note 4; Appendix 5—"Private Abijah Crosby."]
72. Scuttlebutt from army sources indicated that the Army of the Potomac was going to bring Lee and his army to battle in the vicinity of Frederick, Maryland. As so often happens with the military "grapevine," the rumor proved to be false.
73. Probably Charlotte Bradford, a Ladies Aid Society coworker also from Philadelphia.

> We have cut and dispensed four hundred loaves daily, and comforted many.[74]

With her letter finished, the field secretary from Philadelphia saw to its posting, then set about making final arrangements for her departure for Frederick.

The delegation from the Ascension Church in Philadelphia finally reached Gettysburg on Friday, July 10. It had been a tedious and tiring four day trip, and John Y. Foster and the other relief agents were exhausted when they arrived.

> . . . Bridges, railroads, every thing within rebel reach had been destroyed; horses, wagons, and even cattle had been carried off, and travel was difficult. Now and then some dilapidated vehicle crept cautiously along the highway; occasionally a company of returning refugees crowded to join our little caravan; but otherwise the pulses of life seemed to have stopped their beating in all the smitten region. Even sleeping accommodations were scarcely to be had; as we neared our destination every house seemed to be stripped of the most ordinary conveniences.
>
> We arrived at Gettysburg in a drizzling rain, on the evening of Friday, July 10, and reported to the head-quarters of the Christian Commission, were immediately assigned to duty at the Second Army Corps field-hospital, situated on a wooded slope on the Baltimore pike, some four miles from the town.[75]

If these volunteers thought that they had seen devastation along the road from Philadelphia, it was nothing compared to what they saw around them now. Even a full week after the end of battle, desolation and destruction surrounded them as they headed their jaded teams out the Baltimore Pike in the dwindling light of evening.

74. *Report of the Ladies' Aid Society*, pp. 13-14.
75. Foster, "Four Days at Gettysburg," p. 381.

> The scene which presented itself as we proceeded toward our destination no words can depict. Every where the scars and rents of the conflict which had raged along these hills was painfully visible. . . . Every tree was scarred and torn, a chilly blight resting upon its summer crown of beauty. Almost every bush was a lair into which some one had crept for refuge, and found it in agonizing death. Far and near along the hills and in the stretches of lowlands tents stood out against the gathering shadows, revealing where the wounded and dying lay. Here and there great girdles of fire blazoned the slopes, telling of slaughtered animals slowly consuming. Broken caissons, knapsacks, canteens, and small-arms were strewn on every path. Fences were prostrate, and blood sprinkled every tuft of grass which the feet of the contending armies had not trampled down. The houses presented marks of the conflict. One, which was occupied as a hospital, revealed a gaping wound in the second story, where a cannon-ball had gone straight through. . . . Other buildings were riddled in a hundred places; and all, except those used for hospital purposes, were deserted, not a light flashing in the windows, not a child playing on the door-step, not even a dog growling at the gate as we marched on toward our destination through the gathering night.[76]

Awed by the vast and terrible silence, the wagon train pressed on through the outskirts of town, searching for some sign of the Second Corps hospitals.

With some few sketchy directions, and an occasional question of a passerby, the Philadelphia delegation saw the campfires of the Second Corps hospital blazing off to the right of the Pike. They arrived late enough, however, that there was little that could be done in the gathering darkness. The volunteers unhitched and groomed their teams, then sought out some place to stretch out for the night. Saturday morning, July 11, arrived all too soon, and they were soon rubbing the sleep from their eyes, all the while looking around at the

76. *Ibid.*

bustle of activity in the Schwartz farmyard, house, outbuildings, and fields.

> The following morning our labors commenced in earnest. Stores had come up, and their distribution was a duty and a necessity. On all sides the wounded and sick were pleading for help.
>
> "Do carry me to a tent."
>
> "Must we lie here forever?"
>
> "I am *so* weak; can't you give me something to revive me?"
>
> "Please give me a drink of water."
>
> "I want something to eat."
>
> "O, God! must I die here alone?"
>
> Such were the appeals which sounded in our ears.[77]

The situation of the Confederates at the hospital was so grave that Foster and his men were quickly assigned to minister specifically to them.

> Especially were the rebels in need of attention. While Lee, in retreating, had left a detail of men and a number of surgeons to look after his wounded, the necessity of effort was so urgent and immediate that, had they been disposed, they could hardly care for a tenth part of those who were actually suffering. To the care of our enemies, therefore, we devoted our chief attention.[78]

Foster and his companions were struck with the same utter destitution of the captured enemy troops that had so affected Mary Cadwell Fisher when dealing with the Confederates.

> Their condition was horrible. All were dirty, many were filthy, while others were almost absolutely naked, and crouched in their tents, as if ashamed to look into any human face. Almost the first sufferer we encountered was destitute of every article of clothing except a torn shirt; he lay huddled in a heap, striving, in obedience to an irrepressible instinct,

---

77. *Ibid.*, p. 382.
78. *Ibid.*

> to hide his shame and nakedness. Many others we found stretched out upon the ground, silent and helpless, with only blankets flung over them. All lay upon the ground, with pools of water all around them, often with channels the rains had made flowing under them in the hollow of the soil.[79]

John Dooley of the 1st Virginia Infantry stalwartly declared that General Lee had left behind "many hundreds of nurses (from among our private soldiers) and many surgeons of his army to assist and to care for the thousands of the brave men whom he knew could not receive the attention they required from the hands of the enemy." Unfortunately for the almost one thousand Southerners at the Second Corps hospitals, the Confederate commander apparently left behind only those doctors and nurses that could be spared, and many (if not most) were simply not top quality medical men. While primary surgeries were largely finished at the First and Second Divisions, Southern surgeons, aided by some Northern cutters, were still swamped with amputations at the Third Division.[80]

The two-story Schwartz barn, looming over the house and outbuildings of the barnyard, served as a horrifying centerpiece of all the Confederate surgical activity in the First and Second Division hospitals. "In that part of the field to which we were assigned there was a barn, which had been taken as a hospital by the rebel surgeons. The building was broad and strong, but was rather slatternly than otherwise, and by no means, in the manner of cleanliness, what was desirable for hospital use. The rebel surgeons, however, every thing having been removed by the rebel cavalry upon their first appearance, had piled the ground-floor with their wounded, placing them so thickly that it was almost impossible for one to stir without communicating a shock to all."[81]

---

79. *Ibid.*
80. Dooley, *John Dooley*, p. 115; Foster, "Four Days at Gettysburg," p. 382. The exact number of Confederate surgeons and staff left behind in Gettysburg is uncertain. General McLaws' division of Longstreet's corps, one of nine divisions in the Army of Northern Virginia, reported that ten medical officers, two chaplains, and seventy nurses and cooks were left with the division's 576 wounded when General Lee and his troops retreated. Whether this was typical for the other Southern divisions in unknown. [*OR*, vol. 27, pt. 2, pp. 364-65].
81. Foster, "Four Days at Gettysburg," p. 382.

But worse—far, far worse—than the overcrowding in the filthy cattle pens of the barn was the bloody spectacle that dominated the lower floor. "In the centre of the floor the surgeons planted a table for amputating purposes; and there, in full view of hundreds of enfeebled wretches, the process of cutting, and carving, and butchering (for it was nothing else) went on day after day. The scene, as we saw on more than one occasion, was horrible. It was torture for the faint, disheartened wounded to lie, hour after hour, perfectly helpless, compulsory witnesses of the atrocities which these surgeons dignified by the name of 'operations.'"[82]

While their Union counterparts labored around the clock, even to the point of total prostration, to treat the injuries of the wounded, the Confederate surgeons apparently did not work at night. Whether it was due to a lack of lanterns, or simply because they got tired, almost all of the Southern medical team rested nine hours every night before resuming surgery in the morning. "During every minute of fifteen hours every day some sufferer was upon the table. Groans, shrieks, and curses constantly filled the air, the sound of the knife and crash of the saw blending continuously with the din of agony. Legs and arms falling from the table were raked out in armfuls, with every eye fixed on the spectacle, and carried away for burial."[83]

John Y. Foster, for one, was highly derogatory of the Confederate surgeons left behind by General Lee. "It may be said here as elsewhere that much of this distressing condition of the rebel wounded was owing to the neglect and indifference of their own surgeons. Many of these surgeons seemed altogether destitute of those sensibilities which lend a softening influence to the rugged necessities and always forbidding duties of this important office. Some were almost brutal in their treatment of the men left to their care. Indeed, among all the officers and men whom the rebel commanders had intrusted [*sic*] with this work, we saw but a single one—a captain—who appeared to

---

82. *Ibid.* Amputations of this period did indeed look like butchery to civilians unaccustomed to seeing military surgery.

83. *Ibid.*, pp. 382-83. It seems very strange that the Sanitary and Christian Commissions, which fell over backwards supplying every possible need of the hospitals, could not have provided lanterns had the Confederate surgeons requested them. Justin Dwinelle, as surgeon-in-charge of the Second Corps hospitals, was widely known for his equitable treatment of all the wounded, Northern and Southern alike, and would surely have seen that lanterns were supplied if requested by the Confederate surgical team. As hard as it is to imagine, the Confederate doctors left behind seem to have preferred getting sleep at night to treating all of their wounded as quickly as possible.

appreciate the gravity and importance of his office. Night and day, regardless of personal comfort, indifferent to every thing except the welfare of his suffering soldiers, he planned and worked, facing bravely all emergencies, overcoming all obstacles, and so commended himself to those about him that every face kindles at his coming, and all felt the influence of his high example."[84]

For the hopeful wives and sweethearts of wounded Virginians, or Carolinians, or Georgians, having passed through enemy lines, having endured jibes and taunts all the long way to Gettysburg, the grisly spectacle of unearthly screams and severed body parts must have been totally inconceivable. "One circumstance alone which fell under my personal observation will quite suffice, without elaborating further this unpleasant topic, the utter insensibility and want of feeling on the part of the rebel surgeons. The day of our arrival the wife of a rebel officer, who was supposed to have been wounded, rode up to the place we have described, thinking that possibly she might there discover her husband. The groans and screams of agony which saluted her were quite sufficient to fill her mind with dread and sickening fear; but she was doomed to see in a worse form still the barbarous nature of the treatment which might possibly fall to the lot of the one she sought."[85]

"Hardly had she stated to an officer the object of her visit, when a rebel surgeon, with a knife in his hand, leaving a victim on the table, came to the door, and in a loud voice directed one of the hospital detail to 'fetch him a carving-knife,' adding that he would like to have also a razor-strop, as his 'instrument was getting dull.' The scene was too much for the smitten woman. Covering her face, she urged the driver to his quickest pace, and, with the unutterable wail surging in her ears, was hurried away."[86]

Having experienced such unthinking callousness and harsh treatment at the hands of their own surgeons, most wounded Confederates were stunned by the care and compassion shown them by members of the Sanitary Commission, the Christian Commission, the surgeons, and volunteers of the Second Corps. "The effect upon the enemy of the kindly ministrations of the representatives of the

84. *Ibid.*, p. 383.
85. *Ibid.*
86. *Ibid.*

Sanitary and Christian Commission, who thronged the field, in such marked contrast with the treatment of their own nurses, was most marked and palpable. At first many did not seem able to understand it; but when the fact dawned upon them their surprise knew no bounds. They had been taught to regard Northern men as savages; but they found that they had tender hearts, and carried blessings instead of curses in their palms, and for the most part they accepted the kindness frankly and thankfully in the spirit in which it was offered. Scores of men said to us daily, 'We are disappointed in you Northern men; you are doing more for us than we deserve, and much as you are doing, we see that you would gladly do more if you could.'"[87]

All the hopes and dreams of the Southern wounded for a dramatic Confederate victory over demoralized Northern foes had ended ignominiously in captivity behind enemy lines. For many, fierce nationalism and regional pride had crumbled, only to give way to feelings of anger, embarrassment, and confusion. "One short week before they stood in battle array, with 'all the pride, pomp and circumstance of war,' to crush the Northern army. Now prisoners on the invaded soil they lay at the mercy of their captors. They manifested the utmost surprise at the impartial treatment they received at our hands, and could not understand why we fed and clothed them as promptly and willingly as we did our own men."[88]

Mary Cadwell Fisher related one such encounter she had with a group of quizzical Confederate wounded.

> One day, after a very fatiguing morning, I sat down on a stump for a moment's rest among the Southern soldiers. As usual a group of boys gathered around me and one said:
>
> "Madam, I can't understand your treatment of us, Our women would not be so willing to help prisoners from your army, but you are just as kind to us as to your own men."
>
> "Oh," I said, "the reason is that we do not look upon you as enemies. We still regard you as our children, and although you have gone astray we have not given you up and expect you to come back to us, just as a loving mother hopes her wayward boy will repent of his wanderings and disobediences and return again to take his place around the hearthstone. You belong to us yet, and the time will come

87. *Ibid.*
88. Fisher, "A Week on Gettysburg Field."

when we shall again be one people, under a united government."

"Well, boys," said one of the brightest of them, "there is something in that. Now, mar'm, won't you please give us a chaw of tobacker?"[89]

The Confederate death-toll continued to mount. Lee had left behind only the most severely injured men, many with hopeless wounds. Now, even though in the relative care of a corps hospital, these mortally wounded men, in ones and twos, finally succumbed to the effects of their injuries. "Within three hundred yards of the headquarters of the 2d Corps Hospitals, I saw, on Sabbath morning, the 12th inst., twenty-seven bodies of dead confederates, unburied, the food of worms," reported Indiana Military Agent Rev. Isaac W. Monfort to his governor on July 16. "The living, too, in many cases, were found, whose wounds were alive with the maggot. It was not possible, with the supply of surgeons left, to do all that was needed to be done."[90]

But due in large part to the ministrations of the volunteer nurses, coupled with the care and supplies of the Sanitary Commission, Christian Commission, and smaller organizations such as the Baltimore Fireman's Relief Organization and the Germantown Field Hospital Association, many of the Confederates were well on the road to recovery. In spite of the dire circumstances in which they found themselves, the good humor of these seasoned campaigners was slowly returning. Soon even the nurses who had been faithfully caring for their wounds were becoming the target of their good-natured jesting. "What fun we have when the nurses come round to administer 'cornstarch.' About every hour a nurse of the feminine persuasion enters the tent and gives each one about a tea spoonful of this delectable refection. All take it just for the fun of the thing."[91]

Philadelphia, Pennsylvania

It had been a long day for Dr. Theodore Dimon, still on the road from New York. He had arrived late the previous night in Philadelphia; at

89. *Ibid.*
90. *Indianapolis Daily Journal*, July 23, 1863, p. 2.
91. Dooley, *John Dooley*, p. 119.

first light, he was out trying to discover the best way to reach the battlefield. "After inquiring about the condition of the railroad communication with Gettysburg I concluded to take the Pennsylvania Central R. R. to Columbia on the Susquehanna."[92]

Heading northwest to go west was not the straightest way to reach Gettysburg, but Dimon was mostly headed in the right direction. "Accordingly, on the morning of the 11th [of] July I took the cars for Columbia, Pa. The bridge across the Susquehanna had been burned on one of the last days of June to prevent Lee's troops from crossing the river at this point. I was ferried over the river to Wrightsville in a small rowboat. I here found the Northern Central (Pa.) [Rail] Road had been broken up by the Confederate troops and took a private conveyance to York where I got dinner."[93]

After heading southwest to York, Dimon was following in the tracks of both Dr. Bushroad Washington James and his party, as well as Mary Cadwell Fisher and her companions. But instead of walking as had James, Dimon got lucky—this time veering off to the southeast. "By good fortune I soon obtained railroad transportation in a quartermaster train to Hanover Junction and thence by similar means to Hanover, where I was obliged to remain for the night."[94]

As the New York doctor settled in for the night, he had an opportunity to size up his traveling companions. "The carriage from the Junction to Hanover was upon freight cars and the train was crowded with people going to Gettysburg for various reasons. Some out of curiosity to see the battlefield and get trophies, some to take care of wounded friends and relatives, some few to make a profit and business out of the matter, and some to aid in the care of the wounded of their own and other states."[95]

Philadelphia had also seen some very odd correspondence over the last several days, between some of the highest members of the United States Army Medical Department. The cause of all this stir was the unprecedented size of Medical Director Jonathan Letterman's liquor requestion.

92. Dimon, *From Auburn to Antietam.*
93. *Ibid.*
94. *Ibid.*
95. *Ibid.*

Medical Purveyor Murray, in Philadelphia, a stickler for details and a tight-fisted bureaucrat of the old school, had sent off a panicky dispatch to Surgeon General Hammond on July 7: "Sir, I am receiving requisitions every few days for brandy, 100 dozen is required by Surg Letterman for Gettysburg and Frederick. This will take all I have on hand & it is important that I should have some for emergencies. I propose to make a purchase of 800 or 1000 gallons to be put up at the Laboratory, unless you disapprove of it." Apparently, Purveyor Murray did not deem the aftermath of Gettysburg to be an emergency, and was anxious to pass the buck to the surgeon general as quickly as possible.[96]

Surgeon General Hammond's office wrote back three days later, trying to straighten out the boondoggle, but Medical Purveyor Murray was still blustering and fidgeting over the paperwork in his Philadelphia office.

On July 11, the flappable Murray wrote again to Washington: "I have the honor to acknowledge your letter of the 10th inst. in relation to issue of brandy instead of whiskey, & explaining the requirements for my accounts, etc. I am receiving large requisitions from the field in Pa. & Md. & for the Hospitals here, occasionally articles are ordered & approved by the Med Director here which are not on the supply table. Shall I continue to issue these, or ought such requisitions be referred to your office?"[97]

Happily, Doctor Letterman and the Gettysburg hospitals did finally get their brandy, as well as "articles . . . not on the supply table," in spite of the preponderance of military red tape and petty tin despots like Medical Purveyor Murray.

Gettysburg, Pennsylvania

Doctor Dimon and his fellow passengers were up early, all intent on reaching the town of Gettysburg. "At 7 A.M. I left Hanover and arrived in an hour at Gettysburg. . . . At 8 A.M. of the 12th . . . I reported to the Medical Inspector in charge of the general management of the wounded, viz. Dr. [John M.] Cuyler. I found his office on the central square of the town. He said that if I would call again at 9 A.M. he would

---

96. Record Group 112, Office of the Surgeon General, Letters Received, 1818-1870, Box No. 66, Letters Received, July 1, 1863—February 29, 1864, National Archives and Records Administration.

97. *Ibid.*

give me transportation out to the 2nd Corps Field hospital to report to Surgeon Divinelle [*sic*] and to take charge of Confederate wounded who needed assistance there."[98]

At last, there was going to be one administrative person detailed to oversee the care of the Southerners at the bloody barn on the Schwartz Farm. While waiting, Dimon took the opportunity to nose around town and get the feel of Gettysburg. "Meanwhile I deposited my traps at the Purveyor's office and made inquiries so far as possible among people excited and busy with the crowd of unusual occurrences. I found as usual great readiness to convey information among the volunteers and great reticence about the same among the regular medical officers here, while the volunteers appeared to be the most busy and the regulars to have the most liesure [*sic*], and probably for the reason that very much of their business was attended to for them by others."[99]

Finding so many medical men in one place, Dimon asked them how to find the Second Corps hospital. First one, then another shook their heads. Each in turn—every surgeon, assistant surgeon, contract surgeon, and hospital steward—were totally ignorant of the location of the largest Union field hospital at Gettysburg. "The result of my inquiries were nil. I could not ascertain where the 2nd Corps hospital was, nor what chances for eating or sleeping were to be obtained there. Nothing to eat was purchasable in the town."[100]

With such grave need for a qualified surgeon to oversee the care of wounded Southerners at the Second Corps hospitals, the Confederates still waiting to be treated were just going to have to wait a little longer. Unable to locate Surgeon Justin Dwinelle and his facilities, even at the headquarters of the medical department in Gettysburg, Medical Inspector Cuyler finally assigned Doctor Dimon, by default, to care for wounded New Yorkers at a temporary hospital in one of Gettysburg's hotels.[101]

For now, at least, the Second Corps Confederate wounded were just going to have to do without the services of Dr. Theodore Dimon. Throughout Sunday, July 12, the push continued to finish up the

98. Dimon, *From Auburn to Antietam.*
99. *Ibid.*
100. *Ibid.*
101. *Ibid.*

primary surgeries of the wounded Southerners. For the many ministers representing volunteer aid societies, this was going to be another Lord's Day without time to devote to any worship services. Many of the nurses and representatives of various relief organizations rallied in a major effort to feed, clothe, and dress the wounds of those Southerners still awaiting the none-so-gentle attentions of their surgeons.

Not everyone, however, was delighted with the generous treatment accorded to the Second Corps' unwilling guests. Hospital Steward Charles Merrick of the 8th Ohio was extremely irritated by the attention paid to the enemy soldiers laying in the camp. Frustrated and angry, he ended up blowing off steam in a letter to his doctor wife Myra, detailing the apparent injustices he had observed on the part of the various relief agencies laboring at the Second Corps, Third Division hospital:

> Washburn from Elyria and Stanley from Cleve[land] are here.
> Gettysburg, Pa, July 12th, '63
> Dear Wife,
>
> I have been the rounds among my patients and report to you their condition. I have only about twenty left—most of them I have sent away—some of them have died. I have eight very serious cases yet, two of them I have no hope for. Since I wrote to you, two have died, which makes seven since the battle. The two cases I refer to are both shot through the nates—the ball coming out near the os pubis. One has the rectum and bladder both wounded—the other the rectum. We have plenty of help as far as dressers are concerned, but no Surgeon at all to look after the boys.
>
> Our boys are very indignant at the conduct of the "Christian [and] Sanitary Commissions." They devote almost their whole time to the rebels—give them everything to eat and wear—preach and pray with them—but pay very little attention to our men. I have watched them close and bear testimony against them. Not once have they had singing and praying among the Union boys. Is it a compliment to us? Are we so good we do not need their missionary labors? I don't complain on this point, but I do complain that our boys have not had their share of the comforts, the delicacies, the attention they bestow on the rebels. The 14th Ind Sutler sent a lot of wine to their boys. The "Christian Commission" took it and gave every drop to

the rebels. These are facts. They will doctor up the rebels and send them back into their ranks to shoot us down with less mercy than ever.

I went over the battle field yesterday. The citizens are flocking there in crowds, hunting for relics. I counted thirty dead horses in one Battery alone—that is, the Battery we lay in front of. The trees are terribly cut by the storm of shells and solid shot. Gettysburg is a pretty little city. It is not much hurt by cannon, but bullet marks are visible on almost every house and store.

I hope I shall be able to return to the Reg soon, and expect to find a pile of letters then. My health is good.

As ever,
Charles[102]

Others in the three division hospitals of the Second Corps were also wishing they could escape to healthier environs. The polluted water was beginning to take a grave toll on inmates of the camps, both doctors and patients alike.

As for wounded Virginian John Dooley, he stubbornly refused to drink any of the tainted water. While others sickened from the contamination, Dooley gritted his teeth and silently suffered the gnawing pangs of dehydration and extreme thirst. Tough to the very end, he held out "for four days, at the end of which I was so fortunate as to obtain some spring water."[103]

Dr. Bushrod Washington James, surgical representative of the Christian Commission, had not fared nearly as well, however. Intestinal disorders from using the battlefield runoff, even after boiling, were finally forcing the doctor to leave for home. "I watched and toiled among that army of wounded, some from the flower of Lee's routed forces, some from among the noblest and best of the Northern troops, until I became so thoroughly sick and debilitated that I could work no longer!"[104]

---

102. Charles H. Merrick, Letter to his wife, Dr. Myra H. Merrick, July 12, 1863, William P. Palmer Collection, Container 1, Folder 3, MSS 3088, Western Reserve Historical Society, Cleveland, Ohio. All underlining by Merrick.
103. Dooley, *John Dooley*, p. 113.
104. James, *Echoes of Battle*, pp. 103-4, 111.

While someone went out to find transportation for the ailing doctor, James, sickened in body by the water, and sick at heart over all that yet remained to be accomplished at the hospitals, gathered together his few possessions and bade his fellow surgeons and patients a sorrowful good-bye. "With the deepest regret I was compelled to leave the hospital in the woods and start for home, so weak that I could but just crawl to an old hay wagon that was going to the town. . . . The danger of a rough ride in an old hay wagon to the railroad station, about three miles away, was less hazardous and preferable to the risk of remaining in the neighborhood of six or seven thousand wounded men, at the battle-field, after a copious rainstorm, or in the wet forest in which the hospital was situated. All these led me to adopt the plan of trying to reach home."[105]

"The farmer lifted my valise, then helped me up into the springless vehicle, and jolted, bruised and shaken up he conveyed me to the railroad station, and after a tedious railroad trip by way of Baltimore I was enabled to reach home, where I suffered both illness and weariness for weeks before I began to feel the least return of my usual vigor and elasticity."[106]

Dr. Bushrod James survived his brush with destiny in a small Pennsylvania hamlet. What would happen to the men still stranded in Gettysburg, however, still remained to be seen.

---

105. *Ibid.*
106. *Ibid.*

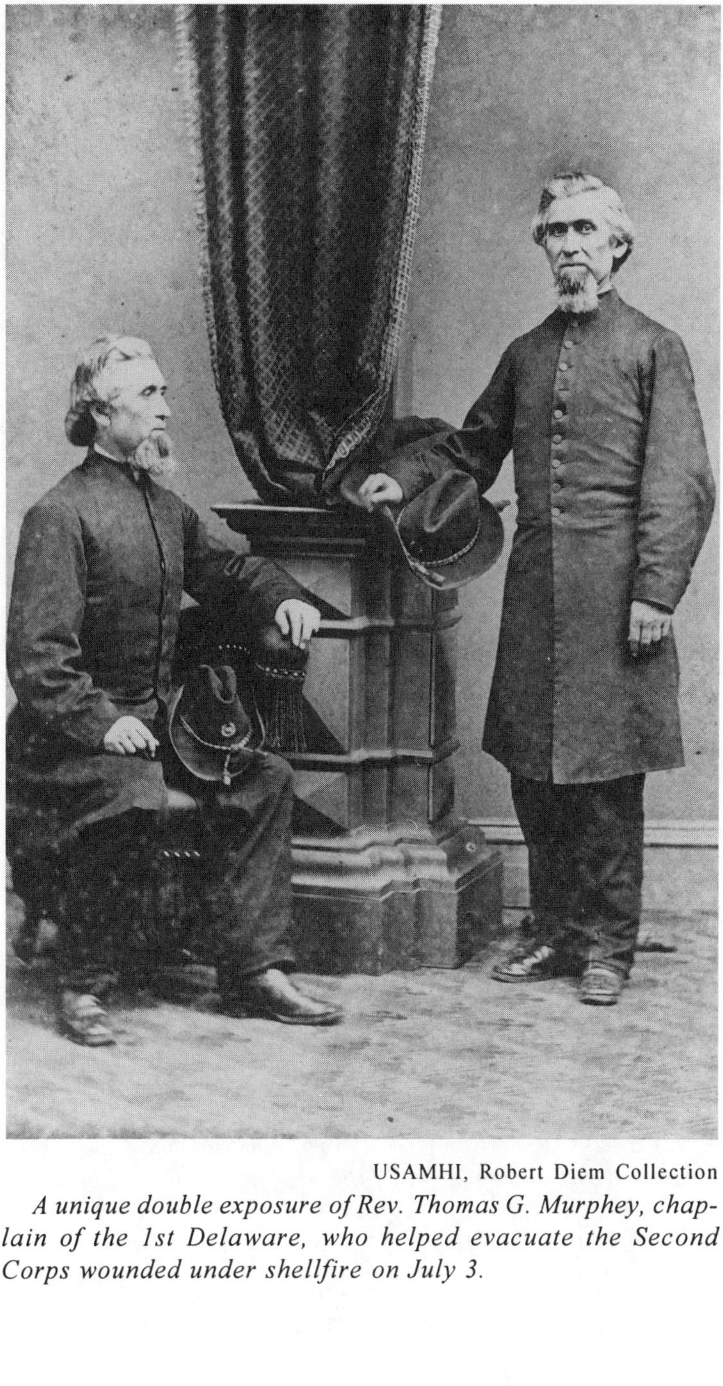

USAMHI, Robert Diem Collection

A unique double exposure of Rev. Thomas G. Murphey, chaplain of the 1st Delaware, who helped evacuate the Second Corps wounded under shellfire on July 3.

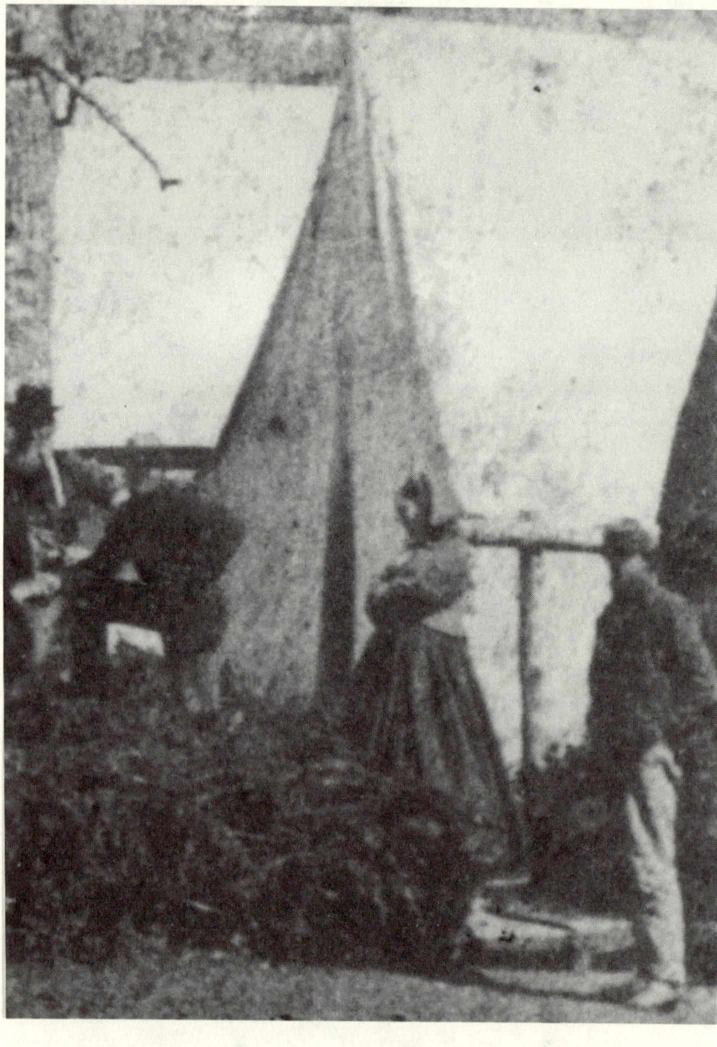

Miller, *Photographic History*, 1911

An extreme enlargement of the Second Corps winter quarters at Brandy Station, Virginia, showing Cornelia Hancock standing outside her quarters just a few months after her experiences at Gettysburg.

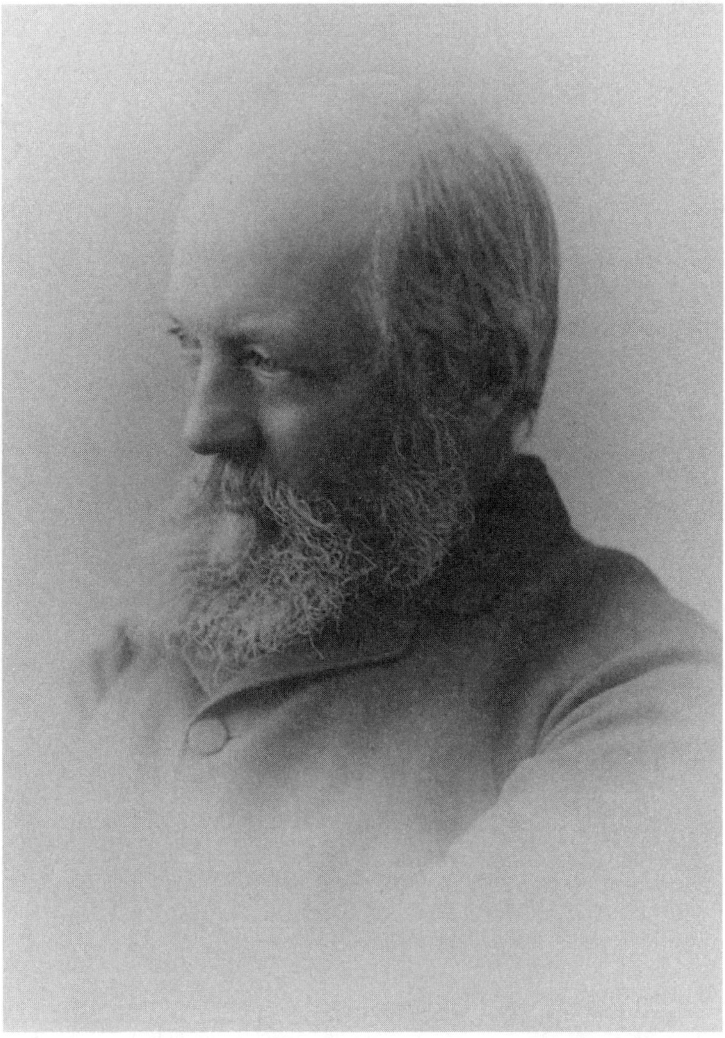

USAMHI

Frederick Law Olmstead, U.S. Sanitary Commission Secretary and opponent of the Christian Commission.

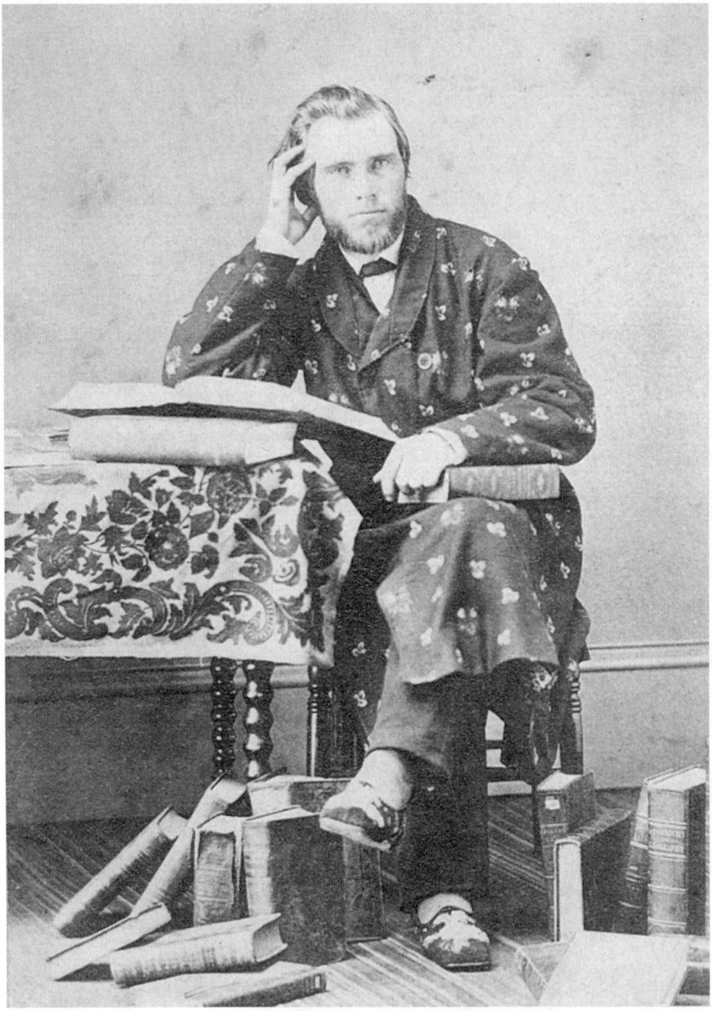

John H. W. Stuckenberg Collection, Special Collections/Musselman Library, Gettysburg College, Gettysburg, Pennsylvania

Chaplain John H. W. Stuckenberg, 145th Pennsylvania, who searched the battlefield after dark on July 2 for the wounded.

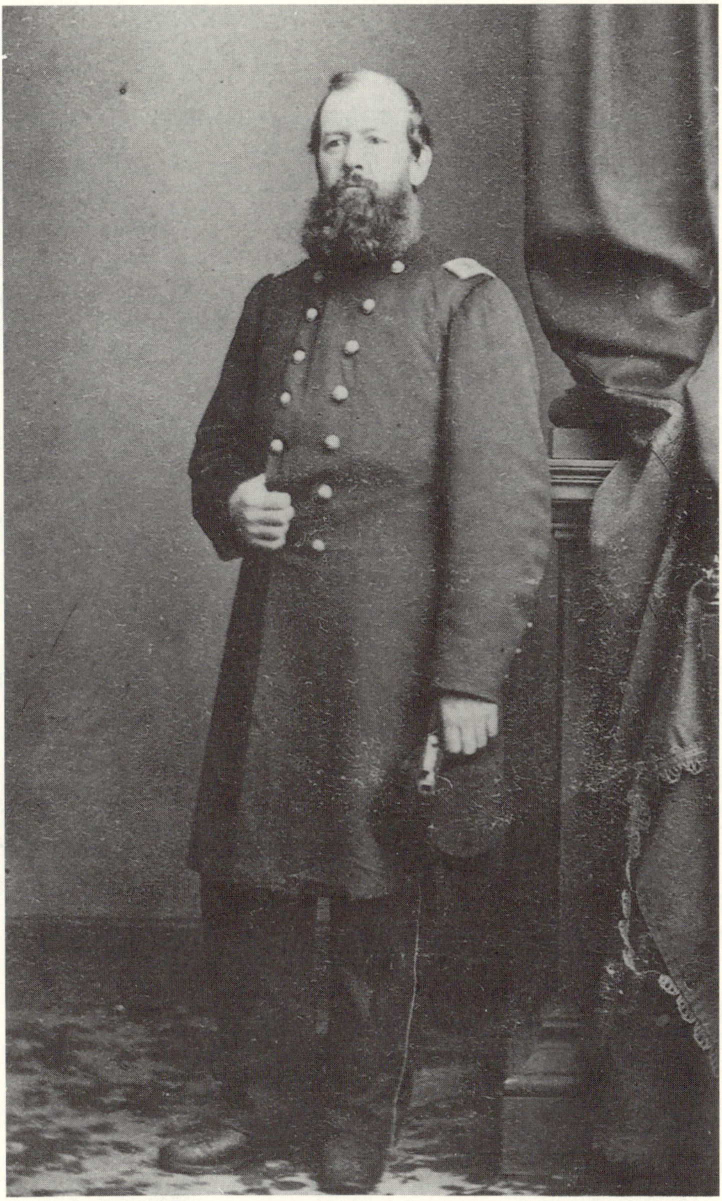

USAMHI, Gil Barrett Collection

Surgeon Justin Dwinelle, 106th Pennsylvania, Surgeon-in-Charge of the Second Division, Second Corps, and Chief Surgeon of the Second Corps Hospital.

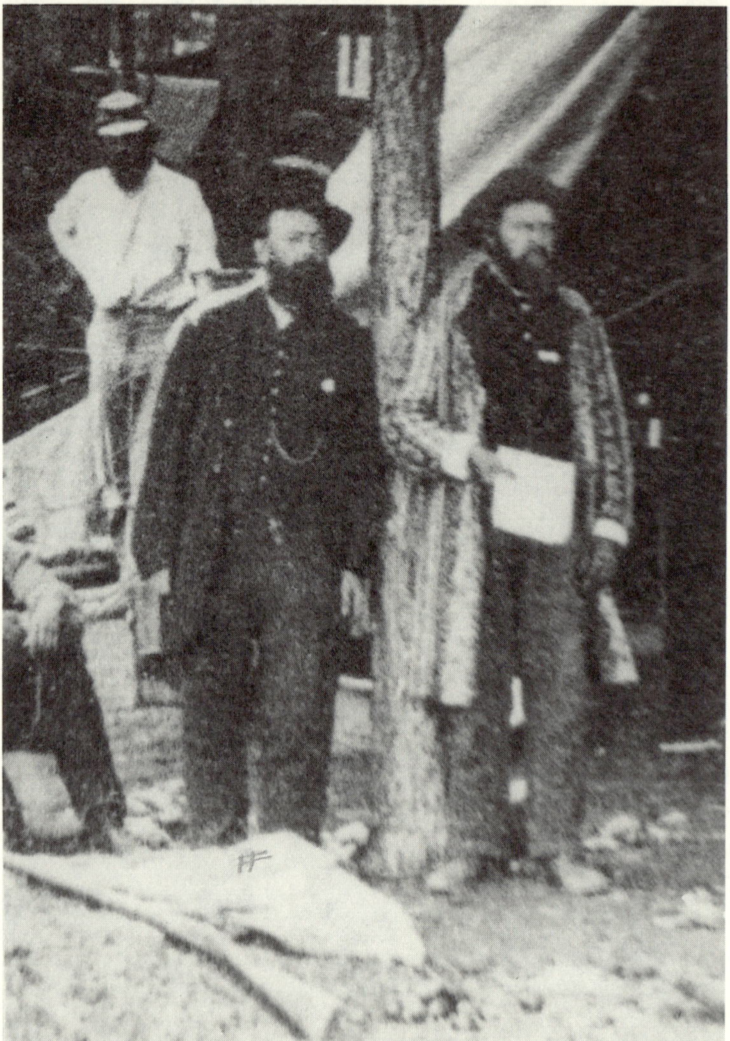

Scott Dwinelle, Alexandria, Virginia

Dr. Justin Dwinelle to the left of the tree, Andrew Cross or Mr. Stilson of the Christian Commission to the right of the tree.

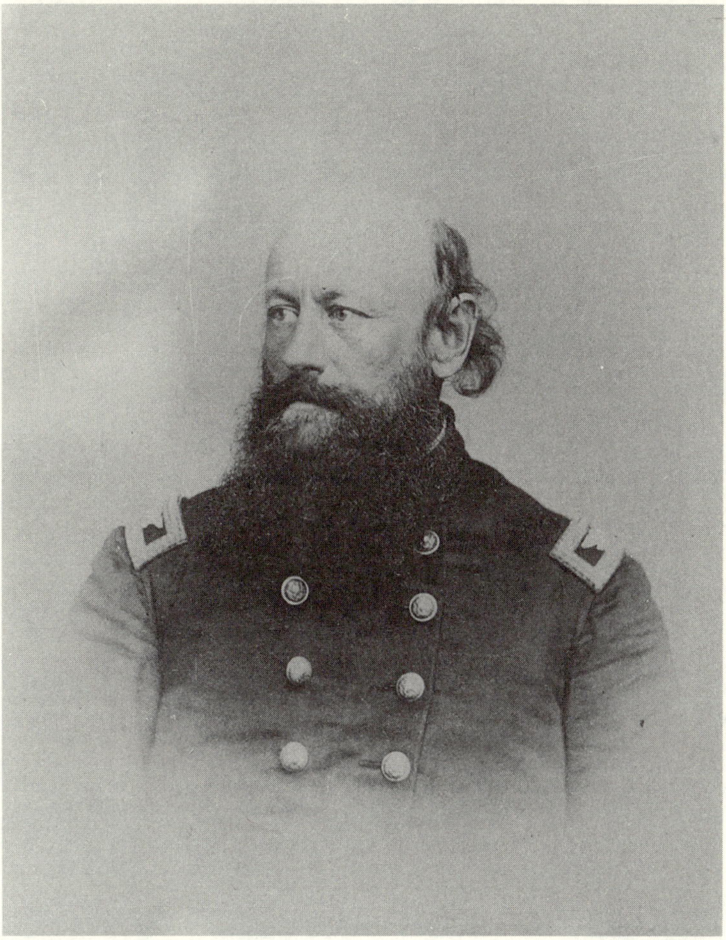

USAMHI

Surgeon Alexander N. Dougherty, U.S. Volunteers, Medical Director of the Second Corps Hospitals at Gettysburg.

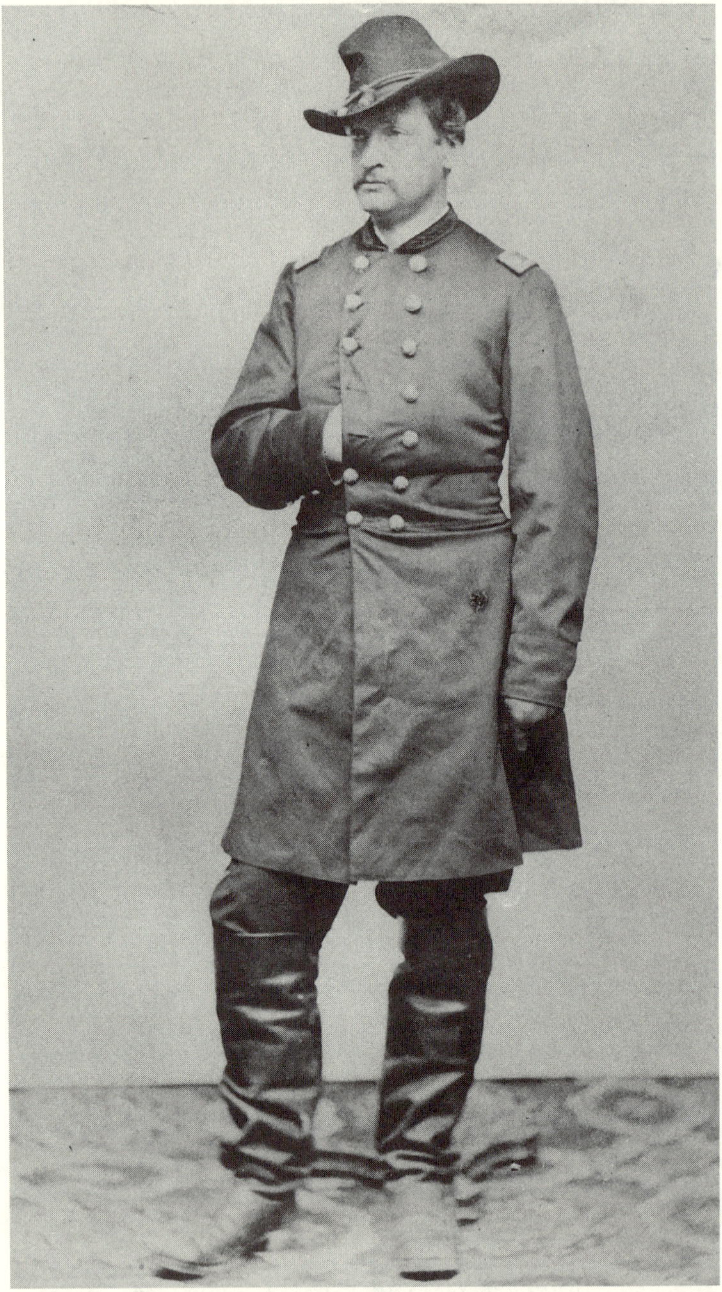

USAMHI

Surgeon Nathan Hayward, 20th Massachusetts, Second Division Chief Operator and one of the most photographed of all Union surgeons, remained with the hospital at the Schwartz Farm when the Army of the Potomac marched away.

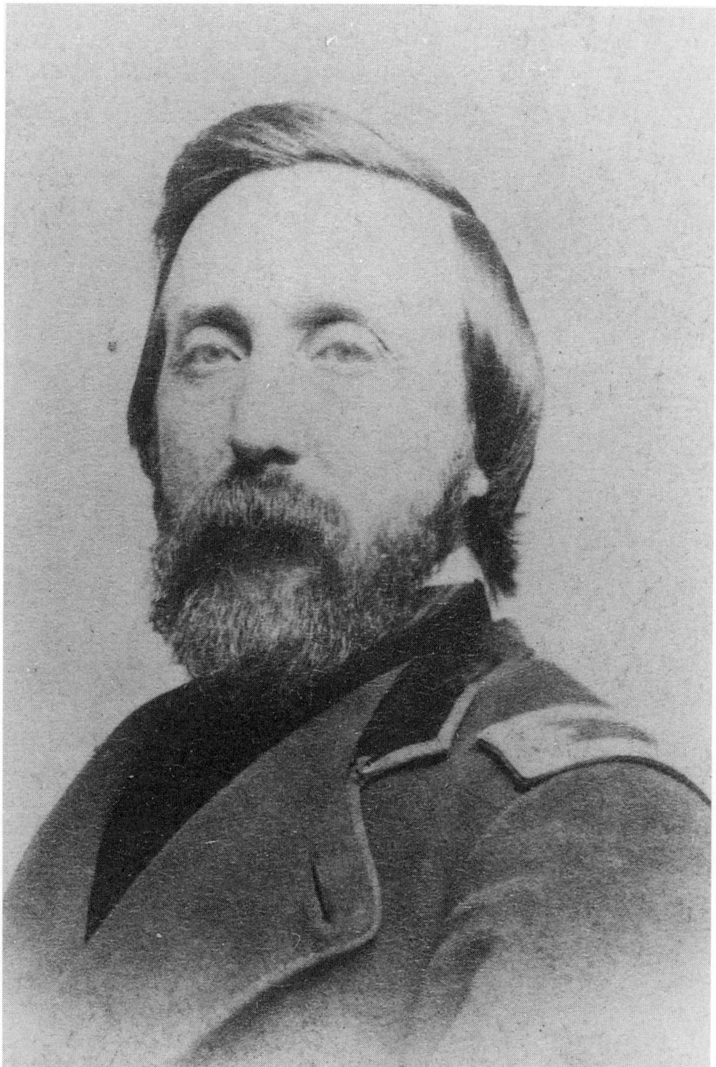

USAMHI, Roger D. Hunt Collection

Surgeon Harry McKindree McAbee, 4th Ohio, Third Division Chief Operator, supervised the primary aid station at the Catherine Guinn Farm.

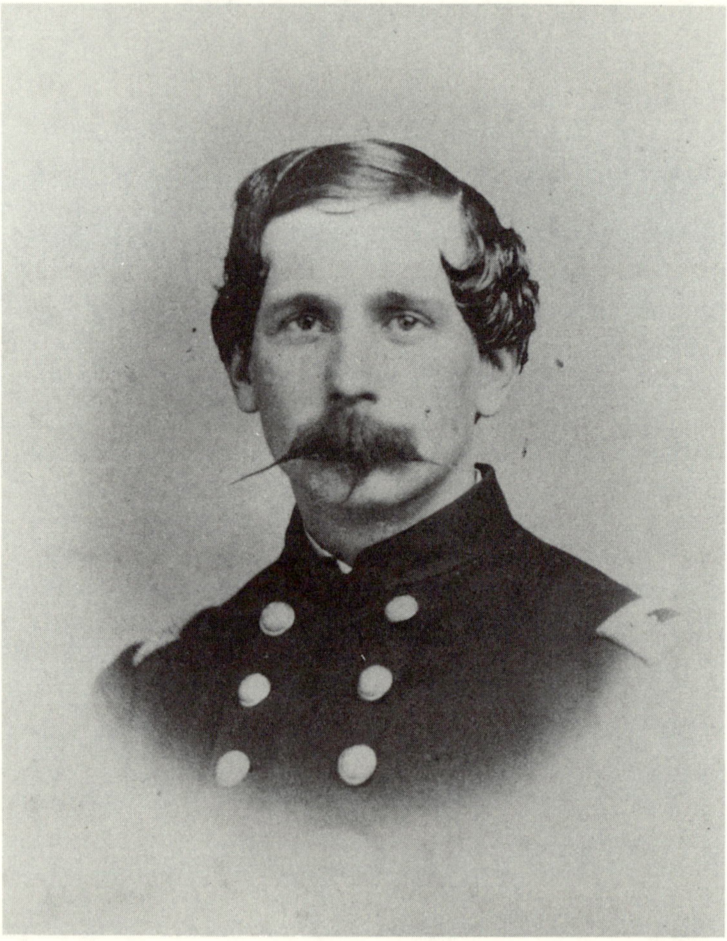

USAMHI, Brent Musser Collection

Surgeon Martin Rizer, 72nd Pennsylvania, was one of the surgeons who marched off with the Second Corps in pursuit of the Confederate forces on July 7.

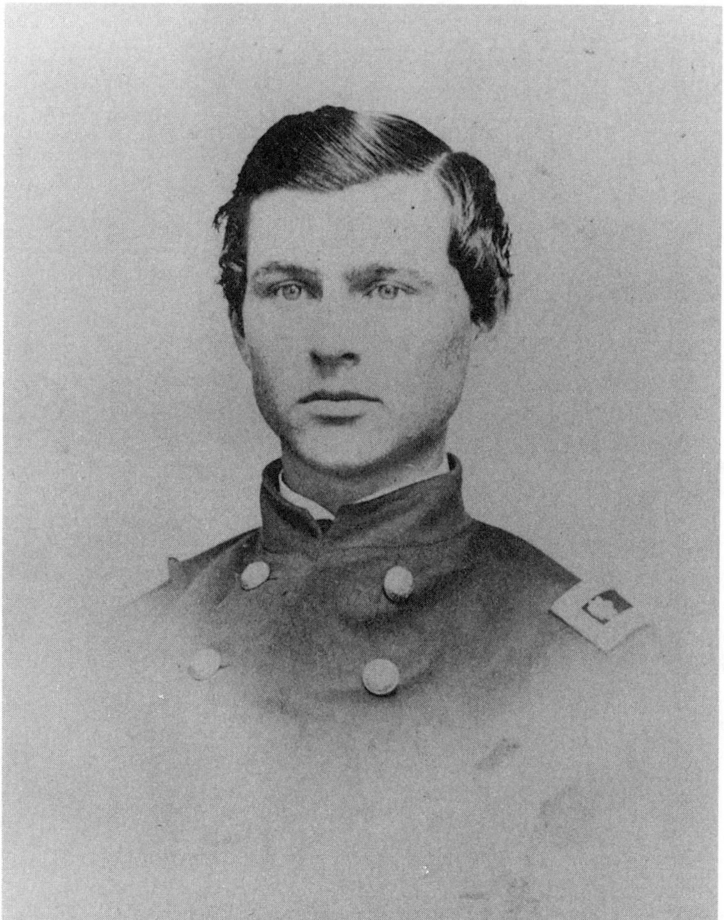

USAMHI, Scott Hann Collection

Surgeon Frederick A. Dudley, 14th Connecticut, was wounded and captured on July 3. Cornelia Hancock mentions him in every letter home until the end of the war.

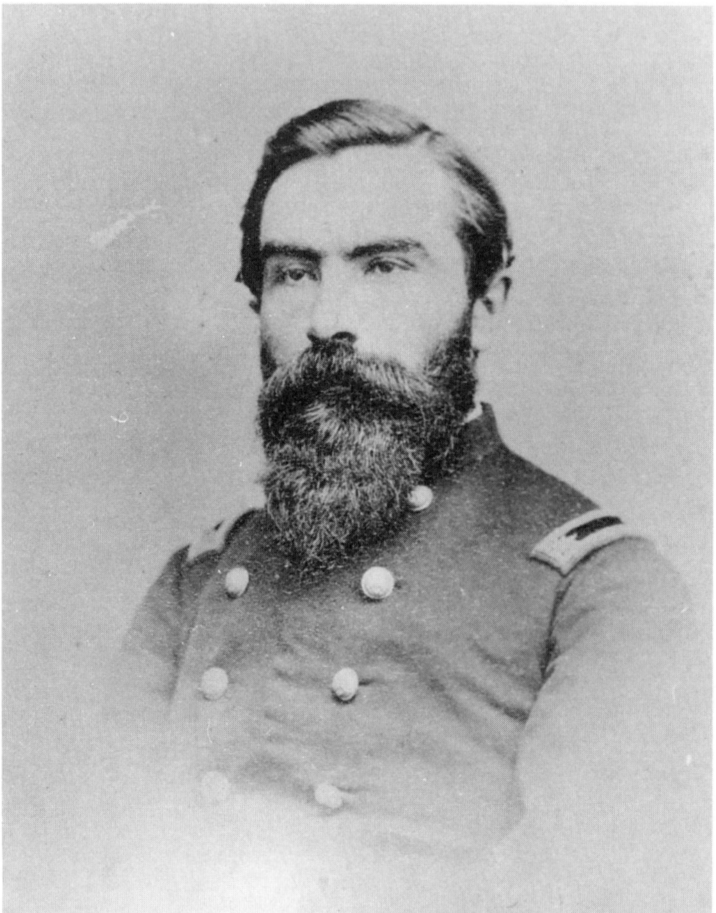

Vermont Historical Society

Surgeon Henry Janes, 5th Vermont, oversaw all field hospitals at Gettysburg after the departure of the Army of the Potomac.

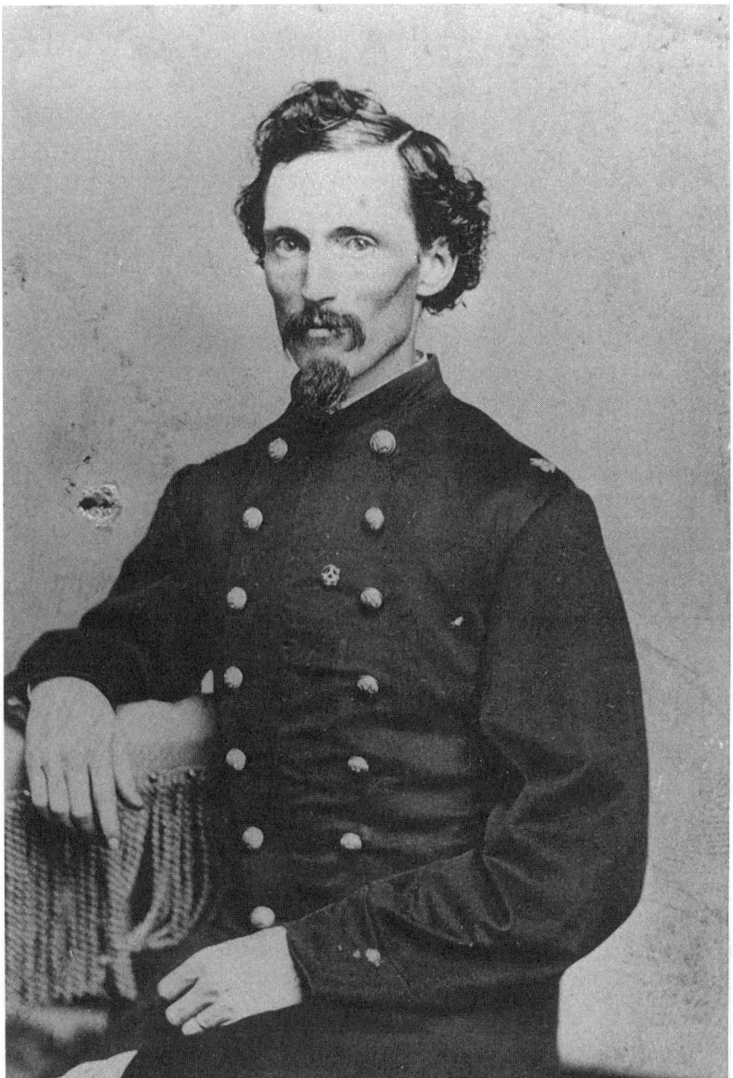

USAMHI

Assistant Surgeon James D. Benton, 111th New York, from Syracuse, New York, worked long hours in the Third Division, Second Corps Hospital.

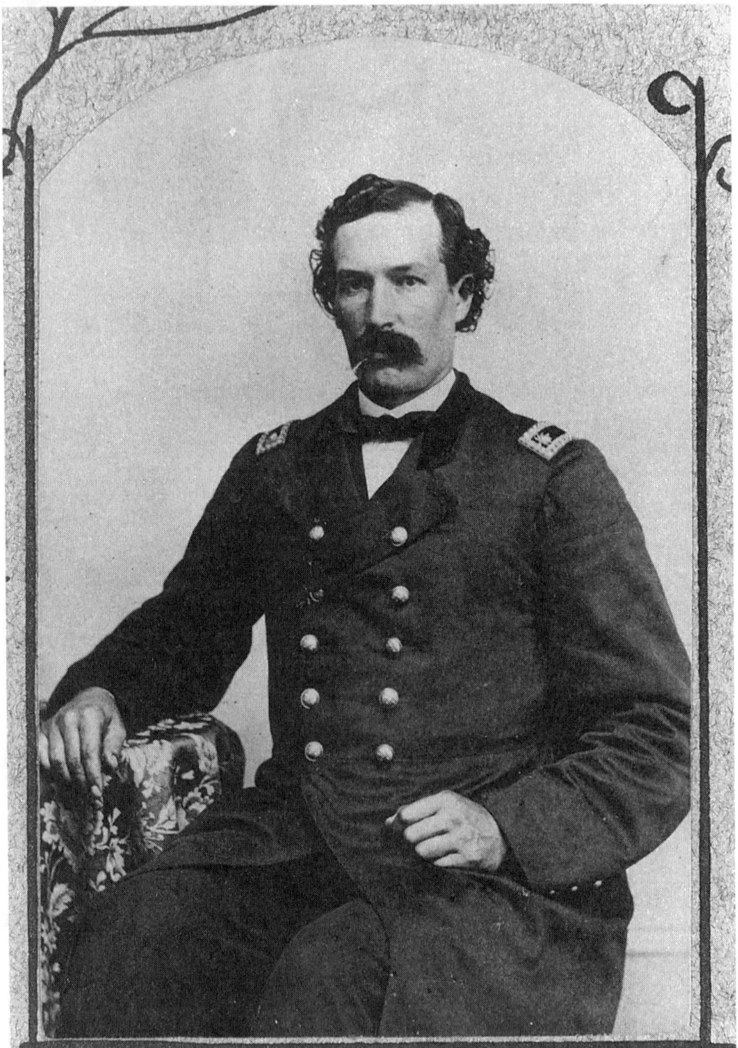

USAMHI

Surgeon John W. Bucknam, 5th New Hampshire, was on the personal staff of Col. Edward E. Cross and attended to him as he lay dying.

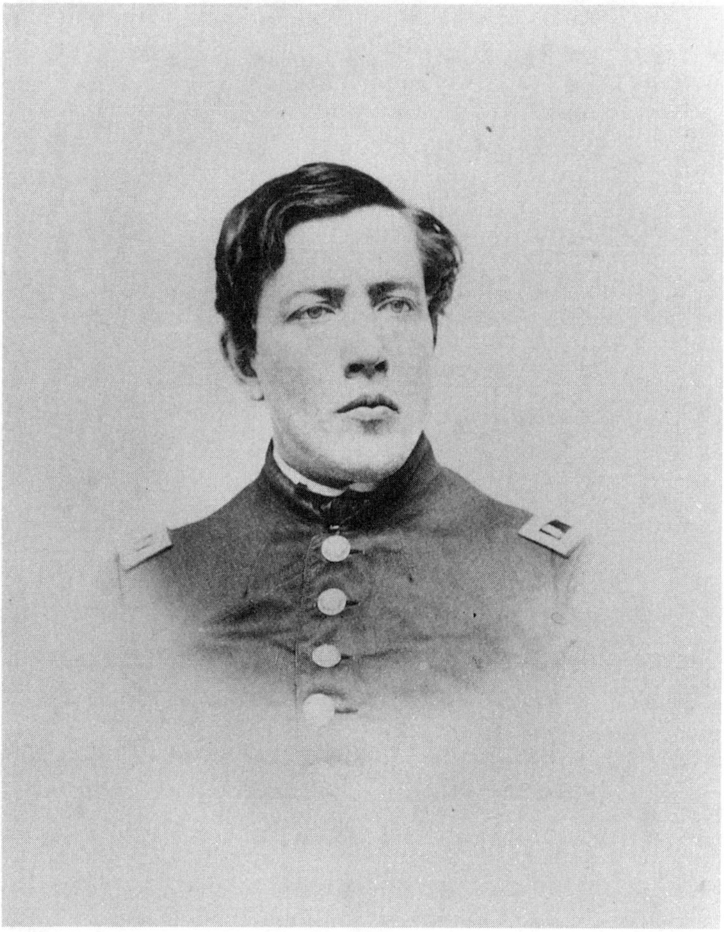

USAMHI

Assistant Surgeon William Child, 5th New Hampshire, was the regimental historian and also attended to Colonel Cross following his mortal wounding on July 2.

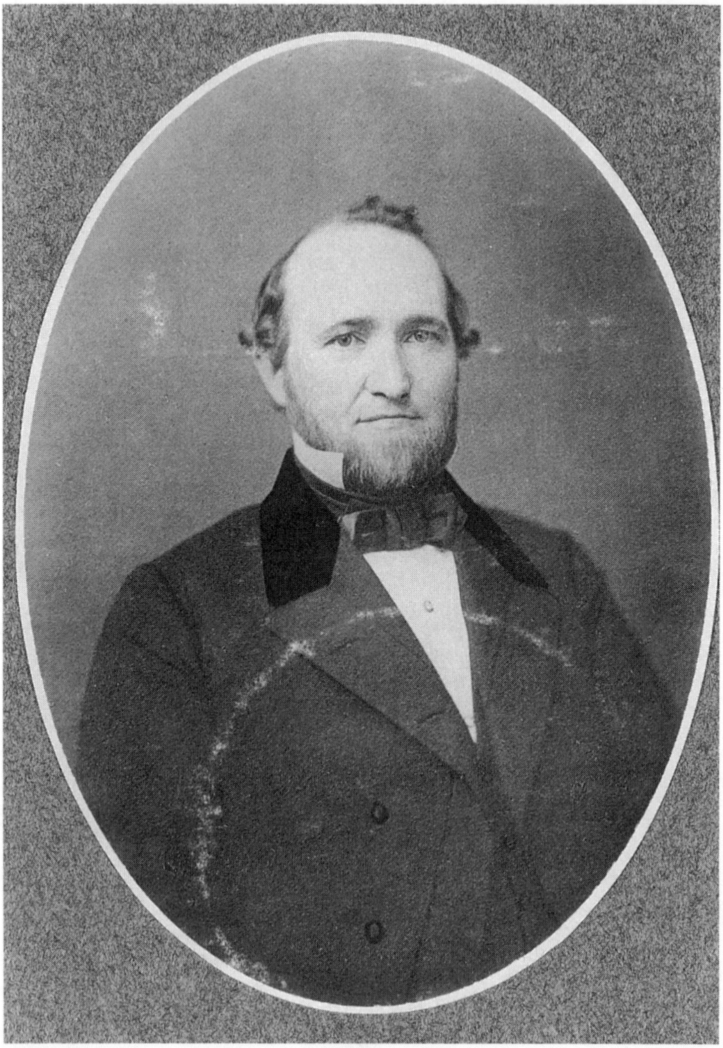

USAMHI

Assistant Surgeon Theodore O. Cornish, 15th Massachusetts, hailed from Boston and was one of a handful of Second Corps surgeons to remain in Gettysburg when the Army of the Potomac marched away in pursuit of General Lee's forces.

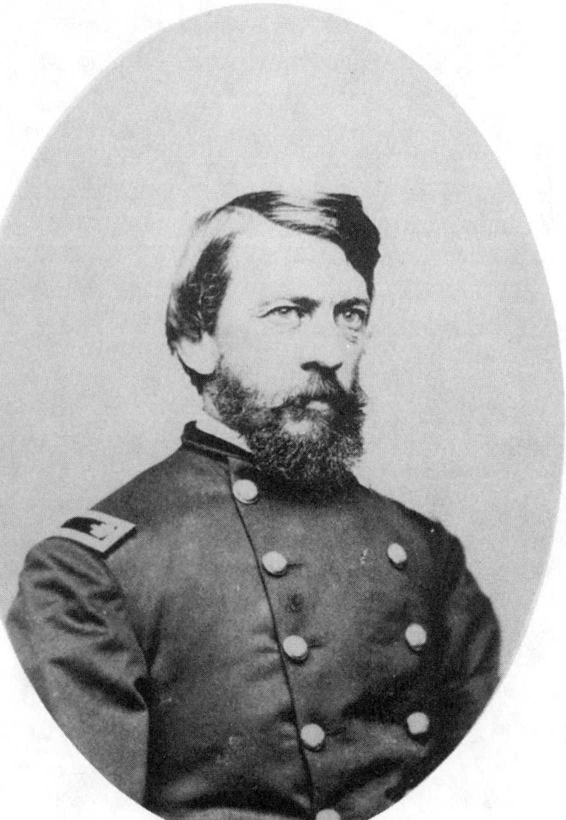

Pennsylvania MOLLUS Collection,
War Library and Museum, Philadelphia

Dr. Jonathan Letterman, Medical Director of the Army of the Potomac.

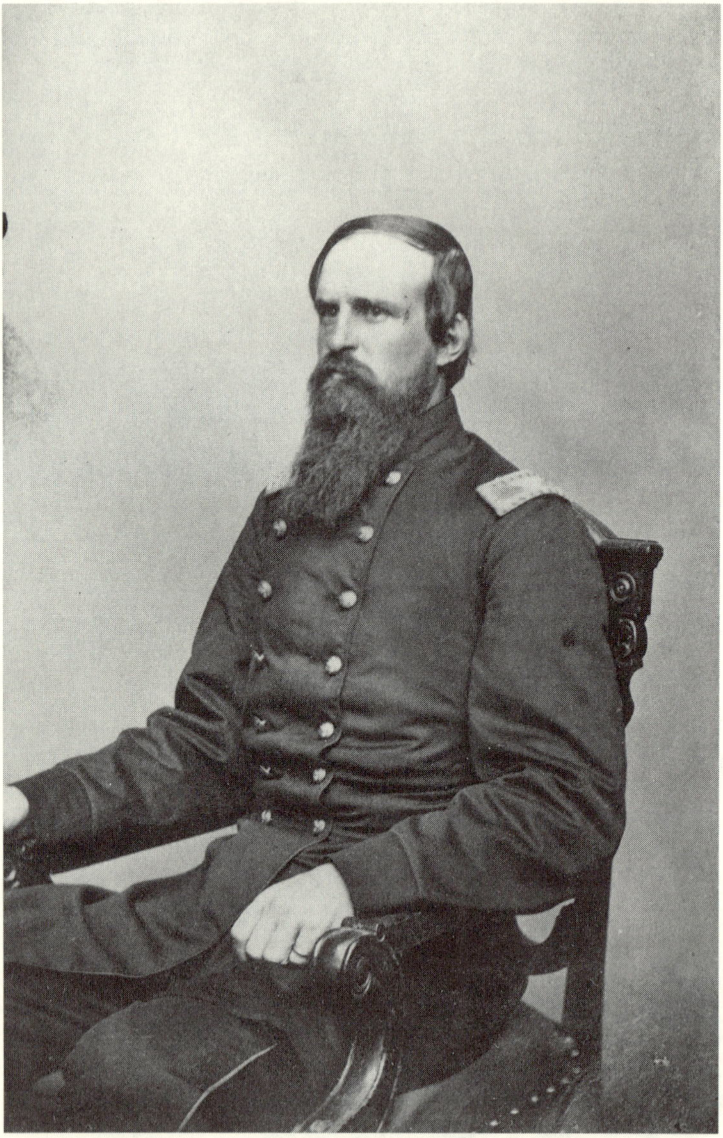

Library of Congress

Col. Edward E. Cross, First Division, First Brigade commander, tried to prevent Lt. Thomas Livermore from becoming Second Corps ambulance chief. Cross was mortally wounded on July 2.

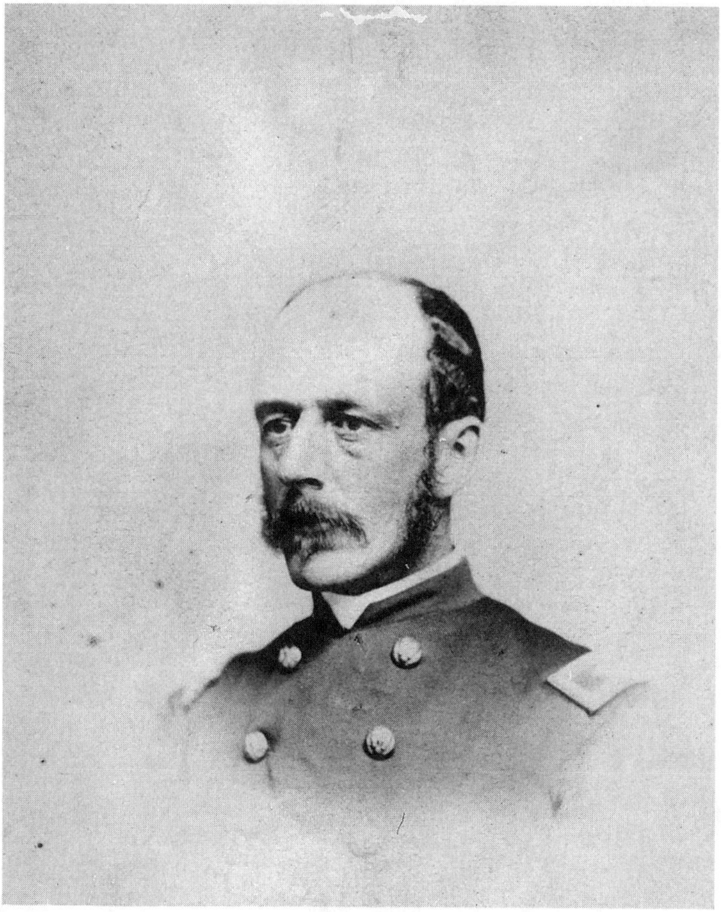

State Historical Society of Wisconsin

Lt. Frank A. Haskell, staff aide to General Gibbon, received a minor leg wound and accompanied Gibbon to Westminster for rail evacuation.

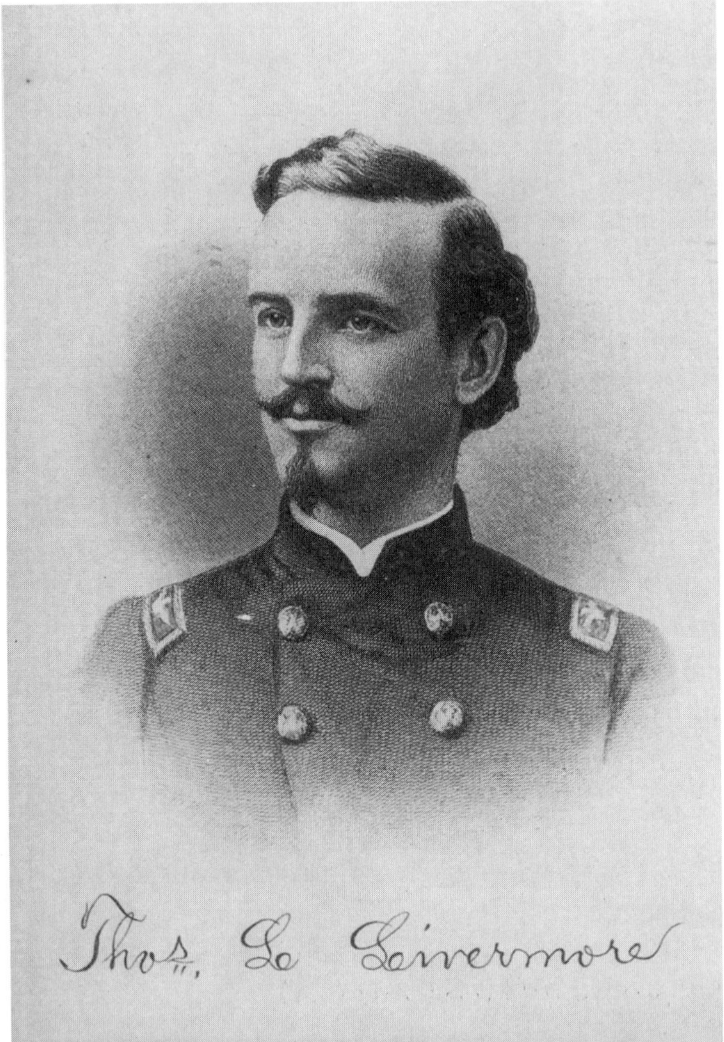

Days and Events, 1861-1866

Capt. Thomas Livermore, the newly appointed chief of the Second Corps Ambulance Corps, personally chose the Rock Creek location for the hospitals.

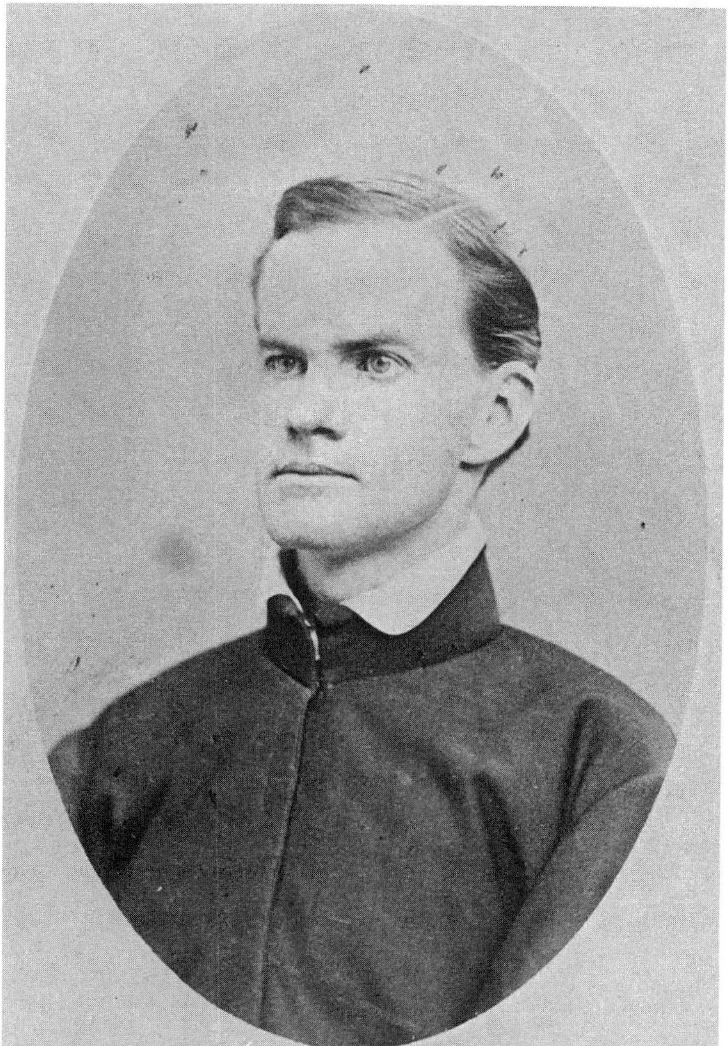

Georgetown University Library, Special Collections
and Archives Division, Washington, D.C.

First Lt. John E. Dooley, Company C, 1st Virginia, was shot through both thighs on July 3, captured, treated at the Second Corps Hospital, and paroled for exchange on February 20, 1865.

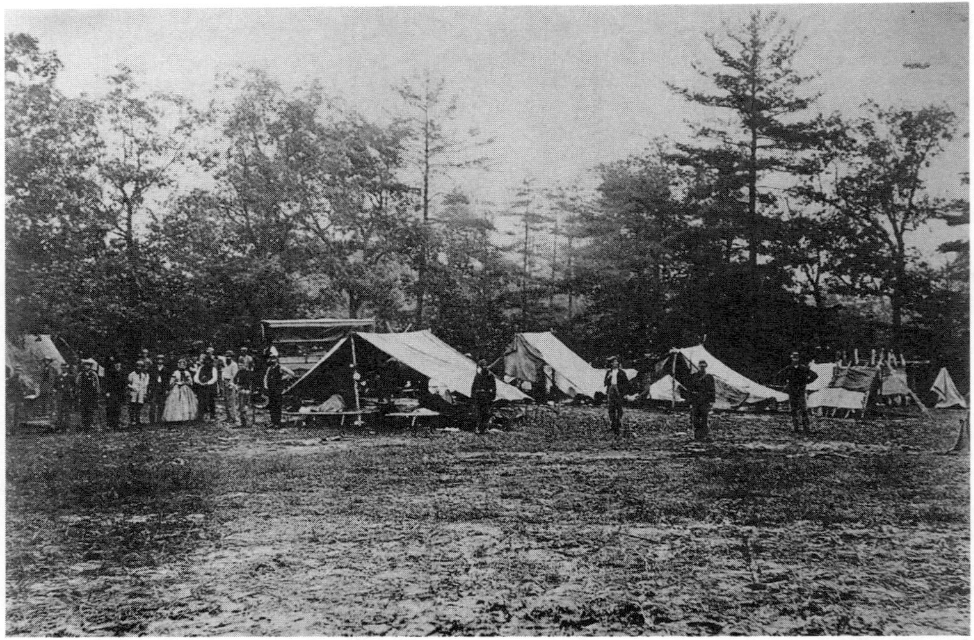

Courtesy of William Frassanito, *Early Photography at Gettysburg*

One of the Frederick Gutekunst photographs of the Second Corps Hospital.

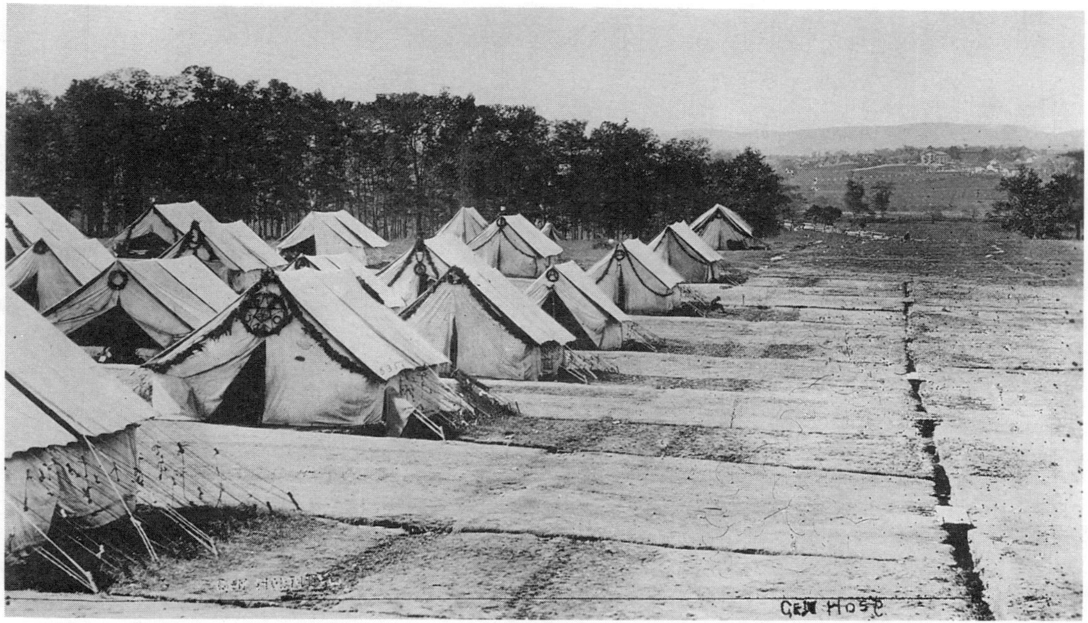

Library of Congress

Camp Letterman General Hospital, Gettysburg, August 1863, where the most seriously wounded were transferred when the Second Corps Hospital closed.

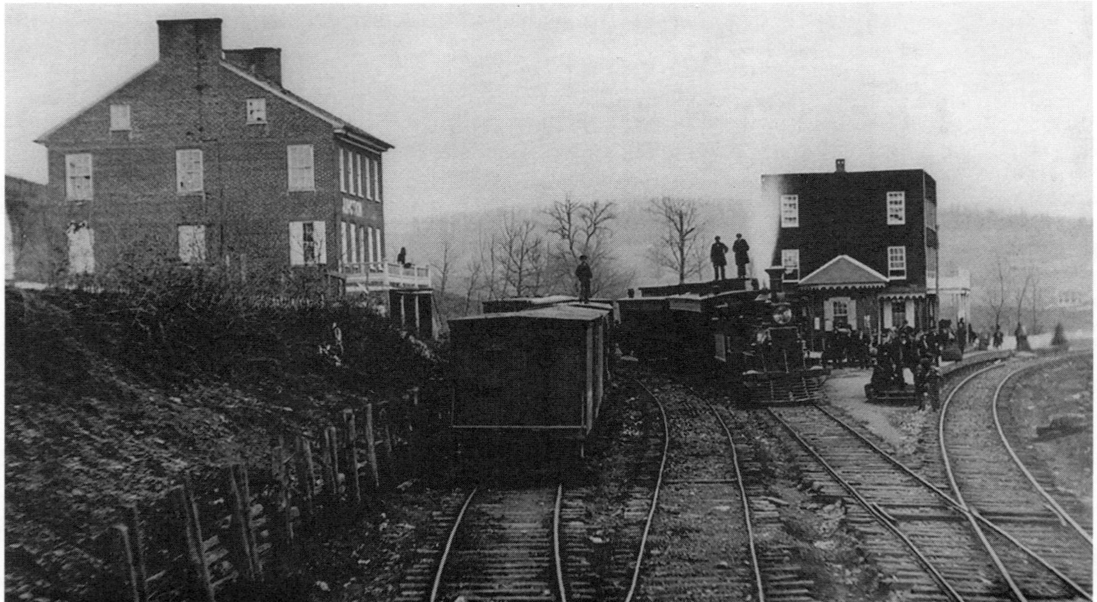

National Archives

Hanover Junction, thirty miles from Gettysburg, was the site of the Christian Commission refreshment station, which Emily Bliss Souder visited while awaiting rail transport to Gettysburg.

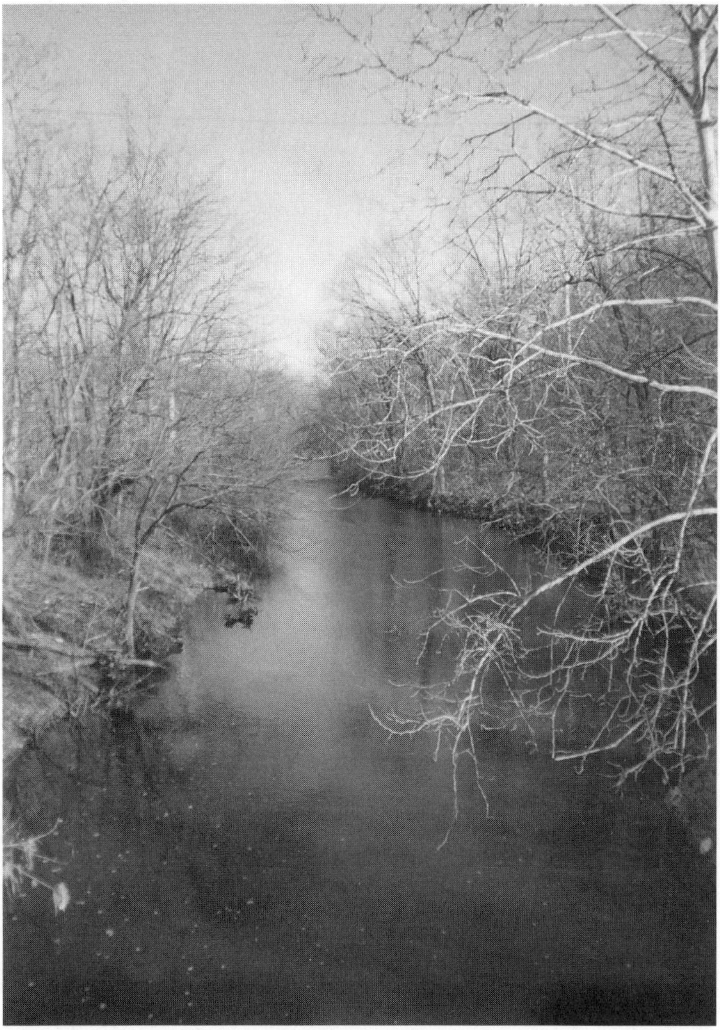

Author's Collection

Rock Creek as it now appears, a short distance from the site chosen by Captain Livermore in the bottomland.

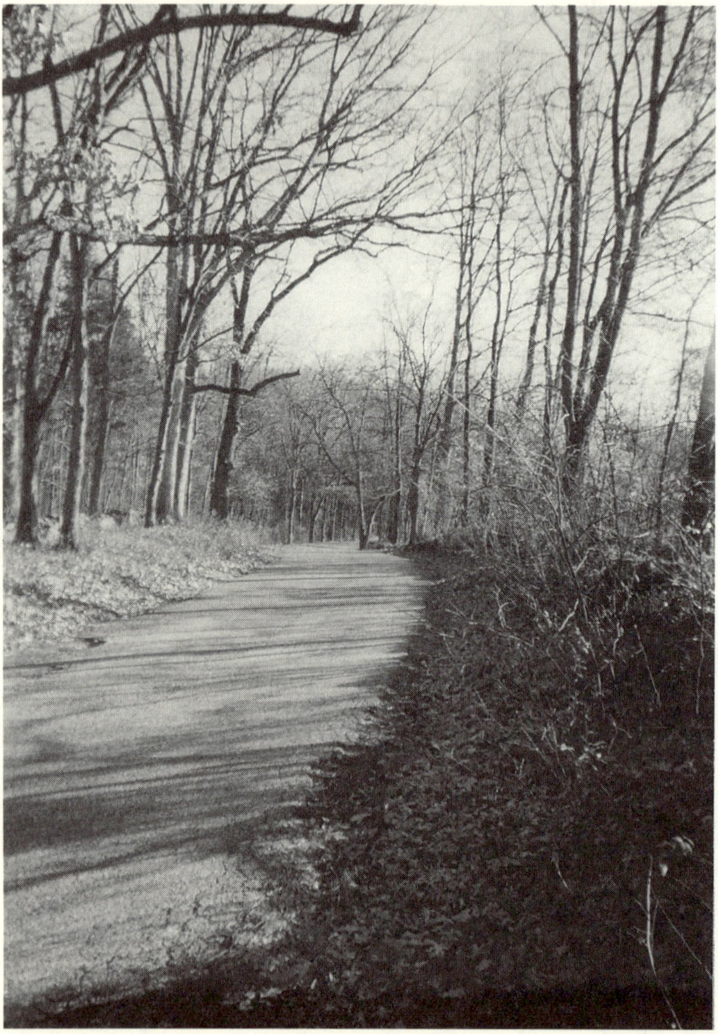

Author's Collection

Granite School House Road, on either side of which were clustered the Second Corps hospitals on July 2 and 3.

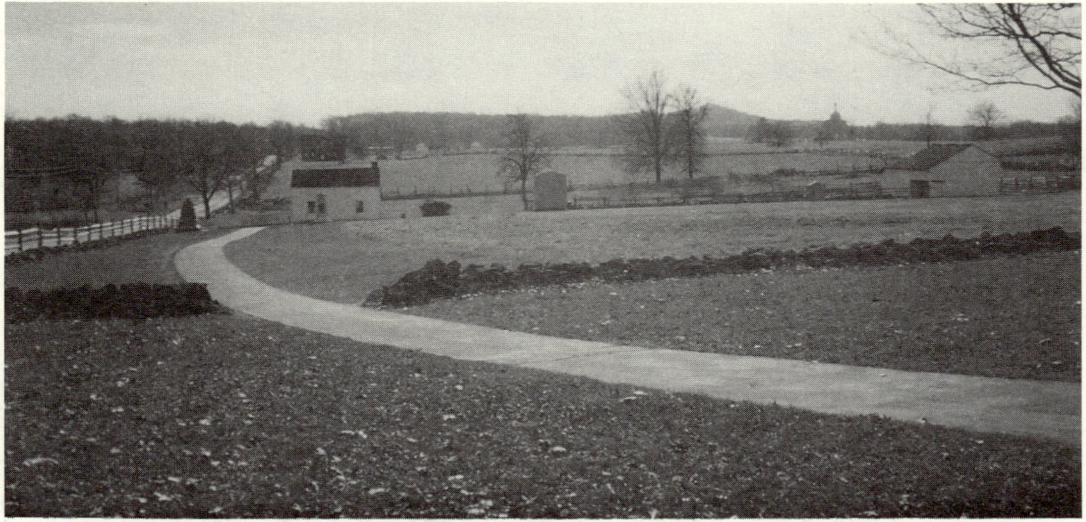

Author's Collection

A view of the aid stations along the Taneytown Road. In the foreground is the Widow Leister House, used by General Meade as his headquarters and hastily evacuated under shell fire on July 3. In the middle distance is the Peter Frey property, where Canadian Dr. Francis Wafer, 108th New York, received the wounded. Barely visible in the distance is the Jacob Hummelbaugh Farm, where Dr. Albert Hamilton, 148th Pennsylvania, set up his regimental aid station.

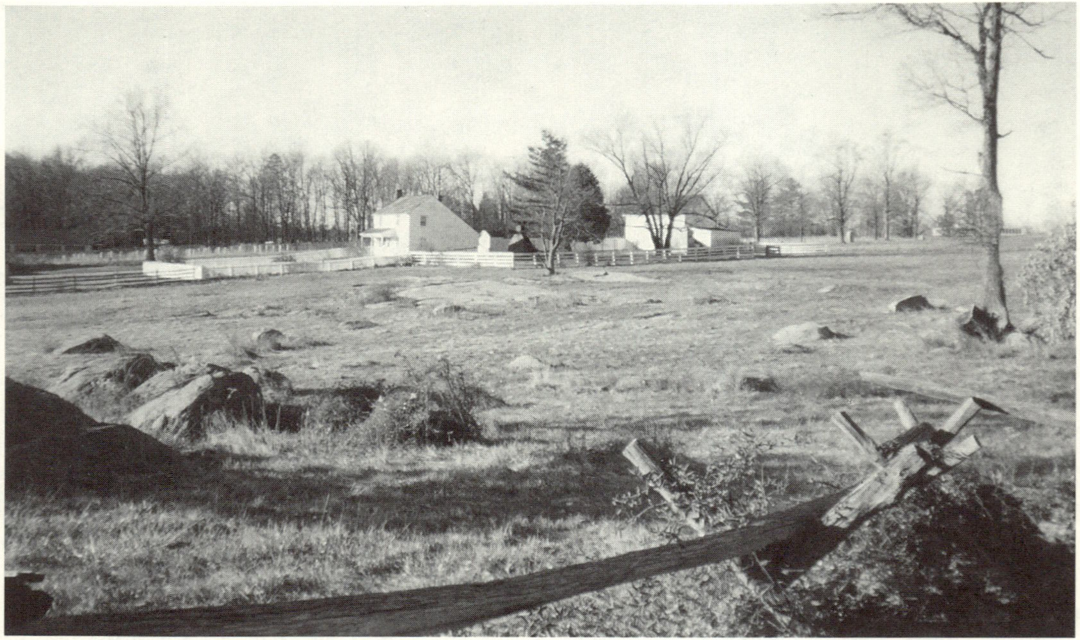

Author's Collection

The Hummelbaugh Farm, 108th New York primary aid station, as seen from the Taneytown Road.

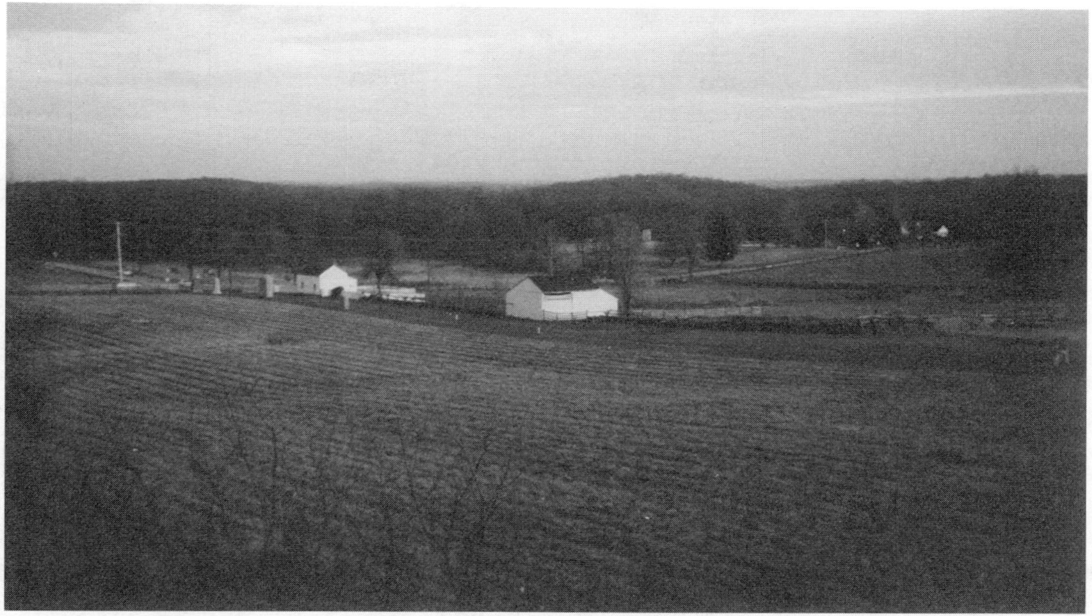

Author's Collection

The Hummelbaugh Farm, 108th New York primary aid station, as it would have been seen by the Second Corps wounded as they headed for the rear.

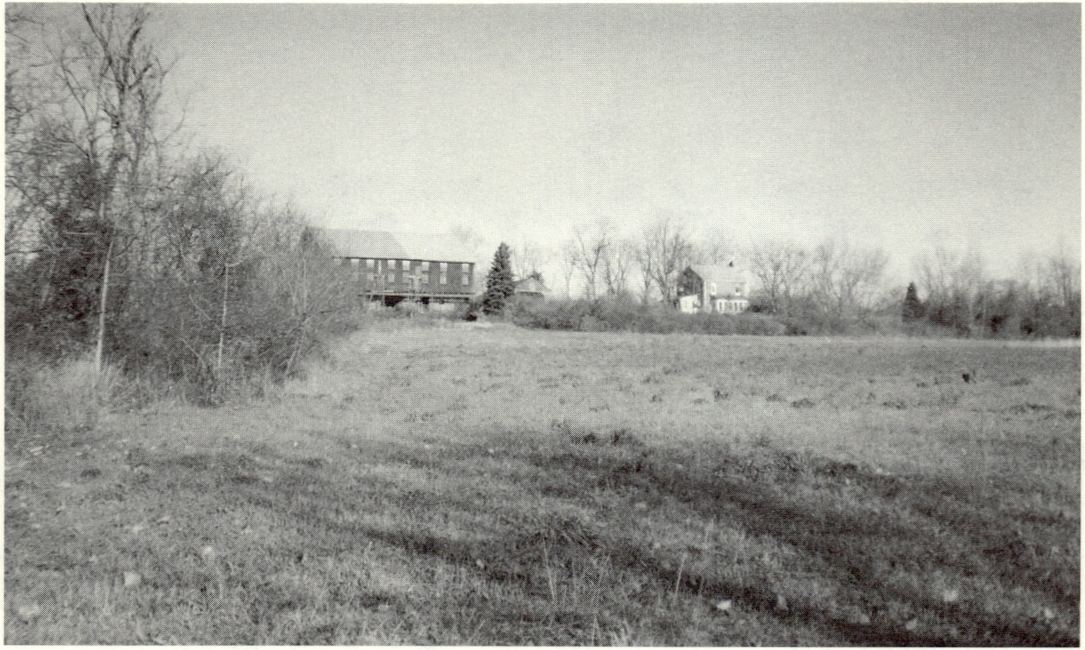

Author's Collection

The Jacob Schwartz Farm, final site of the Second Corps Hospital, as seen from White Run.

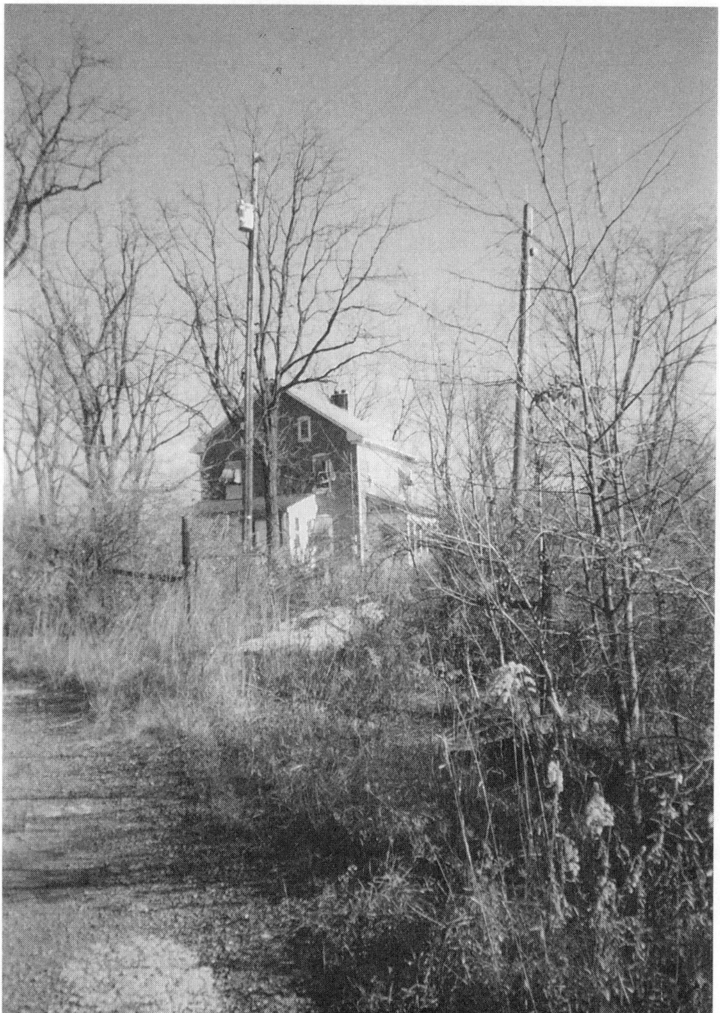

Author's Collection

The Jacob Schwartz farmhouse, probably the one standing in 1863, where Union officers were laid on the porch awaiting treatment.

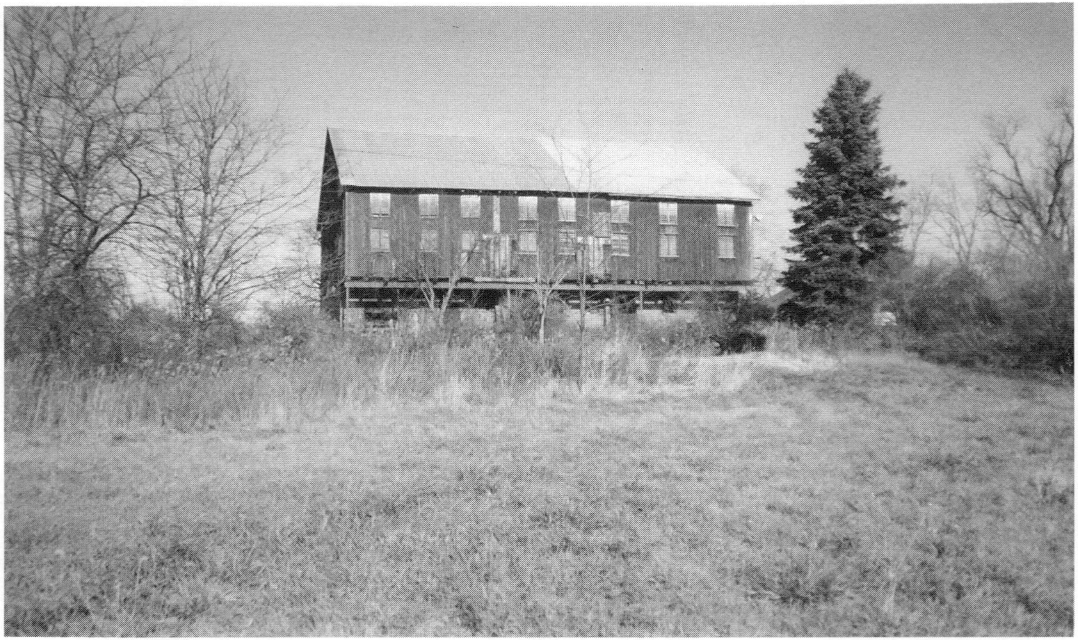

Author's Collection

The original Jacob Schwartz barn, which housed Confederate wounded and where captured Confederate surgeons finally finished operating a week after the battle's end.

Chapter 14

TUESDAY, JULY 7: 5:00 P.M.—WEDNESDAY, JULY 22: 4:00 P.M.

". . . we leave the famous Burgh of Getty. . . ."
Confederate Lt. John Dooley

Gettysburg, Pennsylvania

Gradually at first, and then in ever greater numbers, the wounded were leaving the festering surroundings of the battlefield for healthier locales and more advanced medical care. On foot, by litter, wagon, ambulance, or the rugged jostling of railroad cars, Confederate and Union troops alike were overjoyed to see the town of Gettysburg disappear over the horizon behind them.

Some managed to walk away from Gettysburg. Those considered ambulatory were sent off with the best wishes of the medical staff; with the lesser wounded gone, more time could be allotted to those with grievous wounds. Each man thus released was encouraged to make his way, by whatever means possible, out of town.

Pvt. Austin A. Carr of the 82nd New York Infantry, now on the mend from his glancing shoulder wound and a severe case of hemorrhoids, was discharged (if such a definite word could be used) on July 7. "[I] was there ordered if possible to make my way to Littlestown, Pa." Another invalid, "named Briggs, who had received a flesh wound in the leg, with me started on our painful march to Littlestown, trusting to luck and Providence for something to eat."[1]

For two men just released from the hospital, the going was anything but easy. "We walked slowly, resting frequently, as neither of us were able to walk much, untill [*sic*] about 4 P.M., when we asked and received permission to remain in a barn over night. On the 8th it rain[ed] all day, confining us to the barn, the folks giving us food and drink. On the 9th we reached Littlestown, the citizens there taking the sick and wounded in charge."[2]

After a three day recuperation from the exertions of their short trip, Private Carr and his companion were ready to make the next leg of the journey, this time presumably by train. "On the 12th of July was sent to Baltimore and from there to McDougal Hospital, Fort Schuyler, N.Y., arriving on the 15th. The piles did not bother [me] a great deal while in the Hospital, using only cold water when necessary. I was placed in section B, Ward 8, in care of Doctor Purdy. . . . As soon as I got better, I assisted the nurse to attend the wounded, and helped around what I could."[3]

It was a slow recovery for the New Yorker as he worked at the hospital and helped care for other more seriously wounded men. He eventually did rejoin his regiment on March 2, 1864, apparently none the worse for his Gettysburg adventures.[4]

Fort Schuyler, New York

Other veterans of Gettysburg were also pouring into Fort Schuyler by rail, among them James Moore, Company G, 108th New York. On the day that Carr arrived, Moore wrote to an acquaintance from his hospital bed about his painful ankle wound: "We arrived again as you will see at the old hospital quarters. My wound appears to be stubborn enough. It could not be otherwise. Getting anxious for the last four days. Kept the wounds bleeding all the time. Mine is so now I trust. Some rest will mend it. God grant it may."[5]

---

1. Carr, *A Casualty at Gettysburg and Andersonville*, pp. 11.
2. *Ibid.*
3. *Ibid.*
4. *Ibid.*
5. James Moore, Letter to "My Dear Friend," July 15, 1863, copy in 108th New York Vertical File, Gettysburg Military Park Library, original at University of Rochester.

Some of the wounded escaped the noisome environment of Gettysburg in wagons, often taking matters into their own hands to do so. After more than a week at the Second Corps hospital, and still awaiting an examination of his "fatal" wounds, Capt. John G. B. Adams had finally had enough; he decided it was time to seek treatment elsewhere, whether the doctors would allow it or not. "My mind had been quite active, and I had come to the conclusion that I would move my lodging as soon as possible. One surgeon had said that I would not live twenty-four hours, another that I must remain where I was two weeks. It struck me that to die in twenty-four hours or stay where I was two weeks would neither be pleasant for myself nor those near me."[6]

Being incapacitated by critical wounds left Adams dependent on others to successfully orchestrate his departure from the Schwartz farm hospital. "I talked the matter over with [Duncan] Sherwood. We counted our cash and found we had five dollars each, and we formed a syndicate. We made Mike Scannel our agent, with instructions to bring some kind of conveyance to take us off the field." With the hopeful voices of his wounded comrades ringing in his ears, Scannel was sent on his way.[7]

"The next morning he reported with a citizen, a horse and a side-spring wagon. The whole lot was not worth ten dollars, but we paid our money and were loaded and on our way to Littletown." Nearly ten miles distant from the battlefield stood the hamlet of Littlestown. Living up to its diminutive appellation, the tiny village had been unaffected by both the recent battle and the Confederate forays through the region. As the wounded made their way out the Baltimore Pike away from the scenes of the recent fighting, the citizens graciously threw open their schoolhouse, church, businesses, private homes, and barns as transit hospitals for the wounded. "We arrived in due time, and were driven to a church which had been converted into a temporary hospital. We found it nearly full, but they made room for us. I had a nice place on top of the pews in the broad aisle."[8]

---

6. Adams, *Reminiscences of the Nineteenth Massachusetts*, p. 72.
7. *Ibid.*
8. *Ibid.*; *Indianapolis Daily Journal*, July 23, 1863, p. 2.

Littlestown, Pennsylvania

Having just arrived from the highly regimented order of the Second Corps hospitals, it must have been surprising to Captain Adams just how improvised this makeshift hospital at Littletown was. "There was no organization of the hospital. Two of the town doctors were doing all they could, being assisted by the women. No doubt our Massachusetts women would do the same kind of work should the emergency arise, but I cannot speak in too high praise of the women of Littletown. They would dress the shattered arm of some poor boy, wash the blood from the wounds of another, thinking only of what they could do to relieve suffering. It was like getting home."[9]

Now almost a week and a half after his wounding, Adams' festering, untreated wounds were still oozing, crusted with dried blood and matter, and wriggling with little white worms. "My wounds were in a frightful condition. They had not been dressed, and the maggots were crawling into them. As soon as we were settled the ladies came to see what they could do. They were anxious to dress our wounds, but it required more hospital accommodations than the church afforded, so they washed our hands and faces, and made us as comfortable as possible."[10]

After getting cleaned up, it was time for supper. "A real motherly woman asked what I wanted to eat. I had eaten little except the chicken Billy and Mose brought me, and when she said she had chicken broth, I said, 'Bring me two or three.' As soon as possible she came with a large pan full of broth, but the trouble was I could not sit up to eat it. At my suggestion she brought the prettiest girl in the room, who put her left arm around me and let me lean my head on her shoulder, while she fed me with the broth." While Adams' wounds were considered mortal, his appreciation of beautiful women was still quite alive and well. "Oh, it was nice!" he commented wistfully of that supper.[11]

The Massachusetts captain was beginning to feel decidedly better under the ministrations of his attractive new nurse. "Either the broth or the young lady's presence revived me. My new friend's name was Lucy. She said, 'Don't take breakfast until I come, because I will bring yours from home.' Bright and early Lucy was on hand with a pan of milk toast. She had seen me eat the night before and had brought enough

---

9. Adams, *Reminiscences of the Nineteenth Massachusetts*, pp. 72-73.
10. *Ibid.*, p. 73.
11. *Ibid.*

for six. As she was called away for a few moments, I spoke to the boys who were near, and they soon reduced the surplus."[12]

Still, with those wounds as yet untreated, Captain Adams' condition continued to deteriorate. "We remained here two days. While I had the best care they could give I was growing worse. I had a high fever, and my wounds were getting inflamed. At times I would lie in a stupor for hours. One day I rallied and found the church deserted except Lucy and myself. Soon two men came in."

"'Are you going?' they asked."

"Lucy said, 'No. Mother told me if any were not able to be moved to bring them home, and we would care for them; he is not able, and must not go.'"

"The temptation was strong to stay, but a moment's reflection told me that I required hospital treatment, and I explained the danger to her. The men then carried me to the train and placed me on the floor of a baggage car. Lucy came with us, fixed my head all right, and, as a good sister should, kissed me good-by, and we were off for Baltimore. I was so weak that the *rear* name of Lucy passed out of my mind, and I have never seen her since, but have prayed that the blessings of Heaven be showered upon her, for her constant care the last day in the old church saved me from fever."[13]

The First "Lodge," Rock Creek, outside Gettysburg, Pennsylvania

While some of the lesser wounded (like Austin Carr and his friend Briggs) made their escape on foot, and others (like Captain Adams and Duncan Sherwood) paid to be hauled out of town in the back of a jouncing wagon, the vast majority of the casualties of the July battle picked up the trains at Gettysburg—at first, several miles outside town at the damaged Rock Creek bridge, then later at the site of the town station. "This is the way the thing was managed at first: the surgeons left in care of the wounded three or four miles from the town, went up and down among the men in the morning, and said, 'Any of you boys who can make your way to the cars, can go to Baltimore.' So off start all who think they feel well enough, anything being better than the 'hospitals,' so called, for the first few days after a battle."[14]

The men were still under military control, so they needed to seek out a discharge, or at least verbal authorization, from their surgeons. These

12. *Ibid.*
13. *Ibid.*, pp. 73-74.
14. Woolsey, *Three Weeks at Gettysburg.*

medical officers served as the superior officers of the wounded left under their care at the hospitals. "Once the men have the surgeons' permission to go, they are off; and there may be an interval of a day, or two days, should any of them be too weak to reach the train in time, during which these poor fellows belong to no one, the hospital at the one end, the railroad at the other, with far more chance of falling through between the two."

"For the first few days the worst cases only came down in ambulances from the hospitals; hundreds of fellows hobbled along as best they could in heat and dust, for hours, slowly toiling, and in many hired farmers' wagons, as hard as the farmers' fists themselves, and were jolted down to the railroad, at three and four dollars the man. Think of the disappointment of a soldier, sick, body and heart, to find at the end of this miserable journey, that this effort to get away, into which he had put all his remaining stock of strength, was useless; that 'the cars had gone,' or 'the cars were full'; that while he was coming down others had stepped down before him, and that he must turn all the weary way back again, or sleep on the roadside till the next train 'tomorrow!'"[15]

Into this confusion of stranded casualties, waiting in futility for rail transportation, without doctors, food, or medicines, marooned between a railroad that was not running and hospitals anxious to send away the lesser wounded, stepped the agents of the Sanitary Commission. "The First Lodge," established at Rock Creek where almost two thousand wounded men had walked out of town to awaited rail transportation, was already up and operating when George Anna Woolsey and her mother stepped off the first train to reach the vicinity of the battlefield. "No men were turned back," wrote George Anna in a pamphlet to women's societies scattered throughout the North. "You fed and you sheltered them just when no one else could have done so; and out of the boxes and barrels of good and nourishing things, which you people at home had supplied, we took all that was needed. Some of you sent a stove (that is, the money to get it), some of you the beef stock, some of you the milk and fresh bread; and all of you would have been thankful that you had done so, could you have seen the refreshment and comfort received through these things."[16]

With the trained personnel and sufficient supplies at hand, the Sanitary Commission transit hospital quickly had a quality commissary

---

15. *Ibid.*
16. *Ibid.*

and medical facility up and running, ready to care for the wounded men coming by wagon, ambulance, and stretcher from the corps hospitals to meet the incoming trains. "As soon as the men hobbled up to the tents, good hot soup was given all round and that over, their wounds were dressed—for the gentlemen of the commission are cooks, or surgeons, as occasion demands—and, finally, with their blankets spread over the straw, the men stretched themselves out and were contented till morning, and the next train."[17]

"The lodge, which was established at the temporary terminus of the railway, on Tuesday, was continued there until Friday, when the burned bridge which had prevented the cars from running into town, was replaced by a new structure, and the cars resumed their regular runnings to the station." With the Rock Creek bridge open to rail traffic, the Sanitary Commission immediately began preparations to move their facility into town.[18]

The Christian Commission had also been running an "Eating Saloon," theirs set up at the end of the tracks in Gettysburg; in fact, as one Christian Commission delegate reported, it had been "kept in full operation by us till the Sanitary Commission proposed to take it off our hands. As we had more than we could do to take care of the severely wounded, the offer was gladly accepted. Mr. A. H. Brown and other delegates of the Christian Commission helped the agents of the Sanitary Commission to pitch their tents near the railroad depot, and we thankfully gave over the feeding of hungry soldiers, at this point, into their hands."[19]

"On Thursday, I had a tent and fly erected near the depot," wrote a Sanitary official, "in preparation for the change of terminus of the road, and on Saturday the lodge out of town was discontinued, and the tents used there added to those near the depot. This second lodge was in successful operation on Friday, though it was not generally made use of until Saturday."[20]

The First Lodge out by Rock Creek had done a tremendous amount of work in the less than five days of its existence. "Between Tuesday

17. *Ibid.*
18. *The Sanitary Commission of the United States Army. A Succinct Narrative of Its Works and Purposes*, pp. 155-56.
19. *The United States Christian Commission for the Army and Navy. For the Year 1863. Second Annual Report*, p. 69.
20. *The Sanitary Commission of the United States Army. A Succinct Narrative of Its Works and Purposes*, pp. 155-56.

and Saturday noon, we provided at our first lodge, good beef soup, coffee, and fresh bread, for over 3,000 slightly wounded soldiers, whose injuries did not prevent them from walking to this point, while we sheltered, each night, about fifty more serious cases, which had been brought down by ambulance, and whose wounds required the attention of a surgeon. We were fortunate in having, during these days, the volunteer aid of Dr. [Robert W.] Hooper, from Boston, who devoted himself to this latter work. Mr. Clark, from New Hampshire, Mr. Hawkins, from Media, Pa., and Mr. Shippen, from Pittsburg[h], also lent their assistance, and all these gentlemen materially aided us at this and at the second lodge, until it was fully organized."[21]

The Second "Lodge," Gettysburg, Pennsylvania

"On the day that the [Rock Creek] railroad bridge was repaired, we moved up to the depot, close by town, and had things in perfect order; a first rate camping ground, in a large field directly by the track, with unlimited supply of cool water. Here we set up two stoves, with four large boilers, always kept full of soup and coffee, watched by four or five black men who did the cooking, under our direction, and sang (not under our direction) all day."[22]

Dr. F. W. Cheney was placed in charge of the new facility on July 10. Administration of the the Second Lodge was placed in the hands of seven Sanitary Commission assistants from Canandaigua, New York, two delegates from Baltimore, and four detailed soldiers. "Additional tents were erected, drains made, straw procured, and shelter prepared for 150 men. A store tent was placed near the hospital tents, and given into the charge of two New York ladies [the Woolseys], whose long experience on the Commission's transports, during the Peninsular campaign of last summer, had made them familiar with all of the requirements of this camp. The cars stopped immediately in front of our camp, and distant but a few feet from it."[23]

This was the sight that greeted Surgeon Theodore Dimon as he climbed off the train at Gettysburg on July 12, weary from his long and circuitous trip from New York. "The first thing [I] noticed on arriving at the town was the relief tents of the Sanitary Commission. The station

21. *Ibid.*
22. Woolsey, *Three Weeks at Gettysburg.*
23. *The Sanitary Commission of the United States Army. A Succinct Narrative of Its Works and Purposes*, p. 156.

house of the railroad was burned and as such wounded as could bear transportation were brought to the trains in ambulances, they were subjected to delay before the trains were ready, sometimes even being taken back again to the field hospitals, some miles distant, when they were too late or some occurrence prevented the arrival or departure of the expected train."[24]

"It was made up of five tents; here a surgeon was always to be found to dress wounds; here too was a kitchen and expert cooks, and a large supply tent filled with almost everything necessary and useful; here were tents in which the wearied soldier could sleep and eat; and here, too, caring for all, were to be found the humane ladies whose work is well described in the anonymous pamphlet, entitled 'Three Weeks at Gettysburg.'"[25]

Ambulances and wagons were still at a premium in Gettysburg. The Adams Express Company, with headquarters in Baltimore, maintained a freight office next door to the Gettysburg depot. Moved by the unbelievable amount of suffering in and around Gettysburg, Adams Express Superintendent S. S. Shoemaker came up with a novel way of using his company's resources during this emergency.

In a telegram to Secretary of War Edwin Stanton, Shoemaker suggested that, since "the God of Battles having so far given us the victory, our next care is for the wounded. This company proposes to get a hospital corps of their own—sending men, food, suitable comforts, etc. to the front, with a number of spring wagons to bring in the wounded."[26]

Stanton "heartily approved," adding: "I give you herewith a pass through the lines for your agents and employees." Not to be outdone, the Baltimore Fire Department tendered their services and their vehicles for emergency transpiration. Stanton graciously accepted their offer as well. Soon express wagons, fire equipment, ambulances and medical wagons were plying the streets of Gettysburg, all working

24. Dimon, *From Auburn to Antietam*; Dimon, *Report of the General Agent of the State of New York*, p. 42.

25. Dimon, *From Auburn to Antietam*; Dimon, *Report of the General Agent of the State of New York*, p. 42. Doctor Dimon is, of course, referring to George Anna Woolsey and her mother, Jane Eliza Newton Woolsey.

26. *OR*, vol. 27, pt. 3, p. 521.

together to move the casualties out of town and onto the road to recovery.[27]

"The arrival or departure of the expected train[s]" was a subject much on the mind of Medical Inspector Edward P. Vollum, United States Army. The railroad system that he found upon his arrival in Gettysburg on July 7 was in an extreme state of confusion and disarray. "The railroad authorities were perplexed, and deficient in motive power and rolling stock. The bridges put up since the rebel raids proved too weak excepting for the lightest engines, and for a second time some were carried away by the floods. The telegraph wires were down, and the obstruction to transportation seemed insurmountable."[28]

Compounding the confusion was the fact that Gen. Herman Haupt, who had gotten the railroad back up and running again, had left the Gettysburg area for Washington D.C. Capt. W. G. Rankin, appointed by the chief quartermaster to see to the railroad's operation, had a serious drinking problem, and was way in over his head. He shot off a panicked message to his superior: "There has been great difficulty here in regard to the road . . . and many vexatious delays, owing to a want of men and management. It has not been under my control."[29]

"Out of control" was a better way of putting it. A train would reach the end of the line with a load of desperately needed relief supplies, but there would be no one detailed to unload the freight. Mobbed with wounded men anxious to leave town, the train crew would finally give up in frustration, get up steam, and head back to Hanover without unloading. There was no such thing as a rail schedule. Consequently, there were agonizing delays: "A train of cars loaded with wounded was necessarily detained on the tracks . . . for 24 hours; 600 of them must have suffered the pangs of hunger as well as the faintness of wounds without our succor."[30]

Just when conditions seemed to be most bleak, Chief Quartermaster Rufus Ingalls wired Quartermaster General Montgomery C. Meigs that a "dispatcher with full power" was needed. They got one on July 9—Herman Haupt himself, back from the nation's capital, and breathing

27. *Ibid.*
28. *Ibid.*, vol. 27, pt. 1, p. 26.
29. *Ibid.*, vol. 27, pt. 3, p. 619.
30. *New York Times,* July 16, 1863.

fire over the snafu of the railroad system he had worked so hard to restore.[31]

"Find things in great confusion," snapped Haupt when he arrived; "road blocked; cars not unloaded; stores ordered to Gettysburg, where they stand for a long time, completely preventing all movement there; ordered back without unloading; wounded lying for hours, without ability to carry them off; all because the simple rule of promptly unloading and returning cars is violated." In a matter of hours, he was able to wire the Quartermaster General: "We are about straight again at Gettysburg; I have put the road in the charge of our own men [including Surgeon Henry Janes and Medical Inspector Edward P. Vollum]."[32]

The same day, Captain Rankin smoothly wired his superior that the problem with the railroad "is now corrected, and the road today is working under military authority . . . General Haupt has just been in my office, and railroad matters to this point are arranged so that there will be no confusion hereafter." He neglected to give any details of his meeting with Haupt; the railroad general, never one to be shy, had undoubtedly blistered Ingalls thoroughly for his incompetent handling of the situation.[33]

"General Haupt arrived and assumed military control of the road to Hanover Junction," wrote Vollum. "We then experienced no further delays till the 18th, when an important bridge on the road to Harrisburg gave way under a cattle train, thus diverting, for the following five days, the trains that were intended for New York to Baltimore and York, Pa."[34]

With the arrival of the first trains at the outskirts of town, evacuation of the wounded by rail finally began in earnest, although somewhat haltingly at first. On Tuesday, July 7, three trainloads of Union wounded, bearing a mere 822 men, steamed away from the battlefield—one at 5:00 p.m., another at 7:00 p.m., and a final trainload ten minutes later. On the following day, only one train, loaded with 640 casualties, left town at 1:40 p.m.[35]

31. *OR*, vol. 27, pt. 3, p. 591.
32. Haupt, *Reminiscences of General Herman Haupt*, p. 239; *OR*, vol. 27, pt. 3, pp. 619-20.
33. *OR*, vol. 27, pt. 3, p. 619.
34. *Ibid.*, vol. 27, pt. 1, p. 26.
35. *Ibid.*, p. 27.

Thursday (the day General Haupt resumed control), however, witnessed the first full-scale test of the evacuation system as two packed trains of Northerners pulled ponderously away from Gettysburg—the morning cars carried away 1,012 wounded, while the evening departure was crammed with 1,061 men. By Friday, July 10, the first rush of the lesser wounded had passed; the a.m. and p.m. loads of casualties had dropped to a total of 806 men. After operating for only four days, the railroad had already transported 4,341 wounded Union men, all headed for Baltimore.[36]

Inspector Vollum was shocked by the callous indifference manifested by the railroad officials, which stood in stark contrast to the lavish outpouring of relief from all other quarters. "The period of ten days following the battle of Gettysburg was the occasion of the greatest amount of human suffering known to this nation since its birth, and, as was natural and unavoidable among a Christian people, benevolent societies, Sanitary and Christian Commissions, express companies, fire organizations, bands of generous people of all denominations, and individuals from great distances, all came forward with their offerings, sympathy, and personal services, forming a spectacle at once touching and magnificent, exceeding any similar outburst of sympathy and sacrifice ever witnessed. The railroad companies, who got the only profit of the battle, and who had the greatest opportunities of ameliorating the sufferings of the wounded, alone stood aloof and rendered no aid."[37]

Most horrifying of all to the army medical inspector was the condition of the freight cars sent out by the railroad for the cartage of the wounded soldiers. The transportation officials were pulling every available car from wherever they could be found, rushing them off to Gettysburg without bothering to clean them out after unloading, or adding any human comforts whatsoever. "Their trains were allowed to go off without a single individual attached to them in any way authorized to minister to the wounded. There was no check-line or means of stopping the train in case of necessity; no way provided for passing from car to car. The cars—ordinary stock and freight cars—were always unclean; no one connected with the companies to clean them; the dung of cattle and litter from freight often remained to be removed by any extemporized means at hand. There was no water, or

36. *Ibid.*
37. *Ibid.*, p. 28.

vessels to contain it, no lanterns, no straw—absolutely nothing but the bare cars, filthy from the business of transporting freight and cattle."[38]

Possibly even more disgusting was the thoughtless and mercenary attitude of the few rail employees who did arrive on the scene. The army was paying the railroad by the head count of those transported, and these cold-hearted clerks were interested in one thing, and one thing only—getting the correct tally. "The only agents of the railroad companies that appeared upon this memorable scene were those sent especially to look after their pecuniary interests, and I can testify to their zeal in getting the actual numbers transported and securing the proper certificates therefor, but beyond this they did nothing."[39]

Vollum fired off telegrams to his superiors, and General Haupt promptly stepped in to put a stop to these outrages. The railroad general immediately commandeered that portion of the North Central road and placed it directly under military rule; as a result, the condition of the rail transportation abruptly took a dramatic turn for the better. "Every train of wounded was placed in charge of a medical official detailed by Surg H Janes. Instruments, dressings, stimulants, &c., were furnished him, and he was instructed to announce his coming by telegraph, if possible, and to report in person to the medical director at the place of his destination. Each car was filled with a sufficient quantity of hay, and, on the longer routes, water-coolers, tin cups, bed-pans, and urinals were placed in them, and guarded in route by some agents of the Sanitary Commission. In some instances, these conveniences were furnished by the medical department, but the demand for them by the hospitals often exhausted the supplies at the purveyors."[40]

Inspector Vollum labored all day July 9 with limited resources, struggling to get the evacuation procedures up and moving. In addition to his concerns for the wounded, his superior, United States Army Inspector John M. Cuyler, was due to arrive momentarily. Any anxiety he may have been feeling was unnecessary, however; Cuyler had been experiencing firsthand the frustrating and haphazard nature

38. *Ibid.*
39. *Ibid.*
40. *Ibid.*, p. 26.

of post-battle rail travel that was so sorely testing Inspector Vollum's patience. "I arrived at Gettysburg on the morning of the 10th of July [*sic*], forty hours later than I had hoped to do, in consequence of the irregularities and interruptions on the railways leading to that place."[41]

". . . I reported to him for duty," wrote Vollum to the surgeon general, "and, by mutual arrangement, I continued in immediate charge of the transportation of the wounded, which confined me to the railroad depot and city of Gettysburg." For his part, Cuyler, a Georgian who had remained loyal to the Union, was well pleased with the work that Vollum had accomplished so far. In his report to Surgeon General Hammond, Cuyler wrote of his subordinate: "Immediately on his arrival [he] made arrangements for sending away such of the wounded as were in a condition to be moved in ambulances or on the railroad. Lieutenant-Colonel Vollum had the immediate charge of forwarding the wounded to the general hospitals designated by yourself. In this he was assisted by Dr. [J. D.] Osborne [4th New Jersey], of the Army of the Potomac, a very active and energetic officer. Both of these officers performed the duty assigned them with very great faithfulness and efficiency."[42]

Cuyler's initial inspections at the point of embarkation revealed that everything was moving as smoothly as possible under the less-than-ideal conditions of Gettysburg. "I believe the wounded were received at the railroad depot and placed on the cars with as much care, attention, and comfort as was possible under the circumstances."[43]

Transportation of the wounded to the terminal continued to pose a difficulty for the multiplied thousands of wounded, each one anxious to escape the festering surrounds of the battlefield. "Before the arrival of the fifty ambulances sent from Washington by yourself," wrote Cuyler to his chief several weeks later, "our means of conveying the wounded from the field hospitals to the railroad depot were inadequate, although I am satisfied that as many ambulances were left by the Army of the Potomac as could possibly be spared." Medical Director Jonathan Letterman had initially planned to leave behind six ambulances and four wagons with each corps hospital. In reality, when

---

41. *Ibid.*, p. 24. Cuyler probably arrived on July 11 instead of July 10. Vollum reported that "Medical Inspector Cuyler arrived on the 11th." [*Ibid.*, p. 26], and Cuyler himself reported that Vollum (who arrived on July 8) had "reached Gettysburg some two or three days in advance of me." [*ibid.*, p. 24]
42. *Ibid.*, pp. 26, 24.
43. *Ibid.*, p. 24.

inventoried, only thirty ambulances remained for seven separate corps hospitals when the Army of the Potomac left town. Letterman would defend his gross misjudgment by saying that "I acted on the best information that could be obtained."[44]

With the responsibility of evacuating the wounded left in the capable hands of Medical Inspector Vollum, Inspector Cuyler set out to visit the corps hospitals, personally checking to insure that everything was being handled properly at that end of the process. "The number of medical officers detailed by Medical Director Letterman to remain with the wounded was thought to be sufficient, and probably might have been had not the thousands of the enemy's wounded been thrown unexpectedly on our hands. For some days after the battle, many of the rebel wounded were in a most deplorable condition, being without shelter of any sort, and with an insufficient number of medical officers and nurses of their own army."[45]

Moved by the plight of his fellow Southerners, many of them from his home state, Cuyler, a well qualified surgeon himself, pitched in at the Third Division hospital of the Second Corps, helping finish the case load of Confederate surgeries still pending. His efforts, however, were not viewed with any great admiration by his patients from south of the Mason-Dixon line. "The Yankee surgeon in charge of all the wounds in these parts is a *Georgian!*" wrote Virginian John Dooley in amazement and disgust. "But being educated at W[est] Point he has thought it incumbent on him to deny his native land and join with its enemies."[46]

While working at the Second Corps hospital, Cuyler sustained what could have been a fatal injury. "He is a very fine looking man and has his hand in a sling, for yesterday when operating upon a gangrened wound, the knife with which he was operating cut his finger slightly; and he very sensibly . . . had his finger immediately amputated." Cuyler's response to the injury in a pre-antiseptic era reveals his better-than-average understanding of infection, and his modesty, since he makes no reference to the injury and amputation in his official report of his activities at Gettysburg.[47]

Following his firsthand inspection and participation at the Confederate portion of Second Corps hospitals at the Schwartz Farm,

---

44. *Ibid.*, pp. 25, 198.
45. *Ibid.*, pp. 24-25.
46. Dooley, *John Dooley*, p. 121.
47. *Ibid.*

Cuyler could knowledgeably report that "every effort was made to alleviate the sufferings of these unfortunate men, and as soon as it could be done they were placed under cover or sent away to some general hospital." Some critical shortages, however, still continued to plague the hospitals, even after well over a week following the cessation of fighting: "The scarcity of straw for bedding was seriously felt, and it was not until eight or ten days after the conflict that a sufficient quantity could be obtained."[48]

Cuyler felt true admiration for the surgeons and medical personnel of the corps hospitals whom he observed and worked beside; he glowingly praised both military and civilian doctors alike in his official report of his Gettysburg visit. "As far as my observation extends, the medical officers of the army, and the citizen surgeons who were employed during the emergency, discharged the arduous duties with fidelity and ability. I never saw men work harder and complain less of the difficulties that surrounded them."[49]

Also high on his list of commendation were the ongoing efforts of the voluntary relief agencies to marshal supplies, import foodstuffs and delicacies for the wounded, and physically, emotionally, and spiritually care for the army of broken and bleeding men. "I cannot close this brief report without acknowledging the immense aid afforded by the Sanitary and Christian Commissions. The promptness, energy, and great kindness uniformly exhibited by these benevolent associations doubtless helped to save the lives of many, and gladdened the hearts of thousands, who, with their friends scattered throughout our land, will hold the good and noble deeds in grateful remembrance. To Adams Express we are also greatly indebted for much liberality and kindness extended to the wounded at a time when they were most in need."[50]

With the Rock Creek bridge rebuilt, the trains were now able to travel unimpeded into Gettysburg, rolling to a stop each day opposite the tents of the Sanitary Commission Lodge, adjacent to the burnt depot. More and more commissioners were arriving, each group shepherding their own shipment of supplies; the Lodge quickly was

48. *OR*, vol. 27, pt. 1, p. 25.
49. *Ibid.*
50. *Ibid.*

able to expand its commissary, culinary, and medical operations. "Then we had three large hospital tents, holding about thirty-five each, a large camp-meeting supply tent, where barrels of goods were stored, and our own smaller tent fitted up with tables, where [there were] jelly-pots and bottles of all kinds of good syrups, blackberry and black current. Barrels were ranged round the tent walls; shirts, drawers, dressing-gowns, socks and slippers (I wish we had had more of the latter), rags and bandages, each in its own place on one side; on the other, boxes of tea, coffee, soft crackers, tamarinds, cherry brandy, etc. Over this kitchen, and over this small supply-tent, we women rather reigned, and filled up our wants by requisitions on the Commission's depot. By this time there had arrived a 'delegation' of just the right kind from Canadaiguia, N.Y., with surgeon dressers and attendants, bringing a first-rate supply of necessities and comforts for the wounded, which they handed over to the Commission."[51]

Inspector Vollum frequently came in contact with the workers at the Lodge in his role of supervisor of medical evacuations. He was singularly impressed with the consistent care given to the wounded, without respect to rank or army, by these Sanitary representatives. "Before leaving the wounded were fed and watered by the Sanitary Commission, and often hundreds of wounded, laid over for a night or part of a day, were attended and fed by the Commission, whose agents placed them in the cars."[52]

As soon as General Haupt imposed military control on the railroad, a schedule of departures was put in effect. Timetables varied wildly at first, but, by July 13, the trains were pulling out of Gettysburg regularly at 9:00 a.m. and 3:00 p.m. Knowing that there was an established timetable assisted the corps hospitals to get their evacuees to the Lodge in time to catch the outgoing cars. "Twice a day the train left for Baltimore or Harrisburgh [*sic*], and twice a day we fed all the wounded who arrived for them. Things were systemized now, and the men came down in long ambulance trains to the cars; baggage-cars these were, filled with straw for the wounded to lie in, and broken open at either end to let in the air."[53]

As the caravans of ambulances drew along the tracks, the Sanitary commissioners and all available help turned out to get the wounded on board the rail cars with as little jostling and discomfort as possible.

---

51. Woolsey, *Three Weeks at Gettysburg.*
52. *OR*, vol. 27, pt. 1, p. 26.
53. Woolsey, *Three Weeks at Gettysburg.*

Some stayed behind to carry litters from the Sanitary Commission transit hospital, while still others supported the walking wounded as they hobbled from the trackside tents and clambered on board. "A government surgeon was always present to attend to the careful lifting of the soldiers from ambulance to car. Many of the men could get along very nicely, holding one foot up, and taking great jumps on their crutches. The latter were a great comfort; we had a nice supply at the Lodge, and they traveled up and down from the tents to the cars daily. Only occasionally did we dare let a pair go on with some very lame soldier, who begged for them; we needed them to help with the new arrivals each day, and trust to the men being supplied them at the hospitals at the journey's end. Pads and crutches are a standing want, pads particularly. We manufactured them out of the rags we had, stuffed with saw-dust from brandy boxes, and with half a sheet and some soft straw."[54]

Capt. Benjamin Thompson of the 111th New York Volunteers was also there, showing no ill effects from his wounding about the face from flying rock chips during the July 3 bombardment. He was still suffering from his varicose veins, however, and now he hobbled painfully from wagon to the train as he assisted the loading of his injured friends into the cars. After being sent back to Gettysburg by his regimental surgeon, Thompson had been tireless in caring for the needs of the wounded comrades from his regiment. Like Capt. John G. B. Adams of the 19th Massachusetts and Surgeon Bushrod Washington James, he was forced to hire the services of a local farmer for transportation. "I employed one of them to take the men of my company to the depot. He did it in half a day with one horse and wagon and charged twenty dollars for the service. But it was the best I could do."[55]

Charles Muller of the 1st Minnesota found a bargain, or so he thought at first, when a farmer came by the Second Corps Hospital on July 11 "whit [*sic*] his farmer wagon and said for a dollar each he would take us to the Rail Road Station. I put up my dollar and in company of eight others we were hauled to the Station about 2 miles away."[56]

But getting on the wagon proved easier than getting some food along the way. "On going through Gettysburg we wanted to buy some Bred [*sic*], but they toll [*sic*] us that they wont sell any to the Yankies

54. *Ibid.*

55. Thompson, *Personal Narrative*, p. 49.

56. Charles Muller Papers, Minnesota Historical Society, St. Paul, Minnesota.

[*sic*]." Muller and his companions kept asking along the way, but with the same response. Thoroughly frustrated in their quest to get something to eat, "we had to go to Baltimore whit [*sic*] a growling empty stomach."[57]

Another soldier making his way to the railroad was First Sgt. Levi W. Baker of the 9th Massachusetts Battery, shot in the "hip and shoulder, twice, severe" during the Confederate attack on July 2. He and his companions had received marching orders for "Gettysburg town" at their encampment of walking wounded along Rock Creek on Wednesday, July 7. "We were directed to the Christian Commission room, and coffee and sandwiches refreshed us. About midday it [the rain] began to clear off, and a train of commissary and hospital stores was being unloaded, and was soon filled with wounded. . . . The accomodations were not the best—a box car with a wet floor we had."[58]

With the wounded now on board, the Sanitary personnel did a quick job change from medical assistants to commissary attendants. "When the surgeon had the wounded all placed, with as much comfort as seemed possible under the circumstances, on board the train, our detail of men would go from car to car, with soup made of beef-stock or fresh meat, full of potatoes, turnips, cabbage, and rice, with fresh bread and coffee, and, when stimulants were needed, with ale, milk-punch, or brandy." (It is somewhat uncertain how Charles Muller and his friends from the 1st Minnesota managed to miss out on this snack).[59]

Even with serious wounds, these men were soldiers, and kept thinking like soldiers. Many had lost much, if not most, of their equipment in the course of their wounding, transportation to aid station and field hospital, in the flooding along Rock Creek, and now finally the trip to the train. With few canteens to go around, and no rations in their knapsacks, these veteran campaigners were seriously concerned about having a source of water (both to drink and to pour on their wounds) and food for this rail trip of unknown length. "Water pails were in great demand for use in the cars on the journey, and also empty bottles to take the place of canteens. All our whiskey and brandy bottles were washed and filled up at the spring, and the boys went off carefully hugging their extemporized canteens, from which

57. *Ibid.*
58. Levi W. Baker, *History of the Ninth Massachusetts Battery* (South Farmington, Massachusetts: Lakeview Press, 1888; Lancaster, Ohio: Vanberg Publishing, 1996), pp. 64, 87, 88.
59. Woolsey, *Three Weeks at Gettysburg.*

they would wet their wounds or refresh themselves till the journey ended."[60]

"With each train went a surgeon and attendants in charge of the wounded. Large cans of iced water, bags of crackers, stimulants, &c., were placed on board the cars to supply every necessity. Generally, before leaving, each canteen was filled with water, and each man furnished with an extra cup of coffee, or soup, or with broth, as they desired. This system was continued from the 9th of July till the corps hospitals were relieved of all who were able to be removed to a distance."[61]

With the wounded supplied for the trip and safely on board, the staff of the Lodge would wave them on their way as the couplings snapped tight and the train began rolling away from the tents. With another convoy of wounded heading out of Gettysburg, the Sanitary Commissioners quickly got back to work, preparing for the ambulances that would soon roll to a stop and begin unloading a fresh cargo of transient casualties.

The trip out of Gettysburg was, for many, one of the most memorable aspects of the entire campaign. After several weeks made up solely of hard marches, the swirl of combat, the terror of being wounded, and the agony of trying to survive from day to painful day in the military hospital system, the train trip from Gettysburg took on almost a festive atmosphere, despite the circumstances.

One grievously wounded Massachusetts soldier recalled:

> Early one Sunday morning, soon after the battle, I found myself lying upon one of the platform cars of a long trip. The journey, painful though it was, proved to be the most eventful of my life.
>
> Soon after leaving Gettysburg we began to encounter crowds of sympathetic people at every crossing and station. The kind expressions, the moistened eyes, the uncovered heads, and the showers of hearty "God bless yous" that were rained upon us as we continued on our journey, made a

60. *Ibid.*
61. Wormeley, *The United States Sanitary Commission*, p. 145.

> deep and lasting impression upon every loyal heart upon the train.
>
> I shall never forget that ride nor how the good-hearted Pennsylvania women flocked about the cars at every stopping place and wept over us as if we were their own sons and brothers. "This is a country worth fighting for," exclaimed a New Yorker soldier at my side. The remark expressed the feeling of every one.[62]

No sooner did the train steam its way east over the horizon than a host of latecomers arrived from the corps hospitals. "After each train of cars daily, for the three weeks we were at Gettysburg, trains of ambulances arrived too late, men who must spend the day with us until the 5 p.m. cars went, and men too late for the 5 p.m. train, who must spend the night until the 10 a.m. [*sic*] cars went.[63] All the men who came in this way, under our own immediate and particular attention, were given the best we had of care and food. The surgeon in charge of our camp, with his most faithful dresser and attendants, looked after their wounds, which were often in a most shocking state, particularly among rebels. Often the men would say, 'That feels good. I haven't had my wound dressed so well since I was hurt.' Something cool to drink is the first thing asked for after the long, dusty drive, and pailfuls [*sic*] of tamarinds and water, 'a beautiful drink,' the men used to say, disappeared rapidly among them."[64]

For the men who arrived after the trains left, the Lodge provided the warmth and cleanliness of a woman's touch that many husbands, sons, and brothers had sorely missed during the hard days and weeks of campaigning. "After the men's wounds were attended to, we went round giving them clean clothes; and basins and soap and towels, and followed these with socks, slippers, shirts, drawers, and those coveted dressing-gowns. Such pride as they felt in them! Comparing colors and

62. J. Howard Wert, "In the Hospitals of Gettysburg, July, 1863," No. VI, *Harrisburg Telegraph*, August 16, 1907, p. 7.

63. George Anna was describing the events of July 11-12, the only days when an evening train left at 5:00 p.m., and a morning train departed the next morning at 9:00 a.m. [*OR*, vol. 27, pt. 1, p. 27.]

64. Woolsey, *Three Weeks at Gettysburg*.

smiling all over as they lay in clean and comfortable rows ready for supper, 'on dress parade,' they used to say."[65]

From time to time, when the hurry and bustle of tending to the needs of the wounded had temporarily abated, the workers at the Sanitary Commission Lodge would stop and ponder the tangible delight they felt in bringing order to a very disorderly battlefield, of being able to make a difference in the lives of other people in serious need. "And the milk, particularly if it were boiled and had a little whiskey and sugar, and the bread with *butter* on it, and *jelly* on the butter—how good it all was," wrote George Anna Woolsey reflectively to the many supporters of the Sanitary Commission scattered throughout the North, "and how lucky we felt ourselves in having the immense satisfaction of distributing these things, which all of you, hard at work in villages and cities, were getting ready and sending off, in faith."[66]

One item in particular seemed to temporarily help the wounded, as well as the Commission representatives, mute the nausea and distress produced when prevailing winds swept over the festering battlefield. "Canadaigua [New York] sent cologne with its other supplies, which went right to the noses and the hearts of the men.[67] 'Worth a penny a sniff,' 'that kinder gives one life,' and so on, all round the tents, as we tipped the bottles up on the clean handkerchiefs some one had sent, and when these were gone, over squares of cotton, on which the perfume took the place of them."[68]

The Lodge took special pride in the quality and variety of their cuisine, fueled by the daily freight and ice cars filled with all manner of foodstuffs. Evening meals were a special treat for the wounded, who had so long been forced to endure a diet dominated by hardtack, beans, and salt pork. "We varied our dinners with custard and baked rice puddings, scrambled eggs, codfish hash, corn starch, and always as much soft bread, tea, coffee or milk as they wanted. Two Massachusetts boys I especially remember, for the satisfaction with which they ate their pudding. I carried a second plateful up to the cars, after they had been put in, and fed one of them till he was sure he had had enough. Young fellows they were, lying side by side, one with a right and one with a left arm gone."[69]

---

65. *Ibid.*
66. *Ibid.*
67. Pennyroyal and peppermint oil were also very popular scents in the hospitals.
68. Woolsey, *Three Weeks at Gettysburg.*
69. *Ibid.*

Hanover Junction, Pennsylvania

As the trainloads of casualties were worrying about food and water for their long trip, the Christian Commission already had a system in place to meet the dietary needs of the railroad convoys of wounded men. At various predetermined places along the route of travel, the Commission had set up refreshment stations for the wounded evacuees of Gettysburg. The train would pull to a stop, and each car would in turn be visited by representatives bearing easily digested delicacies such as cold drinks, baked goods, farina, and fruits.

The first refreshment stop after leaving Gettysburg was at Hanover Junction. "At the insistence of Dr. Cuyler, Medical Director, the Commission established a refreshment station, in cars provided for the purpose, at Hanover Junction, thirty miles from Gettysburg and on the main line of railway. Here all the trains of wounded stopped, and nourishing food and drink,—as lemonade, ginger-water, tea and coffee, soft bread, etc., with stimulants for those that needed,—were liberally distributed to the suffering men."[70]

"Lemonade was given to the stronger ones; to those weaker and needing a stimulant, a little brandy or wine. Thus no doubt many were enabled to bear the fatigue of the journey, who but for this would have sunk on the way."[71]

Emily Bliss Souder, a would-be volunteer nurse en route to the battlefield who was stranded at Hanover Junction, described the activity of the relief agency volunteers. Located in a rail car drawn up on a siding, they were busily preparing for the arrival of the next train. "A train of wounded soldiers passed down about an hour ago. A car is stationed here, close to the railroad track, where four ladies from Baltimore prepare lemonade, bread and butter, to refresh the men, beside pies, farina, etc.,—'The Christian Commission Car.' They have three stations on the way."[72]

Bored and restless from the unexpected delay and the oppressive heat, Souder and members of her party walked over to see what the "four ladies from Baltimore" were up to. "We made a visit to this car and saw the ladies at work. Presently, a young man, a member of the Commission, came in with a market basket, filled with loaves of bread,

---

70. Rev. Lemuel Moss, *Annals of the United States Christian Commission* (Philadelphia: J. B. Lippincott & Co., 1868), p. 322.
71. *The United States Christian Commission for the Army and Navy. For the Year 1863. Second Annual Report*, p. 80.
72. Souder, *Leaves from the Battle-field of Gettysburg*, pp. 11-12.

which he had procured from farm-houses not very far distant. I bought a barrel of bread from a baker in Baltimore and could hardly refrain from adding this to their store," confided Mrs. Souder to her husband in a July 14 letter; "but the accounts which we have received of the great necessity for bread in Gettysburg induced me to retain it, as the distance to this point is more easily passed over."[73]

Beside the town church, small businesses, and private homes being used as hospitals, the Christian Commission car proved to be a focal point of local relief activity. "A kind-hearted woman, by the wayside, has been baking sixty pies per day, the materials being furnished to her,—not a trifling service, with the thermometer at ninety degrees or so."[74]

Even the prickly Sanitary Commission was working closely with the Christian Commission to help meet the needs of the wounded as they arrived. "A gentleman belonging to the Sanitary Commission came next, with an anxious face, to inquire if the ladies 'had any way to cook some meat?' The ice in the 'provision car' had melted and he feared that the fresh meat would spoil, the heat was so great and there was so much delay on the road." So the preparation continued for the arrival of the next trainload of wounded.[75]

"Our first stop was Hanover Junction," remembered one veteran of that painful rail evacuation, "and we met a grateful people; good coffee, sandwiches and cakes were brought; old men, women, boys and girls welcomed us. It was late in the afternoon when we left."[76]

After the men had been ministered to, the train rattled out of sight, and the process would begin all over again. "This labor of love was for weeks in the hands of ladies from Baltimore, with such assistance from others as was requisite."[77]

Baltimore, Maryland

"The train stopped at two other places after dark, and we were bountifully supplied," wrote First Sgt. Levi Baker of that surreal rail trip

---

73. *Ibid.*, p. 12.
74. *Ibid.*
75. *Ibid.* The Sanitary Commission was shipping rail cars of refrigerated provisions into Gettysburg, each one cooled by large blocks of ice. Apparently this car was not sufficiently insulated to keep the ice from melting in the torrid July heat.
76. Baker, *History of the Ninth Massachusetts Battery*, p. 88.
77. Moss, *Annals of the United States Christian Commission*, p. 322.

from Gettysburg. As the wounded steamed their way onward from Hanover Junction to each of the other Christian Commission stops, they were drawing ever closer to various central terminals, from which they would then be transferred to public and private hospitals throughout the north. From July 7 through July 16, the 8,345 wounded soldiers evacuated from Gettysburg by rail were all routed to Baltimore. Starting July 17, however, the now greatly reduced numbers of casualties coming from the corps hospitals were also directed to New York, Harrisburg, and York, Pennsylvania.[78]

Volunteer nurses and physicians were on hand at these initial destinations to care for the wounded as they arrived and were carefully unloaded from the trains. Philadelphia-born Mrs. M. J. Boston was living with her inlaws in Baltimore when the city was put on alert for the momentary arrival of an unknown number of Gettysburg wounded. "Orders were sent from headquarters for every hospital to be put in readiness, convalescents were transferred to other points, and a temporary hospital was secured on Central Avenue; while on account of the railroad coming directly from Gettysburg, a long row of two-story houses close at hand was vacated, and here the soldiers could be washed and dressed before being sent to the different hospitals."[79]

Then came the call for doctors, nurses, and anyone who could lend a medical hand. With a brother-in-law on medical discharge after Fredericksburg, and a brother at Gettysburg, the twenty-five-year-old Mrs. Boston was determined to do her part, and volunteered. "An appeal for supplies was next published in the daily papers, and received in hearty response. In a few days everything was in readiness, and some one placed over each department. One took charge of the lint, another of bandages, others the giving of supplies. Some of stronger nerve were the nurses. I was on hand to wash and dress wounds, though wholly inexperienced."[80]

Soon the wounded were arriving by the trainload. "July 4th freight trains loaded with wounded arrived. Oh what a sorrowful scene it was! Guards were stationed at each of those houses, to prevent sightseers from entering. All workers wore a miniature flag, pinned on the left

---

78. Baker, *History of the Ninth Massachusetts Battery*, p. 88; *OR*, vol. 27, pt. 1, p. 27.

79. Mary A. Gardner Holland, comp., *Our Army Nurses: Interesting Sketches, Addresses, and Photographs of Nearly One Hundred of the Noble Women who Served in Hospitals and on Battlefields during Our Civil War.* (Boston: B. Wilkins & Co., 1895), p. 425.

80. *Ibid.*, pp. 425-26.

breast. Three of these were given to each, so if one was lost another was at hand. . . . I am sorry to say there was no one to book the names. Such a thing was not thought of in those hurried and exciting scenes."[81]

She unexpectedly received a promotion in the days just preceding her twenty-sixth birthday.

> A physician came to me on the arrival of the first train and said, "Can you dress wounds?"
>
> "If instructed I can," was my reply.
>
> He then sent me for two buckets of water, two sponges, shirts, drawers, handkerchiefs, stockings, bandages, pins, and lint. Off I went, trembling and nervous at the first sight of the horrors of war, and procured the supplies.
>
> "Now, Mrs. Boston, give particular attention to the cleansing of the wound;" and the doctor showed me just how much blue-stone to drop into a bucket of water. The other bucket was for bathing the face and hands and cleansing the person. Our first patient was wounded on the foot; and when the medical treatment was over and a sheet thrown over him, he thanked me so kindly!
>
> I had an assistant, who was then to bring a sandwich, slice of cake, and a cup of coffee; and while he ate she was to fan him. I thought the men had eaten "salt-horse and hard-tack" long enough to have something better on their arrival in Baltimore.
>
> As we turned away, the doctor said, "Now, Mrs. Boston, I have initiated you into the work." Then to the soldiers awaiting their turn: "I leave you in this lady's care. May God bless you! Now don't any of you fall in love with her, for she has a husband and children." Everything was said to cheer the poor sufferers.
>
> On recovering from my first trial dressing wounds my nerves were strong, and I washed and dressed them as quickly as possible, day and night. Always on leaving a very weak patient I gave him a glass of brandy or wine, bathed his face and hands in bay rum, and put a sheet over the stretcher. With tears in their eyes they would thank me, and ask me to go to see them. I often promised, and meant to go,

---

81. *Ibid.*, p. 426.

> but my time was so occupied I could not, though I sometimes heard from them. They would often inquire my name and residence, and give me theirs; but in my haste I kept no list, though I remembered many a long time.[82]

Now safely away from the horrors of sight, and smell, and hearing of the battlefield and the field hospitals, the "minor" and "less serious" wounds (passed over at the corps hospitals in the necessity of dealing with other more immediately life-threatening injuries) began to take on new, and sometimes fatal, significance. One soldier had a "minor" leg wound, and his brother was called; "soon that brother had to take his lifeless body to his parents." Another was wounded in the side, by a projectile that could not be found and removed, and a telegram was sent off to his wife; "by the time she arrived his remains were in the cemetery." Blood poisoning was doing its deadly work in these pre-antiseptic hospitals, prompting one nurse to muse that "rebel bullets were poison." Quite often, that proved to literally be the case.[83]

Nor were the volunteer doctors and nurses immune from the dangers attendant to caring for the wounded. Mrs. Boston herself contracted an infection in her nasal and sinus cavities: "I assisted a physician in one severe case. A soldier had been without attention for his wounded arm for ten days, and it was in a terribly decomposed condition. As he stood up and I removed the blanket from his shoulders, the odor was something terrible. The doctor cut the flesh from the arm and it fell to the pavement. It soon cleared the crowd away from in front of the hospital. By standing beside the doctor I inhaled the full odor, and was attacked by fainting. The doctor ordered brandy, but I did not take it. A soldier took my place, and I went home a very sick person, but soon returned to my duty, though I continued to feel a stinging sensation in my nose, and it swelled at times. . . . Then followed a very sick time for me; my nose and face were a sight! The doctor attending me said, 'You have contracted blood-poisoning, while dressing wounds, and must stay away now.'" But Mrs. Boston was a stubborn young woman, and she merely moved her relief activities to another hospital.[84]

Infection proved to be fatal for at least one worker in this Baltimore facility. "One of our ladies took her daughter with her, who, having

---

82. *Ibid.*, pp. 426-28.
83. *Ibid.*, pp. 427-29.
84. *Ibid.*, pp. 429-30.

pricked her finger while pinning a bandage, contracted blood-poisoning while washing a wound. The hand was amputated, but to no avail, and she died."[85]

Baltimore, Maryland

Outpourings of love, grief and sympathy followed the train tracks throughout southern Pennsylvania, not surprising in such a staunchly Northern state. But the response in strongly divided Baltimore, Maryland, might be something altogether different. The first hostile shots of the war had been fired in Baltimore, and many of these wounded troops on the evacuation trains remembered that nasty fact all too well.

But if Southern sentiment was in evidence in Baltimore on this summer Sunday, one gravely wounded infantryman from distant Massachusetts saw nothing of it.

> But great as had been the demonstration [of comfort and support] all along the route, we were destined to witness yet greater ones. We arrived in Baltimore just as people were on their way to the churches. The long train with its heavy load of human wreck stopped in the street opposite a building used as a temporary tarrying place for soldiers.
>
> Well-dressed ladies, on their way to a Catholic Church nearby, surrounded us in a moment. Others who had got beyond retraced their steps. Hundreds of others still, who had already entered the sacred edifice, came out; and never in my life did I witness so strange a scene, the women being foremost in everything.
>
> We were tenderly lifted from the cars and as fast as we could be accommodated we were carried in the building. Wounds were dressed and refreshments served. The regular attendants had plenty of willing helpers that day.[86]

For this Bay State native, severely wounded in the groin, the tender ministrations of these church ladies soon turned to caring for his exceptionally intimate wound. When surrounded by men in a

---

85. *Ibid.*, p. 430.
86. Wert, "In the Hospitals of Gettysburg, July, 1863," no. VII, *Harrisburg Telegraph*, August 28, 1907, p. 5.

Gettysburg hospital, changing the dressing of even the most private wound was one thing; however, surrounded by well-dressed women in their Sunday-best in a highly public place, having his wound exposed was something else entirely.

> As I lay upon the sidewalk awaiting my turn an elegantly attired lady leaned over me to inquire if she could do anything to help me. Controlled by embarrassment I declined her profe[rr]ed help with thanks. But she would not leave me; she declared it was her intention to dress my wound. The only way I could see out of it was to tell her the wound's location.
>
> This, I thought, would deter her from any further importunity; but to my surprise it had just the opposite effect. Earnestly, reprovingly, almost indignantly. She declared her disbelief in what she termed sham modesty when human suffering might be relieved. At her command a stretcher was brought and despite my mild remonstrances, I was conveyed to the interior of the building.
>
> Here she performed her friendly service with as much skill and heroism as the most experienced nurse could have commanded; and, when my wound had been cleansed, my appetite satisfied with steaming hot coffee and toast, and I lay comfortable upon a bench while her fan was waving gently to and fro before my face, I fancied there was not a king in the wide world who felt any better and happier than I.[87]

Resting quietly amid the rush and hurried activity of the Baltimore transit hospital, this soldier, sprung from staunch Puritan stock, mused over his encounter with this tender and gracious Roman Catholic matron. "Born and raised in a New England town where Catholics were almost unknown, my religious training had led me to look upon them as somewhat exclusive and shut up within themselves. . . . I had the mistaken idea that all their efforts were in behalf of those of their own faith." All his previous suppositions had proven false in the person of this one Baltimore lady. "I took it all back then and there."[88]

---

87. *Ibid.*
88. *Ibid.*

It did not seem to matter when the trains arrived; there were always reception committees, medical personnel, commissioners, and various volunteers standing by to meet them. "We arrived in Baltimore about 2 A.M., and the Union part of the city was awake," remembered one wounded Northerner. "We were served with coffee, and wounds were washed and dressed; the first time in thirty-six hours. Shops, stores, houses were opened, and we were made welcome; but the hospitals of Baltimore were full already, and we must go further north."[89]

Trains came and went in the two bustling cross-town terminals of Baltimore; while awaiting for an empty train heading north, some men with lesser wounds went in search of injured comrades. "While waiting for the train, some one told me that an officer of a Massachusetts battery was in a hospital near," wrote fellow Bay Stater First Sgt. Levi W. Baker. "Acting at once, I found Lieut. [Alexander H.] Whitaker [of Baker's own 9th Massachusetts Battery] lying in bed with a shattered knee, the first I knew he was wounded. I remember just how he looked: his knee was raised, his face flushed, feverish and restless. I could do nothing, but found a brother Mason and sent to him. Immediately the train started."[90]

Wilmington, Delaware

It seemed almost inconceivable that the word of their coming could have travelled all the way to tiny Delaware. But the indesputable proof was there, right outside the railroad carriages, as far as the eye could see in either direction. "In Wilmington, Delaware, it seemed as if the road for miles was crowded with people who had gathered to comfort us with all that was desirable for food. It was an ovation of edibles and hearty cheer."[91]

Philadelphia, Pennsylvania

While some of the wounded stayed on at Baltimore to convalesce and recuperate, many were shipped north to the immense hospital nexus at Philadelphia. "After a while we were placed again on the cars

---

89. Baker, *History of the Ninth Massachusetts Battery*, p. 88.
90. *Ibid.* It proved to be Sergeant Baker's last kindness to his superior officer; First Lieutenant Whitaker died of his wounds on July 20.
91. "Wounded at Gettysburgh. The War Experiences of Commander Scoville, of Moses Summers Post," *The Syracuse Sunday Herald*, March 8, 1885.

and amid the benedictions of the crowd, now increased to a multitude, the train moved slowly away. All the route to Philadelphia the scenes we had witnessed between Gettysburg and Baltimore were repeated at every town and village. It was worth all we had dared and suffered to receive such an ovation."[92]

With twenty-seven hospitals and over twenty-five thousand beds by war's end, the City of Brotherly Love was the only Northern metropolitan area to rival the nation's capital as a major general hospital center. Wounded troops much preferred the care provided at Philadelphia, with its tasty cooking, widespread generosity of the citizenry, and the compassionate and skillful treatment by Quaker doctors and assistants.[93]

Representative of Philadelphia's hospitals was the mammoth Chestnut Hill general hospital facility, located three miles outside city limits. Chestnut Hill was a permanent hospital consisting of fifty wards, designed to house thirty-six hundred patients, and arranged radially like wheel-spokes around a central courtyard of two and a half acres. The central plaza housed the administrative offices, the six thousand volume circulating library, chapel, reservoir, and other amenities. The hospital even had its own depot on the nearby railroad.

All the luxuries so obviously absent from the corps hospital at Gettysburg were present at this state-of-the-art facility. Hot water was available throughout the wards, piped from the steam boiler beside the laundry. Steam produced by the boilers was used by the kitchen to cook vegetables, and the available menus featured chicken, cakes, various fruits, and ices. The buildings were illuminated at night by gas lights, and the well-stocked dispensary, under the watchful eye of the hospital steward, supplied a wide variety of medicines and hospital stores. Immense storerooms stocked a variety of clothing, laid in to replace the torn and bloody rags of the incoming wounded. Brightly lit operating theatres, complete with observation galleries, were accessible to the surgeons at a moment's notice. Convalescent soldiers posted their mail from the hospital post office, were serenaded under a large rotunda by the hospital band, and slaked their thirst at fountains of ice water scattered throughout the facility.

Many of the wounded from the Second Corps hospitals were received at the depot, where each was carefully weighed, measured,

---

92. Wert, "In the Hospitals of Gettysburg, July, 1863," no. VII, *Harrisburg Telegraph*, August 28, 1907, p. 5.
93. Adams, *Doctors in Blue*, p. 155.

and a complete description compiled. A chart was drawn up, showing the wounded man's name, state, regiment, company, corps, army, civilian occupation, and address of next of kin. Personal effects and clothing were then carefully packed away, and the patient was issued hospital underwear, coat, trousers, and slippers. Finally, a hospital number was assigned to the invalid, as well as a ward and bed number. With all the paperwork completed, the patient was carefully borne off to his new lodging.

Each ward contained sixty-three beds, of which sixty were for patients, two for attendants, and the remaining one for the convalescent ward master. Meals were available to the ambulatory patients in small personal dining rooms at the end of each ward, and were tastefully laid out with china, glassware and table service. Notices were posted that patients were free to eat all that they desired, but not to be wasteful. Bedfast patients had their meals brought to them on trays. At the other end of the ward were the latrines, kept clean and flushed by a constantly flowing stream of water. Opposite the latrine was the lavatory, from which all waste water was carried away by drain pipes running under the raised floors.

The entire facility was administrated by a surgeon-in-charge, with the rank of major. Hands-on medical care was provided by thirty-six assistant surgeons, each one a captain or lieutenant, under the direct supervision of an executive surgeon. Each assistant surgeon was assigned to cover certain wards and beds, with daily reports being filed to the surgeon-in-charge through the executive surgeon. Medical cadets were also quartered at Chestnut Hill, and accompanied the assistant surgeons on their rounds, assisting them as they ministered to the needs of the wounded. Absolutely no amputations were allowed without the express permission of the surgeon-in-charge.[94]

It was here that the train trip ended for George Washington Beidelman, of the 71st Pennsylvania. When he had last written his father, it was from the Second Corps Hospital by Rock Creek. There, he was lying among thousands of desperate, filthy, wounded men,

94. Francois Victor Adolphe de Chanal, "A French Report on Federal Hospitals: Good Order and Cleanliness," *Civil War Times Illustrated*, no. 6 (October 1967): 40-43.

incredibly lucky to have escaped with nothing more serious than a deep gouge plowed into his leg. Now, in totally different surroundings, he picked up his pen again:

> U. S. Hospital, Chestnut Hill
> Phila., July 8, 1863
> Dear Father,
> Arrived here last evening from the "bloody field of Gettysburg." Am not suffering; health and spirits good. The Almighty Disposer of events hath blessed me abundantly.
> I will soon be able to be out, and may probably get to Bloom[sburg, Pennsylvania].
> Having several letters to write. I cannot give you any particulars now.... Please write to me as soon as you receive this.
> Your Affectionate Son—
> George[95]

George was all agog over his new surroundings. A week later, he regaled his father with stories of his close call, and of the wonderful hospital he now enjoyed (more or less):

> To Jacob Beidelman, Esq.
> Ward 37, U. S. A. General Hospital,
> Chestnut Hill, Phila.
> Phila., July 14, 1863
> My Dear Father,
> Yours of the 11th inst. received last evening. Was exceedingly glad to hear from you.
> Am sorry my last letter was not so satisfactory to you as could have been desired; but I think I can give a satisfactory explanation. In the 6th inst. I mailed you a letter which was written on the 4th, at the General Field Hospital of our corps, near the battle field of Gettysburg. That letter informed you that I had been slightly wounded in the battle of the 3rd. by a Minie ball, going through my pants and merely scratching my left leg, while it cut a piece out of my right leg, leaving a

---

95. George Washington Beidelman, ed. Catherine H. Vanderslice, *The Civil War Letters of George Washington Beidelman* (New York: Vantage Press, 1978), p. 179.

furrow about the length, breadth, and half the depth of my thumb; and that isn't very large. My knee, however, made a very narrow escape, the wound being on top, or in front, and only about two inches above the knee-cap.

Well, supposing you had received my first letter, I mentioned nothing of the circumstances of my being wounded, thinking it unnecessary.

I have the pleasure of informing you that my health is good, and I am getting along finely. This is a very good place—splendidly adapted for a hospital, having been built expressly for that purpose. It covers about six acres of ground, and will accomodate about 3,000 patients. "Red tape," however, flourishes here as elsewhere, and the inmates are far too much restricted. There is not enough liberty. A man can get out about 24 hours in a week on the average; and furloughs, I am informed, are out of the question. I doubt if I will be able to obtain a furlough to go to Bloom[sburg]; so you must put off the hope of seeing me for a while longer; in ten months, if I am spared, I will be out of the service. . . .

Your affect. son in Christ—
G. W. Beidelman[96]

Newark, New Jersey

While Chestnut Hill was certainly one of the largest general hospitals in the North, even those of less prestigious size offered much the same care and comforts to the wounded arriving from Gettysburg. While a goodly number of men detrained at Philadelphia, others simply switched trains at the Philadelphia station. Some whiled away the time waiting for the next train by visiting "the old cooper shop" where "we were refreshed." This was the Union Refreshment Saloon, founded by Second Corps volunteer nurse Mary Lee and some of her Philadelphia friends when the war first started. Then it was back on the cars to continue on to less crowded hospitals, or ones closer to their homes.[97]

---

96. *Ibid.*, pp. 179-80. Beidelman was right about the chances of getting a furlough; he was discharged directly back to his regiment on August 21.

97. Baker, *History of the Ninth Massachusetts Battery*, p. 88. For more on the Philadelphia Union Refreshment Saloon, see "Mary Lee, 72nd Pennsylvania nurse" in appendix 3.

Fortunate were the men able to be treated in Baltimore or Philadelphia—the extended rail trip was beginning to take a heavy, sometimes even a fatal, toll on the exhausted Gettysburg survivors. "From Philadelphia to Jersey City the scenes were similar but we were no longer in a condition to appreciate them; for the railroad, as an act of supposed kindness, had given us passenger coaches. No longer having an opportunity to lie down, our sufferings were growing in the extreme. One poor fellow who sat or rather leaned on the seat with me bled to death upon the way."[98]

For First Sgt. Levi W. Baker, lately attached to the 9th Massachusetts Battery, and now on his way to an eastern general hospital, the train trip was a seemingly interminable blur of swaying cars, passing landscapes, and black clouds of soot and cinders. "Again the train is ready and we are rolling north again. All this time I was a passive passenger, going I knew not where. A tedious night passed, and about daylight the train stopped at the Centre street station, Newark, New Jersey."[99]

Baker was helped from the railcar by waiting attendants, and gently escorted to the nearby hospital. "I was assigned to ward six; one end of the room was overlooking the station, the other a wharf on the Passaic, and miles of the river and country beyond. We had a good surgeon and an old soldier of the regular army for nurse. During my stay of six months I could have a pass every day if wanted, and was out a great deal. Within a week a large number were missing, having taken furlough without leave."[100]

Surrounded by such variety in the local scenery, and enjoying the unexpected freedom from the usual military regimen, the wounded cannoneer began to steadily recover from his Gettysburg wounds.

Jersey City, New Jersey

For others, the tedious journey continued on toward Jersey City and the hospitals of New York City and Long Island. Upon arrival, some of the wounded were taken by cart or ambulance to their scattered hospitals; others were ferried across to New York City itself. "At Jersey City our party was divided for different destinations, my

---

98. Wert, "In the Hospitals of Gettysburg, July, 1863," no. VII, *Harrisburg Telegraph*, August 28, 1907, p. 5.
99. Baker, *History of the Ninth Massachusetts Battery*, p. 89.
100. *Ibid.*

own being Bledsoe's Island, where I remained for many weeks," wrote one exhausted survivor of the rail trip. In the setting of the general hospitals, made as cheerful and clean as possible, the wounded and the amputated continued on their long and painful road to recuperation.[101]

As the Union wounded spread outward, carried throughout the North by a web of rail lines, the surgeon general's staff was frantically attempting to find adequate medical facilities to house and treat them. Some regions made it easy by quickly throwing open every facility for their wounded. A message came from the Pittsburgh office of the Sanitary Commission on July 5, addressed to the surgeon general: "Gen. W A Hammond. Send all western Pa. soldiers here for treatment at request of San. Com. J. K. Moorhead."[102]

Others were routed to various hospitals by orders coming directly from the surgeon general's office. Much of the burden of carrying out these orders fell on the shoulders of Surgeon C. W. McDougall, Medical Director of the East. He responded to a telegram received from Surgeon General Hammond on July 10: "Your telegram of today has been received, as follows; 'Wounded are ordered to N. Y.' 'Fill up New England Hospitals.' I presume this to mean that the wounded received shall be sent to those Hospitals; which orders will be carried out, unless otherwise directed." By July 14, McDougall could report that "I have one thousand (1000) vacant beds in the Department, not including David's Island."[103]

On July 23, McDougall sent a detailed telegram to Hammond, cataloging exactly where beds were still available: "Surg General, Have vacant beds as follows [Fort] Schuyler one twenty four (124) Central Park sixty (60) Berward forty nine (49) Portsmouth Grove two twenty two New Haven one fifty two Brattleboro two sixty four."[104]

---

101. Wert, "In the Hospitals of Gettysburg, July, 1863," no. VII, *Harrisburg Telegraph*, August 28, 1907, p. 5.

102. Record Group 112, Office of the Surgeon General, Letters Received, 1818-1870, Box No. 66, Letters Received, July 1, 1863—February 29, 1864, National Archives and Records Administration. Moorhead was head of the Western Pennsylvania Sanitary Commission.

103. *Ibid.* David's Island was a Confederate prisoner of war hospital facility.

104. *Ibid.*

Gradually, the inundation of Northern casualties slowed to a steady stream, and then finally to a trickle as Gettysburg emptied itself of its burden of mangled and dying men. But it would be a long time, a very long time indeed, before those scattered hospitals would finally be cleared of their last Gettysburg patients.

As bodies began to mend, and spirits slowly revived, men began to hanker for home and longed-for family members. Letters began to arrive, in an ever-increasing number, at the office of Surgeon General Hammond, requesting a transfer to some local hospital, one near the wife and children, while convalescing. Joseph Mathews, of Brig. Gen. John Gibbon's Division, wrote directly to the Surgeon General.

> August 31, 1863,
> General,
> I have the honor to make application for a transfer to a hospital in New York City where I can have friends. I have become (for the present) unfit for military duty, by reason of a severe gunshot wound of both thighs received in action at Gettysburg, Pa., July 3d, 1863.
> I am, General, most Respectfully, Your obt Servant, Joseph B. Mathews, Co. B, 15 Mass.[105]

---

105. *Ibid.* Someone else, probably a nurse, wrote the body of the Joseph Mathews letter, while he merely appended his signature and regiment in a shaky and faint hand at the end.

Having heard nothing in over a week, an impatient Joseph B. Mathews mailed off another letter ten days after the first, this one penned by a Mr. W. S. Smith:

> Baltimore, Sept. 10, 63
> Surgeon Genl, Washington, DC
> Dear Sir,
> The application of Joseph B. Mathews, Co. B, 15 Mass. Vol. to be transferred from Camden St. Hospital, Baltimore, to a U.S. Hospital at New York was forwarded to your Headquarters about the 3rd inst. Will you be pleased to say to Dr. Eli Bliss, Surgeon in Charge of Camden St. Hospital, whether the same had been received and granted. Very truly, Joseph B. Mathews.

The transfer was not granted; the medical director felt that "a transfer is not necessary to save life—as he will ultimately recover in this Hospital."

Others thought that they stood a better chance if they could get the clout of elected officials of their home state behind their request. Another enterprising member of the Second Corps tried writing directly to his governor, employing his own unique brand of spelling:

> McClellans Genn. Hospital
> July 14th, 1863
> Gov. Curtain,
> Dear Sir,
> As I am here a wounded soldier, and should like very much to be transfered to the Hospital at Pitsburg, Pa. where I shall have my friends near me to aid and comfort my sufferings. I appeal to you ~~to~~ for information as to whether I can or not. I was informed by the Doctor that by getting an order from you that I could be transfered. And now If you can ~~can~~ do me a favor you will oblidge a Vol. of the 145th Pa. Inf. I would state to you that I have a wife and three children at Pitsburg and it would be gret deal of satisfaction to me to be with them whil endureing the suffering of a very severe wound and it is necessary that I should be with them for their comfort. Ther is nothing more.
> Only I remain Yours Respety,
> Henry Cariher
> Member of the 145th Pa. Vols. Infty.[106]

---

106. *Ibid.* The letter was addressed to his wife with these words: "Dear wife, This you will hand to Govner Curtain." No doubt unable to the reach the governor himself, Mrs. Cariher passed it on to Mr. Moorhead, head of the Western Pennsylvania Sanitary Commission.

Moorhead, in turn, forwarded the letter to Governor Curtin on July 17, with his own note, stating: "Mrs. Cariher, the wife of the writer, has called on me. If you can have her husband transferred to the U.S. Hospital at Pittsburgh, I hope you will do so. We have room and accommodations here for a large number, and would like to have those that belong to this county sent here. Your attention to this will oblige his distressed wife. . . . An early reply is requested. J. K. Moorhead."

Upon receipt of the Cariher and Moorhead letters, Governor Curtin forwarded the transfer request directly to U.S. Surgeon General Hammond on July 20, along with his personal request that it "be complied with if consistent with the Service—By order of the Governor."

Cariher's idea of getting a heavy-hitter to back his transfer seems to have paid off. The surgeon general's office received the request on July 22, and apparently granted the request.

As time gradually closed open wounds and began to heal the handiwork of the surgeons, the nature of the wounds determined where the battered survivors of Gettysburg would go after they were discharged from the general hospital. Those who had endured the agony and confusion of severe amputations usually were given medical discharges when well enough to be released. Others, largely restored in body, but bearing forever after the unseen effects of the wounding, were sent back to their regiments, to there again face the possibility of another ghastly excursion through the military hospital system.

A third group, composed of those that took a terribly long time to recover their stamina and health, went in two different directions. Some remained at the general hospitals as convalescent attendants for the more seriously wounded men. Much bad and very little good was written of these male nurses, who exhibited uneven aptitudes for this type of work. These "nurses by accident" were often in pain themselves, enfeebled, demoralized, and brooding over their own unhealing injuries. They frequently exhibited little compassion or patience toward the helpless wounded men committed to their care. While some did their fumble-fingered best to care for the incoming wounded, many resented being forced to do "women's work," and cared nothing for personal or professional hygiene.[107]

The remainder of the convalescents, sound enough in body to be free of the danger of relapse, were forwarded to special convalescent camps. So widespread was the need for these facilities that one camp alone, in Fairfax, Virginia, four miles from Washington, saw over 170,000 men pass through its gates in 1863 alone. Many of the amenities of the general hospital were still present at these camps, including barracks, promenades, a chapel, library, sutler stores, and separate quarters for officers' families. Under the command of a colonel, the soldiers were armed, and gradually returned to the rigors and disciplines of camp and field duty. When finally well enough to be returned to active duty, the soldier would be issued a fresh uniform, equipment, and weapon, and sent back to his regiment.[108]

107. Adams, *Doctor's in Blue*, pp. 184-86.

108. de Chanal, "A French Report on Federal Hospitals: Good Order and Cleanliness," p. 44.

Those still not well enough to return to duty were assigned to the "Invalid Corps." The Invalid Corps was established in April of 1863, an attempt to keep incapacitated troops in the service, and to improve the hospital guard system. The 161 companies of the corps were drawn by regional residency, and were divided into two units. The first battalion was composed of soldiers still obviously unfit for service in the field, but capable of standing guard and other garrison assignments. The second, the amputee battalion, were able only to be employed as watchmen, or, in some limited instances, as attendants. Distinctive sky blue uniforms were issued to improve esprit de corps, but morale bottomed out. Conscientious soldiers who felt fairly good wanted to be back in the field with their units; those still feeling ill or weak wanted to be sent home. No one wanted to be shunted into this outfit into which, it was rumored, officers were dumping men they wanted to be rid of, or into which healthy men, whom surgeons wanted to keep on as attendants, were transferred.

The concept was a sound one, so the corps was reorganized, this time with exacting safeguards against outside assignment of cowards and personal favorites to its ranks. Under its new designation as the "Veterans' Reserve Corps," it ultimately succeeded, but not by providing hospital attendants. The first battalion gave valuable service in guarding the approaches to the capital during Jubal Early's Confederate raid of Washington in 1864, as well as standing watch at numerous bridges, tunnels, railroads, and government installations. The second battalion, composed of amputees and organized in military companies, worked efficiently with the Medical Department to guard hospitals and to care for the clothing and personal effects of the patients. Prominent in both battalions were survivors of Gettysburg, Union soldiers who had been wounded, and lived to serve others as a result of the care they received at the Second Corps hospitals.[109]

Gettysburg, Pennsylvania

The trip east was not nearly as cordial nor comfortable for the Confederate wounded as for their Union counterparts. The first Southerners were not taken to the railroad until July 11, four full days after the trains began running. Considering the fact that Lee left only his most seriously injured behind when he fell back to Virginia, it is amazing that there were even seventy-six Southern soldiers stable

109. Adams, *Doctors in Blue*, pp. 187-88.

enough to be moved by that time. While the railroad evacuated 4,341 Union wounded in the first four days of operation, only 1,236 Confederates were well enough to be moved out of town by rail from July 11 to July 14.[110]

The day after John Dooley spotted Dr. John M. Cuyler, the United States Army Medical Inspector from Georgia, at work at the Confederate operating tables at the Third Division hospital, the orders came through for his evacuation. "The next morning our party were told to leave Gettysburg, and we could go either to David's Island, New York, or to Baltimore. We preferred Baltimore, but rued our unfortunate choice very bitterly when we learned that every attention, care, and kindness was bestowed upon our fellow prisoners at David's Island, whilst we were treated worse than brute animals and cast into the black hole of Fort McHenry. We could not foresee this difference, however, and approached the Gettysburg depot gaily joking and singing, nor thought of the trouble and suffering awaiting us."[111]

Even here in the North, far distant from Dooley's familiar home in Virginia, friends and acquaintances met by chance with surprising frequency. "As I am getting into the ambulance who should come up but Jack Davis, one of the Sanitaries. Good hearted Jack! His eyes fill with tears when he saw me in such a miserable condition, for I couldn't walk without being assisted, and my pants were stiffened and caked from blood and matter. I am sure that if there had been time and opportunity, Jack would have pulled off his own pants then and there and would have insisted on my taking them."[112]

Accompanied by his friend, Dooley was trundled off in an ambulance to the depot and the tents of the Sanitary Commission. There, at least, all were treated alike, regardless of allegiance, uniform, or dialect. "I do not think that a man of the 16,000 who were transported during our stay went away from Gettysburg without a good meal—rebels and Unionists together, they all had it, and were pleased and satisfied," wrote George Anna Woolsey of their treatment of the wounded. "We had lovely things for the men to eat—as many potatoes and turnips as they wanted, and almost '*too* much cabbages'; and custard pudding, and codfish hash, and jelly an inch high on their bread, and their bread *buttered*—'buttered on both sides,' as the men discovered, greatly to their amusement one night, considering that the

---

110. *OR*, vol. 27, pt. 1, p. 27.
111. Dooley, *John Dooley*, p. 121.
112. *Ibid.*, pp. 121-22.

final touch had been given when *this* followed the clean clothes and cologne,—'cologne worth a penny a sniff.'"[113]

Ambulance schedules and the railroad schedule frequently did not coincide, as George Anna Woolsey could testify. "Late one afternoon—too late for the cars—a train of ambulances arrived at our lodge with over one hundred wounded rebels to be cared for through the night. Only one among them seemed to[o] weak and faint to take anything. He was badly hurt and failing. I went to him after his wound was dressed, and found him lying on his blanket, stretched over the straw, a fair-haired, blue-eyed young lieutenant. . . . I could not think of him as a rebel. He was too near heaven for that. He wanted nothing—had not been willing to eat for days, his comrades said; but I coaxed him to try a little milk gruel, flavored nicely with lemon and brandy; and one of the satisfactions of our three weeks is the remembrance of the empty cup I took away afterwards, and his perfect enjoyment of that supper."[114]

For their parts, the Confederates were bemused and somewhat amazed by the kindliness of these Northern women. "'Have you friends in the army, madam?' a rebel soldier lying on the floor of the car, said to me as I gave him some milk."

"'Yes, my brother is on _________'s staff.'"

"'I thought so, ma'am. You can always tell; when people are good to soldiers, they are sure to have friends in the army.'"

"'We are rebels, you know, ma'am,' another said; 'Do you treat rebels so?'"[115]

For now, at least, in the safe and neutral tents of the Sanitary Commission, away from the fiery rhetoric and the influence of

---

113. Woolsey, *Three Weeks at Gettysburg*; Bacon and Howland, *Letters of a Family During the War for the Union*, pp. 529-30.

114. Moore, *Women of the War*, pp. 140-42. This was Lt. Henry Rauch, of the 14th South Carolina. When Georgy learned that Henry's brother was also wounded, and was scheduled to leave on the next train headed east, she had him removed and placed "by his side on the straw, and for the rest of the day lay in a sort of apathy, without speaking, except to assure himself that he could stay with his brother without risk of being separated from his fellow-prisoners. . . . At sunset I put my hand on the lieutenant's heart to find it still! All night the brother lay close against the coffin, and in the morning he went with his comrades, leaving us to bury Henry, having 'confidence,' but first thanking us for what we had done, and giving us all that he had to show his gratitude—the palmetto ornament from his brother's cap, and a button from his coat." [*Ibid.*, pp. 142-44.]

115. Woolsey, *Three Weeks at Gettysburg*. George Anna consistently called her mother "Mrs." in this semi-anonymous pamphlet.

charismatic leaders, an unofficial truce was declared between the common soldiers of the opposing armies. "It was strange to see the good brotherly feeling come over the soldiers, our own and the rebels, when side by side they lay in our tents. 'Hullo, boys, this is the pleasantest way to meet, isn't it? We are better friends when we are as close as this, than a little farther off.' And they would go over the battles together: 'we were here,' and 'you were there,' in the friendliest way."[116]

Sometimes moments of levity rippled through the ranks of the men—soldier humor, jesting and shared fun of men, blue and grey, who had slept and marched in each others company, or in each others shadow, for many long, weary months. At least one such laugh was at the expense of a local citizen.

> Few good things can be said of the Gettysburg farmers, and I only use Scripture language in calling them "evil beasts." One of this kind came creeping into our camp three weeks after the battle. He lived five miles only from town and had "never seen a rebel." He had heard we had some of them and he came down to see them. "Boys," we said, marching him into the tent which happened to be full of rebels that day waiting for the train, "boys, here's a man who never saw a rebel in his life and wants to look at you," and there he stood with his mouth wide open, and there they lay in rows, laughing at him, stupid old Dutchman.
>
> "And why haven't you seen a rebel?" Mrs. said; "why didn't you take your gun and help drive them out of your town?"
>
> "A feller mightier [*sic*] got hit"—which reply was quite too much for the rebels, they roared with laughter at him, up and down the tent.[117]

When the train did arrive, the Southerners were carried out just as carefully as their erstwhile enemies, and laid gently on the floor of the box cars and baggage vans. Jack Davis, John Dooley's friend, walked with him to the train and saw to his comfort as much as possible. Hasty farewells were said as last minute arrangements were finalized before departure. "But the cars were impatient, and after being tumbled into

116. *Ibid.*
117. *Ibid.*

them like so many horned cattle, I was forced to take leave of my kind hearted friend and class mate, wringing my hand and almost crying because he could not do something for me."[118]

Slowly at first, then gradually picking up speed, the train and its cargo of misery headed east. For the Confederates on board, prisoners-of-war, the only prospect ahead was forced confinement in Northern prisons. For them, the last vestiges of kindness were literally vanishing over the horizon, along with Gettysburg and the tents of the Sanitary Commission.

"Slowly but roughly in our heavy rumbling freight cars we leave the famous Burgh of Getty . . . jolted till every bone and joint in our body was aching and craving relief."[119]

Harrisburg, Pennsylvania

Although there were not crowds standing along the tracks to cheer them on, the Northerners did not prove to be altogether unfriendly to the prisoners-of-war. As the trains stopped to take on fuel or water, people would make their way to the trains, many bearing food and beverages.

"Some of the Confederates passed through Harrisburgh [*sic*] as prisoners, and upon seeing the citizens come out to feed them, one of their chaplains said with tears, 'I thought you would come out and hoot at us; we came here to attack you, and you feed us; this overcomes us more than battle.'"[120]

Baltimore, Maryland

"We arrived about eight o'clock P.M. in the subjugated city of Baltimore. It is Sunday the 12th of July, and my 21st birthday!" mused John Dooley of his very unusual birthday gift.[121]

It was an entirely different reception than that enjoyed by the severely wounded Massachusetts soldier and his friends. While there was quite a turnout upon their arrival in Baltimore, the relief efforts of many Southern sympathizers were severely hampered by Northern troops, anxious to avoid any sectarian unrest in a city already kept firmly in the Union fold by duress. "The depot is crowded by hundreds

---

118. Dooley, *John Dooley*, p. 122.
119. *Ibid.*, p. 123.
120. Dimon, *Report of the General Agent of the State of New York*, p. 47.
121. Dooley, *John Dooley*, p. 123.

who have come to succour the wounded Confederates, and our progress has been intentionally retarded so that their kind hearts, so well disposed toward the enemies of Yankeedom, may be disappointed in seeing us; for as to permitting any of them to come in to talk to us or to serve us, that is out of the question. A rampart of bayonets excludes all assistance which comes not stamped with loyal brand and under loyal approbation."[122]

Despite the best efforts of the military, some undercover Confederates did manage to reach and minister to Dooley and his associates. Most were forced to use subterfuge to gain access to the wounded. "Many however come in bearing upon their best clothes the flag of 'our Union,' but judging from their sly winks and nods we are made to understand that the colors under which they are manoeuvering are not in accord with the feelings of their heart."[123]

Here again were representatives of the Sanitary Commission, bearing welcome food and fresh dressings to bind up the wounds reopened or soiled in the clattering boxcar ride. "They have lint and bandages, etc., and they have hot coffee and crackers which are most acceptable, since the pains of our wounds have by no means assuaged the appetites that within us were ravenous. Still these ministers of health (Sanitary Comm) stayed not with us long, but [were] like busy bees flitting quickly from car to car."[124]

The Union wounded were tenderly offloaded at the row of houses bordering the tracks, there to have their injuries carefully attended to by Mrs. Boston and her fellow nurses; there to be fed, fanned, and fauned over. The Southern delegation from the Second Corps hospital found quite different circumstances attending their care in Baltimore. "We find ourselves soon in darkness in the lonely and deserted depot, and the only noise breaking the stillness of the night the heavy tramp of our bluecoat guard and the distant hum of the large city lulled to its rest."[125]

What tantalizing dreams of escape flitted through their heads that night! Shut up alone in the depot of a pro-Southern city, there to be guarded by only a solitary soldier—was it possible, could it be pulled off? "Can we escape? I remember that Loyola College is but a few blocks off. But suppose we elude the guard? We cannot walk; at least

---

122. *Ibid.*
123. *Ibid.*
124. *Ibid.*
125. *Ibid.*, pp. 123-24.

I cannot, so that renders my case hopeless. So here we lie through the dreary night, slumbering now and awaking, imagining that same excruciating jolting of the long day is still continued and happy to find that we are but dreaming."[126]

Fort McHenry

The morning of July 13 dawned all too soon for the weary prisoners; today they would make the trip to their new home—Fort McHenry. "A wet dreary dawn is chilling us through and through when the coarse voice of a coarser guard awakes us to the consciousness that we must be up and moving; always moving on like poor 'Joe,' and like poor 'Joe' we feel, as we are bundled in every uncomfortable way into ambulances thereby to be removed to Fort McHenry. We are a wretched lot of human beings as, chilled by the rain, depressed in spirits and jolted almost inside out we are rolled along the almost endless streets that lead by the longest route to Fort McHenry. At last we arrive at the veritable fort."[127]

Any illusions carried from Gettysburg of the kind of care to expect were now rudely stripped away, leaving Dooley and his companions aghast at their surroundings. "We who had fondly been picturing to ourselves a large hospital were dismayed to find our ambulances halt before a row of low buildings which appeared somewhat like those in which I have seen cattle quartered. Finally after much delay we are ushered up a filthy staircase into a filthy loft. We are huddled together in this noisome place, filth and vermin in profusion. It is the uppermost story of the yankee guard house of the Yankee garrison quartered here. Col Davis calls it the Black Hole of Calcutta."[128]

With "medical care" nonexistent in this "hospital," the men made themselves as comfortable as possible in these squalid conditions. "Our settling down consists in spreading our blankets on the filthy floor, and although many of us are wounded severely enough to merit beds, but one or two are given even *bunks*, and these are glad enough to leave them to their former occupants—the vermin." After a large iron bucket arrived, filled with something greasy and unidentifiable for lunch, Dooley and his wounded friends bided their time, waiting for night and the forgetfulness of sleep. "Wearily crept this our first day in the guard house. And the night, ah, the night! Mice and roaches

126. *Ibid.*, p. 124.
127. *Ibid.*
128. *Ibid.*

gamboled round our heads, performing feats of wondrous skill to astonish us who were now in this dismal world. No pillows and no blankets to cover up, and then the vermin! And then the fitful sleep of the fagged and wearied wounded."[129]

As for Dooley, his condition still remained quite grave; the bullet had passed through both thighs, and it proved impossible for him to walk unassisted. An abortive attempt to remove the Confederates to Fort Delaware, snarled by the refusal of some Northern women to ride onboard ship with Confederates, left Dooley unconscious on a stretcher borne by four of his companions on July 14. Back again in "the Black Hole," Dooley's wounded companions sang to while away the time—"Cronin sings and McGimpset is singing, and *both* have holes right through their lungs. This is certainly being miserably gay."[130]

Through the efforts of the post surgeon, one Doctor Shepherd, Dooley's wounds were finally swabbed out on July 17. "Today Shepherd who is most kind in his attentions to my wounds extracts *4* maggots and cleanses the wounds thoroughly. They are doing very well now; *I mean my wounds*."[131]

Fort Delaware

John Dooley was finally moved to Fort Delaware, where a new malady began to manifest itself, compounded by his grievous leg wounds. "24th. I only find ease in lying on either side, and have become so chafed and sore that I am threatened with *bedsores* although I have not rested on a *bed* since I left my paternal roof." The next day, further progress is made when "Shepherd extracts from my wound several pieces of my pantaloons that had been carried into my leg by the bullet and which worked themselves back to the surface today, taking twenty-two days to go a distance of 2 inches. Slept well."[132]

On Tuesday, July 28, the Fort Delaware surgeon transferred Dooley and another wounded member of the First Virginia, a Captain [*sic*] Jones, to the Post Hospital, "a clean and quiet building but not adapted to the exigencies of war since it does not accommodate (I think) more than 40 patients. Before being put to bed I am scrubbed well, especially

---

129. *Ibid.*, pp. 124-25.
130. *Ibid.*, pp. 125-26.
131. *Ibid.*, p. 126.
132. *Ibid.*, p. 127.

as to my lower limbs; and the old skin from instep to toe comes off as completely as the slough from a snake, leaving me a *brannew* [*sic*] pair of feet and as delicate and tender as in the days of my infantile oblivion. I am now put to bed in the top story, with the tin roof slanting just over my head and the sun playing fiercely on its metallic covering."[133]

A new enemy—intense, equatorial-like heat—threatened Dooley for the next three days, as the summer sun beat down on the metal roof, making each day hotter than the previous one.

> 31st. Heat and pains increase. The thermometer in this ward is about 92 degrees. . . .
>
> Heat today, Aug. 1st, 94 degrees. Every fibre and muscle are burning and throbbing. No position gives me any relief. Clock goes slower and slower.
>
> Aug. 2nd Heat in my ward 98. But I am finally released from this fiery ordeal and transferred to Ward No. 2 down stairs where it is much cooler and where I suffer less pain. . . .[134]

His move from the attic was timely, since the thermometer peaked at 104 degrees on that Saturday, a full thirty days after his wounding. "Just got away in time to avoid *crisping*," quipped Dooley, who had turned the corner to recovery in his hot upstairs bed. Although he would write that he spent that night "wretchedly sick for several hours and nearly faint from excessive pain," his condition would steadily improve from this point onward. But it would be many more months before the Virginia lieutenant would walk without pain.[135]

---

133. *Ibid.*, pp. 127-28.

134. *Ibid.*, p. 128.

135. *Ibid.*, pp. 128-29. John Dooley survived his hospitalization, and subsequent imprisonment at the Johnson Island, Ohio, officer's prison-of-war camp. He finally arrived home in Richmond on March 6, 1865. The capitol was now a besieged city, and inflation was totally out of control—a pair of shoes was $350, a pair of boots cost $800 to $1500, hats ran $150 to $700, and $5 would purchase a drink of whiskey—"Wonderful prices!," Dooley wryly noted in his ubiquitous diary. [*Ibid.*, p. 173.]

The lieutenant drew $780 in back pay, and waited on parole for exchange; but time had run out for the South, and the Confederacy collapsed in defeat. Dooley traveled through the shambles of his former nation before resuming his interrupted studies at Georgetown University.

Sadly, his dream of becoming a Catholic priest were never to be realized. He died prematurely on May 8, 1873, just nine months short of his ordination. [*Ibid.*, p. 216.]

New York, New York

For those Confederate prisoners being transported into New England, the trip was proving exceedingly difficult. Vicious draft riots were sweeping through New York City in July, resulting in widespread burning, looting, and vandalism. Blacks especially were singled out by the bloodthirsty horde; those unfortunate enough to be captured by the rampaging mob were severely beaten and many lynched, left hanging on nearby trees and lamp posts.

Regiments from the Army of the Potomac were eventually needed to restore order in the streets. As a result of the civil unrest, however, rail travel was severely disrupted, throwing a major curve into the transportation of captured Confederates.

On July 15, Medical Director of the East Charles W. McDougall wired Surgeon General Hammond from New York City, bringing him up to date with news of the extraordinary measures that were now necessary in order to convey prisoners of war to their internment camps:

> General, The New Jersey railroad Company having refused to transport the rebel wounded to this city on account of the threats of the mob, I would advise that those not yet forwarded be sent by sea.
>
> The six hundred detained in Philadelphia yesterday by this decision of the company will be brought by water; the Steamer *Commodore* having been dispatched last night, for this purpose.
>
> I telegraphed Surg. Swift today, to fill this steamer to its capacity with any rebel wounded remaining, destined for New York.
>
> Very Respectfully, &c
> C. W. McDougall
> Med. Director
> Dept. East[136]

---

136. Record Group 112, Office of the Surgeon General, Letters Received, 1818-1870, Box No. 66, Letters Received, July 1, 1863—February 29, 1864, National Archives and Records Administration.

David's Island, New York

The influx of thousands of captured Confederates stretched the Northern prison camp system to its very limit. Instead of dribbling in in groups of hundreds from skirmishes and small battles scattered here and there throughout several theaters of war, a deluge of Southern prisoners of war, many of them seriously wounded, threatened to inundate the few facilities capable of caring for their highly specialized needs—providing both medical care and secure confinement.

David's Island, New York, was a prime example. At 2:30 p.m. on Monday, July 13, the medical director of the East telegraphed Surgeon General Hammond with the following report: "Surg General, I have about five hundred (500) vacant beds left after receiving David's Island for Rebel wounded."[137]

McDougall worked his staff hard that week, preparing for the expected glut of enemy casualties. As the wounded Confederates began to arrive in force, the medical director took the next step to house the incoming Southerners, as he reported on the evening of Tuesday, July 21: "Surg Genl, Ordered several days since all the tents to be put up at David's Island[;] will accomodate eighteen hundred[,] four hundred now. The remainder by Saturday next."[138]

By Thursday, July 23, the crunch was really being felt at David's Island. McDougall's report to Surgeon General Hammond reveals a prisoner of war camp growing at an astronomical rate: "General, I have the honor to report . . . that David's Island is being crowded with rebel wounded, and that they are coming forward much more rapidly than anticipated with some temporary inconvenience. The carpenters are at work erecting the tents and nineteen hundred beds were ordered up today. Bedsteads for immediate use were lacking, but will be supplied. Surgeon Simon was ordered by telegraph to be prompt in sending his requisitions for whatever was required. I presume that by tonight there will be there twenty two hundred rebel wounded." He confirmed that 2200 Confederates were indeed present in the facility later that same evening.[139]

While David's Island may not have been, as John Dooley optimistically described it, a garden spot where "every attention, care, and kindness was bestowed upon our fellow prisoners," Medical

---

137. *Ibid.*
138. *Ibid.*
139. *Ibid.*

Director McDougall and his staff continued to scramble to adequately house, clothe, and feed the flood of bloody and bandaged Southerners arriving from Pennsylvania.[140]

Gettysburg, Pennsylvania

And still they kept coming from Gettysburg. Northerner and Southerner, Union and Confederate, wearing uniforms (or the ripped and mutilated tatters of what were once uniforms) of blue and grey—each one bearing in his body the marks of the ferocious three day conflict. Each one also bore in his face the marks, the lines, the shadows of his struggle to live, to survive this obscene violation of living and vital flesh with filthy bits of metal, wood, and other foreign substances.

But the floodtides of evacuation had begun to slow now. In the first frantic week of moving the wounded away from the putrid battlefield, 7,382 injured men had been transported by rail to Baltimore. By July 22, when records were no longer kept, a staggering 11,425 had been moved in just over two weeks, with 8,653 of them being routed to or through Baltimore from Gettysburg. An additional 4,000 were sent into Baltimore from both Littlestown, Pennsylvania, and Westminster, Maryland.

While 3,817 wounded Confederates had been removed east to military hospitals and prisoner of war camps, 2,922 still remained in the corps hospitals outside Gettysburg on July 22. For them, it was still a bitter, ongoing battle to cheat death.[141]

---

140. Dooley, *John Dooley*, p. 121.
141. *OR*, vol. 27, pt. 1, p. 27.

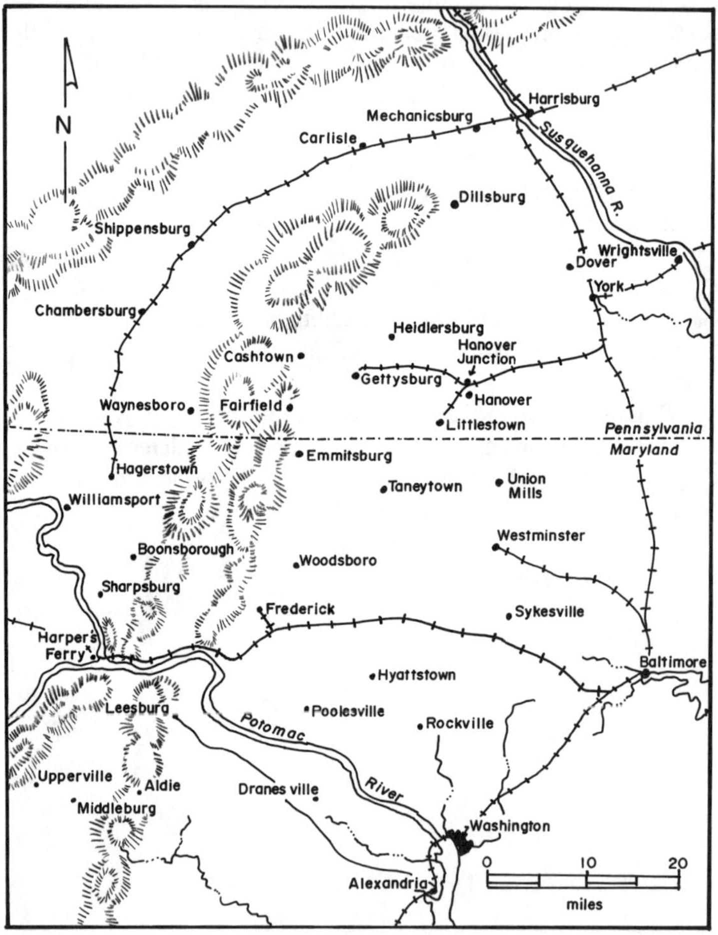

Map by John Heiser

Rail system to evacuate the wounded from Gettysburg.

CHAPTER 15

THURSDAY, JULY 2: DUSK—FRIDAY, AUGUST 8

". . . a young man whose face . . . seemed that of one of my own kindred. . . ."

Emily Bliss Souder
Volunteer Nurse from Philadelphia

THE CONFEDERATE WOUNDED OF THE SECOND CORPS HOSPITAL

Gettysburg, Pennsylvania

As Lt. John Dooley and his injured comrades steamed their way out of Gettysburg, they were only the vanguard of the Confederate wounded to leave the Second Corps hospital. Most of the 952 wounded Southerners still lay in tents, or in the big bank barn out on the Schwartz Farm, too fragile from wounds or traumatized by surgery to be evacuated. These men were more, however, than just numbers of captured enemy troops, or statistics in a military ledger. Each man had a name, a family, his own personality—each had his own unique story of Civil War life, and death.

Second Lt. Giles H. Cooper, 24th Virginia Infantry

One of the wounded men laying near Lieutenant Dooley at the Second Corps hospital was Lt. Giles H. Cooper, an officer of Company D of the 24th Virginia Infantry. Felled by a severe wound to the leg during the Southern assault on July 3, he was carried to the hospital after laying overnight on the field near the Emmitsburg Road. There the seriousness of his wound led to prompt amputation at the lower third of his left thigh.[1]

"About two yards from me on the other side of the road is a Virginia Lieut., 24th Va. His leg is torn and mangled fearfully; it is now amputated between the thigh and knee. There he reclines with his back against a stump and his wounded stump of a leg dragging heavily on the ground, clumsily bound up and portions of flesh exposed and bedraggled in the mud."[2]

Having little to occupy his time other than scribbling in his diary, Dooley had numerous opportunities to record his observations of this fellow lieutenant from his home state. In an army of hard talking, hard drinking, and hard living troops, this Virginian seemed to possess a quiet dignity and reserved manner unlike many of his companions. "I have watched this officer pretty closely and although I have seen much pain and agony in his expression, I haven't heard a single word of complaint or impatient exclamation break from his lips. Only once I heard him ask some negro camp attendant in a tone of piteous expostulation to make a little fire near him, for the rain was chilling him to the very marrow of the bones. No fires were made however, for whether it was against orders or the result of neglect, we suffered a great deal from rain and the chilling night air."[3]

Moved with compassion by the quiet agonies of his neighbor, Dooley tried to make him as comfortable as possible. "My poor friend appeared to suffer so much that after a selfish contest with my better impulses I sent him over my oil-cloth, that being doubled up and placed under his amputated member it might free him from much pain and distress. This gave him much relief and he appeared much grateful; and now we were both equal in regard to exposure to the weather, for neither of us had any covering except our clothes."[4]

After Dooley's departure for Baltimore, Lieutenant Cooper's condition began to steadily deteriorate. The seriousness of the thigh amputation, compounded by exposure to the drenching rain and chill dampness, had significantly weakened him. Despite a tenacious battle for life, he finally succumbed to the effects of his wound on July 27. He

---

1. Kathleen Georg Harrison and John W. Busey, *Nothing But Glory: Pickett's Division at Gettysburg* (Gettysburg, Pennsylvania: Thomas Publications, 1993), p. 246.
2. Dooley, *John Dooley*, pp. 112-13.
3. *Ibid.*
4. *Ibid.*

was buried under a walnut tree in Yard B, on a hillside of the Schwartz Farm, at some distance from the farm buildings in the direction of the neighboring George Bushman Farm. On June 13, 1872, his remains were exhumed with the other Southern dead buried at the Schwartz Farm, and shipped to Richmond in Box #202, where they were interred in Hollywood Cemetery, this time with full military honors.[5]

When the war was only a distant memory, Lieutenant Dooley would pause and muse about that officer on the muddy hillside at Gettysburg. "Long have I remembered this noble example of patience, and although I don't know what became of my Virginia friend, I have often recalled his quiet suffering form to my mind and described to others his unexampled equanimity."[6]

Lt. Francis A. Timberlake, Company B, 7th Tennessee Infantry

Also placed on the ground near Dooley and Cooper was yet a third lieutenant—Francis A. Timberlake of Company B, 7th Tennessee Infantry. Timberlake was a native of Smith County, Tennessee, and his kinsman Fountain P. Timberlake, also from Smith County, served in the same regiment. He had shown conspicuous gallantry at Fredericksburg, holding ground against overwhelming odds, and charging the enemy when his ammunition was exhausted. Even though he was officially named Francis, he was hearty and robust, and everyone simply called him "Frank."[7]

The bullet that brought him down had richocheted around inside him, causing severe injuries within his abdominal cavity; Dooley noted that his neighbor was "wounded through the body and suffering continual and acute pain. The bullet had entered just to the right of the stomach but instead of piercing through, it had been turned from its course by muscle or cartilage, or something which it followed, and came out near the back bone."[8]

One look at the wound was enough for a swift diagnosis by one of the Second Corps doctors. "A Yankee surgeon examined his wound at this hospital and told him there were no hopes of his surviving over 48 hrs." The response of his gravely-injured patient must have amazed the examining physician. "Timberlake laughed (only weakly but

---

5. Coco, *Wasted Valor*, p. 127; Harrison and Busey, *Nothing But Glory*, p. 246.
6. Dooley, *John Dooley*, pp. 113.
7. John Gross, e-letter to Roland R. Maust, March 5, 1997.
8. Dooley, *John Dooley*, p. 117.

cheerfully) and told the surgeon he didn't feel quite prepared for death and would like to live a little longer. The Doctor insisted that he was in earnest, and Timberlake (who had a very strong will) told him he was *determined not to die.*"[9]

Sometimes survival truly was a case of mind over matter, and Lieutenant Timberlake was adamantly determined to physically prove that adage to be true. "He didn't die, either," noted Dooley, with some wonder, in his ever-present diary, "but for more than a year after that he was in prison with me; he was suffering continually and very painfully, for his wound would close only to reopen again. How well I remember his manly face with his long flowing beard."[10]

But although he did survive his wound, the Tennessee officer paid a high price in the long-term agony he was forced to endure due to the invasive wound to his abdomen. "How patient in all his sufferings!" marveled Dooley. "For, though suffering month after month and day after day, he tried to smile and be cheerful all the time."[11]

Frank Timberlake proved to be a comrade of unflinching morality and personal integrity. "I love to recall his high tone of honor and gentle but sensitive manner. I recollect as if but yesterday that I received some money in prison. He knew of it for I told him. He was unable to do anything for himself, not even to pay for his washing. He was suffering very much on this account and would not ask me to lend him a cent. I knew his wants and begged him to let me lend him some of my little store. He blushed almost to his very eyes and refused positively to accept of a loan because he might not be able to repay it. I insisted and he grew almost angry, so that I forced the money into his pocket and ran off."[12]

In spite of his painful condition, the Volunteer Stater was a practical joker of some note. Months later, with autumn steadily giving way to the onset of frigid winter at windblown Johnson Island Prison in Lake Erie, off the coast of Sandusky, Ohio, a still-recovering Dooley would record the humorous antics of his friend. "Today I feel well enough to assist in cooking dinner and supper. Whilst about making my coffee, Timberlake comes over to annoy me, and hides the coffee, then runs off."[13]

---

9. *Ibid.*, pp. 117-18.
10. *Ibid.*, p. 118.
11. *Ibid.*
12. *Ibid.*
13. *Ibid.*, p. 147.

The fondness and respect of the Virginia officer for his Tennessee friend clearly comes through in the pages of his diary. "He was as gentle as a child and spoke most sweetly and affably to all his friends. But when wrong and outrage were mentioned, or insult or injury offered to himself, his high forehead would crimson to the very roots of his hair and one might well imagine he had a lion to deal with instead of the gaily laughing and agreeable companion of a few minutes before."[14]

Col. Lewis Burwell Williams, Jr., 1st Virginia Infantry

John Dooley's commanding officer, Lewis B. Williams, had also fallen before the Yankee battle lines in the ill-fated Southern advance of July 3. Born September 13, 1833, Williams was an 1855 graduate of the Virginia Military Institute. He went on to make a successful career as a lawyer, only to finally return to his alma mater as a professor. The Virginia bachelor entered the Confederate service as a captain of Company A, 13th Virginia Volunteer Infantry, in April of 1861. A rapid rise through the ranks catapulted Williams to lieutenant colonelcy in less than two months, and brought a transfer to the 7th Virginia Volunteer Infantry. Still another move in April of 1862 returned Williams to the venerable 1st Infantry, this time as its colonel rather than a mere captain.[15]

William's had already been wounded once in the war, suffering a painful injury which led to his capture at the Battle of Williamsburg in 1862. A strict disciplinarian, Williams had staunchly willed himself to survive the long and debilitating period of rehabilitation, and eventually returned to duty at the head of his beloved regiment.[16]

The colonel was one of sixteen officers who advanced on horseback in the disastrous Friday afternoon advance. Struck in the shoulder, he toppled from his horse, further injuring himself by falling on his own drawn saber, according to an eye-witness account. Lieutenant Dooley ministered to his senior officer for the rest of July 3, following the Confederate repulse, and on throughout July 4, trying his best to make his commander comfortable. This time, he was critically

---

14. *Ibid.*, p. 118.
15. Harrison and Busey, *Nothing But Glory*, p. 181; Dooley, *John Dooley*, p. 108; Robert K. Krick, *Lee's Colonel's: A Biographical Register of the Field Officers of the Army of Northern Virginia* (Dayton, Ohio: Morningside Bookshop, 1979), p. 371; Coco, *Wasted Valor*, p. 127.
16. Dooley, *John Dooley*, p. 108.

wounded; a round had struck Williams in the neck, then traced its way down his spinal column. "He suffers continual and intense agony," noted Dooley in his diary. The proffered assistance of a Northern officer was tartly rebuffed by Williams, who preferred the heavy-handed, but well meant, ministrations of the painfully wounded Dooley.[17]

Dooley implored the ambulance officers who were overseeing the evacuation of the wounded to transport Colonel Williams to a Union hospital for medical assistance, and received their solemn promise that they would remove him as soon as possible. "Towards the middle of the day I have the satisfaction of knowing he had been removed," noted Dooley in his diary, to one of the Second Corps hospitals.[18]

Further details of Williams treatment and death are sketchy at best. "I never saw him afterwards," continued Dooley; "he died after 4 or 5 days' intense suffering." The colonel's remains were shipped for interment to Greenmount Cemetery in Baltimore, Maryland. After laying undisturbed for over thirty years, Lewis Burwell Williams, Jr. made his final journey home to Virginia, where he was reburied, with appropriate military honors, in Hollywood Cemetery on February 16, 1896.[19]

Sgt. William S. Jinkins, 7th North Carolina

Colonel Williams was fortunate to survive long enough to be evacuated to the corps hospitals in the rear of the Union army. Many of the men who fell in the Pickett-Pettigrew-Trimble attack of July 3, lacerated and punctured by Northern lead and shrapnel, lay mortally wounded on the battlefield and died in Union aid stations strung along the back of the Army of the Potomac's defensive line.

Thirty-four-year-old Jinkins had been severely wounded in the torso during the advance, and had been carried back to the primary station at the Peter Frey Farm. A Union officer, Lt. Abner R. Small, happened upon the stricken sergeant as he was assisting the wounded on July 4 during his off-duty hours.

> My duties permitting, I went among the wounded in a grove on the left of our position, where lay many hurt

---

17. *Ibid.*, p. 109; Coco, *Wasted Valor*, p. 127.
18. Dooley, *John Dooley*, p. 109. Contrary to Dooley's account, both Harrison and Busey [p. 181] and Krick [p. 371] record Williams as killed in action, not wounded.
19. *Ibid.*; Harrison and Busey, *Nothing But Glory*, p. 181.

survivors of the rebel attacking force; men of Pickett's division, and Heth's, and Pender's. I proffered what assistance I could. I remember stopping beside one poor fellow who was shot through the body. His wants were few.

"Only a drink of water," muttered the wounded Southerner. "I'm cold; so cold. Won't you cover me up?"

Then his mind wandered, and he murmured something about his mother. Then he had a clear sense of his condition. Would I write to his home, and say how he loved them, and how he died?

"Tell them all about it, won't you? Father's name is Robert Jenkins [*sic*]. My name is Will."

I thought I heard him say that he belonged to the 7th North Carolina and came from Chatham County. His words faltered into silence. I covered his face.[20]

The Northern lieutenant stuffed the paper and stubby pencil back in his pocket, and moved on to the next casualty.

Unlike so many of his comrades, however, Jinkins was not destined to occupy one of the mass graves of nameless corpses being trenched out beyond the Union battlelines. The Carolinian was carefully buried in the Frey orchard, just south of the stone farm house on the west side of the Taneytown Road. There his solitary grave was visible to passersby on the nearby thoroughfare during the years following the battle.

In the 1870s, as the land began to heal from the scars and ravages of the passage of two hostile armies, removal of the Southern remains was underway, spearheaded by efforts of local doctor Samuel Weaver. Sadly, the identity of a number of the Southern dead was lost or effaced in the transfer to Southern cemeteries; among these now-unknown dead were all that remained of North Carolinian William S. Jinkins. The sergeant's final resting place is at present still unknown.[21]

Second Lt. John R. Presgraves, 8th Virginia Infantry

Often the very first experience in a new location or on a new job makes an indelible impression on a person's memory. So it was with Clarissa Fellows Jones, a Philadelphia school teacher doing volunteer

20. Small, *Road to Richmond*, p. 107.
21. Coco, *Wasted Valor*, p. 117.

work as a nurse to wounded Confederates. "I will never forget my first case. He was a young fellow, lying on a rock, and suffering intensely from lockjaw. Beside him was his brother, nursing and caring for him. The anxious brother did not even have a handkerchief; he was bathing the boy's wounds with a piece of paper. I was burdened with handkerchiefs at that time, so I gave the rebel a few, and my, he was so glad to get them. I stayed with him some time, bandaged his wounds and did what I could for him, and his brother told me his story."[22]

Four brothers—George, William, James, and John—had all joined the same regiment, and gone off together to experience the excitement of war. "Their name was PRESGRAVES, and they lived on the James River. He said that he had two other brothers in the battle, and he feared that they both had been killed. When he [Pvt. George W. Presgraves] saw this brother [Second Lt. John R. Presgraves, Company I, 8th Virginia] fall, he allowed himself to be taken prisoner, purposely, so that he could be with him. When he had told this much of the story, he looked up at me with his big tear-filled eyes, for he knew his brother was going to die. 'How am I going [to go] back to my father and tell him of this, and that, in all probability, his other two boys have been killed in this same battle? I am afraid that I am the only one left. My poor father! He was more like a big brother to us, and you don't know how much we loved him.'"[23]

Actually, the two remaining Presgraves brothers had been captured, not killed, during the battle. All four brothers had been serving in Company I of the 8th—George W. and William T. were still buck privates, while brother James had a leg up in rank as third corporal. Ranking them all was John R., who, as a second lieutenant, now laying infected and dying from the tetanus he had contracted, either from the bullet that had fractured his left leg, or else from the ground upon which he had been laid. Surgeon Charles S. Wood, 66th New York, amputated the infected limb on July 13, but the tetanus continued its deadly grip on young Presgraves.[24]

---

22. Clarissa Fellows Jones, "Nursed the Confederates at Gettysburg," *Philadelphia North American*, Sunday, June 29, 1913, special section, p. 4.
23. *Ibid.*
24. *Ibid.*; Harrison and Busey, *Nothing But Glory*, pp. 268-69. All three of the captured brothers miraculously survived their prison experiences and were exchanged. William and James were exchanged on the very same day (May 25, 1865) at the same location (Conrad's Ferry, Maryland), indicating that they had probably been imprisoned together. George, on the other hand, was exchanged from a different place (Fort Delaware) on a different day (June

Clarissa Jones was deeply moved by the story of the Presgraves brothers, and the gentle young Virginian as he cared for his dying brother. "The tears came to my own eyes. I did everything I possibly could do for that poor boy. He was so affectionate to his brother and waited on him night and day."[25]

A case of tetanus was a certain death sentence—all anyone could do was to wait for the inevitable end to arrive, and to make the patient as comfortable as possible until the death rattle sounded. Nurse Jane Boswell Moore also remembered the young Virginia lieutenant, and the long tedious days spent with him awaiting death. "A lieutenant from Virginia, dying from lockjaw, having lain out in the rain after his leg was amputated, seemed exceedingly happy, and took great delight in hymns, which, he said, just expressed his feelings. He told his brother, who leaned over him in an agony of grief, to tell his mother and sisters to meet him in heaven."[26]

Nurse Moore racked her memory for the words of every hymn that she knew in order to console the dying Virginian. "Taking his brother's place, I said, while fanning him, 'Lieutenant, do you remember that beautiful hymn, "There is a fountain filled with blood?"' His eyes lighted as I slowly repeated it, and 'Jesus, lover of my soul,' pausing after each to see that he was neither dead nor sleeping. I then repeated that sublime hymn 'Rock of ages, cleft for me,' and as I was then obliged to leave him, read the closing verse, endeavoring to throw into those glorious words all their full strength and force of meaning."[27]

The young lieutenant from the James River valley was deeply moved by the comforting words of those familiar hymns. "It is impossible to describe the beam of glory, unearthly and beautiful beyond all that I have seen, which lit his face as I proceeded. His eyes shone with brilliant lustre; he pressed my hands affectionately, seeking to detain me, laid his for a moment on my breast, and then pointed upward, as though he would have contrasted here and THERE."[28]

20, 1865), indicating that George was probably the brother who cared for his dying sibling at the Second Corps hospital. [Typescript copy of the *Philadelphia North American* in Newspaper Files, Gettysburg National Military Park, with critical notes by Kathleen Georg Harrison.]

25. Jones, "Nursed the Confederates at Gettysburg," p. 4.

26. Jane Boswell Moore, "An Incident in Gettysburg," in *The United States Christian Commission. Second Report of the Committee of Maryland, September 1863*, p. 107.

27. *Ibid.*

28. *Ibid.*

After nearly two weeks of ceaseless agony, Lt. John R. Presgraves died on July 15. "His brother asked if he could not go into Gettysburg and buy a pine coffin, for he intended to come back after the war and bring the body home. He was given permission and, instead of being buried in a blanket, as was the case with the great majority, this one boy had a pine coffin."[29]

A pitifully small handful of onlookers turned out for the brief graveside ceremony, a combined service for all who had died during the previous day in the division hospital. It would be a burial at the hands of strangers, far from home and kin, in a strange and hostile northern soil. "Major Holstein and his wife read the burial service each day over the long stretch of the dead, and Mrs. Moore and I always accompanied them," recalled Clarissa Fellows Jones. "But at this particular time, Major Holstein did not have his glasses with him, and he could not read without them." The appropriate words and prayers would have to be bypassed today. After all, it was just so many more lifeless corpses, each having become anonymous and alien in death, stiff with rigor mortis and caked blood in the harsh light of day.[30]

Pvt. George W. Presgraves was appalled that his brother should just be dumped in the ground, like a load of discarded fieldstone, without any real thought or mourning. "As soon as the brother realized this, he sat on a log and cried as though his heart would break. Finally he regained his composure and, looking up, said: 'Is there not somebody who will say a word over my brother? Must I go home and say that he was buried like a dog, without even a prayer for him?'"[31]

Once again, Clarissa Fellows Jones was touched by the fierce loyalty of the surviving brother, even with the blood ties now tenuated in death. "Miss Moore and I could not resist this appeal. Major Holstein let us have his book, and we read the burial service. We all felt intensely sorry for this poor boy, he was so much affected by his loss." The burial service completed, young John Presgraves was laid to rest west of the Schwartz farmhouse near Yard C, in the shade of the woods on the ridge above Rock Creek.[32]

For his part, George Presgraves was determined to carry out his pledge concerning his brother, and, emboldened by their care for his brother, he shared his plans with Miss Jones and Miss Moore. "He

---

29. Jones, "Nursed the Confederates at Gettysburg," p. 4.
30. *Ibid.*
31. *Ibid.*
32. *Ibid.*; Harrison and Busey, *Nothing But Glory*, p. 269.

told us that he was going to escape—told us how he was going to do it and how he was going back to his father. We all knew about it, but we said nothing. We let him go. So, of course, we were not surprised when we heard that he was missing; but no one told on the poor fellow or what course he had taken."[33]

The Presgraves honor and family loyalty continued as steadfast in death as it had been in life. Sometime between 1865 and 1870, before the general disinterments began, the Presgraves brothers returned to Gettysburg, as quietly and unobtrusively as George had left the blighted town in 1863. In the simplicity and depth of familial grief, a crumbling pine coffin containing the body of Second Lt. John R. Presgraves, 8th Virginia Infantry, was carefully removed from the Pennsylvania soil and solemnly returned to the James River land where John had grown to young manhood.[34]

Col. John Bowie Magruder, 57th Virginia Infantry

The musket balls caught John B. Magruder at chest height. Magruder was stepping over the stone wall on Cemetery Ridge during the July 3 Confederate assault, making a beeline for Cushing's abandoned cannon that sat a tantalizing twenty steps away. "They are ours," bellowed the youthful officer, his eye on the coveted prize; "they are ours!" Just at that moment he was shot twice, one bullet from a 72nd Pennsylvania musket slamming into the left side of his chest, the other, fired by an infantryman from the 69th Pennsylvania, tearing through his upper right arm, then passing into the ribcage. The two projectiles bored crisscrossing paths through the colonel's chest cavity, miraculously missing any vital organs, and each other, along the way.[35]

At twenty-four, Magruder was a great success story back home. Born in Scottsville, Virginia, November 14, 1839, he had grown up in nearby Keswick Depot, and set out from there for the Virginia Military Institute. Magruder moved to Culpeper as a school teacher after graduating from the University of Virginia. Entering the service in July of 1861 as captain of Company H, 57th Virginia, he had steadily and persistently risen through the ranks—major, early 1862; lieutenant colonel, July 1862; full colonel, January 1863. Now Colonel Magruder

---

33. Jones, "Nursed the Confederates at Gettysburg," p. 4.
34. Coco, *Wasted Valor*, p. 117.
35. Harrison and Busey, *Nothing But Glory*, p. 418.

had been shot down at the head of his regiment, with his face toward his Yankee enemies in an obscure Northern town named Gettysburg.[36]

Having fallen so close to the Union lines, the colonel was moved back to the Second Corps Hospitals on July 4. There he was tenderly cared for in the Rock Creek lowlands by Catherine Wert, one of the neighbors of the Schwartz's, and mother of J. Howard Wert, a local young man who made frequent visits to the Second Corps Hospital.[37]

Colonel Magruder knew from the experience of other battlefields that his wound was a mortal one. "I am sinking. I will never leave this Northern land alive," he confided to Mrs. Wert. "Some day, when peace is restored, my friends in Virginia will carry my bones to the ancestral burying ground. But I will never more join the family or social circle. Death is creeping up on me. The surgeons are very kind and try to encourage me, but I feel my race is run. I have faced my duty as I saw it like a man, and I have no regrets."[38]

With the nearness of death, Magruder's thoughts turned to concern for his soul. "But now, when the shadows of death are closing around me, I fear, madam, I may not have been earnest in the discharge of religious duties as I should have been. I must soon face my maker. Madam," the dying Confederate officer looked up at Katy Wert, "will you pray for me?" Mrs. Wert wrapped her warm hands around the clammy ones of the officer, and lifted her voice in prayer for the dying man, who had strangely become more like a son to her than an invader.[39]

The vigorous health of young manhood withstood the effects of the fatal wound longer than was initially expected by the surgeons. As the hours passed, Katy Wert returned again and again to hold the hands of the steadily failing man in hers and to pray with him. After she had finished, the Virginian would always smile wanly at his faithful nurse, and speak quietly in his slow, gentle drawl. "'Madam,' said the Colonel, as he warmly grasped the hand of the woman, 'I have followed you. I have understood all your pleadings at the throne. I have seen a new light. I now know that I am nothing, and that Jesus and his redemption is everything. I am ready to die in peace. I thank you,

---

36. *Ibid.*
37. Harrison and Busey contend that Magruder was treated at the Twelfth Corps, not the Second Corps, hospital [p. 418].
38. J. Howard Wert, "Twas Fifty Years Ago," #12, *Harrisburg Telegraph*, July 5, 1913, p. 10.
39. *Ibid.*

madam; oh! I thank you.'" On July 5, Mrs. Wert walked over to the Second Corps hospital to find that the ever-polite young colonel had finally lost the battle for life. His body had been put out for the burial detail, and he was laid to rest in one of the graveyards in Farmer Schwartz's fields.[40]

The Southern colonel did not need to wait for the re-establishment of peace to be removed to his "ancestral burying ground." His body was disinterred in October, while the scars of battle and bloodshed were still harshly visible on the Pennsylvania landscape, and transferred under flag of truce to Richmond. An Epsilon Alpha fraternity brother saw to it that his remains and personal effects were carefully placed in a metallic coffin before finally being reburied in the warm, friendly soil of the South.[41]

Col. Hugh Reid Miller, 42nd Mississippi Infantry

The complicated and frustrating struggle to return home during wartime dominates the story of the distinguished commander of the 42nd Mississippi. Hugh R. Miller, born in 1812, was a native South Carolinian. By 1840, however, he had uprooted himself and moved to distant Mississippi, where he followed a notable career as a circuit judge. As a state legislator, Miller was an instrumental player in the Mississippi State Secession Convention. Backing his words with suitable actions, Miller enlisted as an infantry captain in 1861, and served at the First Battle of Manassas. His natural leadership skills were immediately evident, and by May 14, 1862, he had risen through the ranks to become colonel of the 42nd. Well known and respected, he was at the head of his command, on the right flank of Brig. Gen. Joseph Davis' brigade, when they stepped off from their Seminary Ridge staging area on July 3.[42]

Severely wounded in front of the Second Corps lines, he was carried back to the Rock Creek hospital site. In all the hurry and bustle of moving the wounded from the battlefield to the new location of the hospital, the Confederate officer was unloaded from the ambulance and unceremoniously laid in the midst of Union, not Confederate, wounded. There Christian Commissioner Andrew Cross and his associates found him on July 5. "In a fence corner just above us,

---

40. *Ibid.*
41. Harrison and Busey, *Nothing But Glory*, p. 41; Coco, *Wasted Valor*, p. 129.
42. Krick, *Lee's Colonels*, p. 250.

among our men, lay Colonel Hugh R. Miller, of Pontotoc, Mississippi, of the 42d Mississippi Regiment, an eminent lawyer and judge of that State, shot through the left breast and right knee. We gave him a little wine and a cracker, which he took with great modesty, saying he was not dangerously wounded but thankful for our offer to write to his wife, Mrs. Susan G. Miller, at Sunnyside, Cumberland Co., Virginia. The Surgeon told us his case was dangerous."[43]

Cross and his men circulated through the swelling crowd of wounded and dying men, and soon found themselves again at the crowded fence corner. "Calling again after a short time to see if he would have anything, he modestly said: 'I am very much obliged to you, but give it to those around, who are worse, and need it more.'"[44]

Sometime after July 5, the seriously injured officer was transferred from the Second Corps facility to a private home in town, where he was tenderly cared for by a sympathetic family. It was from there that an urgent summons was dispatched to Chaplain Thomas D. Witherspoon of the 42nd Mississippi, who had remained behind in Gettysburg to help attend to the many Southern wounded unable to be evacuated to Confederate hospitals by the retreating Army of Northern Virginia. "On the very day before the order came to break up our field-hospital [July 19], tidings had come to us that the Colonel of the regiment in which I served, Colonel Hugh R. Miller, was lying mortally wounded at a private residence in Gettysburg, and had expressed a desire to see me. I reached his bedside just in time to receive his dying expression of his faith in Christ and his readiness to depart."[45]

Witherspoon immediately set about making all the necessary arrangements for his former commander. "Through the generosity of the kind family (a Maryland family) at whose home Colonel Miller had been so assiduously and tenderly cared for, the services of an embalmer were secured, and the body skilfully [*sic*] embalmed and inclosed [*sic*] in a metallic case."[46]

Next, it was necessary to obtain proper military transit permits to ship the sad cargo south. "The Commandant of the Post at Gettysburg, whose name I do not recall, but who was a true gentleman as well as [a] true soldier, on application being made to him to send the remains

43. Cross, *The War and the Christian Commission*, pp. 14-15.

44. *Ibid.*, p. 15.

45. Thomas D. Witherspoon, "Prison Life at Fort McHenry," Paper 1, in *SHSP*, 8:77.

46. *Ibid.*

through the lines by flag of truce, did all he could to further this end.[47] For he not only sent the remains to Baltimore in charge of one of the members of his staff, but he allowed Edwin Miller, the youthful son of the Colonel, and myself, his chaplain to accompany the remains as escort with a letter to General Schenck, the Commandant at Baltimore, requesting that we should be permitted to accompany the remains by flag of truce to Richmond."[48]

At Baltimore, however, the grieving pair of Confederates ran afoul of the anti-southern sentiment evinced by some Northern officers stationed in this rancorous city.

> The scene on arrival at General Schenck's headquarters in Baltimore was one that beggars description. The polite and gentlemanly Lieutenant who had accompanied us presented the letter from his superior officer, and it was handed to Colonel Fish, General Schenck's Adjutant. He read it, and asked, "Where is the body?"
>
> The Lieutenant produced the receipt of the Adams Express Company, who had it in charge, and the Colonel, receiving it, handed it to one of his subordinates, and said, "Go and get that body and have it buried."
>
> "Where shall I bury it?" asked the surprised official—to which the answer was in substance that he did not care where, so as the body was put out of the way, adding that he had stood all that he was going to stand of this paying honors to Rebel dead.[49]

The chaplain and his young charge were outraged at the cavalier treatment, so contrary to the civilized ways of war.

> Edwin Miller, overwhelmed with the thought of the dishonor about to be done to his father's remains, pleaded most earnestly to be permitted to accompany the officer and see the remains interred, and it was only after a long interval, and through the intercession of friends of Colonel Fish, who were the witnesses of the boy's agony, that he was

---

47. Colonel Alleman was post commander of the 36th Pennsylvania Militia stationed at Gettysburg following the battle.
48. Witherspoon, "Prison Life at Fort McHenry," pp. 77-78.
49. *Ibid.*, p. 78.

permitted to accompany the remains to their sepulture [*sic*], and have them placed in a vault instead of being buried in the ground.

When the question of the disposition of the body had been finally settled, the Lieutenant in charge of us asked, "What shall I do with these men?" referring to Edwin Miller and myself. To which the reply was, "Let them go down to the guard-room."[50]

The two hapless Confederates were unceremoniously thrust into a basement room filled with drunken soldiers, deserters, bummers, and Southern sympathizers, and the iron door slammed behind them. Following a night punctuated by nationalistic braggadocio, traded oaths, and impromptu fist fights, Chaplain Witherspoon was shipped off to Fort McHenry, and the younger Miller released.[51]

The remains were finally removed from their temporary resting place, passed south through the Union lines under flag of truce, and completed their journey to Richmond. There, in the First Presbyterian Church, the colonel's military funeral was conducted on July 29. The widow, Susan Gray Walton Miller, was composed at the graveside, but, within six months almost to the day, she herself was laid to rest alongside her deceased husband.[52]

The only known official communication to pass under flag of truce through the battlelines at Gettysburg concerned the fate of Colonel Miller. The July 4 communiqué, addressed to General Meade, and signed by Robert E. Lee himself, requested Meade (as a personal favor to Lee) to ascertain the condition of Miller. Considering the resolution of the situation at Baltimore, it seems quite likely that this wish was indeed honored.[53]

Col. William Gibson, 48th Georgia Infantry

One of the most extraordinary stories of wounded Confederates at the Second Corps hospital involved Colonel Gibson and the incredibly loyal troops of his 48th Georgia Infantry. During General Longstreet's

50. *Ibid.*
51. *Ibid.*
52. Krick, *Lee's Colonels*, p. 250.
53. Robert E. Lee, Letter to George G. Meade, July 4, 1863, formerly in the collection of Ted and Mary Sutphen, Gettysburg, Pennsylvania.

July 2 offensive, the 48th Georgia, part of Wright's brigade of Hill's Third Army Corps, occupied the property of the Codori family near the Emmitsburg Road. This proved to be an ideal spot for sniping at the Federals on Cemetery Ridge, so the 106th Pennsylvania Volunteer Infantry was sent out to roust the Confederates from the protective cover of the large frame barn and brick house.[54]

As they approached the farm, Capt. R. H. Ford of Company I spotted a Southern officer emerge from the buildings, frantically waving a pocket handkerchief. Ford pointed the officer out to his superior, Lt. Col. William L. Curry, and Curry immediately dispatched Ford and his company to meet the Confederate. Lacking a white handkerchief, someone pulled out an old newspaper and stuck it on the end of a bayonet as a sign of temporary truce. Then the little command marched out to the Codori house, feeling strangely conspicuous under the watching eyes of both their own men and the enemy regiment.[55]

The officer they approached was Capt. Claiborne Snead of the 48th Georgia. Snead informed his Union counterpart that his colonel, William Gibson, was gravely wounded, and in need of immediate medical attention. Nearly the whole regiment was there in the buildings behind him, he said, and they desired to spare their colonel's life, even if it meant his captivity. Could the 106th Pennsylvania see to the instant transportation of the critically injured Gibson to the nearest Union hospital?[56]

Born on March 10, 1822, in Warren County Georgia, Gibson had been a lawyer of some note in Augusta, serving also as judge and state senator before the war. Colonel Gibson was something of a prodigy in an army of citizen soldiers and military men where promotions were frequently meteoric—he enlisted as a private in Company C, 48th Georgia on March 3, 1862, and soared to the colonelcy in just three weeks. Never one to be shy, he wrote to President Jefferson Davis on March 22, 1863, seeking promotion to brigadier general in light of having commanded Wright's brigade at Antietam, and his four conspicuous battlefield wounds. Now he lay dangerously wounded at the Codori Farm, *hors de combat* for a fifth time, with a ball through the thigh.[57]

---

54. Ward, *History of the One Hundred and Sixth Pennsylvania*, p. 193.
55. *Ibid.*
56. *Ibid.*
57. *Ibid.*; Allen D. Candler and Clement A. Evans, eds., *Cyclopedia of Georgia*, vol. 2 (Atlanta, Georgia: State Historical Society, 1906), p. 120;

Thinking quickly, Captain Ford gladly agreed to see that Colonel Gibson be given the care that he needed . . . provided that the entire Georgia regiment surrendered as well. Captain Snead protested indignantly—all they wanted was medical care for their commander, not wholesale capitulation of the entire regiment. He and the remainder of the Georgia troops should be allowed to return to their lines. But Ford remained adamant; surrender the entire regiment and Colonel Gibson would be sure to receive the best treatment possible.[58]

The Southern captain was backed into a corner, and knew it. Objecting vehemently and repeatedly, Snead finally had no choice but to acquiesce to Captain Ford's demands. Colonel Gibson was gently carried through Union lines and on to the nearest aid station by some of his men. As the litter made its way toward the Union lines, the rest of the Georgia regiment began pouring out of Farmer Codori's buildings—five captains, fifteen lieutenants, and two hundred and fifty enlisted men reluctantly came out with hands up and muskets inverted, handed over their weapons, and glumly marched to the rear as prisoners of war. Captain Ford staggered back to Lieutenant Colonel Curry of the 106th Pennsylvania, arms full of captured officers' swords. Handing over his trophies, Ford returned to his regiment and continued on toward the Emmitsburg Road. Soon afterwards, lack of support forced the Pennsylvania men to withdraw back to the relative safety of their own lines.[59]

When word reached Brig. Gen. Alexander Webb of his regiment's spectacular accomplishment and its distinguished captive, he arranged for immediate ambulance transportation of Colonel Gibson to the Second Corps hospital. There he received prompt and personal medical care from the surgeon of the 106th Pennsylvania, Dr. Justin Dwinelle himself. Gibson had a robust constitution, and was soon recuperating nicely; in fact, he regained strength so completely that he soon attempted to escape the hospital and rejoin what was left of his

---

Confederate Military History, extended edition (Wilmington, North Carolina: Broadfoot Publishing Company, 1987), pp. 122-23; Nicholson, *Pennsylvania at Gettysburg*, p. 544; Smith, *History of the Nineteenth Maine*, p. 74; Charles H. Banes, *History of the Philadelphia Brigade* (Philadelphia: J. B. Lippincott & Co., 1876), p. 183; William D. Robertson, "My Enemy, My Brother, Mason Wounded at Gettysburg Treated as a Brother Mason," *California Freemason*, June, 1992, pp. 7-8.

58. Ward, *History of the One Hundred and Sixth Pennsylvania*, p. 193.

59. *Ibid.*, pp. 193-94; *OR*, vol. 27, pt. 1, p. 434. Lieutenant Colonel Curry backs up Captain Ford's claims of capturing 250 Georgians in his after-action report.

shrunken regiment. Unlike George W. Presgraves, however, Gibson was recaptured before he could reach Confederate lines and returned under armed guard to the hospital.[60]

Medical Inspector John M. Cuyler, a Georgian who had remained loyal to the Union when the war came, struck up an acquaintance with Colonel Gibson while assisting with Confederate surgeries at the Second Corps Hospital. Just before returning to his office in the Capital to make his official report, he dashed off a hasty note to Doctor Dwinelle, asking for special care to be given to his newfound friends:

> Gettysburg, July 24th
> My dr. Doct.,
>
> I leave tomorrow for Washington and may return in a few days. Will you please see if Col. Gibson and the Georgia officers with him are in need of any thing & let them have what you approve of and I will be responsible for the amount. Tell them this for me.
>
> Very truly,
> Jnothn Cuyler[61]

Although "the Georgia officers," especially Captain Snead, may have rankled under their forced surrender, Colonel Gibson had nothing but good things to say of his captor and his care at the Second Corps Hospital. Taking up pen and paper before being shipped off to prison camp, Gibson jotted a gracious note to Captain Ford of the 106th Pennsylvania:

> Hospital Camp, 2nd Army Corps July 30th, 1863
> Captain R. H. Ford
> Dear Capt,
>
> I had hoped to meet you again to express to you my thanks for the kindness and attention shown me by you on the 2nd Inst, yet circumstances have prevented, & I regret to learn that on the next day you were wounded. Yet I am much gratified to know you are fast recovering & hope you will soon be fully restored to health.

60. Ward, *History of the One Hundred and Sixth Pennsylvania*, p. 194.
61. Union Field Hospitals Vertical File, Gettysburg National Military Park Library.

I now think that I shall recover myself, & trust that peace may soon be restored to our unhappy people & that I may have an opportunity of expressing my thanks to you in a manner more agreeable & pleasant to us both.

Dr. Dwinell[e] has done all for me that I could wish & his kindness to me will never be forgotten. He has the will & the sense to do his whole duty to his fellow man, & is an upright, just, & honorable gentleman.

Hoping to meet soon again & as friends & Brothers would meet. I am, Captain, very Respectfully & truly your obt servant.
Wm. Gibson
Colonel, 48th Georgia Regiment, Augusta, Ga.[62]

Colonel Gibson was transferred to Camp Letterman General Hospital when the Second Corps Hospital folded up their tents on August 10, 1863. Staying there until that General Hospital closed in mid-November, he was forwarded to the Old Capitol Prison in Washington, D.C. on November 30, 1863. Then, when he was well enough to endure normal prisoner-of-war treatment, it was off to Fort McHenry, Maryland on January 12, 1864, and yet another move to Point Lookout, Maryland on January 23, 1864. The peripatetic colonel was finally exchanged on March 10, 1864.[63]

His intense quest for promotion absorbed most of his remaining time in Confederate service. Letters traveled to Richmond again and again, but all to no avail. Finally, in disgust, Gibson resigned his commission as colonel of the 48th Georgia on November 12, 1864. He died in Macon, Georgia, on April 5, 1893.[64]

---

62. Ward, *History of the One Hundred and Sixth Pennsylvania*, p. 194. All underlining by Colonel Gibson. The original letter is owned by William D. Robertson of Napa, California. Robertson, a Mason, "realized that certain words in the letter were underlined in a random fashion. This led him to believe that William Gibson was a Mason, as during the Civil War Masons did this as a kind of code that only fellow Masons would recognize." (William Gibson was indeed a Mason, a member of Webb Lodge No. 166, Augusta, Georgia, from 1856 to 1872). Since most of the underlining is in the section mentioning Doctor Dwinelle, it is assumed that the doctor was a Mason as well (his son and three grandsons were Masons). [Scott Michael Dwinelle, letter to the author, March 28, 1994].
63. Candler and Evans, *Cyclopedia of Georgia*, vol. 2, p. 120; *Confederate Military History*, pp, 122-23; Robertson, *My Enemy, My Brother*, pp. 7-8.
64. Candler and Evans, *Cyclopedia of Georgia*, vol. 2, p. 120; *Confederate Military History*, pp, 122-23; Robertson, *My Enemy, My Brother*, pp. 7-8.

Pvt. William P. Yearger, 22nd Georgia Infantry

William Yearger was also a part of General Wright's hapless July 2 initiative; unfortunately, this Georgian did not fare as well as Colonel Gibson of his sister regiment. A Northern projectile had done irreparable damage to his left leg, and resulted ultimately in its amputation at the Second Corps hospital. It was there that John Y. Foster, a civilian volunteer nurse from Philadelphia, found the young private on July 10, housed with the other Confederates in a recently erected hospital tent.

"A soldier from Georgia was brought to our hospital greatly prostrated from the loss of his left leg. We saw at once that his case was hopeless, and bestowed upon him the closest care possible under the circumstances."[65]

The young man was terribly homesick, nostalgically longing for the care of friends and family and the missed fellowship around the family dinner table. "From the first his mind seemed full of images of home, and he talked of little else beside his relatives. 'I have an old father at home,' he would say, 'and brothers and sisters; oh, if I could only go to them and sit in their midst once more!'"[66]

Interspersed with his fond reminiscences of home were violent self-recriminations over having ever become a soldier in the first place. "Then his thoughts would seem to go back to the beginning of the war, and he would bemoan his folly in having entered the army, declaring, with a despairing voice, that his heart had never been in the contest—that he would give years of his life if he could only go back again and be as he was before he took up arms. 'You can never know,' he said, 'what we have suffered in our army. We thought when we enlisted that the life of a soldier was full of charms—even those of us who volunteered purely in obedience to popular clamor and not from any principle, thought we should not after all be so very badly off, but we have long ago found out our mistake.'"[67]

Private Yearger's condition continued to deteriorate, and it soon became necessary for someone to tell the young man of his impending death. Foster was as close to the Georgian as anyone, so he tried to gently break the news to the dying Confederate in an indirect manner. "William, you have often spoken of your home and friends; if you have

65. Foster, "Four Days at Gettysburg," p. 383.
66. *Ibid.*
67. *Ibid.*

any thing to say to them, I think you had better write them as soon as you can." Up to this point, Yearger had apparently been totally unaware of the seriousness of his wound; "he comprehended in a moment what I meant. For the first time the thought that he might die presented itself distinctly to his consciousness."[68]

"'You mean, then, that I must die?'" The question hung ominously in the fetid air of the hospital tent. "I answered him that such was the opinion of the surgeon, adding that probably he could survive but a day or two at furthest. Then I asked him if he were ready to die."[69]

"'Oh, no!,' he cried, with a great sob. 'I am not prepared to go. My mother taught me, long years ago, my duty to God; she died praying for me, but I have forgotten it all, and now I am to die and be shut forever from her presence.'"[70]

Foster continued to quietly talk with him, reassuring him that there was still time to change his ways, still time to make his peace with God. "I told him that life was still his, and it was not yet too late. Then prayers were offered, and the exhausted soldier lay for a time perfectly silent."[71]

"After a while he roused himself and begged me to write what he should dictate." As Yearger formulated what he knew would be his final words to his family, "all the love in his heart poured forth. He told his father how he had suffered on the field; how he had been wounded and cared for by strangers and enemies; how he was dying with no hands but theirs to soothe and minister to him. Then he implored the father never to permit his younger brothers to go to the field, telling him they would but go to their death, and it would be in vain; victory could never be theirs. Then, when all else was said, he bade me write words of farewell to each of the dear ones by name, concluding with: 'Father, brothers, sisters, I hope to meet you in heaven'—a sob lying between each word as he gave them to me to write."[72]

When Foster stopped by to visit early the next day, it was clear that young Yearger had but a short time left to live. Foster stayed by Yearger's side, talking with the young soldier, unwilling to let him die alone so far away from home. "During all the morning, tightly clasping my hand in his as if afraid of losing a friend in that last hour, he talked

---

68. *Ibid.*, pp. 383-84.
69. *Ibid.*, p. 384.
70. *Ibid.*
71. *Ibid.*
72. *Ibid.*

of death and the judgment, weeping over his wayward life. . . . Toward noon, as he lay calm and silent for a moment, a lady visiting the tent came to his side and soothed him with her gentle speech, bidding him lay hold upon the Hand that carries the keys to the Celestial City." The young Georgia private continued to cling tenaciously to life. "The afternoon faded down the slopes and grew dim in the valleys, and the night crept up starless and grim." Still the long deathwatch continued.[73]

Finally, as midnight approached, Yearger became increasingly aware of his own imminent demise. "Clasping my hand closely still, he whispered, 'Turn me over, please, and put me on my knees.'" It was a struggle for Foster, wrestling the feeble man with one leg off the cot, trying to prevent inflicting still further agony upon him. "I did as requested, holding him as best I could, so that the stump of his leg might not touch the ground. The movement must have pained him, but he seemed unconscious now of suffering." As Yearger struggled to breathe, weakened by suffering, "half erect, leaning on my arms, he stretched out his own, spreading his palms heavenward, [and] lifted his eyes with an inexpressible longing upward, as if he would appease, in one last absolute surrender, divine justice; and so, without a word, he died, his head falling on his breast, his hands dropping limp and prone, life going out as softly as a summer dream flits its wing over the sleep of a baby." Foster would pensively confide later that, even "though dead, the pressure of that hand lies still in my palm."[74]

Foster gently laid the lifeless body back on the bunk, adjusted the worn and tattered uniform, folded the clammy hands and closed the sightless eyes. "I clipped a lock of hair, as he had requested, from his pallid temples, wrote upon it the day and hour of his decease, and sent it with his small effects, by an officer of his regiment, to the friends he was never again to see." Having done all he could for William P. Yearger, late of the 22nd Georgia Infantry, John Foster moved out into the pitch darkness of an overcast Pennsylvania night, took a deep breath of fresh air, then headed off to his own tent.[75]

Several of Private Yearger's regimental comrades were buried in the graveyards of the Second Corps hospital. But when the Schwartz Farm was surveyed between 1866 and 1870, preparatory to the removal of the Confederate dead, William P. Yearger's body was not among the

---

73. *Ibid.*
74. *Ibid.*
75. *Ibid.*

identified remains.[76] Perhaps the few passing years had served to efface Yearger's identity from his gravesite; or perhaps the father, brothers, and sisters had come to the Schwartz Farm, come to mourn young William, the reluctant soldier, and take him home again.

Lt. James M. Seals, 42nd Mississippi Infantry

While John Y. Foster took ministering to Confederate wounded easily in stride, other Northerners struggled to overcome strong anti-Southern sentiments when dealing with these needy men. Emily Bliss Souder, like Foster, was a volunteer nurse from the City of Brotherly Love, but her view of Southerners was harsh and extremely critical. "The rebels bear their sufferings very differently from our men," she wrote on July 20, a few days after arriving at the Second Corps hospital. "Some of them, their officers, are intelligent and gentlemanly; but the privates are for the most part perfectly abject. They whine, and cry, and complain; and their own men, who have been detailed as nurses, *will not* wait on them. They may well be called 'white trash,' for they are lacking in nearly all those qualities that we respect and value."[77]

Mrs. Souder came face to face with her prejudices on her very first full day at the Second Corps medical facility. "I wrote a letter yesterday [July 19] for Lieut Seal[s], of the 42d Mississippi, a very interesting young man," she admitted with some surprise. "On Wednesday morning last [July 15], we first visited the camp hospital of the Second Corps. We came to do what we could for our suffering soldiers,—for the martyr-heroes who had stood between us and death. We had scarcely entered the field of labor when some one came and begged me to see a young Mississippi lieutenant."[78]

"A momentary conflict arose in my mind. 'He is a rebel,' I said, 'and I had not felt as if I could do anything for a rebel.'"[79]

"'I think he is a fine young man,' was the answer, 'and he is going to die.'"[80]

The revelation that the man was facing death seemed to melt some of the frost from Mrs. Souder's heart. "I could hesitate no longer, but signified my willingness to go. Lying on the ground, in front of one of

76. Coco, *Wasted Valor*, p. 132.
77. Souder, *Leaves from the Battle-field of Gettysburg*, p. 34.
78. *Ibid.*, pp. 34-35.
79. *Ibid.*, p. 35.
80. *Ibid.*

the large hospital tents, was a young man, whose face, as I looked at him, seemed that of one of my own kindred; the same blue eyes, brown hair, and light complexion. With sorrow, I spoke of his coming North *on the wrong side*. A Massachusetts man in the tent eagerly answered for him: 'He could not help it; he is a good Union man at heart.' This was Lieutenant Seal[s]."[81]

What could she do for him? asked the Pennsylvania volunteer nurse. "In reply to my offer of service, he said I could do nothing for him. He was groaning in spirit, and suffering greatly, having been wounded in five places, and had also suffered amputation. He wished to be raised from the ground. I told him that the surgeons were supplying stretchers as fast as they received them, and doing all in their power to make the men comfortable." So ended Emily Bliss Souder's first encounter with a Southern patient.[82]

The pressures of trying to meet the physical, medical, emotional, and spiritual needs of thousands of wounded men kept Mrs. Souder and Lieutenant Seals apart for the next several days. "For a day or two I missed him, and thought he was gone, but he lingered on. Yesterday [July19], I wrote his farewell message to his wife, which he was scarcely able to utter, even in a faint whisper."[83]

Seals expended his remaining strength on his final farewell letter; within hours, the blue-eyed, brown-haired man so like Emily Souder's "own kindred" was dead. The Mississippi lieutenant was buried in the second row of Yard B between the Jacob Schwartz and George Bushman farms. Sadly, within ten years, his grave was lost, and his unidentified bones traveled south between 1871 and 1873, in the somber company of 3,320 other Confederate remains.[84]

Pvt. Dawson W. Arnold, 5th Florida Infantry

Facing death was something that every Civil War soldier considered from time to time, especially when advancing against well entrenched enemy troops who were firing musket volleys and artillery shells. But the thought of becoming a museum specimen was something that probably never crossed the mind of young Pvt. Dawson W. Arnold of Florida, even in his most terrifying nightmares.

---

81. *Ibid.*
82. *Ibid.*, pp. 35-36.
83. *Ibid.*, p. 36.
84. Coco, *Wasted Valor*, p. 113.

Eighteen-year-old Dawson was advancing in the Pickett-Pettigrew-Trimble assault of July 3, intent on reaching and overrunning the Northern lines on the distant, smoky heights, when he found himself toppled by a hammer blow to his left leg. Looking down in shock, Dawson saw blood pouring from a mangled gash in the front of his trousers; a conoidal musket ball had ripped into his thigh, shattering the upper third of his left femur. Dawson could only lie there helplessly, a sidelined spectator watching his regiment's advance to and be repulsed from the deadly heights of Cemetery Ridge.

After spending an agonizing night on the field, young Arnold waited anxiously until stretcher-bearers collected him and sent him off to the Union Second Corps hospital. Examination by the attending surgeon left no doubt that a immediate and radical amputation was the only appropriate treatment for Dawson's grievous wound. The surgery was carried out, and the young Floridian was given a cot and blanket in the amputation ward. It was optimistically hoped that his youth and stamina would give him sufficient will and ability to survive.

Yet Dawson did not regain his vitality. The severity of the wound, the shock, horror and exposure of lying all night on a battlefield of screaming wounded and mutilated men, the grinding pain and ghostly sensations from toes now gone, and the sapping tedium of fighting for life in a strange land and among enemies were taking their inevitable toll on young Dawson Arnold.

By early August, the Second Corps hospital was ready to break down their facility and catch up to their corps. Among the few remaining patients still being attended was an ashen and drawn Dawson Arnold. On August 5, the young soldier was tenderly transported from the Schwartz Farm to the new Letterman General Hospital out on the York Pike. His admission records tell the stark story of his failing health: profuse suppuration, overall emaciation, and large bedsores on his back.

By August 12, his condition was compounded by the onset of chronic diarrhea. Try as they might, the hospital staff could not seem to help young Dawson regain his strength. His stump was not healing properly, and the large foliaceous masses of callus uniting the fragments were extremely delicate and brittle. Dawson's health continued to deteriorate, until, on September 15, the tenacious soldier from Florida finally lost his fight with exhaustion. His remains were interred in the Letterman cemetery, adjacent to the medical facility.

Unknown to Private Dawson, an Army Medical Museum had been set up in Washington, a facility that would display unusual pathological and surgical specimens from the field. These samples were to be contributed by army surgeons in field hospital practice for the purpose of clinical instruction. Pvt. Dawson W. Arnold's shattered femur was of such interest to the Second Corps surgeon performing the amputation that he preserved the extremity, and shipped it off to Washington at the first opportunity. The only known surviving remains of Private Arnold are specimen #1938 in the Surgical Section of the Museum, a ghastly dry and brittle reminder of the very real pain, suffering, and anguish of one young boy from Florida.[85]

Sgt. Matthew Goodson, 52nd North Carolina Infantry

Invasive wounds of the chest cavity were almost universally fatal during the Civil War. By 1863, an experimental treatment of chest wounds was being advocated—the terrifying breathlessness (dyspnoea) experienced by chest wound patients was significantly relieved by hermetically sealing the wound with a plug of charpie and lint made airtight by coatings of collodion. Unfortunately, the mortality rate remained about the same, whether the wounds were sealed or not.[86]

When Sgt. Matthew Goodson toppled to the ground with a bullet through his chest during the Pickett-Pettigrew-Trimble assault of July 3, he must have known that his chances of survival were extremely slim. The projectile had pierced both lungs, then exited through his left side. As Goodson desperately struggled to catch his breath, his regiment was repulsed with severe losses and the sergeant was captured. The gasping North Carolina officer was removed to the Second Corps hospital for treatment.

Unfortunately, there was no doctoring that would be able to save the life of this North Carolinian. He slowly weakened with each passing day, painfully wheezing and gasping for each breath. His suffering finally came to an end on July 12. The remains of the sergeant were interred in the second row of Yard D, in Farmer Schwartz's cornfield. But the travels of Matthew Goodson were far from over.

In January of 1866, a compassionate Gettysburg resident named Hiram Warren wrote to tell Goodson's widow, Catharon J. Young Goodson, that he had discovered her husband's grave. He promised to see that Goodson's body would be moved to Evergreen Cemetery,

85. *Ibid.*, pp. 113-14; Adams, *Doctors in Blue*, pp. 34, 37, 42.
86. Adams, *Doctors in Blue*, pp. 136-37.

where he would personally mark the gravesite, and see to its perpetual care.

In late January 1866, the Evergreen Cemetery Board resolved that a portion of "Area E be set aside for the burial of the Rebel dead, beginning west of Ivy Rock and extending continuously westward and southward as far as possible or may be necessary." On January 29, 1866, a grave was prepared for Sergeant Goodson in Lot #169, Section E, and Hiram Warren carefully saw to the removal of the North Carolina native to his new resting place.

Then, unexpectedly, the Evergreen Cemetery Board reversed itself a year and a half later. In August of 1867, they unilaterally decided to "move the Rebel dead buried in Ever Green Cemetery to a more secluded spot." During the complicated process of disinterment, transportation, and reinterment, all record of Sergeant Goodson's whereabouts were lost.

In 1914, a purposeful delegation of Goodson progeny descended on Gettysburg, intent on tracking down their lost ancestor. Intensive research turned up no clues, and the Goodsons dejectedly returned home empty-handed. Sixty-five years and several generations later, a new delegation of Goodsons returned to Gettysburg in 1979, hoping that computerization and better research methods would help them accomplish their goal this time. They, too, left with the same frustrating lack of results.

Today, in a quiet corner of the Memorial Garden of First Presbyterian Church in Concord, North Carolina, there stands a modest grave marker bearing the name "Goodson." However, there is no body to accompany the simple stone, and beneath the sod there rests no coffin. It stands in mute testimony of the unexpected goodwill of a Northern stranger, and to the hope that, one day, still another generation of Goodsons will finally return to the ground of North Carolina the few moldering remains of Sgt. Matthew Goodson, 52nd North Carolina Infantry, from the "secluded spot" where they now rest in lonely anonymity in or near Gettysburg's Evergreen Cemetery.[87]

Pvt. Samuel Parrish, 28th Virginia Infantry and/or Pvt. Samuel Parish, 57th Virginia Infantry

Who was Private Sam Parrish (or Parish)? Was he from Company E of the 28th Virginia, or was he actually from the 57th Virginia Infantry?

87. Paul Lentz, Concord, North Carolina *Tribune*, May 11, 1986.

The more one researches the strange life and death of Samuel Parrish/ Parish, the more one wonders whether this is one single person, or actually two. A pair of separate and totally unrelated stories recall the wounding and subsequent deaths of the shadowy Privates Parrish/ Parish at the Schwartz Farm.[88]

Jane Boswell Moore had accompanied her mother from Baltimore, both ladies intent on serving as volunteer nurses at the Union Second Corps hospital.[89] Jane meticulously kept a chronicle of the people she encountered while serving at Gettysburg. "Among the many touching incidents, I find in my journal a hurried record of one especially to which I now look back with a feeling of mournful satisfaction. It was that of Samuel Parrish, of the 28th (Rebel) Virginia Regiment."[90]

She first came in contact with Parrish, a young Southerner deeply concerned about his spiritual well-being, following the first week of feverish struggle to get the wounded treated, fed, sheltered, and clothed. Now that the big medical tents were up and regular hospital routines established, the Moores found themselves with an ever-increasing amount of time to attend to the social amenities of life. "We were one afternoon on our way to take a cup of coffee with the Surgeon of the 72d Pennsylvania [A. Stokes Jones], when a citizen came from the Rebel encampment, on a gentle slope of ground directly back of our tent and beyond the hollow, and mentioned the fact that a Rebel boy who was in a dying condition wanted some one to talk with him about Jesus."[91]

Jane Boswell Moore was deeply moved by the heartfelt request, and set out immediately to see to the needs of the wounded Confederate. "In a shelter-tent on some straw, his gray blanket thrown

88. Even researchers disagree as to exactly who Samuel Parrish was. Robert Krick's *Gettysburg Death Roster* does not list him as killed, but does mention a Samuel Parrish of the 57th Virginia Infantry who died as a result of the battle. On the other hand, Kathleen Georg Harrison and John Busey's *Nothing But Glory* show no Samuel Parrish in the 57th Virginia, but instead list a Samuel Parrish in Company E of the 28th Virginia, who enlisted near Richmond in 1862, and was wounded and subsequently killed. To further confuse the issue, the National Archives and Records Administration have no records of any Samuel Parrish for either regiment.
89. Moore, *Women of the War*, p. 554.
90. Moore, "An Incident in Gettysburg," p. 105.
91. *Ibid.*

aside, lay a lad of nineteen, shot through the lungs, and breathing with great difficulty." The local citizen stuck his head into the tent, and

> said he had found some one who would talk with him. "I am very glad," he said, turning to me, "that you have come."
>
> Seating myself on a log in front of his tent, I began by making some inquiries as to his condition and history. He told me that he had been in the army twelve months; that whilst away at Suffolk his mother had died, but he spoke of a sister to whom some one had written. He had never been wounded before, and when I remarked, "This will about end your battle—are you aware of it?" he answered, "Oh, yes, I know that before to-morrow's sun rises I shall be gone, and I should be glad to rest if I were quite sure I would go to heaven."
>
> "And why should you not be sure? . . . the way is very clear—the Saviour makes no hard condition, but as the hymn says, "Tis only look and live." Now tell me what it is that troubles you and let me see if I can do you any good? You do not doubt the Saviour's word, do you?"
>
> "Oh, no, ma'am, but it's temptation. . . . I think, yesterday, I felt as if I was saved and happy, but to-day something says you don't feel just as you ought, and so I am clouded and unhappy."
>
> Fixing my eyes on him earnestly, I said, "Samuel, what is it that saves us—is it our feelings or anything that we have done or can do?"
>
> "Oh, no, but I am tempted to believe I am not so great a sinner and then I don't feel my sins as I ought."
>
> "And probably in your weak, dying state you never will feel them so. None of us realize such things as we should, but it is a blessed thing that the Lord Jesus does not require of us any thing more than to feel our need of Him and be willing and ready to take him as our Saviour. Feelings are little to be depended on. What you want now is simple faith—faith in the power of the Lord Jesus to save you, and faith in His willingness to do so; but let me read to you a little narrative of the death of a soldier whom I knew, and I trust his happy words may be yours."[92]

92. *Ibid.*

Many such evangelistic tracts were freely distributed by the Christian Commission throughout the hospital system, to patients and staff alike. Young men, facing sudden and unexpected death, were often ready to hear and respond to the Gospel message of these pamphlets. Reaching in her pocket, she drew out one of the small brochures that she carried with her for just such situations as this.

> I then read the little soldier's tract, "He is my Christ." At the words "Remorse, grief, and tears will not save you," he said, "Oh, no!" and when I read further, "Will you not have this Christ for your Saviour?" he almost sprang from his humble couch, exclaiming in a deeply fervent tone, and with an emphasis I never shall forget, "I will!," then, adding in broken sentences, "Oh Lord, receive me! Oh, Lord, accept me at once—just right away—let me feel it now! Be with me when trouble is near."
>
> I explained to him more fully the plan of salvation, its wonderful freeness, the helplessness and guilt of the sinner, saying you must just go to Christ because you are weak, and He is strong, you must trust in His righteousness because you are sinful and He is holy. . . . That is all that is needed; now trust your soul with Jesus and feel happy in Him. You know that His word can never be broken; and it says, "Believe on the Lord Jesus, and thou shalt be saved."
>
> "But," he replied, "it troubles me to think I can't pray. I can't even think a sentence, and if I do, it's all wrong."
>
> "Well, you can say, 'Lord, forgive my sins, and save me for Christ's sake,' and if you can't do that, trust your soul on Him. He never cast out any poor soul that came to Him, and He never will. You remember reading, 'He is able and willing to save unto the uttermost all that come unto God by Him.'"
>
> "No, ma'am, I never had any schooling. I worked with my father and brother-in-law harvesting, for we were very poor, and I had a hard time of it; so we calculated that I would get my schooling when I was above size; but then this war broke out, and now that's all done with."
>
> I asked if he remembered that sweetest of hymns, "There is a fountain filled with blood," which seems to express the penitent emotions of the believer in all ages, and his eye brightened as I said, "What a comfort it is to know that this fountain is open for you, and that you can lose all your

guilty stains." He then asked me to draw his socks on his feet, as the fleas troubled him, making me promise to come again that afternoon.[93]

The youthful Maryland nurse then moved on to other Confederate tents, spending time in encouraging the sufferers, and giving them something to eat or drink.

> Later in the afternoon I again saw Samuel, and read to him the tract called "Sick Soldier," and also prayers and verses from the Soldier's Manual of Devotion. His lips moved as I read, and most fervently at the close did his voice join in the words "for Christ's sake." He listened most attentively, not wishing me to begin until he had adjusted every fold of his blanket, "because," he said, "I want to hear it all."
>
> On leaving him, he said, "I shall be gone in the morning."
>
> I hope not, but if so I trust you will be with Jesus. I want you to give yourself to Him, and not think about feelings or anything else that will cause you to doubt.
>
> "I will," he said, and bidding me "good night," covered himself with his blanket, and turned over for that long last sleep, from which, if I see him on waking, it will be on the resurrection morning.[94]

Yet, surprisingly, both Parrish's and Moore's predictions were wrong. "Next day I came again, . . . and I saw a group around Samuel's tent. They told me he was dead, but I saw he was perfectly unconscious and dying, slowly struggling for breath, which he continued to do nearly all day." But as the ruddy shades of evening began to color the skies, the 28th Virginia Infantryman gasped his last shuddering breath and died. Samuel Parrish had gone to see Jesus.[95]

J. Howard Wert tells the story of a vastly different Samuel Parish. Young Howard lived on the family farm, about a mile east of the Schwartz's, with his father Adam and mother Catherine. Catherine,

---

93. *Ibid.*, pp. 105-6.
94. *Ibid.*, p. 106.
95. *Ibid.*

affectionately known among the Second Corps wounded as "Aunt Katy," spent her waking hours during that sultry July attending to the needs of the thousands of wounded scattered in hospital tents around the pasturelands of her neighbor's homestead. Of the many she ministered to in those dark days, "above and beyond all others her love went out to a poor illiterate orphan boy—Sam Parish of Botetourt County, Virginia, one of the thousands who had fallen in Pickett's Charge."[96]

Young Sam immediately took to the warm and motherly "Aunt Katy," and in no time was sharing the hard details of his life. This Sam Parish had been orphaned early in life. "My parents died when I was a baby. I cannot remember either of them." He was shunted off to an uncle who would take him in and raise him; unfortunately, as happened so often, Sam became the whipping boy of his relative's family. "I was beaten, and bruised, and kicked, and cuffed, and starved. Oh! mam, it was a hard, hard life. I often wished I was dead."[97]

His only friend during those years of abuse was his older sister, who had been passed off to yet another relative. "Her life was nearly as hard as mine. Here is her picture." Parish fished something out of his pocket and proudly showed the likeness to "Aunt Katy." It was a "homely, old-fashioned ambrotype of a pleasant-faced buxom girl, which he had carried with him through campaigns and battles; and which, with pleading he had saved when the rags of gray were shorn from his body to prepare him for the hospital cot."[98]

For the Sam Parish of Botetourt County, Virginia, the war proved to be a welcome escape from the unrelenting brutality of his home life. At first, it was uncertain whether the fifteen-year-old could manage to wrangle his way into the army. "I was so glad when they agreed to take me," he once told his devoted nurse. "My uncle was very angry, but an officer threatened to arrest him for opposing the Southern cause that needed soldiers and that made him slink away." The rigors and privations of military life agreed remarkably well with the underprivileged teen. "In the army I had enough to eat most of the time and was treated like a man. I always tried to do my duty, but now this ends it all."[99]

---

96. Wert, "Twas Fifty Years Ago," *Harrisburg Telegraph*, July 5, 1913, no. 12, p. 10.
97. *Ibid.*
98. *Ibid.*
99. *Ibid.*

His one great regret in facing death was leaving behind his sister. "I only wish I could see my sister again. She'll be very lonely. I didn't see her very often; she lived in another county but she'll be lonier [*sic*] than ever when I never come back."[100]

Mrs. Wert carefully tended to the needs of the dying Virginian youth, much as she did for Col. John Bowie Magruder as he lay dying. (Colonel Magruder would have been Parish's commanding officer if Parish were indeed a member of the 57th Virginia Infantry).

J. Howard thought young Parish to be "an absolute heathen in a Christian land." Any attention to his spiritual needs would certainly not go amiss, because it was clear that the gaunt teenager from far-off Virginia would never see his twentieth birthday. When asked about his religious life, young Parish was painfully candid. "No, mam, I never prayer [*sic*]. I never knew there was anyone to pray to. No, I never went to school. I cannot read or write. I never went to Sunday School or church."[101]

A devout Methodist who "never lost an opportunity to say a word about the life boynd [*sic*] this transient scene," Aunt Katy asked the young man if she could pray for him. "Yes, mam, pray for me and I thank you. . . . I know that I need it. I don't know nothing about God or the place I am going to. I hope he won't be very hard with me for I was never taught anything." Slipping to her knees there in the close confines of the hospital tent, "Aunt Katy" earnestly prayed for the dying man who "was never taught anything."[102]

When she finished, she rose to her feet, and, just before leaving to attend to other patients, she paused to teach young Parish the words of the Lord's Prayer. She would slowly say a phrase, and then the Virginian would haltingly repeat after her:

> Our Father, which art in Heaven . . .
> Hallowed be thy Name . . .
> Thy kingdom come . . .
> Thy will be done on Earth . . .
> As it is in Heaven . . .
> Give us this day our daily bread . . .
> And forgive us our trespasses . . .
> As we forgive those who trespass against us . . .

---

100. *Ibid.*
101. *Ibid.*
102. *Ibid.*

And lead us not into temptation . . .
But deliver us from evil . . .
For thine is the Kingdom . . .
And the Power . . .
And the Glory . . .
For ever and ever . . .
Amen.[103]

By the time she finished, every man in the tent had joined in, some feebly mouthing the words, others mumbling or gasping out the text, each one pouring out this heartfelt prayer to God.

Young Parish did inevitably succumb to the effects of his wound, and was laid out in the gruesome daily collection of dead bodies awaiting burial. J. Howard Wert happened on the interment that day, and vividly recalled the details fifty years later. There was Private Parish in the midst of a ghastly phalanx of wasted corpses, an orphan now in death as well as in life. What immediately caught young Wert's attention was that "there was a smile of content, almost of gladness on his pain-drawn and wasted features. I saw his body wrapped in a blanket and placed with twenty others in one of the trenches that dotted the fields of the Schwartz farm, and, as men in blue hurriedly filled in the ground, mine were the only tears that fell for the orphan waif."[104]

One Parrish or two? Postmortem records of the illusive Virginian(s) Samuel Par(r)ish are equally as scarce as solid data from his life (or lives).

Dr. J. W. C. O'Neal's disinterment journal lists a "Samuel Parrish, 57th Virginia" as buried in Yard D at the Schwartz Farm, in the first row of the cornfield cemetery. His remains, however, were never positively identified, and the moldering fragments of bone and tissue once known as Samuel Parrish were shipped off to Richmond in one of the thirteen boxes from the Second Corps graveyards at the Schwartz Farm, each marked with a large "S."[105]

---

103. *Ibid.*
104. *Ibid.*
105. Detailed roster of known Confederate dead, compiled by Kathleen Georg Harrison from the handbook and burial lists of Dr. John W. C. O'Neal, J. G. Frey, the Weaver family and others, Gettysburg National Battlefield Park.

No burial records have ever been discovered for a Samuel Parrish of Company E, 28th Virginia Infantry. Perhaps some forgotten notation will turn up one day that will finally set the record straight concerning two young Virginians, joined forever at the hip in death by their name.

Third Lt. Edward B. Harvey, 18th Virginia

Any relationship maintained between husbands and wives, lovers and sweethearts, fathers and children during the Civil War years, apart from sporadic furloughs or absences without official leave, was subject to the capricious whims of the army mail system. The on again-off again diary of Third Lt. Edward B. Harvey, Company H, 18th Virginia Infantry, coupled with his wife Betty's letters and diary, bears grim witness to the heartbreaking nature of wartime correspondence.

Edward and Betty lived a quiet antebellum existence in Evergreen, Virginia. He had enlisted in the 18th Virginia in Appomattox County, Virginia, March 8, 1862, still early enough in the struggle that the war was something of a romantic adventure not to be missed. The thirty-four year old laborer promptly began a steady climb up the promotional ladder—in three short weeks he had worked his way up to third lieutenant of Company H, the "Appomattox Grays."

Throughout the marches and campaigns, letters laboriously made their way back and forth between Edward and Betty, often crisscrossing in the ponderous military mails. Both jotted down the dates of their correspondence in their own private diaries. Edward noted only four letters written to his wife during the ten months from September of 1862 until the Battle of Gettysburg. Betty, on the other hand, showered her spouse with nineteen letters from March to August of 1863. While Edward was enduring the difficult march to Gettysburg, Betty faithfully posted a letter to him on June 28 "by Lt. [T.] Gilliam."

The Confederate advance of July 3 wreaked havoc on the command structure of the "Appomattox Greys." Capt. William T. Johnson was shot in the left groin and captured. First Lt. James G. Harvey was killed outright, as were Third Sgt. Hugh B. Swan and Fifth Sgt. James M. Hamlet. Thigh wounds were especially rampant in this regiment—First Sgt. William R. Elam, Second Sgt. George M. Pollard and Third Lt. Edward Harvey were all shot in the right thigh and left incapacitated on the field, only to be captured later.

Lieutenant Harvey almost certainly ended up at the camps of the Union Second Corps Hospital, with many of his fellow soldiers from the 18th. Although there is no record of the surgery, it is likely that he lost his right leg on a Second Corps amputation table. While he was recuperating in a Union wall tent, Betty conscientiously mailed off still another communication to Edward, thoughtfully addressing this one to Richmond so that it would be awaiting her lieutenant husband when he returned with the retreating Confederate forces.

The lieutenant's condition was still serious enough that he was transferred to the newly-erected Camp Letterman when the Second Corps Hospital broke camp in early August. It was there that he finally lost his life to a prostration fever and secondary hemorrhage on August 6. He was buried in Section 3, Grave #13 of the Camp Letterman Hospital cemetery.

News that Edward had fallen at Gettysburg, probably received from other wounded and furloughed members of the regiment, must have finally reached Betty in distant Evergreen. She picked up her pen once again to write a letter to her fallen hero. She sent it off "to Gettysburg Pa" on August 26. The notation in her diary opposite that date tells the bitter conclusion of the story: "the last one I ever wrote him and he was dead all the time."[106]

Edward finally did return with his comrades to Virginia—not in victorious marching ranks, but when he was finally disinterred on June 13, 1872. His earthly remains were placed in Box #45 for the long trip home.[107]

Pvt. James M. Burchett, Company K, 8th Virginia

Not every Confederate was a rebel by choice. For some, it was a direct result of intense peer pressure, sometimes excessive and even to the point of life-threatening. Such was the case of Pvt. James M. Burchett of Company K, 8th Virginia Infantry, and fifty-nine of his friends. "A nephew of President [Andrew] Johnson, named Burchett, was also a Union man among rebels; with a number of others, they were attempting to come into our lines when captured."[108]

Burchett proved to be a fiery proponent of the Union, a sentiment that understandably went over very poorly with most members of his

106. Harrison and Busey, *Nothing But Glory*, p. 284; typed transcript of the fragmentary diaries of Edward B. and Betty A. Harvey, courtesy of the Appomattox Court House National History Park.
107. Harrison and Busey, *Nothing But Glory*, p. 284.
108. Holstein, *Three Years in Field Hospitals*, p. 45.

regiment. Nevertheless, his nationalistic zeal attracted others of like bent in the 8th Virginia. Staunch secessionist officers decided to make a bloody and decisive example of these traitors to the South. "The rebels told them they would be put in the front ranks, and when they came to Gettysburg, carrying out their threat, they were made breastworks of."[109]

In the swirling maelstrom at the height of the Pickett-Pettigrew-Trimble Charge, Private Burchett and his friends attempted to get over the wall and into the safety of the Union lines. It proved to be a difficult day to attempt desertion. "None of the sixty escaped unhurt."[110]

Private Burchett went down with a serious wound to the lower third of his left leg, but only after having his shoulder dislocated in the close-in fighting around the wall. "Burchett lost a leg, and one arm permanently disabled."[111]

Even at the Second Corps Hospital, the rabble-rousing Burchett incited the other Confederates. "He was a free-spoken Union man among them, and seemed to be no favorite with the rebs on that account."[112]

Despite his pro-Northern sentiment, he still felt strongly the responsibilities to his family living in the South. In a move that no doubt put his life in jeopardy, "he remained a prisoner, hoping in the exchange to be sent to Richmond, that he might save some property belonging to his father, who had lost everything in Kentucky."[113]

On November 17, 1863, Pvt. James M. Burchett did indeed succeed in getting exchanged from West's Buildings Hospital, a transit hospital in Baltimore for the processing of wounded Confederates. There is little doubt that he immediately headed for Richmond, to attend to the needs of his family.[114]

Nephew of Jefferson Davis

Battlefield wounds were no respecter of age, rank, or prestige—both young and old, generals and privates, the well-known and the obscure fell in the fight and ended up at Second Corps Hospital. "We

---

109. *Ibid.*
110. *Ibid.*
111. *Ibid.*; Harrison and Busey, *Nothing But Glory*, p. 270.
112. Holstein, *Three Years in Field Hospitals*, p. 45.
113. *Ibid.*
114. Harrison and Busey, *Nothing But Glory*, p. 270.

had a nephew of Jefferson Davis in our camp," remembered Clarissa Fellows Jones, thirty-one-year-old Philadelphia schoolteacher turned volunteer nurse. "Poor fellow, he suffered terribly. A special chair was rigged up for him because his back was injured; but he begged so hard to be taken out of it that the doctors finally consented. But no matter in what position he was placed, he was not satisfied."[115]

He proved to be a difficult patient throughout his entire tenure at the Second Corps Hospital.

> When the orders came to take the men who were not dying to Camp Letterman, the Union men had considerable trouble lifting him into the wagon, he suffered so intensely.
>
> Finally, one gruff soldier said, "That's what you get for fighting against us,"
>
> But the poor fellow answered in a kindly tone of voice "I fought against you only once, and I'll never fight again. And remember, my dear man, the Lord says that you must forgive, if they fight seventy times seven."[116]

There is no indication of whether the harried teamster truly felt any real forgiveness or not. As for the Philadelphia nurse, "that was the last I ever saw or heard of him."[117]

The Nameless Confederate Wounded

Many Southern wounded lived and died at the Union Second Corps Hospital without leaving behind a record of their identity. In the race to save lives and minister to as many as possible, names were of only secondary importance to the lives in need of rescuing. The stories of these men, even anonymously, reveal much of the life and death of unique individuals following the battle of Gettysburg.

"Day before yesterday it rained very hard," jotted Jane Boswell Moore in her pocket notebook, undoubtedly describing the torrential downpour that flooded Rock Creek on July 6; "I took a bottle of brandy

115. Jones, "Nursed the Confederates at Gettysburg," p. 4.
116. *Ibid.*
117. *Ibid.*

and tin cup and went down the hill-side, where the wounded Rebels lay exposed to the storm, giving to each a small quantity of brandy and water. They were thinly clad and excessively cold, but they knew that many of our own men were suffering as much, and were very thankful."

"I went up to one, whose face was partially covered with a blanket, I thought to protect him from the rain; 'Friend, won't you have a little of this to keep you from feeling the cold?' He made no reply, and I repeated the question, but drawing the cover away saw that life had fled." Nurse Moore carefully replaced the blanket covering, and moved on to the next wounded man.[118]

"In one of our rambles over the field we found a soldier who, although not apparently a severe sufferer, was anxious to rehearse his ills," recalled John Y. Foster in 1864. "The surgeon of our party, after some cursory examination of his wounds, remarked, 'You must have that limb examined, my good fellow; I will send for you to-morrow and have you brought up.'"[119]

Foster, a member of a volunteer delegation sent out from the Ascension Church in Philadelphia, had come to the battlefield to render aid with "garments, delicacies and medicines" produced by the generous members of the congregation, along with "a large money collection." Foster and his associates were assigned the portion of the hospital grounds reserved for the care of the Confederate wounded.[120]

"A look of unutterable longing came into the soldier's face. He knew the thought of the surgeon's mind; that examination meant amputation, and he exclaimed, half-savagely, but with a childish entreaty mellowing the defiance of his voice, 'I can't lose that leg—I can't, I can't!'"

"'But why?' we said."

"He paused a moment, and a startled look passed over his face, as if in a flash he had thought of his dear ones at home and their dependence on him, and his possible inability to care for them in the

118. Moore, "An Incident in Gettysburg," p. 109. This account is consistent with the record of events immediately after the flooding, since the Confederates were not yet under cover at the Schwartz barn, but rather "down the hill-side" along Rock Creek.

119. Foster, "Four Days at Gettysburg," p. 383.

120. *Ibid.*, p. 381.

future. Then he answered haltingly, 'Because, because, Sir, I have use for it.'"[121]

The overwhelming glut of patients needing amputations meant that some would, of necessity, have to wait days before having their wounds attended. This was especially true since the Union wounded were treated first. Such was the case with one casualty of the Picket-Pettigrew-Trimble charge of July 3.

"One evening we found a fair-faced young Virginian lying apart from the main hospital, who had received a ball through the knee. He was suffering terribly, and an examination of the wound showed that amputation ought not to be a moment delayed."[122]

John Foster and his companions immediately secured a stretcher. "He was carried to a tent and laid upon a table, the surgeons preparing meanwhile for the operation. Further examination, however, induced the belief that he was too greatly enfeebled to undergo the operation at that time, and it was accordingly determined to postpone it until tomorrow."[123]

Foster attempted to make the wounded Rebel as comfortable as possible for the night on the hard surface of the operating table. "Placing a rude pillow under his head, and folding a blanket over his person, the poor fellow was left on the table to gather strength in repose, none of us doubting that he would rally and finally be restored."[124]

As it turned out, the decision to delay the surgery had been a fateful one. "The next morning, expecting confidently to find him better and stronger, we called again at the tent, passed in, and lifted the bloodstained blanket—he was dead."[125]

---

121. *Ibid.*, p. 383. Foster does not tell whether this soldier's leg was indeed amputated the next day or whether he survived the experience. All of Foster's experiences took place between July 10 and July 14.

122. *Ibid.*, p. 386.

123. *Ibid.*

124. *Ibid.*

125. *Ibid.*

Frequently, there simply were no surgical techniques known to contemporary medical science that could fix some of the battlefield injuries. In the Confederate ward, John Foster and the Philadelphian delegation were brought up short by that horrible reality.

"In a little tent, as we pursued our investigations, we found a dead soldier, lying on his face, his hands clenched, his eyes set, the earth all about him clotted with blood. Immediately in the centre of his back, just below the shoulders, was a ghastly wound made by a shell which had carried away a solid mass of flesh, and left exposed the vital parts."[126]

Skin grafts and tissue transplants were still unknown techniques; there was no adequate treatment possible, so someone had improvised. "A rebel surgeon had attempted to dress the hurt by spreading over it a great batch of sticking plaster, but this had loosened, leaving the sore more ragged than before; the blood had poured out afresh; the agony had become too great to bear, and, with none to help, the poor sufferer had died by inches."[127]

The intensity of his death pains, laying alone and afraid in the torpid heat of that shelter tent, is almost impossible to imagine. "In his agony he had clutched and loosened the earth as far as he could reach; and there, with his face fallen into the pit his own hands had made, he lay on the field where he had hoped, perhaps, to win distinction, and whence, it may be, he had expected to send news of victory." As he died by slow degrees, in incomprehensible agony, he had literally begun to dig his own grave.[128]

Jane Boswell Moore had received a box of printed material and other goods from the Baltimore Christian Commission in late July, and from it she endeavored "to supply every man in our hospital with a little book, which the rebels said are now very scarce in the south. One, a fine intelligent fellow, asked me to take a piece of ticking, and make a little bag like a haversack, in which he could carry *his* home. This man has been a member of the Methodist church for ten years, and greatly enjoyed the hymns in the soldier's hymn-book."[129]

126. *Ibid.*
127. *Ibid.*
128. *Ibid.*
129. Jane Boswell Moore, "Letter from Gettysburg," *Lutheran Observer*, August 21, 1863.

By the end of July, the unbridled outpouring of relief aid to the shattered patients at Gettysburg had peaked and begun to wane. Luxury supplies, and even staples, were harder to obtain, even with the untiring efforts of the Sanitary Commission, Christian Commission, Adams Express Company, and a host of other volunteer relief agencies. "Oranges have been very scarce," wrote Miss Moore to her benefactors back in Baltimore on July 26. "Yesterday we gave one to a poor rebel, who had been craving one all day. He afterwards showed it to a friend, saying that he would not take a dollar for it."[130]

A close encounter with death and dying made the convalescent wounded far more introspective about their eternal destiny, and sometimes led them to reevaluate questionable lifestyles and habits. Rev. J. B. Poerner, representing the Christian Commission, took every opportunity to hand out tracts and Bibles throughout the Confederate section of the hospital. "While unpacking and distributing the Testaments, a soldier of the 14th Virginia Regiment came to me and said, 'Chaplain, will you accept this book? (reaching out in his hand a pack of well worn cards) and give me a Testament for it?'"

"'Certainly,' I answered. 'I am thankful for it and will take it to Baltimore and show it to the Committee of the U. S. C. C., as proof of your firm resolution to serve henceforth the Lord.'"[131]

For every card-sharp, for every foul mouth, womanizer, or heavy drinker in the Confederate ranks, there were also deeply devout men who regularly read their Bibles, and lived a life of quiet devotion. As John Y. Foster from Philadelphia discovered, "there were many among them who seemed to be hearty, genuine Christians. Frequently they would be found at prayer or humming hymns in a subdued way."[132]

In the most ghastly surroundings imaginable, one young Confederate, even though dangerously wounded himself, was able to minister to every single person within earshot. "One brawny fellow,

130. *Ibid.*

131. Rev. J. B. Poerner, "A Good Exchange," in *The United States Christian Commission. Second Report of the Committee of Maryland, September 1863*, p. 109.

132. Foster, "Four Days at Gettysburg," p. 385.

who occupied a place on the floor of the barn already mentioned, sang for hours together, apparently wholly unconscious of what was passing right under his eyes, his strong clear voice of praise piercing like a bugle-note, even the tumult of the shrieking sufferers who were piled like so many bullocks all around him."[133]

As life ebbed and slowly faded for dying Southerners, as surgeons shook their heads in exhaustion and frustration, as nurses futilely tried to speak at least a word to every man, the hymns of far-off churches and homey parlors brought unspeakable comfort and encouragement, like a breath of fresh air, in the midst of death and disaster.

Surrounded by historic events and the massive movement of men and materiel, the exchange of small kindnesses often prove to be the most memorable things of all. One volunteer nurse from Philadelphia remembered the impact that new underwear, an old pipe, and a worn dollar bill had on one young Confederate.

> One day, falling in with a sprightly, pleasant fellow—a mere boy in years, but intelligent beyond the average, who had sustained an injury compelling quiet, but not in any sense dangerous—he entreated me to find him some clean under-clothing, saying he was sure his hurts would mend much more rapidly if he could be provided with such a change. His request was at once complied with; and a happier, more delighted being I never saw. Indeed, one found it almost impossible to comprehend how so small a thing should occasion such exuberant rejoicing as this poor child exhibited over the acquisition of a simple pair of drawers and a shirt.
>
> "Isn't this grand!" he exclaimed, again and again, as he smoothed the sleeve of his shirt; "it makes a fellow feel like a king." Then, as the sense of possession grew upon him, he insisted upon giving some tangible form to his gratitude. "I have an old pipe," he said; "it is all I have; it has gone with me all through the campaign; won't you take it and keep it in proof that I am grateful for your kindness?"

133. *Ibid.*

I made light, of course, of my services, told him I had done nothing at all; that I didn't want to rob him of a comforter; but he insisted, absolutely entreated indeed, that I should accept his offering.

There was no getting away from importunity like this. I had in my pocket a meerschaum that had seen long service, and was about as worthless as the soldier's; so finally I consented to an exchange, which occasioned the young fellow renewed satisfaction, since now, as he said, he "would have something to remember me by." His pipe I have still; mine he put in his shoe on the spot, that being the safest place, he said, to carry it; and to-day, for all I know, at some rebel camp-fire or lonely picket-station he may be using it, seeing perhaps in its puffs of smoke pictures of that sultry day at Gettysburg.[134]

But the delights of this day were still not over for the Confederate—another member of John Foster's group stopped to chat with the freshly-attired patient.

Upon parting with the light-hearted boy, who came from Columbia County, Georgia, one of the party, ascertaining that he was penniless, gave him a "greenback," the bare appearance of which, without regard to its value, seemed to excite the liveliest emotions. Turning the bill over again and again, and examining it closely in all its parts, he exclaimed, "Isn't it nice, though? And this is the money you have in these parts?" Then, with another look, "We never see any thing as handsome as that down our way. Our money is dirty and ragged, and sometimes the more you have of it the worse you are off."[135]

I have said that the rebel wounded displayed the warmest appreciation of the efforts in their behalf. In most cases it was a pleasure to contribute to their comfort. One day, in

134. *Ibid.*

135. *Ibid.* "Greenbacks" had just been issued by the Federal government as a measure to help finance the war effort.

walking over the field, we heard a weak, pitiful voice calling us to stop; we turned aside, and in a little hollow discovered an old man, with long white hair, lying upon his back with a sharp, splintered rail for his pillow.

"I have waited *so* long," he said, with an emphasis on the "so," as we bent over him, "for some one to come to my help; but all have seemed too busy to listen." Then, half-apologetically, he added, "It isn't much I want; only that you will get something soft to put under my head: this rail is *so* hard it has almost worn off my poor scalp."

Of course so little a service was most cheerfully performed. One of us, after a diligent search, obtained a quantity of old rags, and these were fashioned into a sort of pillow, and lifting his head, thrust the support beneath.

"Oh, that is paradise!" he said, and folding his hands and closing his eyes he was in a minute in a profound and peaceful slumber.[136]

Mary Fisher Cadwell, her son, and the two ladies accompanying the wagonload of spirituous relief supplies and "necessaries of all kinds" from York, Pennsylvania, found plenty to do among the wounded Confederates at the Second Corps Hospital.

One morning, soon after I began my work, one of the Southern boys came and begged me to go to a comrade of his, who had been shot in the head. The lower part of his face was entirely gone. He could not speak, was suffering intense agony, but no one could understand what he wanted.

I gave him a pencil and card. He wrote, "I am dying for a drink!" It was impossible for him to swallow anything with his mutilated face, but a lady provided a cup with a tube and gave him some lemonade, which afforded him relief. Nothing could be done to alleviate his suffering. His wound could be dressed only by repeating cloths wet with cold water. The raw flesh was alive with vermin. His companion, who attended him with the utmost devotion, told me he was a "good fellow." They always called him the "praying boy."

136. *Ibid.*, p. 384.

> He showed me the little Bible which contained his mother's name and a prayer for her darling's safety. He wanted us to write and tell her where and how he had died. After giving him all the time I could spare I left, promising to go and see him the next day. When I went back the next morning his place was vacant. His mother's prayers were answered. He was safe at home in the house with many mansions which God had prepared for his children.[137]

Patients suffering from the excruciating agony of tetanus also craved the ability to take a long draft of something cool. With the slow-flying bullets picking up debris in their flight, and with amputees and men with open wounds laid out on the bare ground of farmyards and in fields generously fertilized by manure, it is amazing that there were not far more cases than those recorded.

Jane Boswell Moore and her mother, who had cared for Second Lt. John R. Presgraves of the 8th Virginia Infantry, ministered to another Confederate with lockjaw.

> A North Carolinian, whose leg had been amputated, and who was now suffering with lock-jaw, was very anxious for a drink, and also to be turned over. We tried in vain to get a bottle or glass to his mouth; his teeth were set and his agony fearful, but he continued feebly to articulate, "Oh, do get the doctor to come here a minute, and I will do anything for you."
>
> The nurse said the man could not be moved, but would probably die before morning.[138] I have witnessed much suffering, but thought then that I had never seen anything so truly heart-rending. That piteous agonized face, shall I ever forget?—His breast heaving convulsively with the death struggle.[139]

The nurses needed to move on to other patients; was there someone who could stay with the North Carolinian? "He spoke of a

137. Fisher, "A Week on Gettysburg Field."

138. Probably Clarissa Fellows Jones, who was assigned to nurse the Confederates.

139. Moore, "An Incident at Gettysburg," p. 106.

chaplain who had been there and was gone; so I went for one of the Christian Commission, who remained with him."

The duties of the day kept the mother-daughter team from returning to the bedside of the man with locked jaws. "Next day I came again, but the poor North Carolinian was dead." Nameless, he was laid out for burial in the expanding cemeteries surrounding the Second Corps Hospital.[140]

> Among the men were all classes, creeds and colors. In one of my errands in a remote part of the field, I was called to see a most distressing case. Long before I reached the designated spot I heard the most agonizing groans and appeals for mercy, a constant repetition of "Oh, God! have mercy upon me; Oh! God have mercy upon my lost soul."
>
> Again was the cry lifted up in pitiful tones! "Oh, God, save me from my sins!" I found on reaching him one of the hopelessly wounded cases, a poor fellow who had been left to die, being past all aid. I approached him and asked what I could do for him. He turned his eloquent dark eyes, lustrous and beautiful, even in his dying agony, upon me.
>
> I shall never forget the impression he made upon me. A man of powerful physique and remarkable personal beauty, with a rich, dark olive complexion. Every lineament of his face spoke of intellect, pride and great magnetic power. Oh, what anguish was depicted there. He reminded me of some great creature brought to bay, with no way of escape. Such terror! Such fear! The like I never before saw painted on the face of man.
>
> He shook his head and said in reply to my question: "You can do nothing. I must die. I only ask for death. Oh, this dreadful, dreadful suffering! Oh, my soul!! Oh, God, have mercy on my poor soul!"
>
> I inquired about him of a man lying near, who told me he had seven gunshot wounds through his body, that he could not be moved, and nothing could alleviate his pain. Of his former life or history nothing was known. They had fought side by side in several battles. Until then he had seemed to

140. *Ibid.*

bear a charmed life; possessed of incredible strength and bravery, his tall form was ever to be seen in the thickest of the fight. He was always a reserved and moody man, evidently far superior in intellect, education, and position to most of the soldiers, with whom he never fraternized.

As he lay there his eyes riveted to my face, as though he would fain derive some comfort, I tried to soothe him by pointing out to him the way to obtain the mercy he so eagerly craved and repeated to him the old, yet ever new story of Him who suffered greater agony than he endured, even the burden of the guilt of all mankind, and died on the cross that he and all men might live eternally.

He listened with despairing eagerness, then turning away with a groan, replied: "Oh! madam, my Saviour has not yet come. I must die without seeing Him. I am a Jew."

Again, I tried to tell him of the infinite love and compassion, that even at the eleventh hour, he might believe and lay his sins on the "Lamb of God that taketh away the sins of the world." He mournfully shook his head and said: "Oh! I have heard all those sayings before, but my Christ has not come. Oh! God of Abraham, hear me." He begged for death to end his miseries. I left him, to send some opiate which I hoped might reduce him to blessed unconsciousness.

Two days after I was near the same part of the ground and heard his faint voice still uttering the same prayer to the "God of his fathers," but I did not approach him. It was too painful to witness such distress with no power of relief.[141]

---

129. Fisher, "A Week on Gettysburg Field."

Chapter 16

THURSDAY, JULY 2: DUSK—FRIDAY, AUGUST 8

"Kiss me, lady, before I die."

Mary Cadwell Fisher
Volunteer Nurse from York

THE UNION WOUNDED OF THE SECOND CORPS HOSPITAL

Gettysburg, Pennsylvania

By far the largest contingent of wounded at the Second Corps Hospital were from north of the Mason-Dixon Line. While they were collected from the battlefield before their Confederate opponents, and received preferential treatment in terms of surgery, care, and shelter, many were in just as grievous conditions as the Rebel wounded confined in the Schwartz barn. Each Union patient had a different story of tenacious survival or eventual death in the hospital system that extended from the battlefield to the primary aid station, then on through the division hospital and the corps hospital to the final destination of the general hospital.

Pvt. Rowland L. Ormsby, Company G, 64th New York Volunteer Infantry

Hailing from optimistically-named Wellsville, New York, twenty-one-year-old Pvt. Rowland L. Ormsby was in the prime of his life when he charged into the maelstrom of the Wheatfield as part of the July 2 stopgap measure to slow the Confederate breakthrough of Sickles' Third Corps. In the savage swirl of battle, a bullet came in low, and the

New Yorker was carried off the field with a gaping hole blown through his right leg. The slug had shattered the bone in its passage, necessitating amputation at the upper third of the thighbone.[1]

Ormsby was placed in the amputee ward to convalesce, but slowly began to fail in the face of the overwhelming violence done to his body. It was there that Emily Bliss Souder, foregoing her usual summer vacation on the seacoast to nurse mutilated men at Gettysburg, encountered the dying young man. She tenderly nursed him, but on July 17, young Ormsby's life came to an excruciating end. He was interred with other Northerners in the cornfield at the Schwartz Farm.

The next day, Mrs. Souder sat down to complete some correspondence in the cool of the late July evening:

> July 18, 1863.
> Dear__________,
>
> I was truly rejoiced to receive your letter with its enclosure. It is past eleven o'clock at night, and I have just finished a letter to the mother of a young man, of the New York 64th Volunteers, who died yesterday, and from whose head I cut a beautiful lock of black hair, which I enclosed with three oak leaves plucked from a branch which grew directly over his tent. We constantly witness heartbreaking scenes, but the Lord has endued us with strength to bear them.[2]

The letter, wisp of hair, and the cluster of leaves mailed to Ormsby's mother were barely on their way to Wellsville before Ormsby's father arrived at the Second Corps Hospital. The elder Ormsby had been methodically scouring the medical facilities around Gettysburg in search of his wounded son. His painstaking search finally brought him to the Schwartz Farm, and the heartrending news of his son's death just two days previously. In another letter, dashed off to "Friends" during a noontime lull on July 22, the faithful nurse commented on the tragic visit:

---

1. Gregory A. Coco, *Killed In Action: Eyewitness Accounts of the Last Moments of 100 Union Soldiers who Died at Gettysburg* (Gettysburg, Pennsylvania: Thomas Publications, 1992), p. 48.
2. Souder, *Leaves from the Battle-field of Gettysburg*, pp. 30-31.

> I cut a beautiful locket of black hair from the head of a young man belonging to the New York 64th Regiment, Rowland Ormsby, and sent it with an oak leaf that grew directly over his tent. Two days after, the father came, but we did not see him.[3]

Just how long young Ormsby's father stayed in Gettysburg to mourn his lost son and visit his gravesite is unknown. However, when he returned with heavy heart to New York, Ormsby's remains were left behind in the ruined cornfield of Farmer Schwartz. Pvt. Rowland L. Ormsby, Company G, 64th New York Volunteer Infantry, was ultimately moved to the National Cemetery in Gettysburg, where he rests with his fellow New Yorkers, men who had lived together, charged together, and fell together in an obscure wheatfield in Pennsylvania.[4]

Pvt. Alfred G. Gardner, Battery B, 1st Rhode Island Light, Second Corps Artillery Brigade

Infantrymen were not the only ones falling in the vicious Gettysburg fight. Artillerymen were doing their very best to blow each other up with well-placed anti-battery fire, whether sending over explosive rounds, or solid shot designed to dismount the big field pieces. One such charge played havoc on the men of Battery B, 1st Rhode Island Light, of the Second Corps Artillery Brigade, as they were smoothly working through the numbered system of loading their weapon during the enemy bombardment on July 3.

> During the cannonade, one of the guns of Battery B was struck by a rebel shell, which exploded, killing two cannoneers who were in the act of loading. No. 1, William Jones, had stepped to his place in front, between the muzzle of the piece and wheel on the right side, and, having swabbed the gun, stood with sponge staff reversed (which is also the rammer) waiting for the charge to be inserted by No. 2. Alfred G. Gardner, No. 2, had stepped to his place, between the muzzle of the piece and wheel on the left side, and, taking the ammunition from No. 5, was in the act of

3. *Ibid.*, p. 53.
4. Coco, *Killed In Action*, p. 48.

inserting the charge when a shell struck the face of the muzzle, left side of the bore, and exploded.

No. 1 was killed instantly by a fragment of the shell, which cut the top of the left side of his head completely off. He fell with his head toward the enemy, while the sponge staff was thrown two or three yards beyond him.[5]

The effects were just as spectacular for Private Gardner, although the outcome was not as immediate. "Alfred Gardner was struck in the left shoulder, almost tearing his arm off. He lived a few minutes, and died shouting: 'Glory to God! I am happy! Hallelujah!' His sergeant and friend bent over him to receive his dying message; which was, to tell his wife that he died happy, and send her his Bible."[6]

"Old Mr. Gardner," as he was known by his younger messmates, was quite well-known as an intense student of the Bible. Sgt. Albert Straight wrote of him: "He was a pious man, and he and I had been tenting together on this march." Hailing from Middletown, Rhode Island, he had not yet been in the military a full year, having mustered into Federal service on August 12, 1862. His extremely unusual response to being wounded was no doubt a direct response to the overwhelming shock of seeing his arm almost torn off, coupled with his hope of soon experiencing the things which he had just been reading about in his morning devotions.[7]

With the bombardment raining death all around, evacuation by ambulance was utterly impossible, and any medical assistance might as well have been a million miles away. Not that it would have helped—an arm torn off at the shoulder was a virtual death sentence. His body was interred on the grounds of the Michael Fiscel Farm (a neighbor of Jacob Schwartz to the south), just east of the house, about a mile south of his artillery position. When the National Cemetery was established, his remains were gently removed there, and now lie in the Rhode Island section.[8]

In the meantime, the battle roared on. "Sergt. Albert Straight, and the remaining cannoneers, tried to load the piece, but, in placing a charge in the muzzle of the gun, they found it impossible to ram it home. Again and again, with rammer and an axe, they endeavored to drive in the shot, but their efforts were futile, as the depression of the muzzle

5. Rhodes, *The History of Battery B*, pp. 209-10.
6. *Ibid.*
7. *Ibid.*, pp. 209-10.
8. Coco, *Killed in Action*, p. 92.

was too great, and the attempt had to be abandoned. As the piece cooled off, the shot became firmly fixed in the bore of the gun."[9]

A touching memorial still exists to Private Gardner and his friends of the Battery B, 1st Rhode Island Light guncrew. At the State House in Providence, Rhode Island, a twelve pound smoothbore is on display. Called the "Gettysburg Gun," it carries on its scarred carriage and weathered tube the evidence of that hot July afternoon, when a Confederate round hit it dead on at the muzzle. Wedged and fused into the mouth of the field piece is a twelve pound cannon ball, the very last thing that Private Alfred G. Gardner ever handled before receiving his fatal wound.

Pvt. Gustavus Ritter, Company D, 111th New York Volunteer Infantry

There was no hiding from the July 3 artillery fire. Even though the Confederate cannonade was landing considerably further to the rear than the gunners had intended, some stray shots were falling within the battlelines of blue-clad troops. Even those seeking shelter behind barricades or buildings were not safe from the incoming rounds.

When the bombardment unexpectedly began raining down on the Union line, Capt. Benjamin Thompson of the 111th New York Volunteers remembered

> most of our men made straight for a designated line in front of our cannon, where, being over the hill and lower than its crest, they would be much less likely to be injured and would be in line for repelling a charge which we felt would follow the cannonade.
>
> Some, however, were foolish enough to huddle behind a small house near the line. Seeing them, Gen Hays sent me to drive them out. Returning with them we passed in rear of a small stable and here I got my first knock down. A round shot, going through the stable, brought away a board entire, and this, flying through the air, took me fair upon the nose and laid me flat. This excited a hearty laugh notwithstanding our peril.[10]

---

9. Rhodes, *The History of Battery B*, pp. 209-10.
10. Thompson, *Personal Narrative*. This would have been the Bryan house and stable.

Captain Thompson was lucky that it was only his nose that was damaged at the Bryan barn. Pvt. Gustavus Ritter of Company D was not nearly as fortunate. Lt. Samuel B. McIntyre of Company A relates the terrifying ordeal that Private Ritter endured:

> Some three or four men thought there was some safety behind the barn, until a shell ripped through it, tearing off a board and killed some of them, when they speedily returned to the regiment. A man of Co. D, whose name I now forget, had both his legs taken off below the knee. His comrades placed him just at our right, behind this barn, and he remained there until he died, holding up his poor bleeding stumps by his arms under his legs.[11]

Private Ritter's burial site has never been found. Perhaps his comrades in the 111th simply dug his grave near where he lay behind the shot-torn barn, just one of the more than 163 Second Corps burials in the triangle prescribed by the Bryan Farm, the Peter Frey farmstead, and the Hummelbaugh place. The Lyons, New York, native was just thirty-three years old when he bled to death on the battlefield, completely out of reach of medical care due to the severity of the enemy shelling.

Pvt. Luther White, Company K, 20th Massachusetts Volunteer Infantry

Of all the soldiers carried off to the cemeteries of the Second Corps, there is record of only one who ever came back again. "His name was Luther White, Co K, 20th Massachusetts, from Boston; he was wounded by a piece of shell, which tore off part of his ear, and shattering his jaw, laid bare one side of the throat. After the battle, he remained for three days unconscious, then rallied; and again sank away until he died—as it was thought, and carried to the grave."[12]

Anna Holstein remembered the unforgettable graveside ceremony:

---

11. Samuel B. McIntyre, Letter, Bachelder Papers Collection, Gettysburg National Military Park Library; Coco, *Killed In Action*, pp. 90-91.
12. Anna Morris Ellis Holstein, *Three Years in Field Hospitals of the Army of the Potomac* (Philadelphia: J. B. Lippincott & Co., 1867), p. 42.

> I recall a burial where three were at one time taken to the little spot we called a cemetery. One sultry afternoon in July the stretcher-bearers came tramping wearily, bearing three bodies of those who had given their lives for *freedom*; as the last reached the place, the men dropped with a rough, jolting motion the army couch whereon he rested.
>
> The impatient effort to be rid of their burden was probably the means of saving a precious life; for the man—*dead*, as they supposed—raising his head, called in a clear voice: "Boys, what are you doing?"
>
> The response as prompt: "We came to bury you, Whitey."
>
> His calm reply was: "I don't see it, boys; give me a drink of water, and carry me back." Then glancing into the open grave: "I won't be buried by this raw recruit!" The raw recruit was a lieutenant of his own regiment.
>
> Not many stand so near the "dark valley" that they look into their own graves, and *live*. The "boys" did carry him back; and with the greatest care, his life *was* saved.[13]

Dr. Theodore Dimon, General Agent of the State of New York for the Relief of Sick, Wounded, and Discharged Soldiers, encountered the resurrected Private White during his inspection tour of the Second Corps Hospitals. The reanimated Bay Stater was making the most of his recent notoriety, and Dimon was struck by "the humor of a Massachusetts soldier who was shot through the head—the ball making a clean furrow, taking bone and brains."[14]

"He was 'sitting up' under a little dog tent, 'entertaining visitors,' who were informed that he had been given up—as upon all ordinary calculations he ought to have been—and his grave made for him and he about to be placed into it, but he added with a decided expression about his mouth and a comical look in his eye, that 'he could not see it.'"[15]

White continued his slow and painful recovery, and was eventually shipped out of the Second Corps Hospital. The plucky Boston soldier,

12. *Ibid.*, pp. 41-42.
13. Dimon, *Report of the General Agent of the State of New York*, p. 48. Holstein thought it was a shell that injured White, while Dimon said it was a "ball." Perhaps White was struck twice.
14. *Ibid.*

however, managed to keep in touch with his former nurse. "Months afterwards he was sent to 'Chestnut Hill Hospital,' Philadelphia; from there he wrote to me to say that his surgeon thought he would recover."[16]

Color Cpl. Enoch K. Miller, Company F, 108th New York Volunteer Infantry

One of the most difficult things for any military commander, whether captain of a company or major general of an army, was to personally witness how his direct orders played out in the lives of his troops, to see men that he had come to know and admire laying dead on the field, or being carted away in fleets of ambulances. Lt. Col. Francis Edwin Pierce, of the 108th New York, the "Rochester Regiment," wrote to a friend following the battle, describing the emotions that raced through his mind as he watched men whom he had personally commanded being removed from the field following the ill-fated Confederate attack on July 3: "I saw four of my old company in an ambulance, that came to the front [for the] wounded after the firing had ceased. [Enoch] Miller, [Daniel] Schout, [Darwin] Skinner and [John] Swager. I rode alongside and bade them good bye."[17]

Pierce must have been sobered as he looked down into the open rear of that ambulance; blood flowed from open wounds, injuries were hastily bound up in gory bandages, and extremities lay skewed and swollen by the passage of ball or shell fragment. "I remember how they looked and what they said. One of them said 'Good bye, Col., they caught me this time,' another, 'good bye, Col., be back soon,' another 'goodbye; if I don't come back, I know that what few are left can take care of our old flags, be careful and not get hit."[18]

But the color corporal of the 108th was so weak that no flip remarks came readily from his lips. "Poor Enoch Miller could just raise his head and, looking very pale, just whisper 'good bye, Col.,' and then he gurgled something in his throat that I couldn't understand, and I would not pain him to ask him again what he said." And then the ambulance trundled away, and Pierce turned back to his regiment.[19]

---

16. Holstein, *Three Years in Field Hospitals*, p. 42.
17. Lt. Col. Francis E. Pierce, Letter to Edward D. Chapin, July 27, 1863, in Blake McKelvey, ed., "Rochester in the Civil War," Rochester Historical Society, vol. 22 (1944): 171.
18. *Ibid.*
19. *Ibid.*

Over three weeks after the battle, he would look back on that scene and write: "Two of them I did not expect to live an hour, but both I understand are doing well. Such scenes completely unman me. I can stand up and fight, but cannot endure the sight of suffering, particularly of our own men."[20]

Pierce heeded his soldier's parting injunction; he was careful "not to get hit," and retired a career officer in 1880. Three of the four desperately wounded men did survive to fight another day. But Miller was mortally wounded, as he probably suspected when he gasped out his farewells from the back of the ambulance. Although his exact date of death in the Second Corps Hospital is uncertain, he lays today in the New York section of the National Cemetery at Gettysburg.

While every wound on the battlefield of Gettysburg was potentially life-threatening, many men escaped by a hairs-breadth, bearing witness to the closest of close calls. Here are three typical stories of passing brushes with death or grievous wounds during the swirling insanity of battle.

Lt. Isaac Plumb, Company C, 61st New York Volunteer Infantry

Lieutenant Plumb was charging through the swirling smoke and nasty in-fighting of the Wheatfield when the impact of a Confederate slug slammed him to the ground. Convinced that he was mortally wounded, he tightly clamped his hand over the site of his abdominal "wound." Finally, daring a quick look, the New Yorker found no blood oozing between his fingers. The perilous circumstances of the battle prevented a closer examination, so he got up, dusted himself off, and rushed back into the meleé.

Later that evening, when the bullets had finally stopped flying in his general vicinity, Plumb carefully inventoried his person to see if he could determine what had happened. He found that a slug had hit his sword belt plate squarely, but, rather than plowing on into his intestinal tract, had glanced under the plate and ricocheted into his vest pocket. There, a large ring of keys had stopped the chunk of deadly lead; it had mashed itself around the keys and the ring, badly

20. *Ibid.*

damaging some of his keys, but sparing his abdominal cavity a mortal wound. Plumb would live to celebrate the Fourth of July.[21]

Pvt. Tom Gardner, Company H, 14th Connecticut Volunteer Infantry

With the bullets flying thick and fast during the Confederate attack on July 3, the wonder is that anyone escaped the deadly projectiles. Pvt. Tom Gardner had as close a call as anyone could have, and still walk away. In the deadly free-for-all that developed along the Second Corps lines, a Rebel took aim at the Connecticut infantryman's head and squeezed the trigger. The detonation snapped the rifled musket back fractionally, and the enemy slug, rather than blowing a huge hole in Gardener's face, plowed a deep furrow right across the top of his skull.

Gardner would suffer some incredible headaches in the following days, and have a permanent new contour to his skull, but he lived to fight another day.[22]

Pvt. Frederick Frey, Company F, 108th New York Volunteer Infantry

Many soldiers, in the early days of the war, dreamed of glorious wounds, something that would draw admiring and adoring glances from the ladies, and envious looks and scowls from the menfolk. A wound that was a conversation piece; a badge of honor, proving that he had faced the enemy and borne the consequences. A battlefield injury that gave him bragging rights, although not too painful, nor disfiguring, and certainly not fatal.

Real battle had proven to be something else entirely. The reality was that men were disemboweled by flying shrapnel, were decapitated by

---

21. Gregory A. Coco, *On the Bloodstained Field* (Gettysburg, Pennsylvania: Thomas Publications, 1987), p. 45. Sadly, Lieutenant Plumb would not survive another Independence Day. He was seriously wounded on the picket line at Cold Harbor on June 3, 1864. Company C, comprised of students, teachers, and alumni of Madison College (now Colgate), would lose their friend, who passed away on July 4 in a Washington, D.C. hospital. Lt. Charles Fuller, who had lost a leg on a Second Corps operating table at Gettysburg, wrote the eulogy and led the delegation of citizens who welcomed Plumb's remains home to Norwich. [William D. Johnson, letter to Roland R. Maust, December 1, 2000.]
22. *Ibid.*

premature detonations of their own artillery shells, brave men screamed shrilling as they held on to the stump of an arm or leg, whistled wetly as air sucked in and out of chest wounds, or drowned in their own blood.

War could also be cruel and quirky in the wounds it handed out. Such was the case of Fred Frey of the 108th New York Volunteer Infantry. Having the gun shot out of his hand was perfectly fine; it showed that he had been in the heat of the battle, and survived. But the ultimate indignity, a lasting memento of a chance encounter with a passing rebel bullet, he would carry prominently for the rest of his life. Although Private Frey escaped with his life, somewhere in the thick of the battle, he had felt the heat of a passing bullet, and reached up to find that the very end of his nose had been shot clean away.[23]

Col. Edward Ephraim Cross, 5th New Hampshire Volunteer Infantry

Few men came to Gettysburg with such a vast wealth of experience as did Col. Edward Ephraim Cross, whose snappish temperament almost kept Capt. Thomas Livermore from the command of the Second Corps Ambulance Corps at Gettysburg.[24]

Born in Lancaster, New Hampshire, on April 21, 1831, he early developed into an avid reader, taking full advantage of all the educational opportunities of his New England community, attending both public schools and private academies. His tenacity was evident early in life—he steadily worked his way up from apprentice to shop foreman of the *Coos Democrat*, the local newspaper.[25]

Wanderlust seemed to be ingrained into Edward Cross, and his experiences before the Civil War bear record of his quest for adventure and excitement. Quitting the small town newspaper business, Cross spent a summer in Canada with his father, Col. Ephraim Cross,

---

23. *Ibid.*
24. Cross was christened Edward Ephraim Cross, his middle name that of his father, but he frequently used his mother's maiden name Everett as his middle name instead.
25. Background details of Cross' life are from an photostatic copy of Colonel Cross' unidentified obituary, almost certainly from the *Coos Democrat*, the small Lancaster, New Hampshire newspaper covering activities in Coos County in Northern New Hampshire; *The Coos Republican*, July 14, 1863; and Child, *A History of the Fifth New Hampshire*, pp. 218-25, 311-14. Child records Cross' birthdate as April 22 [Child, *A History of the Fifth New Hampshire*, p. 311].

constructing a steamboat on Memphramagog Lake. After assisting several local survey parties, he packed his bags and set out for Ohio.

His experience with the *Coos Democrat* came in handy when Cross reached Cincinnati. At only twenty years of age, he quickly found employment with the Cincinnati *Atlas* and the Cincinnati *Daily Times*, again working his way up from journeyman to local editor, then principal editor, and finally to traveling correspondent. As a free-wheeling journalist, Cross toured Indian Country around the Great Lakes, trapping, buffalo hunting, and fighting the native population when he was not writing. Under the pen name "Richard Everett," his "poems, prose sketches and illustrated articles" provided thrilling reading for the residents of the Queen City and were soon picked up by other newspapers.

After a winter spent in Washington, D.C., where he further expanded his readership by working as a "special" for the *New York Herald* and other papers, Cross was offered the editorship of the *Cincinnati Times*. But the tedium of a big city newspaper office was not for the freewheeling Cross; he declined the offer, bought a small press and printing equipment, and headed west.

Cross and his party of pioneers set off for the distant territories in 1858, bringing along "the first steam engine and printing press ever transported across the Rocky Mountains." Finally settling in frontier Arizona Territory, Cross soon organized the Santa Rita Mining Company, intent on stripping silver from the ore-laden southwestern hills, as well as making a name for himself in the process. On the side, he published the first newspaper in the Territory.

Whatever time was left over from mining and publishing went to fighting Indians. No doubt claiming knowledge of Indians from his newspaper coverage of the Great Lakes tribes, Cross often volunteered his services to government expeditions, or simply organized his own independent companies to pursue the rampaging Apaches. And with his very own newspaper, he unabashedly published stories of his derring-do in the wilds of the Gila and across the Mexican border.

But, beside living a life reminiscent of a "penny-dreadful" plot, Cross proved himself to be a careful student of his surroundings, and an early ethnographer and linguist. In his travels, "extensive notes upon the character of the roving Indian tribes were carefully prepared, and included five vocabularies."[26]

---

26. Child, *A History of the Fifth New Hampshire*, pp. 311-12.

As if all this were not enough excitement for one man, the New Englander also presided on a semi-regular basis in the Lynch Courts. His prickly personality made him the principal in several duels, a local one fought with rifles, and another one south of the border with swords. With typical élan, he survived them both, and lost nothing in the printed retelling. Throughout his years in Arizona, the only thing that lured him back to the placid lifestyle of the east coast was the chance to receive the Masonic Degrees in the old Lodge at Lancaster, New Hampshire.

The coming of the Civil War sent its far-ranging ripples throughout the country, even to the remote Southwest. When Federal troops were pulled from the Territory, the Indians promptly took full advantage of the situation to stage daring raids and armed forays against the white settlers. In the ensuing attacks, tribal raiders swept down on the mine, destroying the mining equipment and slaughtering most of the employees. Cross once again escaped unscathed. After burying any salvageable machinery, he dissolved the mining company, and headed south to serve as *Chef de Battalion* with the militia of Mexico's Liberal party.

But the siren call of impending civil war in America was too strong—the enterprising miner/newspaperman/adventurer soon tendered his resignation, and headed home to New Hampshire. Cross lost no time in making his way to the capitol in Concord. There he personally offered his services to Governor Berry, and was soon commissioned colonel of the 5th New Hampshire Regiment.

Now thirty-one, and a full bird colonel like his father and namesake, Cross was an imposing man with a full tawny beard who sat tall and erect in the saddle, "lithe like an Indian." The colonel was fiercely devoted to his men—he saw to it that they were fed and clothed well, and he taught them to aim carefully when they fired their weapons. He instilled strict military discipline in his regiment, advocating unwavering obedience to orders as the highest virtue, while discounting the idea of ever retreating. Unlike so many other army commanders, his frontier experience had taught him the value of good camp sanitation and policing, and he relentlessly drilled the concept of personal hygiene into his men.[27]

---

27. Cross obituary; Child, *A History of the Fifth New Hampshire*, pp. 311-12; Thomas Livermore, *Days and Events*, p. 256; Charles A. Hale, "With Colonel Cross at the Wheatfield," Brooke Papers, Historical Society of Pennsylvania, Philadelphia, Pennsylvania, reprinted in *Civil War Times Illustrated*, vol. 13, no. 5 (August 1974): 35.

After so many years of rugged independence, Colonel Cross was a man used to getting his own way; as a team player in a military hierarchy, he definitely left much to be desired. He was highly critical by nature, and jumped readily and often to unwarranted conclusions. His blunt outspokenness, especially when discussing politics in general and certain politicians in particular, most probably retarded his climb up the promotional ladder.[28]

But while viewed with varying degrees of respect, anger or loathing by members of his command and various acquaintances, there was never any question of his personal bravery under fire. Shot through the thigh at the Battle of Fair Oaks, he weathered the painful wound, only to be severely wounded again at Antietam. Hardly worthy of mention were a medley of lesser wounds sustained along the way.[29]

One of the notable aspects of the Civil War was the great number of soldiers who experienced strong premonitions of their own impending death. On June 28, as the Army of the Potomac marched north in pursuit of Lee's forces, Cross was riding alongside a newly minted brigade staff aide, nineteen-year-old Second Lt. Charles A. Hale of the 5th New Hampshire. When talk turned to thoughts about the upcoming fight, Cross candidly stated: "It will be my last battle." He then went on to give detailed instructions to Hale concerning the disposition of his possessions after his demise.[30]

A few days later, while in line of battle on July 2, Cross was "walking back and forth in his quick, nervous way, hands clasped behind his back" as he watched Confederate troops smash into Sickles' Third Corps line along the Emmitsburg Road. After years of exposure to the blazing heat of the west, Cross habitually wore a jaunty red handkerchief on his head as a bandanna during muggy summer days. Now Lieutenant Hale was horrified to see his colonel pull instead "from an inside pocket a large, new, black silk handkerchief," asking that Hale help him snug up the knots. When General Winfield Scott Hancock, commander of the Second Corps, rode up and exclaimed: "Colonel Cross, this day will bring you a star," the New Hampshire newspaperman and Western adventurer slowly shook his head. "No, General," he replied gravely, his glossy beard fluttering in the desultory breeze, "this is my last battle."[31]

---

28. Cross obituary; Livermore, *Days and Events*, pp. 756-57.
29. Cross obituary.
30. Hale, "With Colonel Cross at the Wheatfield," p. 32.
31. *Ibid.*, pp.. 34-35.

So firmly was his impending death fixed in his mind that the colonel called over Assistant Surgeon William Child as he passed through the troops just before they charged into battle on July 2. Cross entrusted to Doctor Child's care "a massive gold ring, some valuable papers, a pocketbook, and some other valuables. He said, 'Good-by! It will be an awful day. Take care of yourself, I must go into the fight, and I fear I shall be killed. Good-by!' and away he rushed to lead his command."[32]

All of Cross' premonitions proved to be correct. Ordered into the breach to shore up General Sickles' crumbling line, Cross, serving as brigade commander that day, promptly moved his men up and into the area of the Confederate breakthrough. After getting the troops into position, the colonel passed on foot through a stand of woods to check on the right flank of his brigade. As he walked along, a Southern marksman perched on top of a boulder spied him, took careful aim, and fired.

The bullet stuck Cross directly in the torso, tearing through his abdominal cavity and exiting near the spine. One of Cross' men witnessed the shooting, and within minutes one of the 5th New Hampshire men circled the boulder and shot the Confederate marksman dead.[33]

> Thus wounded he was carried about one mile to a locality directly in the rear of the right wing of the army, near Culp's hill, into the midst of a wheatfield.[34] The crop had just been cut and bound into sheaves. A good number of these were gathered by his attendants and a comfortable bed was formed upon which the noble form of the dying hero and patriot was tenderly laid. The gloom of a deep darkness covered all. Some camp-fires crackled and glimmered, flashed and cast weird shadows around the group of friends and attendants. Now and then a shell went screeching across the sky, bursting with a sudden flash and stunning report.

---

32. Child, *A History of the Fifth New Hampshire*, p. 217.
33. Hale, "With Colonel Cross at the Wheatfield," p. 36; "With Colonel Cross," pp. x, xiii, Brooke Papers, Historical Society of Pennsylvania, Philadelphia.
34. At this stage of the battle, with so much confusion surrounding the Third Corps collapse and massive shifting of the Second Corps units, it is difficult to pinpoint the exact location of this primary station. Since Sergeant Meyers and his squad of pioneers from the 148th Pennsylvania, also a Second Corps unit, visited the site to bury the dead, this must have been a Second Corps station at the extreme right rear of their positions.

Many of his regiment, men who had followed him in a score of battles, were around. His brother, Major [Richard E.] Cross, was bending low by his side; his surgeon, Major J. W. Bucknam, rendered skillful medical aid and friendly comfort. Assistant-Surgeon [William] Child silently watched the colonel whom he so much admired and respected. Standing nearby were the officers and men who had so often followed him into battle. All faces were sad, all hearts were sorrowful. The dying warrior had a kind word for all. To his officers and men, he sent messages of love, of respect, of encouragement.[35] To his brother he gave messages of love to his sisters and brothers, and with tears and sighs urged his brother to care for the mother and to convey to her his tenderest respect and love. Shells were bursting near; spiteful picket firing was in every direction. Life was drawing to an end in that noble form. He constantly murmured, "My brave men."

In pain he lived on another hour and still another, until at 12:30 midnight that brave spirit went out on the great battle-field.[36]

Captain Livermore and his staff were so inundated with wounded awaiting transport to the Second Corps Hospitals that it was impossible to get away until the ambulance chief had everything well under control.

. . . I found myself unable to go to him until midnight, when I rode to the spot where he lay. It was a little dell, possibly one through which a little stream ran, between the Taneytown road and the Baltimore road, and from a quarter to half a mile from my [ambulance] park going toward Gettysburg. Here under the shelter of some boulders lay a

---

35. Capt. Thomas Livermore received one of Cross' missives, but was too busy with the Ambulance Corps to come immediately [see Chapter 4].

36. Child, *A History of the Fifth New Hampshire*, pp. 211-12. While this sounds like a very stoic and noble end to Colonel Cross' life, Drummer John B. Hollowell from Company B, 148th Pennsylvania Volunteers, tells of a more anguished passing of the colonel: "He was taken to the rear, and his sufferings were so great, during the night, that he begged for someone to shoot him so he might be relieved from his great suffering. Before morning death relieved him." [Muffly, *The Story of Our Regiment*, p. 331.]

large number of our wounded and dead who had been brought from the field. They lay upon the ground covered with their blankets, and the living were nearly all silent, having fallen asleep from fatigue. I picked my way among their prostrate forms to the spot where the colonel lay, and inquiring of an officer of my regiment, whom I saw, which was the colonel, he pointed him out to me, indicating that he was dead.

I went to him and turned the blanket back from his face, and saw that it was true that he was dead. The moonlight or starlight enabled me to see his features distinctly. They were placid and exceedingly lifelike, and it was hard to persuade myself that the flush of life had gone from them. His lofty forehead was smooth, his long, silky beard lay upon his breast undisheveled, and he looked more as he would if he slept than seemed possible. I was told that he had called those of his regiment who were about him and told them that he did not regret death, except that he had hoped to see the rebellion suppressed; that he hoped they would be good soldiers and keep up the discipline and good conduct of the regiment. He sent for various members of the regiment, myself included, and also my little boy Charlie, to bid us farewell.[37] . . . I was oppressed with great regret that I had failed to see Colonel Cross before he died, but I took his sending for me as proof that my course had not given such offense to him as to forfeit his friendship.

Sitting beside the colonel listening to what the officer told me about him at midnight, surrounded by many wounded, was a sad experience and one which can never forsake my memory.[38]

In the wee hours of July 3, when everyone attending Cross' body had either wandered away or nodded off, a detail of pioneers under the command of Sgt. T. P. Meyers of the 148th Pennsylvania arrived to bury the dead. Meyers wrote that "some of my men carried out the

---

37. "The boy, Charlie Fullerton, . . . had come to serve my lieutenant and myself at Falmouth, and had remained with us until I left the regiment, chose to go with me to the staff, so that I was provided with a very good servant." [Livermore, *Days and Events*, p. 274.]

38. Livermore, *Days and Events*, pp. 254-55.

dead and laid them in rows, heads all one way, and the one against the other. About the third man carried out was the tyrant commander of our Brigade, Colonel Cross, of the 5th New Hampshire Regiment, killed in the woods near the wheat field. We did not bury him."[39]

Second Lt. Charles A. Hale of the 5th New Hampshire, left behind the lines to guard some captured Confederate skirmishers when the colonel walked off into those fateful woods, never saw his commander again. "Along after two o'clock, word came from the hospital that Colonel Cross had died at midnight and that his body had been carried back towards Baltimore." There Cross' body was embalmed and sent home to Lancaster, New Hampshire, accompanied by staff aide Capt. Welcome A. Crafts, arriving Tuesday evening, July 7. His casket, draped with the U.S. flag, on which rested his cap and sword, lay in state on the wide covered porch at his family's home.[40]

Cross always immensely enjoyed his infrequent visits home to the gently rolling hills of New Hampshire. He frequently expressed the desire that, wherever he died, he might be finally laid to rest in the old familiar cemetery near his home. The flamboyant Col. Edward Ephraim (and/or Everett) Cross was interred by North Star Lodge, No. 8, Ancient, Free and Accepted Masons, of Lancaster, "in the presence of an immense concourse of people, on Thursday [July 9] at 6 P.M.; the national flags dropped at half mast; the band played solemn dirges; the fraternity, in large numbers, assisted in the solemn ceremonies, and amid a throng of friends who had known him from boyhood, the brave soldier, the true friend, the impulsive and honorable man was borne to his final resting place in the valley he loved so well amid all his wanderings, where he now sleeps, unmindful of the din of battle or the shouts over that victory for which he laid down his valient [*sic*] life."[41]

Capt. Ephraim Wood, Company H, 125th New York Volunteer Infantry

An abdominal wound very similar to Colonel Cross' felled the "old man" of Company H, 125th New York, forty-five-year-old Capt.

39. Child, *A History of the Fifth New Hampshire*, p. 211; Muffly, *The Story of Our Regiment*, p. 461. The pioneers were well aware that ranking officers received special treatment, in death as well as in life.
40. Hale, "With Colonel Cross at the Wheatfield," p. 38; Child, *A History of the Fifth New Hampshire*, pp. 212-13.
41. Cross obituary.

Ephraim Wood. The real tragedy of Captain Wood's injury was that the battle of Gettysburg was, for most intents and purposes, almost over.

The Pickett-Pettigrew-Trimble charge of July 3 had crested on the Union lines in front of the 125th New York line of battle, just north of the angle in the low stone wall and just south of the Ziegler Grove. The broken Rebel attack was beginning to ebb back toward the distant Confederate lines, and the less cautious members of the 125th stood up in the spattering gunfire to observe the retreat.

Wood, born May 14, 1818, had always possessed an avid interest in military affairs, having served with the Troy City Artillery company before the war. Now, as the greatest charge of the war roared to a crescendo and then started to subside, the New York captain could not resist the impulse to watch the waning moments of the attack. "Bravely standing behind that historic stone wall was . . . captain . . . [Wood], who scorned the defense of even a low field-marking fence, and with needless boldness faced death," remembered his regimental chaplain almost forty years later. "And death came. A bullet pierced his abdomen."[42]

The wound was not immediately fatal. "Willard D. Green, of H Company, saw him the moment he was struck." His comrades, including Pvt. Charles W. Belknap, gathered him up and transported him over the ridge to the Widow Leister home, now a riddled and shot-torn wreck of what had been, just a few hours earlier, General Meade's army headquarters. Private Belknap solicitously remained with him until he was finally placed in a Second Corps ambulance.[43]

"He was borne from the field to the hospital at Rock Creek, there—the next day—to die," continued Chaplain Ezra D. Simons. "Sergeant Jacob Houch and the writer kneeled at the brave dying man's side, who, after intense suffering, passed away, speaking with last breath the name of his wife." Beyond his soldierly qualities, Simons admired the captain as a man of unwavering integrity. Simon's concluded that "his short career with the regiment, displayed, in all of its phases, from Harper's Ferry to Gettysburg, the qualities of a true man and a brave soldier. He died a true Christian.[44]

---

42. *New York at Gettysburg*, 2:890.
43. *Ibid.* Charles W. Belknap, copy of his unpublished diary in the Camp Letterman Papers, Gettysburg National Military Park Library, Gettysburg National Military Park.
44. *New York at Gettysburg*, 2:890.

Private Belknap, in far more terse language, simply recorded in his diary that Wood died at 6:00 a.m., July 4, at the Third Division, Second Corps Hospital. Curiosity did indeed prove fatal to the "old man" of Company H.[45]

Capt. John C. Hilton, Company, 145th Pennsylvania Volunteer Infantry

Captain Hilton had taken a nasty wound to the leg in the severe fighting on July 3. The thigh had been shattered, and he was racked with pain as he awaited medical treatment. As the Second Corps Hospital hurriedly evacuated their facilities along the Taneytown Road on the afternoon of July 3 in the face of intense Confederate shellfire, Hilton refused to go. Convinced that he was a goner, it seemed just as easy to die in a deafening explosion as to linger painfully for days or even weeks in the hospital.

In the midst of showers of hot shrapnel and mass pandemonium, a familiar specter appeared out of the dust and flying debris—Chaplain J. H. W. Stuckenberg of Hilton's regiment. "The captain [Stuckenberg] was moving among the wounded, giving them nourishment, and writing letters for those in a dying condition, the enemies shells came screeching and crashing through the trees," wrote Captain Hilton over forty years later. "It became necessary to hastily remove back to a safer position. When they came for me I refused to allow them to remove me as I was told I could not live, and by this time I was in excruciating pain."[46]

Stuckenberg picks up the story: "I saw Capt J. C. Hilton near the spot where the hospital was in the morning. He was wounded in [the] thigh, the bone being shattered up to the hip joint, and the surgeons said there was no hope of his recovery. I was informed of these facts and requested to announce them to him. He was lying on the ground, under the shade of a tree, by the side of a brook, attended to by one of his men. My task was a delicate, unpleasant and sad one. When I told him that probably his wound would be fatal, he told me he had feared it, but it seemed he never so fully realized it as then. His eyes filled with

45. Charles W. Belknap, copy of his unpublished diary in the Camp Letterman Papers, Gettysburg National Military Park Library, Gettysburg National Military Park.

46. John C. Hilton, Letter to Mrs. J. H. W. Stuckenberg, June 7, 1906, Stuckenberg Collection, Musselman Library, Gettysburg College.

tears, deep emotions were traced on his youthful countenance, he cast a glance upward and lay silent."[47]

With the prospect of imminent death ahead, Hilton's thoughts turned to concern for his spiritual condition. "'Chaplain, what does it take to constitute a Christian?'" asked the critically wounded soldier. "He was very anxious about his soul. He had been piously trained, had been a good boy, it seemed, but for some years had been rather careless. After conversing awhile on the subject of religion, he spoke about his mother and sisters. Were it not for them death would be easy. He loved them tenderly and wanted to live for their sakes."[48]

"His deep feeling moved me deeply," wrote Stuckenberg, "he was overwhelmed with emotion—he, his servant, and I all of us wept. He said he did not want to be taken to the hospital—he must die anyhow and would as soon die where he was as anywhere else. 'Bury me,' he said, in utter hopelessness of recovery, 'under this tree.'"[49]

Stuckenberg, however, was not content to leave it at that. Hilton continues the story: "For an hour or two I remained alone, when the Capt [Stuckenberg] came back with four stalwart men and pointed me out, and without paying attention to my remonstrations, raised my stretcher on their shoulders, and 'taking step' hurried me to the rear amid the bursting of shells."[50]

Chaplain Stuckenberg himself wrote the postlude to Hilton's battlefield story: "His leg has since been amputated and strong hopes are entertained of his recovery." The leg came off on a Second Corps operating table, right at the hip. The odds were incredibly long that he would ever survive.[51]

Yet, he utterly astonished the entire medical staff by recovering from the traumatic surgery. "Captain J. C. H[ilton], of the 145th Pennsylvania Vols., from Erie . . . was suffering from a thigh amputation, the only one of nineteen similar cases, performed at the same time, that lived."[52]

Hilton not only "lived," but actually counted the loss as a small price to pay for the Union victory at Gettysburg. "A young man from Erie, a Captain in the 145th Regiment P. V., when speaking of the loss of

---

47. Stuckenberg, *I'm Surrounded By Methodists*, pp. 80-81.
48. *Ibid.*, p. 81.
49. *Ibid.*
50. Hilton to Stuckenberg, June 7, 1906.
51. Stuckenberg, *I'm Surrounded By Methodists*, p. 81.
52. Holstein, *Three Years in Field Hospitals*, p. 44.

his leg, remarked with a flashing eye, that he would willingly have lost his arm also, if Lee's army had been utterly routed and destroyed."[53]

When he was moved to Camp Letterman Hospital in early August, he was recovered enough to regain much of his old combative nature. In fact, so incensed was he that a Rebel officer had been placed in the back of his tent that, in a major huff, "he instantly ordered the nurses to carry him, upon his bed, under a tree which stood near—and there he remained nearly all day, until the surgeon in charge settled the difficulty by removing the rebel."[54]

Anyone with that kind of fire was sure to survive, even with one leg entirely gone. Survive he did, even returning to serve again with the 145th as a brevet major with an artificial limb. And he would come back to Gettysburg at least one more time, many years later, as full of vim and vigor and war stories as ever, for the unveiling of the 145th Pennsylvania Regiment monument.

Cpl. William Schultz, Company I, 71st Pennsylvania Volunteer Infantry

While some cheated the odds of mortality, others lingered interminably in an purgatory of anguish before dying, even with "wonder drugs" like morphine. William Schultz, a twenty-one-year-old bachelor, was wounded in both thighs during the vicious fighting on July 2. After being treated at the Second Corps Hospital, he was tenderly transported to Letterman General Hospital, where he gradually began to fail.

"The only [remaining] child of a widowed mother,[55] from Montgomery County, Penna., lay from July until October, calmly bearing untold agony from a wound which he certainly knew must result in death; yet his one anxious thought, constantly expressed, was: 'Mother, do not grieve; it is best, and right; bury me with my comrades on the field.'"[56]

---

53. Souder, *Leaves from the Battle-field of Gettysburg*, p. 51.
54. *Ibid.*
55. "Mrs. Schultz of Norristown, Penna." handwritten notation in margin of Holstein, *Three Years in Field Hospitals*, p. 46, copy in USAMHI.
56. Holstein, *Three Years in Field Hospitals*, pp. 46-47. Actually, William died on September 29, 1863. A statement like "Mother, do not grieve; it is best, and right; bury me with my comrades on the field" sounds strange to our ears. But with death as a constant reality in the era of high infant, childhood, and even adult mortality, there was an almost universal emphasis of dying a "good death," at home and surrounded by mourning family and friends.

"So, at sunrise one bright autumn morning, his soul went up to God." At first temporarily interred at the General Hospital, the remains of Corporal Schultz were finally "laid to rest among the nation's honored dead in Gettysburg Cemetery."[57]

"This bereaved mother, who gave her *all* for her country,—her eldest upon Antietam's hard-fought field, Willie at Gettysburg,—with the thousands of others who have made the same precious offering, are names to be gratefully remembered and cherished while the record of this war endures."[58]

Pvt. Alvin L. Greenlee, Company F, 140th Pennsylvania Volunteer Infantry

Civil War surgeons, like the M.A.S.H. doctors who followed in their footsteps, were convinced that primary surgery was the proper time to correct as much as could possibly be corrected—within the time allotted. Then it was on to another patient.

Secondary surgical procedures were more dicey. Compounded by hospital fevers, hemorrhaging, laudable pus, and the effects of septic shock, going in again was often a risky procedure, and only to be pursued when all else had failed. But sometimes it was the only option to save a life that was rapidly slipping away.

This was the prospect facing Pvt. Alvin L. Greenlee of Company F, 140th Pennsylvania Volunteer Infantry. A bullet had fractured his thigh on July 2, and he immediately began a desperate battle for his life. He was transported to the Second Corps Hospitals; the minié ball must have just grazed the femur, for the broken bones were set, and he began his long and painful convalescence.

Considering the seriousness of his injury, Private Greenlee was moved to Camp Letterman General Hospital, rather than shipped off by rattling railcar to general hospitals further east. His mother, like Mrs. Schultz, had been notified, and she, too, rushed to his side to care for his every need. While in town, she boarded with the James Pierce family, whose home still stands at the corner of Baltimore and Breckenridge Streets. Their daughter, Matilda (but known to all as "Tillie"), wrote of her houseguests.

57. *Ibid.*, p. 47.
58. *Ibid.*

> The friends and relatives who came to minister to the wounded were, on account of the crowded conditions of the hotels, compelled to ask accommodations from private citizens. In this manner quite a number were taken into our home. Most of their time was spent at the hospital, some coming back to us in the evening, and leaving as soon as possible the next morning.
>
> I was frequently invited to accompany these visitors, and in this way often found myself by the bedside of the wounded. One lady who was stopping at our house, I remember in particular; a Mrs. Greenly [*sic*]. Her son lay suffering at the hospital, and in company we frequently visited him.[59]

The suspense of not knowing if a son, or brother, or father would live or die was terribly wearing on visiting family members. The hours from dusk to dawn, when all non-camp personnel were required to leave the hospital grounds, were especially traumatic. It seemed so easy for patients to surrender to death's siren call in the stillness of the night. "I shall never forget the anxious suspense of that mother," wrote Tillie Pierce in later years. "Whilst absent from her loved one, even for a few hours, her spirit knew no rest, and as soon as possible she would hurry back."[60]

Sadly, Private Greenlee's recuperation was not going well at all; in fact, he was steadily deteriorating. "One day, when he was very low, it was concluded that by amputating his limb his life might be spared. After the operation had been performed her son sank rapidly."[61]

August 3 dawned ominously for the Greenlee family. "At last came the words: 'Mother! Dear Mother!—Good bye!—Good!—Mother!'—and all was over. Her darling boy lay before her in the embrace of death; but a mother's tender love had traced a smile upon his countenance. As the life went out from that [w]racked body hope and joy forsook that fond mother's heart."[62]

Now the familiar Gettysburg ritual of securing a casket, arranging transportation for the body, sending off telegrams and letters notifying hometown relatives and distant relations, and repacking bags for the

---

59. Pierce, *At Gettysburg*, p. 110.
60. *Ibid.*
61. *Ibid.*
62. *Ibid.*

difficult trip was begun anew. "Oh! that sad face and bleeding spirit, as she bade us farewell to follow the coffined remains to her far off home."[63]

Brig. Gen. Samuel Koskiusko Zook, First Division, Third Brigade, Second Corps

When a general fell, everyone paid attention. Full bird colonels had clout, but generals were the nearest thing to God in the Army of the Potomac. Even young ones like Samuel Koskiusko Zook.[64]

But long before he was ever a brigadier general, Samuel Kurtz Zook was growing up with a sense of history and destiny all around him. Born on March 27, 1821, in Chester County, Pennsylvania, his folks packed him off at an early age to the home of his maternal grandmother. There he lived and played right in and around General Washington's winter encampment, where he "enjoyed commanding his schoolmates on the fortifications at Valley Forge around his home, even to the point of 'arresting' his sister for failure to obey an order."[65]

Growing up with childhood influences like that, it came as no surprise that he gravitated to the military. He could always be found hanging around the militia units from Chester, Delaware, and Montgomery counties, asking endless questions, and watching the drilling, the pageantry and the parades. His persistence finally paid off—at nineteen, he managed to wrangle an appointment as adjutant of the 100th Pennsylvania.

Young Sam Zook proved himself to be relentlessly driven to succeed. Realizing that he could progress further and faster outside the peace-time army, he temporarily sidelined his interest in the military, and began working for the Washington and New York Telegraph Company in 1846. He was very proficient at the keys, and

---

63. *Ibid.*
64. General biographical data of Samuel Zook is from Ezra Warner, *Generals in Blue: Lives of the Union Commanders.* (Baton Rouge: Louisiana State University Press, 1964; reprint, 1991), pp. 576-77, and Brad Eide and Robert Lawrence, "Samuel Zook," *The Gettysburg Discussion Group Web Site*, February 28, 1999, www.gdg.org/szook.html. Like Col. Edward Cross, Zook was simply not content to leave his middle name alone. Although christened Samuel Kurtz Zook, he later adopted the name of the Polish general Thadeus Koskiusko, emigre hero of the Revolutionary War, as his own.
65. Eide and Lawrence, "Samuel Zook."

also worked as a lineman, stringing telegraph wire between Norristown and Philadelphia. As telegraphy steadily expanded westward, Zook traveled with it.

His ambition eventually helped him climb the corporate ladder, all the way to the superintendent's office. With his rise to the boardroom came a move to New York City, and the chance to once again dabble in martial affairs. He was soon moonlighting with the militia again, this time as lieutenant colonel of the 6th New York Militia, the "Governor's Guard."

His enterprising nature began to assert itself again, and Lieutenant Colonel Zook, telegraphy magnate, having conquered all that was within reach in the communications industry, left the business and turned his attentions elsewhere. By 1855, he was hard at work in a local brokerage firm.

As war fever swept through the North, Lieutenant Colonel Zook abandoned his financial office, and traveled with his regiment to Annapolis, serving there as military governor during the First Bull Run Campaign. Zook immediately started looking to the future; he contacted friends, wrote letters, and campaigned aggressively with every influential person he knew who could help him obtain an independent command.

The three month enlistment period of the 6th New York Militia expired on July 31, 1861, with the war barely begun. So it was back to New York for the forty-year-old Pennsylvanian, this time to recruit a new regiment of his very own. The former business executive knew very well how to excite and inspire men, and Zook was soon on his way back to the front, this time as colonel of a good-looking new regiment, the 57th New York. It was late in the year, and the regiment was sent off to Washington, D.C., to join Brig. Gen. William H. French's brigade of Brig. Gen. Edwin V. Sumner's division in winter quarters.

In the exotically-named Camp California, the colonel's time was spent largely in whipping his raw recruits into some kind of military shape. Zook showed himself to be a firm disciplinarian, blunt even to the point of severity, a man who vehemently hated cowardice, but, under all the military trapping, was a commander with a good heart. Those long hours of his youth, spent in observing drilling bodies of troops, paid off handsomely now, and the 57th, now known variously as the "National Guard Rifles," the "Clinton Rifles," and "Zook's Voltiguers," soon took on a cohesiveness born of many days spent suffering together in the ranks. In his off-hours, Zook turned his attention on his next objective—securing a general's star.

A series of deadly battles soon transformed Zook's flatfooted greenhorns into a crack veteran regiment. The Peninsula Campaign was more grueling than bloody for the New Yorkers, but allowed Zook to shine in a daring reconnaissance behind enemy lines. On June 27, with Lee moving against McClellan at Gaines' Mill, Zook discovered a well-orchestrated deception of massive troop activity by a minimum of actual soldiers, all coordinated by Confederate General Magruder:

"Colonel Zook, who was field officer of the day, came in and reported most of the enemy's force in front had disappeared." Creeping out beyond the skirmish line, he had been able to observe the enemy's subterfuge—legions of slaves were being paraded round and round, "beating drums, and making a great noise; with true military instinct he concluded the enemy in front had gone to join in the attack on Porter and immediately rode in to General Sumner and demanded permission to lead an attack." Sadly, Sumner "was afraid to act on his own responsibility, but sent an aide to General McClellan to report the colonel's conclusion, and that was the last we heard about the matter. Zook was greatly chagrined and amazed at the want of activity on Sumner's part, feeling certain we could have got into Richmond or into the rear of Lee's army."[66]

Despite his initiative and audacity in the face of the enemy, the 57th was forced to fight at Sharpsburg without Colonel Zook. Though only forty-one years old, the Pennsylvanian was afflicted with severe rheumatism, sometimes even having difficulty getting out of his own cot when he awoke in the morning. Absent on medical leave when the battle developed, the colonel of the 57th New York was taking treatments for his condition at the Russian vapor-baths in New York. In order to stay in the field, he took massive doses of colchicine, which compounded his health problems by irritating his intestinal tract.

Regardless of his infirmity, it was Zook who commanded the entire division at the bloodbath of Fredericksburg, losing 527 men assaulting Marye's Heights. Zook himself fell in the ugly attack, and he was excited at the prospect of receiving a general's commission as a result of his leadership. "Now by God!," he expostulated in a letter to a friend; "if I don't get my star, I'm coming home." General Hancock's warm commendation did indeed net him a promotion to brigadier general.[67]

---

66. Favill, *Diary of a Young Officer*, p. 131.
67. S. K. Zook, Letter to E. I. Wade, a friend in New York, December 16, 1862, in Eide and Lawrence, "Samuel Zook."

Zook was deeply moved by the grisly experience of Fredericksburg: "I walked over the field, close under the enemy's picket line, last night about 3 o'clock. The ground was strewn thickly with corpses of the heroes who perished there on Saturday. I never realized before what war was. I never before felt so horribly since I was born. To see men dashed to pieces by shot & torn into shreds by shells during the heat and crash of battle is bad enough, God knows, but to walk alone amongst slaughtered brave in the 'still small hours' of the night would make the bravest man living 'blue.' God grant I may never have to repeat my last night's experience."[68]

With time off for recuperation, he was soon back on the march again, this time to Chancellorsville as a brigade commander. On the road, Generals Hancock and Zook got into a shouting match over some supposed wrong. Hancock was widely known for his unbelievable vulgarity of speech, but, despite his Mennonite heritage, Zook "always gives as good as he gets without fear of consequences," wrote his personal aide-de-camp. The incident "took place between Hancock and Zook while the 140th was on the march to U. S. Ford, destined for Chancellorsville. . . . It was the greatest cursing match I ever listened to," wrote one stupefied bystander from the 140th Pennsylvania. "Zook took advantage of Hancock, by waiting until the latter got out of breath, and then he opened his pipe organ, and the air was very blue."[69]

Although General Zook played only a limited role at Chancellorsville, he was instrumental in moving badly-needed troops up to the battlelines. In the rearguard action following the battle, he gave orders to men of the 140th Pennsylvania to help the 5th Maine Battery escape from Lee's pincers. "We advanced in double line of battle," remembered the regimental historian, ". . . at such a pace that General Zook, who superintended our part of the advance in person, could hardly keep his place ahead of the line."[70]

Following the Union debacle at Chancellorsville, Zook took leave in Washington. When he returned, his brigade was already on the road, moving north toward Pennsylvania. Despite the past string of Northern battlefield failures, Zook was confident that his brigade was primed to trounce the Confederates this time. He wrote his father on

---

68. *Ibid.*
69. Favill, *Diary of a Young Officer*, p. 223; T. Henry, Letter to J. Ray, January 29, 1902, in Eide and Lawrence, "Samuel Zook."
70. Stewart, *History of the One Hundred and Fortieth Pennsylvania*, p. 69.

June 28th: "The men are in good spirits, and will fight splendidly. If Ewell is not reinforced before we reach him, he'll get warmed."[71]

Second Corps Surgeon William Warren Potter encountered his former commander in the 57th New York during the grueling march to Gettysburg. "We halted for a rest between 11 and 12 o'clock, and I sat down upon a hay-cock in a field. Gen'l Zook soon joined me, sitting upon the hay beside me, and we entered into conversation about the importance of the work before us."[72]

As Doctor Potter remembered it, "the general had bought a horse in Maryland that day, for which he paid $250. It was a handsome animal, and he said it was a good purchase if he lived through the impending battle; but if he should be killed not so and, in that event, he desired the horse sold. I inferred that he felt apprehensive for his own welfare, and that he might not survive; so I cheered him with a few encouraging words, reminding him of his previous good fortune in battle, etc."[73]

Sadly, his premonitions were well-founded. On July 2, as the ill-advised position of General Sickles' Third Corps started to crumble and collapse under the intense Confederate attack, Hancock ordered up General Zook's Third Brigade of the First Division, to plug the hole in the Federal line. "At or about 3 o'clock P. M. the fatal bullet went crashing through his body." His aide, Captain Favill, picks up the story: "While trying to keep the lines as efficient as possible, watching the situation in this pandemonium of death, I saw Zook a little towards the left, riding to the rear, supported by [Capt. C. H. H.] Broom and a mounted orderly. I rode up to him instantly, when he looked up with an expression I shall never forget, and said: 'It's all up with me, Favill.'"[74]

Battles don't stop, even for wounded general officers, so

> I told Broom I would turn over the command to [Col. Orlando Harriman] Morris [of the 66th New York] and join him as soon as I could, but Morris was not to be found readily in the great confusion of the battle.[75] [Col. Richard Petit] Roberts of the One Hundred and Fortieth [Pennsylvania] was killed, and the troops by this time were sadly mixed up with other

71. Eide and Lawrence, "Samuel Zook."
72. Potter, *Three Years with the Army of the Potomac*, p. 58.
73. *Ibid.*
74. *Philadelphia Times*, January 6, 1864; Favill, *Diary of a Young Officer*, p. 246.
75. Unknown to Captain Favill, Colonel Morris had also fallen in the vicious fighting.

> commands. I found [Lt. Col. John] Frazer [*sic*], however, the lieutenant-colonel of the One Hundred and Fortieth Pennsylvania, next in rank, and notified him of the death of Zook, and directed him to assume command. He wished me to remain, but I was personal aide-de-camp to Zook, and my duty was to him, and therefore I declined. Just then [Col. John R.] Brooke [commander of the Fourth Brigade] came up and took command of the whole line, and relieved the situation completely.
>
> I rode off the field and overtook the general with Broom, riding very slowly toward the Baltimore pike. The General was in great pain, and Broom told me he was shot through the bowels. I went ahead to find an ambulance, but before I returned they had fallen in with one, and were driven to the field hospital.[76]

The ambulance pulled in to the First Division Hospital, "in an oak opening east of the Taneytown Road, between it and the Baltimore Pike." Located near the Stone Schoolhouse on Schoolhouse Road, the medical facility was already in the process of moving to a safer location further to the rear. As a general officer, Zook warranted immediate examination by Divisional Chief Operator Charles Squire Wood. "Surgeon Wood, one of our best doctors, after examining the wound, told us that it was fatal, and nothing could be done."[77]

The reason for evacuating the hospital quickly became evident to Captains Favill and Broom during the hasty examination. "There being no shelter there, and the enemy's shot frequently reaching the spot, we took the general on a stretcher, and carried him to a small house some distance in the rear on the Baltimore road, close to a bridge crossing a small creek."[78]

The battle had been raging for two days now, and, general or no general, all the houses in the vicinity were crowded with wounded and suffering humanity. "The house was already filled with men severely wounded, and the sight was most distressing; the howls of pain from

---

76. Favill, *Diary of a Young Officer*, pp. 246-47.

77. Potter, *Three Years with the Army of the Potomac*, p. 58; Favill, *Diary of a Young Officer*, p. 247.

78. Favill, *Diary of a Young Officer*, p. 247. From Favill's description, this was probably the Hoke Toll House, a small stone building which served as a toll booth for the Baltimore Pike. It stood on the north side of the pike, just after it crossed the Rock Creek bridge.

the men in the hall and front room were so dreadful that we moved the general back into a small room cut off from the others, and here we spent the night, doing what we could to make our dear commander comfortable."[79]

Dr. William Warren Potter, First Division surgeon-in-chief, learned of the wounding of General Zook sometime later in the day, as he was engaged in caring for the First Division wounded. "While busily engaged in their care, I received word that Gen'l Zook had been grievously wounded, and was being moved to a farm house on the Baltimore Pike. I immediately repaired to the place and discovered at once that he was fatally shot, a shell having torn open his left shoulder and chest, exposing the heartbeat to observation. I remained with the general until about 11 o'clock p.m., and left word with Lieut. Favill, of Zook's staff, that I would come again in the morning should he survive the night, which now looked very improbable."[80]

It would prove to be a difficult night to get any sleep, despite the grinding exhaustion following a day of strenuous battle. "I went out several times during the night," recalled the aide-de-camp, "and looked at the ghastly scenes on the floors of the hall and parlor. As many men as could lay side by side completely covered the floors, which were streaming with blood, and the poor fellows seemed to give way completely in their misfortunes. Over twenty of them died and were carried into the yard during the night. Zook was calm, serene, and dignified, speaking occasionally, but never of himself, and apparently suffering but little pain."[81]

But even the longest nights eventually come to an end, and the sun reluctantly rose above the scarred horizon to witness another day of ghastly bloodshed.

> At daylight we concluded to move still further to the rear, as the cannon balls sometimes reached even this dreadful spot, so we took up the stretcher, and moved down the road amidst a motley crowd of ambulances, ammunition trains,

---

79. *Ibid.*

80. Potter, *Three Years with the Army of the Potomac*, pp. 59-60. Both Favill and Broom clearly discuss the general's wound as being shot through the bowels. To his credit, however, the doctor penned his reminiscence some twenty-five years after the battle. After all that time, it is not surprising that Potter may have been a bit sketchy on his remembrance of one particular case, even that of a former commanding officer.

81. Favill, *Diary of a Young Officer*, p. 247.

> and disorganized men, making it very difficult to get along; about a mile down the road we turned to the right, and took possession of a comfortable house; it was occupied by several women, who were scared out of their wits, and glad to have us in the house.
>
> We placed the general on the stretcher in the front room on the left of entering, and had the women make some chicken soup or broth. I asked the general if he would like to see Dwight, the noted chaplain of the Sixty-sixth, a special favorite of his, but he declined, saying it was too late. He signified his wishes in respect to his private affairs, and requested me to attend to everything for him, then calmly awaited the end.[82]

It was here that the irrepressible Doctor Potter, eager to personally care for his prominent patient, again found General Zook and the two aides. "I once more repaired to Gen'l Zook's side finding him still alive, but rapidly sinking."[83]

"At times he brightened up and spoke with considerable animation," noted Favill of the general, "so that we began to think that the doctor might be mistaken, and tried to make him think so, too, but he shook his head, and said there was no hope. We had frequently amongst ourselves discussed the nature of various wounds, and were all well aware that a shot through the intestines was considered necessarily fatal. He drank a little whiskey at times, and some broth that the women made for him. . . ."[84]

"He was cool and composed to the last moment of his life. About fifteen minutes before his death he quietly inquired of his attending physician how long he had to live, having previously requested his adjutant general to ascertain and advise him how the battle was going. Just at this moment Captain Favill reported 'that the bands had been ordered to the front, flags were flying and the enemy were in retreat.' 'Then I am perfectly satisfied,' said the General, 'and ready to die.'"[85]

---

82. *Ibid.*
83. Potter, *Three Years with the Army of the Potomac*, p. 60.
84. Favill, *Diary of a Young Officer*, pp. 247-48.
85. Douglas D. Zook, "A Biographical Sketch of Samuel K. Zook," *The Bulletin of the Historical Society of Montgomery County* [Pennsylvania], vol. 23, no. 2 (Spring 1982): 121.

"He lingered, however, until near two o'clock p.m., passing away without a murmur or complaint, and in the full possession of all his mental activity," remembered Doctor Potter, who was, by his own claim, at the general's side until the end. "The famous cannonade, the prelude to Pickett's heroic charge, was in full blast at this hour, and Zook breathed out his life amidst the uproar and mad clamor of two hundred guns. . . . As soon as the general breathed his last, I made haste for the front, where I knew my services were needed."[86]

When the forty-two-year-old general with the receding hairline and no-nonsense beard breathed his last, the race against decomposition immediately began. Both staff aides were quite well aware that the clock was ticking. "Broom wrote [Maj. William G.] Mitchell, of Hancock's staff, a line notifying him of the general's death, and asking for passes, so that we could take the body home, which were immediately sent to us."[87]

Broom and Favill busied themselves with the others preparations that needed to be made for the upcoming trip, packed their belongings, and turned over staff duties to other officers. "Early the following morning, July 4th, we secured some ice, packed the remains in a rude box, and sent them over to the railway station in an ambulance."[88]

The ambulance, with coffin and the two aides, must have driven east to meet the incoming trains, out beyond the destroyed Rock Creek bridge, although Favill does not mention it. "Broom and I rode upon the box containing the general's remains, in a freight car crowded with corpses, and the stench was prodigious. Several others were in the car, there being no passenger cars on the trains for some reason. We moved very slowly and did not arrive in Baltimore till seven o'clock the following morning [July 5]."[89]

---

86. Potter, *Three Years with the Army of the Potomac*, p. 60. The time of his death is reported variously as "soon after midnight" [Warner, *Generals in Blue*, p. 577], "near two o'clock p.m. [Potter, *Three Years with the Army of the Potomac*, p. 60], to "shortly before 5:00 p.m." [Zook, "A Biographical Sketch of Samuel K. Zook," p. 121]. If it was that difficult to verify the exact time of death for a brigadier general, think of the problems encountered by the average fighting man as he faced death at Gettysburg.

87. Favill, *Diary of a Young Officer*, p. 248.

88. *Ibid.* One cannot help but wonder where the two enterprising staff members "secured some ice." The First Division Hospital of the Second Corps, one would suspect.

89. *Ibid.*, p. 249.

It was now two days since General Zook passed away, two long, miserable, muggy days with very little ice to slow the relentless forces of nature. "The weather was fearfully hot and our position most distressing. As soon as we arrived, in company with David, the general's brother, we went to an undertaker and had the body embalmed, carefully dressed, and enclosed in a heavy casket." With the body now properly prepared, the actual job of mourning could finally begin.[90]

"The following day [July 6] we took the remains to Port Kennedy, Pennsylvania, his father's home; here we remained two days [July 6-7], a continuous crowd of people flocking in from all the surrounding country to view the remains. During this time Broom and I relieved each other in standing guard, and in answering a thousand curious questions." But if Josiah M. Favill thought that his duties to his commander were drawing a close, he was quite mistaken.[91]

"In the meantime, the family received a telegram from the Mayor of New York City, asking that the remains be sent on to that city to receive a public funeral." The former militia aficionado and telegraph executive had made a big impression on his adopted hometown, and now New York wanted to repay the favor. The two aides repacked their bags, and prepared the general's body for still another lengthy trip.[92]

"The family consenting, on the 7th of July, in a special car sent by the Mayor of New York City, the remains in our charge, together with a large funeral party, left for that place, where we were received on arrival, by a detachment of militia and several very gorgeous staff officers, who escorted the party to the city hall; where the coffin was placed in the governor's room, and there remained until Monday, July 10th, visited by thousands of people. The room was heavily draped in mourning, and either Broom or I, together with a guard from the city militia, was always on duty."[93]

New York City was not exactly putting its best foot forward—draft riots had broken out, the city was on fire in several places, looters were on an insane rampage, and lynch mobs wandered the streets in search of helpless black victims. "Everywhere lives and property were in danger, and the civil authorities temporarily helpless."[94]

---

90. *Ibid.*
91. *Ibid.*
92. *Ibid.*
93. *Ibid.*
94. *Ibid.*, pp. 249-50.

After laying grandly in state for several days, the grief-stricken population wept its anguish over the fallen hero as the body of Samuel Koskiusko Zook was laid to rest in Greenwood Cemetery. Ever the efficient officers, "as soon as the obsequies of General Zook were over," Broom and Favill "reported to the military commander of the district, General Dix."[95] Every trained soldier was surely needed in such a time of crisis.

But even in death, General Zook seemingly could not remain long in one place. Even though the setting was magnificent, a place where friends and acquaintances could come easily and often to mourn, it was still not the friendly graveyard of home. Eventually, when all the hoopla had passed, and attention turned to other fallen heroes, the general was quietly returned to his family burial plot in Montgomery Cemetery in Norristown, Pennsylvania.[96]

For his conspicuous gallantry under fire, Brigadier General Zook was breveted posthumously to the rank of major general of United States Volunteers. But, when all was said and done, his mother and family would always remember him as that little boy, now grown up and gone, who had been endlessly fascinated with all the pomp and splendor of the military.

The Nameless Union Wounded

Even though they did not receive the attention lavished on a fallen general, it seems difficult to imagine that some of the Union men died nameless and faceless in the midst of a Union hospital, surrounded by Union army surgeons and hospital staff, cared for by volunteer nurses from throughout the North, and ensconced in a bureaucratic hospital system that recorded every patient's name, rank, unit, nature of injury, and other vital statistics. Sadly, the overwhelming glut of wounded soldiers thrown at the Second Corps Hospital allowed some Northern wounded to simply slip through the cracks of the bureaucracy. The following stories reveal the agonizing struggle for life among these nameless men, remembered only by those whose lives they briefly touched.

95. *Ibid.*, p. 250.
96. Zook, "A Biographical Sketch of Samuel K. Zook," p. 121.

Drummer John B. Holloway of Company D, 148th Pennsylvania, saw much suffering and anguish when he was detailed to work with the Second Corps Hospital.

> Perhaps the most distressing case of suffering I saw was at this battle, in the case of a man who was shot through the throat from side to side, and his throat was swelling shut. He was at the field hospital in the woods by the hillside. He would roll and crawl and tumble about on the ground, then get up and walk back and forth, beckoning with both of his hands to all who were about him.
>
> This continued until a surgeon, I think Dr. Vishart, went to him, laid him on the ground, run an instrument into his throat and windpipe, and insert a silver tube. The man was relieved of his great suffering, but he died in a short time.[97]

Emily Bliss Souder wrote home to her sister on July 22.

> A Maine boy died yesterday, quite near to the spot where the ladies' tents are pitched. I stood by a fine, intelligent-looking Massachusetts man a day or two ago, whose life was ebbing away, and after repeating some passages of Scripture, I was able to sing,
>
> "There is a happy land!"
>
> Ah! how little were the surroundings like those of a New England home![98]

Sgt. T. P. Meyer was one tough soldier, a man who had seen it all as a pioneer in the 148th Pennsylvania Volunteers. But even tough guys could sometimes be deeply moved, especially by the personal tragedy of one young man in the Second Corps Hospital.

---

97. Muffly, *The Story of Our Regiment*, pp. 331-32. Hollowell is referring to Surgeon J. W. Wishart, 140th Pennsylvania Volunteers who performed an emergency field tracheotomy procedure.
98. Souder, *Leaves from the Battle-Field of Gettysburg*, p. 48.

Here occurred one of the most pathetic incidents of the War. A young soldier, a mere boy, who was brought to the hospital carried on a stretcher while a soldier walked alongside and with his hand held a wound in the thigh near the body. He said he was entirely free from pain.

A surgeon examined the wound and said, "Nothing can be done for you; you must die; if you have any word or message to send home, attend to it at once; you will die within a few moments after your comrade takes his hand from your wound and that must be soon."

He asked for paper and pen which were quickly furnished. He wrote a letter to his mother, stated his condition and that a comrade was holding the wound while he wrote to her, saying that as soon as he finished the letter his comrade would let go and he would bleed to death in a few minutes.

The letter was finished, he let himself fall back, hesitated a moment, then said, "Now you may let go," and Levi Smith, of Company A, 148th [Pennsylvania], who held the wound withdrew his hand, and in a few minutes life had gone out.[99]

Sometimes death was not the enemy. Death was often a precious friend, a dearly anticipated harbinger of ultimate cessation of the gnawing and irreparable agony of shattered limbs, perforated abdominal cavities, devastating cranial wounds, and the blazing consumption of infection. "A captain from Indiana, with closed eyes, was earnestly praying aloud, 'Jesus, take me to thy home! Jesus, take me to thy bosom! Lord, have mercy on me!'" Jane Boswell Moore, deeply moved by the continual impassioned pleas of the suffering Hoosier, could only write that "before the morning breaks the bosom of Jesus will be his last and blessed resting place."[100]

---

99. Muffly, *The Story of Our Regiment*, p. 468. Apparently, the bullet had nicked an artery close up to the trunk of the body. Amputations that high on the leg had an extremely low success rate; with arterial bleeding, there simply would have not been sufficient time to complete the surgery before the patient bled to death.

100. Moore, "An Incident at Gettysburg," p. 103.

Death was no respecter of age, or even of means. Mary Cadwell Fisher from York, Pennsylvania remembered one young man who was dying, but not of battlefield wounds.

> One beautiful evening, after a long day's hard work, one of my boys came to me and said: "There is a 'little chap' out there who has heard there was a woman from his home and he wants to see you." I found him at the farthest extremity of the hospital, with a half dozen other hopeless cases. He was a lovely boy, scarcely more than a child, who had run away from his home in Providence, Rhode Island. He was a brave boy and a great pet among the soldiers, who nursed him as tenderly as possible, but could but poorly supply a mother's loving care. How he longed for one more look of her dear face and once again to hear her sweet words of love! He was so frail and slight it was a marvel how he could have endured the fatigue and privation so long. He was not disfigured by wounds, but constant marches, insufficient food and often sleepless nights had exhausted his strength and he had not vitality to resist the sharp attack of fever. He was perfectly conscious, but too weak to say much. I asked the poor child what I could do for him.
>
> "Oh, I want my mother!," replied the boy.
>
> I sat down on the ground and taking him in my arms tried to comfort him. He turned his face to me, saying, "I am so tired," laid his head against me and appeared to sleep. The last rays of the sun touched the lovely features of the dying boy. The long-drawn shadows vanished in the gathering darkness. Silence, unbroken save by the plaintive moans of some poor victims, succeeded the hum of the busy day. The pitying dews shed a balm upon his brow.
>
> Fainter and fainter grew the breath and more feeble the clasp of the little hand, when suddenly rousing he opened his eyes, glazed in death, and looking long and earnestly in my face, said: "Kiss me, lady, before I die!" Clinging still closer to the stranger who could but faintly represent the fond mother's tenderness he so craved, he dropped his heavy lids and slept away his brief life as peacefully as a child goes to sleep in its mother's arms. I gently laid the

lifeless form down on the hard earth and left him to a soldier's burial and a nameless grave.[101]

So far from home, and surrounded by the no-nonsense, pragmatic approach of the military, women volunteer nurses were frequently the only representatives of propriety, decorum, and human dignity in the entire camp. "A young man from the 19th Maine died last Tuesday," recorded Emily Bliss Souder on July 27.

> Everything that day was hurry and bustle, as the encampment was being removed to a new spot at some distance from the former one. I prevailed, however, on the nurse, with the authority of the ward-master, to put a clean shirt and drawers on him, and they promised to let me know when he was buried.
>
> When called, Mrs. Curtis, Mrs. Campion and Miss [Anna] Raymond went with me to the spot where the body of this Maine boy lay, in a wide, shallow grave, beside a Pennsylvanian, each wrapped in his blanket, and the name of each written on paper pinned to his breast. I returned to camp, the men detailed for the duty agreeing to wait, and found Rev. Mr. Parvin, who performed the burial service.[102]

It was not much in the way of dignity, but a few appropriate words and a clean set of clothes was all the respect available when death came wholesale at the Second Corps Hospital.

Not all of the patients at the Second Corps Hospital were wounded. Army life, and its mix of poor diet and poorer sanitation, still put men in the hospital with intestinal disorders, fevers, and other camp ills. "On my arrival at the surgeon's headquarters one morning, one of the surgeons desired me to look after some sick boys who had been placed in a separate tent the day before. The presence of those who had been

---

101. Mrs. Mary Cadwell Fisher, "A Week on Gettysburg Field," *The Philadelphia Times*, Saturday, December 23, 1882.
102. Souder, *Leaves from the Battle-Field of Gettysburg*, pp. 64-65.

badly wounded was very unfavorable to the sick and seemed to retard their recovery."[103]

Volunteer nurse Mary Cadwell Fisher from York, Pennsylvania, immediately went to check on these invalids.

> There were about half a dozen of them who needed nursing and special diet. I had just begun to inquire into the wants and needs, when I heard a faint voice say: "Come here."
>
> As I went over to the cot its occupant said: "Don't you know me?" I carefully studied his wasted lineaments, but could not discover one familiar feature.
>
> "Don't you remember Charley M-----------, who lived in the little brown house on the hill in N--------?"
>
> He was the son of a poor widow in my native town, whom I had often seen in my girlhood days, but who until then had passed from my notice. He was so happy to find some one to whom he could talk about his mother and his home.
>
> He directed me where to find a number of boys from the neighboring towns, all of whom were delighted to once more see a Northern woman, even though a stranger. I spent most of my time with them after that, writing to their friends and attending to their wants.[104]

Sometimes the kindness of strangers was manifest in the most mundane and routine of activities; activities now suddenly rendered impossible by changing circumstances. Christian Commissioner Rev. George Bringhurst, from Philadelphia, remembered the profound difference that a simple question made to one patient.

> One very dark night I met a soldier whose arms had both been shot away. He was getting to his tent, and I asked what I could do for him.
>
> "Oh, nothing, Chaplain," he said, cheerfully; "unless you would tie my shoes for me. They have been bothering me a good deal."[105]

103. Fisher, "A Week on Gettysburg Field."

104. *Ibid.*

105. Smith, *Incidents of the United States Christian Commission*, p. 162.

Choking back tears at the simple request that presaged a lifetime of severe disability, Rev. Bringhurst knelt down and carefully tied tight loops in the soldier's brogans. When he rose to his feet, it was with an entirely new appreciation of the simple things of life. "The little deed became a joy."[106]

> Occasionally some of the wounded Unionists on the trains leaving Gettysburg received kindness not intended for them. All along the border [of Pennsylvania and Maryland] there were men and women whose whole sympathy was with the South. It was this class that presented faces wreathed in smiles when news came of a Union defeat; but after Federal victories had countenances elongated as the office boy who can't get off to see a double header baseball game. . . ."
>
> One morning, near the close of the hospital period, the train from Gettysburg contained a considerable number of soldier convlescents [*sic*]. In fact that was the case on almost every train. Now the clothing in which the wounded were sent out from the hospital was of so nondescript a character that a prominent citizen on the train concluded two of the men were Confederates.
>
> Taking a seat near them, he inquired after their welfare, at the same time informing them how ardently he sympathized with the South and how confident he felt of its ultimate triumph. He was a man of means, and, as he slipped a five dollar greenback into the hands of each, inquired from what part of the Confederacy they came, the money was pocketed very promptly.
>
> "I am from Maine" said the one with a merry twinkle of the eye.
>
> "I am from Vermont" said the other with a sarcastic laugh.
>
> Several persons had overheard the conversation and they gave the citizen so loud a guffaw that he fled to the little stuffy combination baggage and smoking car. As soon as Hanover was reached he jumped from the train, although

106. *Ibid.*

York had been his destination, and made rapid tracks away from the depot as jeer after jeer followed him.[107]

As health returned to traumatized bodies, the full range of human emotions returned as well. This was immediately evident to Charlotte McKay when she was requested to make a very unusual visit to a couple of wounded soldiers.

"A soldier, greatly excited, rushed, one day, into my tent, and begged me to come a little distance down a hillside, and stop a fight between two men, where, if something of the kind was not quickly done, there was likely to be a murder. Without a moment's thought I ran to the spot, where was the humiliating spectacle of two of our men, their faces already bloody and swollen, grappling and fisty-cuffing [*sic*] each other with the fury of wild beasts, while a dozen or more of their comrades, standing around, were urging on the fight."[108]

One can only imagine the shaming effect of coming face to face with a motherly-looking woman, hands planted firmly on her hips, in the midst of a boyish free-for-all. The brawlers never stood a chance. "No sooner had I laid my hand on one, and uttered a few words of surprise and shame at their unsoldierly conduct, than they drew off from one another, and relinquished the fight, though not without mutterings of future vengeance."[109]

After being hooted and catcalled by their spectating companions, the bruised combatants slunk off in different directions, mumbling ominously under their breath. "I afterwards heard that one of them deprecated the interference of *the woman*, which prevented the full punishment he was intending. I attribute the success of this effort solely to the fact of my being a woman, and believe that it was not so much my personal presence as the suggestion of some mother, wife, or sister, far away, that tamed their ferocity, and shamed them out of their bloody purpose." She also failed to credit the overwhelming effect of *"the look"* which she bestowed on the embarrassed rowdies.[110]

107. Wert, "In the Hospitals of Gettysburg, July, 1863," no. VII, *Harrisburg Telegraph*, August 28, 1907, p. 5.
108. McKay, *Stories of Hospital and Camp*, pp. 53-54.
109. *Ibid.*, p. 54.
110. *Ibid.*

CHAPTER 17

MONDAY, JULY 13: DAWN—FRIDAY, AUGUST 8: MIDNIGHT

"This hospital is to be moved down to Gettysburg."

Cornelia Hancock
New Jersey Volunteer Nurse

Gettysburg, Pennsylvania
Monday, July 13, 1863

Things at the Union Second Corps divisional hospitals were finally beginning to run more like a regularly established medical facility. Staff and volunteers alike now had sufficient time to look around, take stock of their surroundings, and write down their observations.

"The Ladies old and young take hold with a hearty good will," commented 8th Ohio Volunteer Infantry Hospital Steward Charles Merrick, late on July 13, in a quick note home to his wife Myra. "One, Miss Hancock, is deserving of especial praise. She is a frail looking woman, although possessed of a ruddy pretty face. She is on the go all the time. How she endures it I cannot understand. She is chatty and cheerful and the only one I have noticed yet who is not everlastingly asking that indelicate question of the men: 'Where are you wounded?'"[1]

Politicians, whether blatantly on the campaign trail or sincerely concerned over the fate of their constituency, continued to put in an appearance at the hospital grounds. "[Pennsylvania] Gov. [Andrew] Curtin was here yesterday. He was around to see the boys and give the

1. Charles H. Merrick, Letter to his wife, Dr. Myra H. Merrick, July 13, 1863.

boys a chance to see him. He is social and makes himself quite popular by his ease and freedom with the boys, and the sympathy he manifests for the wounded. He is a young looking man."[2]

As the number of patients steadily shrank, there was now enough spare time to take sightseeing excursions to Gettysburg and the battlefield. Steward Merrick, accompanied by a visiting newspaperman from Elyria, Ohio, made a second visit to the scarred town and its surrounds on July 13: "I have been down through the Burg again to day. There is scarcely a house in the whole City but has bullet marks. Gracious! it must have hailed lead bullet all over the City. But few cannon shots are to be seen. Washburn wants me to go over the battle field with him tomorrow and explain the position of our men and the rebs—the position of our Regiment, etc. I can tell him as far as our Corps is concerned, but know little of the other Corps."[3]

But even as it diminished in size, the Second Corps Hospital continued on as a full-blown emergency ward, filled with critically injured men. Although the death rate had significantly slowed after ten days, men still continued to sink and die from the overwhelming effects of trauma, infection, and exhaustion. The increasing orderliness of the hospital simply meant that they could now die recognized and remembered, rather than anonymous and alone. "Another of our boys died last night which makes eight since the battle. I have only eight more to care for; two of them, beside Capt. Nickerson, I consider almost past hope. The Doctors are of the opinion that Capt. Nickerson cannot live. His father is here. . . . We have an abundance of help now and plenty to eat."[4]

Having "plenty to eat" at the Second Corps Hospitals did not mean that the local farmers were becoming more generous with their produce. If anything, they seemed to grow more parsimonious with every passing day. News of their tight-fisted profiteering had already spread to other parts of the state, where it was reported with open contempt in local newspapers. Under the heading "Shameless Conduct of Citizens of Adams County," the July 13 edition of the *Lancaster Daily Express* described the prevailing situation this way:

2. *Ibid.*
3. *Ibid.*
4. *Ibid.*

Here is a farmer who has twelve stray cows, all of which he has milked daily, in addition to his own, whose farm and crops have been protected from the hands of the despoiler, by the blood of the slain, and whose barn is filled with 200 bleeding, dying patriots. Does he give them milk when they ask and plead for it? Yes. At five cents a pint! Does he give them one loaf of bread when they have saved for him 10,000? Yes. At forty cents a loaf. Here is another who has been driven from his home by the invading hosts, who bought tobacco at eight cents a plug and sells it to the wounded at 15. Bought letter paper at a cent per sheet and taking advantage of their misfortune, sells it to the disabled at five—all because they have unfortunately fell defending his home. They seem to be proud of the opportunity, and laugh at their cunning in counting their gains—it is not cunning, it is something less than duplicity.

This is sufficient to dampen the patriotism of any soldier, and woe, woe I say unto the soldier who falls among friends, if these are our friends.[5]

Tuesday, July 14, 1863

Even though the surgeons at the Third Division Hospital were convinced that Capt. Azor Nickerson "cannot live," Nickerson had definitely not subscribed to their morbid diagnosis. In fact, he and a wounded friend were quietly collaborating, jointly battling the odds and the ever-present specter of sepsis and disease, with nothing but sheer grit and two bottles of wine. Nickerson wrote:

> While I was on duty in the Shenandoah Valley and in the Pennsylvania campaign, I had become much attached to the adjutant of an Indiana regiment that belonged to our brigade, [John J. P. Blinn]. About the time we left the Peninsula, in August, 1862, he had resigned in a miff about

---

5. *Lancaster Daily Express*, July 13, 1863. Despite these stories of money-grubbing local farmers, the author has discovered no report that Jacob Schwartz or his family indulged in any schemes to gouge the wounded soldiers at any time during the hospital's tenure on their property. In fact, there are no stories concerning the Schwartzs at all, leaving one to surmise that they moved to the home of father Moses, or perhaps stayed during July and early August with one of Jacob's brothers.

> some real or imagined slight in the way of promotion and I had lost sight of him.
>
> On the evening of the second day's battle, as I was about to take charge of my detachment for the skirmish line, an officer rode up and tapped me on the shoulder. I turned, and there was my old friend in the uniform of an adjutant-general. We had little time for exchange of greetings, but he told me he had been assigned to the staff of the general commanding a brigade in the division of my corps next on our left. Just then the adjutant announced that my companies were ready, my friend and I shook hands; he returned to his division, and I went down to the skirmish line.
>
> One day, when the Reverend Adams was visiting me, he casually remarked upon the similarity of my case with that of another officer in the Second Division hospital, in whom he was also greatly interested, and he mentioned B[linn]'s name. I then found that my friend was also so badly wounded that it was not thought possible for him to recover. Mr. Adams said he was so anxious to live, at least until his widowed mother, who had been telegraphed for, came.[6]

Captain Blinn had fallen near the now-famous Copse of Trees, with a bullet-shattered hip. On July 4, he dictated two letters to his Indiana family; immediately upon the letters arrival in Terre Haute, his mother made arrangements to go to her son's side.

Azor Nickerson was deeply moved by the determination of his Hoosier friend, and he came up with a novel way to encourage him, even though almost a mile separated the camps of the Second and Third Division Hospitals. "I then sent a message to B[linn], that if I were alive at ten the next morning, I would join him in a glass of wine, at least, we could each take one at the same moment."[7]

The will to survive now centered on a daily libation—something so common in the military as to be hardly worth noting, but now a white-knuckled battle for life itself for the two horribly wounded men. Each day, at the stroke of ten, Nickerson and his friend, even though wracked with pain and bed-ridden, solemnly drank to each other's health as they celebrated another ever-so-precious day of life. "We

---

6. Nickerson, "Personal Recollections of Two Visits to Gettysburg," p. 25.
7. *Ibid.*

continued this long-distance greeting for several mornings, . . ." remembered the Ohio captain.[8]

"One day, just before the time for my glass with B[linn], a message came to my father. Instead of opening the bottle of wine for me as had been his custom, he came over to my bunk, laid his hand gently on my forehead, and looking sadly out across the green fields toward the hospital of the Second Division, he said: 'Poor Captain B[linn] can't drink with you this morning; he is dead.'"[9]

Fortunately, Captain Blinn's mother Dorthea had arrived the day before he died (either July 14, as remembered by his mother, or July 18, the date on his military records).[10] William Harrow wrote in his battle report: "My own assistant adjutant-general, Capt. John P. Blinn, throughout both days manifested himself a thorough soldier and patriot. He fell, mortally wounded, on the 3d, while gallantly cheering on the men of the command to which he was attached. No tribute can now reach him, but a worthier man and soldier has not died for his country."[11]

Scuttlebutt around the camp had it that Hospital Steward Charles Merrick and the walking wounded of the 8th Ohio would soon be released to return to the Army of the Potomac. Since the patients in his care were all stable, Merrick seized his one last opportunity to take a more leisurely tour of the battlefield. Again accompanied by his journalist friend, they spent the entire day walking through what had once been the lush fields of rural Pennsylvania, picking up souvenirs and mementos like so many others visitors.

> We went over a good portion of both lines to see the effect of artillery on both sides. He loaded himself with various relics of the field, and took notes of many remarkable things. It is evident enough that our artillery was far more destructive than theirs. We made better shots and on the line of the rebel batteries we found but four unburst shells,

8. *Ibid.*
9. *Ibid.*
10. Coco, *Killed in Action*, pp. 103-6.
11. *OR*, vol. 27, pt. 1, p. 421. The Hoosier adjutant general's body was shipped home to Terre Haute, Indiana, and interred in Woodlawn Cemetery.

> while on our side the shells of the rebels lay by the dozens. We measured one tree for [the] "fun of it" which one of our balls had gone clear through twenty two inches of green oak, and the tree [I] recollect nearly a mile from our Battery. Washburn could hardly believe it.
>
> Another good sized tree near one of their Batteries was hit 19 times. So you must know it must have been rather dangerous working their guns. But O, such piles of dead men and horses. The whole plain beyond their battle line is one vast grave—"My God!" says Washburn. "Lee must have sacrificed half his army here."[12]

But unlike so many of the thrillseekers visiting the sight of the recent battle, the two Ohioans sought out not only scenes of glory, but also the lonely burial sites of mutual friends. "I went with him to the grave of Hayden and others of our Regiment. Lieut. Hayden sacrificed himself almost foolishly and did not use ordinary caution, but to give our men courage imposed himself needlessly. So of Capt. Nickerson. He was shot while trying to enforce an unimportant order."[13]

As darkness set in, Merrick and Washburn headed back to the Second Corps, Third Division Hospital. It had been a long, full day, and they chatted about all the things they had seen on the battlefield. Washburn, a newspaperman through and through, could hardly wait to get home. "He will publish an account of the visit and said he would send it to me, but I fear it will not reach me. He gave me a kind invitation to write for his paper."[14]

Henry Janes, surgeon-in-charge at Gettysburg, took time out of his busy schedule on Tuesday evening to pen a few lines to his chief, Medical Director Jonathan Letterman of the Army of the Potomac. He was anxious to keep him up-to-date on the progress of evacuating the wounded, supplying the hospitals, and plans for the new general hospital to be located at Gettysburg.

12. Charles H. Merrick, Letter to his wife, Dr. Myra H. Merrick, July 15, 1863.
13. *Ibid.*
14. *Ibid.*

GETTYSBURG, July 14, 1863—6 p.m.
JONATHAN LETTERMAN,
Medical Director, Headquarters Army of the Potomac:

Five thousand eight hundred Union and 1,500 Confederates have been sent from here, besides 4,000 supposed to have gone from Littlestown and Westminster.

I think about 3,000 Union and 6,000 Confederates remain. Probably 3,000 cannot be moved. Dr. Brinton has plenty of the kind of supplies sent from Philadelphia, but, at the request of Dr. Cuyler, has made requisition on Dr. [Christopher C.] Cox for some articles. Dr. Cuyler is here; also General Thomas, who has power to act for the Secretary of War.

Have selected a fine site for the camp. Am anxiously awaiting the tents.

HENRY JANES,
Surgeon in Charge[15]

Wednesday, July 15, 1863

One by one, and in small bands, the walking wounded and the remaining convalescents were being discharged back to the care of their respective regiments. As the division hospitals steadily dwindled in size, less and less staff were needed to keep the corps hospital functioning smoothly. As surgeon-in-charge Dr. Justin Dwinelle released them from hospital duty, surgeons, stewards, and other regimental staff frequently shepherded men from their own regiments or brigades as they set off in search of the Army of the Potomac.

For Hospital Steward Charles H. Merrick of the 8th Ohio Volunteer Infantry, the time had indeed come to head back to his regiment. He dashed off an excited letter to his wife Myra while awaiting final orders to leave the Second Corps Hospital. "Dear Wife, At last I am on my way to the Regiment. I gathered all belonging to our Reg not wanted for nurses and reported to Dr. Guynell [Justin Dwinelle], who will forward us to the Regiment. We are now halted in the woods near our Hospital waiting his order. I hope we shall [not] be held long here, for I am impatient to reach the Regiment."[16]

---

15. *OR*, vol. 27, pt. 3, pp. 699-700.
16. Merrick, Letter to his wife, Dr. Myra H. Merrick, July 15, 1863.

There was no set routine for returning from hospital to army camp—it was a come-as-you-please, make-it-up-as-you-go type of thing, as Merrick was well aware. "I think we shall take the 'overland route' afoot. Some of us think we shall take the cars and go to Washington, thence to the Regiment; but in either case we anticipate a pleasant time. They are in my charge, and if we foot it across the country, you may be sure I shall not order any forced marches. We shall take our own time and depend upon the farmers for rations. There is nine of us of the 8th and six of the other Regiments in our Brigade."[17]

One last medical note for his doctor-wife on the condition of his charges: "Our boys are doing very well. None have died since I wrote last. Capt. Nickerson is some better, and there is some hopes of his recovery. Washburn will remain until the case is decided one way or the other."[18]

The post was ready to go out, and final clearance from Doctor Dwinelle was on the way: "I have a chance to send this and close abruptly. Charles"[19]

A reporter from the *Philadelphia Public Ledger* wrote a somber dispatch to his readers on July 15:

> Let no one come to this place for the simple purpose of seeing. To come here, merely to look at the wounded and dying, exhibits a most vitiated and disgusting taste. Besides, every such visitor is a consumer, and adds to the misery of the sick, by subtracting from the means that should be given exclusively to them. Let all that come, come with stores for the sick, and ready to work for them, but let all mere sightseers stay at home.[20]

Emily Bliss Souder, for one, had come with "stores for the sick, and ready to work." But having just arrived in town after foregoing her annual seaside vacation, Emily and her party quickly learned that a good night's sleep was a rare commodity in Gettysburg. "We were

17. *Ibid.*
18. *Ibid.*
19. *Ibid.*
20. *Philadelphia Public Ledger,* July 15, 1863.

aroused from sleep very early by the sound of ambulances driving past on their way to the camps for the wounded, and also by the perpetually passing wagons loaded with coffins, either going empty to the battle-fields, or returning with their sad freight."[21]

The wounded who were stable enough to be evacuated by rail from Gettysburg continued to be moved by ambulance from the Second Corps Hospital to the town depot. Emily Souder and her party, awaiting transportation out at the Second Corps Hospital, found that the wounded were making their way to them, instead of the other way around. "While we were waiting, as the ambulances passed on their way to the depot, we handed the poor soldiers a drink from the doorstep."[22]

Although twelve days had passed since the battle, and great strides had been made in supplying and caring for the wounded, Gettysburg and its outskirts were still a ghastly spectacle for the unprepared visitor.

> We saw the rifle-pits, the dead horses, the shattered windows and the stone walls, all scattered and many soldiers' graves. Chloride of lime has been freely used in the broad streets of the town and to-day the hospital was much improved by the same means; but it is needful to close the eyes on sights of horror and to shut the ears against the sounds of anguish and to extinguish, as far as possible, the sense of smelling.
>
> We rode in an ambulance to the hospital of the Second Corps. The sights and the sounds beggar description. There is a great need for bandages. Almost every man has lost either an arm or a leg. The groans, the cries, the shrieks of anguish, are awful indeed to hear. We heard them all day in the field, and last night I buried my head in my pillow to shut out the sounds which reached us, from a church quite near, where the wounded are lying. We could only try to hear as though we heard not, for it requires strong effort to be able to attend to the various calls for aid.[23]

---

21. Souder, *Leaves from the Battle-Field of Gettysburg*, p. 22.
22. *Ibid.*, p. 16.
23. *Ibid.*, pp. 17, 22-23.

The Sanitary and Christian Commissions, as well as many other smaller but no less dedicated organizations, had been moving massive quantities of foodstuffs and medical supplies into the area. Emily Bliss Souder found a vastly different scenario at the Second Corps Hospital than had Cornelia Hancock just a week previous.

> We dispensed buckets of milk punch and quantities of corn-starch, nicely prepared with condensed milk and brandy, besides sundry cups of tea, an unwonted luxury, and broth made of beef jelly condensed, with many other services and a little chat occasionally with some poor fellow. . . . There are perpetual calls for "something for a wounded soldier who can't eat anything hard,"—"milk punch," "a cup of tea," or "a cup of coffee with milk."[24]

Soft diets continued as a critical need at the Second Corps Hospital, and the creativity of the relief organizations was evident in the variety of specialty foods available to the patients.

> The condensed milk is invaluable. The corn-starch, farina, and milk punch are eagerly partaken of, and a cup of chocolate is greatly relished. A poor fellow with a broken jaw seemed to appeal, though mutely, for special attention. I beat up two or three eggs, added a spoonful of brandy and a cup of scalding hot milk, which he managed to draw through his scarcely opened lips, and at once seemed revived.
>
> Two or three desperately wounded men beg for *ice*, with an earnestness of agonized entreaty which could brook no denial. I promised, if possible, to obtain it; but found that the surgeon had absolutely forbidden that the ice should be touched, as the lives of many men depended upon their having it. You may judge how painful it was to carry this message in lieu of the cooling morsel of which I hoped to be the bearer.[25]

Meal times were always an adventure at the hospital—there was no telling who might sit down at the lunch or dinner table. "Many surgeons came to our table which we arranged to-day," wrote Emily

---

24. *Ibid.*, pp. 17, 18.
25. *Ibid.*, pp. 24, 18.

Bliss Souder to a friend, "asking for a cup of coffee and we had a distinguished party to dine, Adjutant-General Thomas and his son, with a surgeon or two. Another visitor we had, well-known to fame, a distinguished Copperhead from New York. . . . He did not wait to partake of coffee with General Thomas. Indeed the ladies said they had no refreshments for Copperheads and he should get nothing from them."[26]

Sixty hospital sites now lay scattered throughout Gettysburg and the outlying areas. To Surgeon Henry Janes, whose unenviable job it was to supervise all of the field hospitals following the battle, it was a logistical nightmare of monumental proportions. Providing sufficient surgical and domestic supplies, and assuring adequate medical care, were becoming an ever-increasing problem. To make matters worse, Janes had only thirty ambulances to move the thousands of wounded men from widely dispersed field hospitals to the railroad depot. A more efficient system desperately needed to be developed, and quickly, to streamline this makeshift hospital situation.

In a radical departure from the standard military procedure, Janes and his staff (and, possibly, the absent Doctor Letterman as well) had been considering the novel possibility of establishing a general hospital at the battlefield itself, instead of transporting the wounded to general hospitals in distant cities. Janes, accompanied by United States Medical Inspectors Edward P. Vollum and George K. Johnston, scoured the rolling country around Gettysburg, looking for a suitable location for the new hospital.

The site the team ultimately agreed upon was part of George Wolf's sprawling farm property out along the York Pike. The "Wolf Woods," as they were locally known, was a popular picnic spot, and featured a large grove of oak and hickory trees that grew up near a bubbling fresh-water spring. The ground was on a rise to the east of Gettysburg, and was mostly well-drained. Due to its elevation, breezes moved freely through the trees, and could carry away the foul stench of decaying flesh and bodily discharges from infected wounds. And the railroad tracks lay only 150 yards away from the proposed site—a fact not lost on the medical men.

---

26. *Ibid.*, pp. 18-19.

Doctor Janes had immediately put in requisitions for a number of large medical tents and all kinds of hospital stores. On July 15, the tents arrived, and were shipped out to the new facility; in a move of political astuteness, the new hospital would henceforth be known as "Letterman General Hospital."[27]

With all the equipment and supplies being requisitioned for the new general hospital, one would think that a single cookstove should have been a fairly easy request to fill. Unfortunately, that simple appliance started a bitter squabble between Doctor Janes and Second Corps nurse Charlotte Elizabeth McKay.

"My chief embarrassment at Gettysburg was the want of a stove," remembered McKay, "and all suitable means of cooking. My only resort in that line, with the exception of a chafing-dish, heated with a spirit-lamp, that I had brought from Washington, was to a fire in the open air on the hillside, over which were stretched long poles, resting at the ends on upright stakes. On the poles were suspended great camp-kettles and caldrons, where were cooked rations for from a thousand to fifteen hundred men. In my distress at seeing so many wants in the way of special diet that could not be met, I went to the town. . . ."[28]

Of course, she was dealing with the army bureaucracy, so the stove would have to be requisitioned through proper channels. "Having found that a nice stove could be purchased there, I made application to the quartermaster of the post, and received from him a promise to buy the stove, and furnish for it immediate transportation, provided I would send him a requisition to that effect from the surgeon-in-chief of the division, approved by the chief medical officer of the corps hospital. This was easily done, and I was rejoicing in the hope of this valuable acquisition, when, to my dismay, the requisition was returned disapproved by the medical director of the post."[29]

Charlotte McKay was not one to take rejection easily. Rather than giving up, she went in search of Doctor Janes, the medical director overseeing the wounded at Gettysburg. "I then went to this officer,

27. Report of Medical Inspector Edward P. Vollum, U.S. Army, *OR*, vol. 27, pt. 1, p. 27.
28. McKay, *Stories of Hospital and Camp*, p. 54.
29. *Ibid.*, pp. 54-55.

represented our great need, and begged him to approve the requisition."[30]

Doctor Janes was looking at the bigger picture—setting up a unified general hospital at the battlefield. He was adamant in his priorities. "But I might as well have appealed to a rock. He was going, he said, to receive some stoves from Baltimore for the general hospital, which was to be established at Gettysburg, and he would loan me one of them. . . ."[31]

Somewhat mollified, Charlotte reluctantly accepted his offer of one of the Maryland stoves. "But when the stoves came they were not adapted to our use, and so time and opportunity slipped by, while scores of our men were dying daily, and my tent filled with supplies which could not be suitably cooked. Another effort to purchase a stove from our hospital fund was frustrated in the same manner."[32]

Stymied in her pursuit of an adequate cookstove, Charlotte McKay turned her attention to another serious concern in the hospital wards. "Our men were also suffering for want of sheets, the coarse army blankets being their only defence [*sic*] against the flies, and these were terrible on their wounds in the hot weather. I have seen men, with both hands disabled, crying in helpless agony from the tortures of these merciless little insects."[33]

Moved by the severe discomfort of her patients, Mrs. McKay went to Gettysburg in search of linen sheets . . . and ended up once again in the office of Doctor Janes. No, there were no sheets available. "When I entreated the medical director to furnish us some sheets from the Government stores, he put me off with the excuse that he would need them all for the new hospital which was to be; and not a sheet could be obtained for our division hospital save a few that I begged from the Sanitary and Christian Commissions."[34]

Charlotte McKay was genuinely perturbed by the cavalier treatment she received at the hands of Doctor Janes. "I do not mention this conduct of the chief medical officer at Gettysburg as an illustration of the way in which our efforts to alleviate the sufferings of our wounded soldiers were generally seconded by surgeons and other officers, for the majority, so far as my observation extended, were kind-hearted and sympathizing, appreciating the difficulties we had to

---

30. *Ibid.*, p. 55.
31. *Ibid.*
32. *Ibid.*
33. *Ibid.*, pp. 55-56.
34. *Ibid.*, p. 56.

encounter, and aiding us as they could,—but it does illustrate a phase of the difficulties to which women working in our military hospitals were *liable*."[35]

Thursday, July 16, 1863

Bright and early Thursday morning, work crews set out from town along the York Pike, teams drawing wagons heavily loaded with tools, supplies, and tents. They met at the Wolf Woods, unloaded their equipment, and set to work. One observer noted that "the medical officers of the Government had already on the 16th of July, commenced establishing a temporary General Hospital in tents on the York road, some two miles from Gettysburg."[36]

Even though all primary amputations were finished by July 10, the work at the operating tables continued on. Secondary amputations of gangrenous limbs needed to be done, as well as repair work on patients with severe hemorrhaging. Emily Souder never did get inured to it like Cornelia Hancock. "The amputation table is plainly in view from our tents. I never trust myself to look toward it."[37]

Even with increasing numbers of volunteers streaming into the area, "the necessity of more help is terrible. The men are dying all around us and there is no time to say more than a friendly word, as one is called from tent to tent and requested to prepare 'milk punch for eight men,' or 'cornstarch,' or 'tea,' 'a portion for seven and also for eight.' What can we do, when these poor souls, who have just undergone amputation, require nourishing and stimulating food to keep the life in them at all? We cannot stop to talk with them. We can only labor assiduously with our hands."[38]

There simply were not enough hours in the day to accomplish everything that needed to be done at the hospital. "I provided myself before leaving home with a large quantity of paper, stamps, etc., expecting to write many letters for the soldiers, but thus far, have not

35. *Ibid.*
36. Dimon, *Report of the General Agent of the State of New York*, p. 56.
37. Souder, *Leaves from the Battle-Field of Gettysburg*, p. 26.
38. *Ibid.*, pp. 26-27.

found time and many that were alive yesterday are gone to-day and several that we saw to-day, I fear we shall see no more forever."[39]

Some were willing to get quite huffy about semantics, even in the midst of suffering and dying on a massive scale. "We had quite an argument with a minister from Maryland, who, standing on the street, happened to overhear a remark made by one of us to Mr. Bringhurst, as he sat in a carriage, on his way to the field, in regard to the question of nursing the rebels. This gentleman felt it to be his duty to walk into our boarding-house and take us to task, strangers as we were. . . . He charged us with taking a very unchristian view of the matter. We told him that we took care of them as suffering men and not as rebels. We learned afterwards that this gentleman was well known as a secessionist."[40]

The Sanitary Commission, headquartered at the Fahnestock Store in downtown Gettysburg, had, by now, perfected the movement of supplies into Gettysburg and throughout the surrounding area. Dr. Henry W. Bellows, president of the Commission, and a man who "likes to see his usefulness made manifest in newspapers," wrote in the July 16 *New York Times*: "Every day since Tuesday, a car-load of delicacies, costing $2,000 in Baltimore and containing 1,000 pounds of mutton, 1,000 pounds of chicken, 1,200 dozen eggs, 1,500 loaves of soft bread, with condensed milk, beef stock, etc. had been ordered forward and distributed." He also expounded on the "ceaseless wagonloads" of hospital clothing that were rolling into town.[41]

Although it looked great in print, and sizable donations of money were being made to the Commission itself, funds were rushing out far faster than they were coming in. By July 23, only $75,000 would remain in Commission accounts. In a cost-cutting measure, Dr. Cornelius R. Agnew, a member of the Commission's Executive Committee, sent out a personal memorandum to the agents in charge at Gettysburg, quietly urging them "to take in sail."[42]

39. *Ibid.*, p. 27.
40. *Ibid.*, p. 26.
41. Strong, *Diary of the Civil War*, p. 425; *New York Times*, July 16, 1863.
42. William Quentin Maxwell, *Lincoln's Fifth Wheel: The Political History of the United States Sanitary Commission.* (New York: Longmans, Green, 1956), p. 212.

Dr. Theodore Dimon still had not managed to make it to the Second Corps Hospital. Dispatched by the army to Gettysburg from his New York home, he arrived on July 12, and immediately reported to Medical Inspector Cuyler.[43]

Cuyler was delighted to see him, and promised to send him within the hour to oversee the Confederate wounded out at the Second Corps Hospital. Sadly, no one in Medical Director Janes' office seemed to have the foggiest notion, now over a week after the battle's end, as to where Doctor Dwinelle and his hospital were to be found. But there was no shortage of needy hospitals, so the New Yorker and his bags were promptly shunted over to the United States Hotel.[44]

Dimon found the hotel packed with about 200 wounded, well staffed, but "every part and parcel of the premises were disorderly and filthy inside and outside of the building." The situation was further complicated by a supervising surgeon who spent most of his time "concocting iced drinks for himself and visiting friends and in exclaiming against the women" nursing staff. Doctor Dimon would brook no interference from this bumbler; he immediately set about correcting these deficiencies. By July 15, when the hotel hospital was consolidated with another facility, it was running smoothly under Dimon's watchful eye.[45]

Dimon may have simply been moved to another hospital had it not been for a dispatch dated July 16, 1863, with a unique job offer:

> Surgeon Theodore Dimon
> Dear Sir,
>
> I desire to obtain your attention and care and as far as may be permitted your surgical skill and experience for the wounded soldiers of the State of New York now in the hospitals in and about Gettysburg. Whatever is necessary for their health and comfort you are authorized to procure for them.
>
> If any soldier of our state is neglected or improperly treated you will call the attention of his surgeon to the case.

43. Dimon, *From Auburn to Antietam.*
44. *Ibid.*
45. *Ibid.*

If this does not remedy the evil, then the facts of the case should be reported to his superior officer.

You will also use your influence to render the transportation of the soldiers as comfortably as possible.

For these and other purposes which may be necessary for the care and comfort of the soldiers from the State of New York, you are authorized to hire and pay for such materials and assistance as you may find necessary. The couriers of the New York State Soldiers' Depot at No. 50 Howard Street, New York City, will report to you and be subject to your orders and you may employ additional couriers if necessary.

A record should be made of the names and places of burial of the soldiers who may die and a map should be drawn indicating the localities of their graves. When the headboards at graves of N. Y. State soldiers are not marked or are insufficiently marked, you will please have them well marked with black paint.

You are authorized to draw on me for such means as you may need to carry out the instructions of this letter (if the draft now given you does not prove sufficient) but if the amount of your draft will exceed the amount of my draft you will advise me before you draw it.

You will report to me at No. 50 Howard St., New York, New York, once in two weeks. This report you will please make as detailed as possible showing the care and attention given the soldiers.

I am of the opinion that no appropriation has been made by the legislature of New York for coffins or any funeral expenses of soldiers. These should be furnished by the General Government. I will examine this matter and advise with the Governor on my return to New York and telegraph you the result.

Truly Yours,
John F. Seymour
General Agent of the State of New York[46]

A hefty job description—head a governmental fact-finding mission, personally visit every hospital treating New York patients in the entire Gettysburg area, provide any needs of the Empire State

---

46. *Ibid.*

wounded, locate all known graves of New York troops, draw a detailed plat map of the interment sites, ensure that all graves found were legibly marked, make a master list of all New York fatalities, and oversee the transportation of any New Yorkers as they travel home. Even armed with financial carte blache and the massive authority of New York State, Dimon was definitely going to need all the "additional couriers" he could lay his hands on.

It looked as though Doctor Dimon would get to visit the Second Corps Hospital after all.

Friday, July 17, 1863

Overwhelmed with the pressures of constantly being available to minister to the needs of thousands of men at the Second Corps Hospital, Emily Bliss Souder took a few moments to get away. "Mrs. Campion and I, allowing ourselves a little space for taking an observation of a portion of our surroundings, walked a few yards from the border of the encampment, and visited the slaty ridge where our Union soldiers belonging to this corps are buried [Yard C]. We read the names with sad interest."[47]

Rather than the clean and neatly manicured environs of a community cemetery, the two ladies found a trashy quagmire following the recent showers. Cracker-box grave markers, with personal data almost washed clean in the inclement weather, canted dangerously in every direction, making the burial yard more reminiscent of a scrapyard than a graveyard. "The ground all around is thickly strewn with the debris of the battle. We picked up a tourniquet, with which, we are told, all the New Hampshire boys are supplied; an open Testament, still perfect, though wet and somewhat soiled, with 'H. K. Campbell, 145th Re. P. V.,' written in pencil on the blank leaf,—tin cartridge boxes, minnie balls, belt clasps, etc.—These we shall carefully preserve as mementoes."[48]

Refreshed emotionally, if not rested physically, by their visit to the cemetery, the ladies returned to the bustle and noise of the hospital. It was shaping up to be another grinding day of pain, loss, and agony. "We are very busy, from seven in the morning till seven at night. Twelve poor souls passed . . . to their final account, six Union soldiers and six rebels."[49]

---

47. Souder, *Leaves from the Battle-Field of Gettysburg*, p. 28.
48. *Ibid.*, pp. 28-29.
49. *Ibid.*, p. 29.

"Supplies are abundant. The distress and suffering are beyond description, but there is a great change for the better since we came, and these continuous showers are, the surgeons say, the best possible thing. . . . Rags, pads, and pillows are much wanted; no danger of too many of them." However, the muggy weather was playing havoc on some of the fresh supplies. "Lemons are spoiling; so many have been sent."[50]

"We sleep in town, riding out in the morning and returning at night. Both going and returning, we pass the Cemetery which must henceforth be so interesting to all loyal Americans, but we have not allowed ourselves time to enter the gateway."[51]

Saturday, July 18, 1863

> This day is the first without rain since we came here. The camp ground is so wet and muddy that we can scarcely get on, even with India rubbers. The cool wet weather has been extremely favorable, for both the men, who have almost all suffered amputation, and for the citizens also, as it washes off the ground and relieves the surface by absorption. There has been a great change since we came in this respect.
>
> This morning the ride to the camp was quite comfortable by comparison, except when we were passing those places where the dead horses poison the atmosphere. It seems strange that they were not destroyed, but by degrees they are being consumed by fire. We have not had time to visit the battle-ground or the Cemetery. We go to the camp early, and are busy to the utmost all day.[52]

Despite rubbing shoulders with both Union and Confederate wounded, Emily Souder's aversion to dealing one-on-one with Rebel soldiers was never very far below the surface.

> Today, at Doctor Morris's request, I went to the rebel camp, and wrote several letters. I found the office very uncongenial in every respect, and hardly think I shall attempt it again. Mrs. ----- and Mrs. ----- have devoted

50. *Ibid.*, p. 30.
51. *Ibid.*, p. 29.
52. *Ibid.*, p. 32.

> themselves to this branch of the service with great assiduity.[53] The rebels are truly wretched for the most part, without fortitude or much else that makes a man what he should be. . . .
>
> The stores of almost everything are wonderfully abundant, but the necessity is frightful. The surgeon in charge said to me today, "We cannot have too many pads." Mrs. Turley received about one hundred to-day. They were gone directly, and I had to go to the Christian Commission tent, to hunt up two or three for a poor fellow from Massachusetts, who said he was suffering terribly. About eight inches square is a good size. Bran is the article most used for stuffing them. These pads have to be renewed almost daily, as everything becomes horribly offensive.[54]

Camp Letterman General Hospital was starting to fill up, even though it was not scheduled to open officially until Tuesday, July 22. Sixteen hundred wounded had already been carted or carried out of town to Wolf's Woods, mostly from the smaller house hospitals of Gettysburg. Now situated in the new general hospital, they were under the careful supervision of four hundred doctors and attendants. Southern surgeons were moved out to the new facility to care for their own wounded. By July 18, the farflung Gettysburg hospitals were rapidly emptied of their patients, leaving only the Public School, the Lutheran Seminary, the Buehler Warehouse, and a few private homes serving as convalescent hospitals.[55]

Sunday, July 19, 1863

By now, the relief services offered by Mrs. Souder and her associates had been pared down to an exact science. Their tents were set up in a small enclave, convenient to supplies and to the rest of the hospital complex. "The Christian Commission have a tent on the ground. Very near that is Mrs. Curtis's tent, and Mrs. Campion and Anna Raymond are there. Immediately adjoining is another tent, where

53. Probably Jane Boswell Moore and her mother, Mrs. Moore.

54. Souder, *Leaves from the Battle-Field of Gettysburg*, p. 31.

55. *Adams Sentinel & General Advertiser*, August 18, 1863.

Mrs. Turley, Mrs. Chaplain, and Mrs. J. L. Claghorn are chiefly to be found, while I do anything that comes to hand in either one, and go to the Commission tent for anything that is needful."[56]

"The supplies are most abundant of everything except pads and pillows. Pads eight inches square, made of the poorest materials possible, and filled with bran or sawdust, or soft hay, are more needed than any other thing. They are thrown away daily, or ought to be, and they '*cannot have too many.*'" In addition, as the general health of the patients improved, a new craving was developing: "'Butter!' is the cry of the soldiers."[57]

Though "butter" may have been on their lips, survival was the entire focus of their thoughts. The flesh wounds and those with easily stabilized injuries were long gone, already evacuated to general hospitals throughout the east. Now only the most seriously wounded remained: "desperate cases of amputation, compound fracture, and penetrating wounds of the chest and pelvis." "Six to eight men lie in almost every tent, and scarcely one of these who has not lost an arm at the shoulder, or else his leg. Ghastly suffering stares you in the face, and while many are cheerful and hopeful, many others are wan and downhearted. It is wonderful how the eyes of these poor fellows will brighten at a friendly word from a woman."[58]

"I was surprised and much interested to find the Colonel [William Colvill] of the First Minnesota, and [Second] Lieutenant [Charles] Mason and several of their regiment, in the same tent. I promised to take them under my especial charge. . . . I was glad to be able to give to each of them an orange, a luxury much craved and difficult to obtain at this season, and took them some chicken soup, which they thought very comfortable. I have seen a number of Minnesota boys, but have not their names, and am sorry to add, have seen also the graves of many Minnesotans."[59]

The close association in the amputation ward, between Northerners and Southerners who had lost at least one or more limbs, seemed to have finally broken down most of the walls of animosity so prevalent the previous week. "In almost every tent the Union soldiers and the rebels lie side by side, friendly as brothers. I said to some of them

---

56. Souder, *Leaves from the Battle-Field of Gettysburg*, p. 37.
57. *Ibid.*
58. Wormeley, *The United States Sanitary Commission*, p. 145; Souder, *Leaves from the Battle-Field of Gettysburg*, pp. 33-34.
59. Souder, *Leaves from the Battle-Field of Gettysburg*, pp. 39-40.

yesterday, that the North and the South would surely know each other better than ever before, when this war was over."[60]

As the hospital developed a daily routine, Sundays were again becoming days of worship and contemplation. "On Sunday morning, a plain-looking woman arrived from Michigan, to find her only brother had been buried ten days. We gave her some refreshment, and she joined in a short religious service at our tent. Rev. Mr. Adams of Maine was present. We sang 'Coronation,' 'Soldiers of Christ, arise!' and 'Rock of Ages.' . . . Rev. Mr. Morris, from Germantown, officiated."[61]

Grieving mothers, wives, and sisters continued to show up at the tents of the Second Corps, searching for a wounded son, or father, or brother, or friend. More often than not, it was already too late.

> Mrs. H[ughes] arrived from Michigan to find that her only brother was already buried. Two days before, Mrs. Reynolds, from Philadelphia, came to find her husband, already buried. I gave to each some refreshment, and then begged them to assist me, for surely nothing helps us forget our own sorrows like trying to relieve the sorrows of others.
>
> They each helped me prepare a whole barrel of bread for toasting, and Mrs. Reynolds and I dipped toast, till you would surely have thought that every man was supplied. I told several of the soldiers that we were going to toast the Army of the Potomac. They are delighted to have a little home cooking. We made delicious farina and corn-starch, with plenty of brandy in it, for these amputated cases require stimulating food. It is wonderful how much of the aspect of nearly all has improved since we have been here.
>
> Three or four soldiers are detailed to wait upon the ladies. One calls himself Bridget, and washes dishes all day. Another splits wood and attends to the stoves, of which we have three. How grateful our soldiers are to the ladies for their labors of love, you can hardly imagine. You can see their eyes brighten, when we pause at the door of a tent to inquire how they are thriving.[62]

---

60. *Ibid.*, p. 36.
61. *Ibid.*, pp. 49, 37.
62. *Ibid.*, pp. 37-38, 49.

Monday, July 20, 1863

With so many mouths to feed, and relying mostly on perishable supplies, some days were spent living hand to mouth. "Monday morning there was no bread, none in the ladies' tents, none in the Christian Commission tent, none in the Commissary's stores; but directly a wagon drove up loaded with supplies, brought by two kind damsels,—mammoth loaves of homemade bread, fresh eggs, and a pot of butter . . . pies . . . and other comfortable things. . . . We must adopt for our motto, 'The Lord will provide.'"[63]

Exciting news reached Emily Bliss Souder and her party when they returned from working at the hospital. "On Monday evening . . . after tea, we received a telegram, and found on opening it that four gentlemen were at Hanover Junction, and would be here during the evening. We were all quite astonished, as we had not an idea of seeing our better halves at this time. The next day they made a tour of the battle-field, the Cemetery, the Seminary, the College, and Round Top, and then rode to the camp to see us at work."[64]

Mrs. Hanness, volunteer nurse from central New York, she of the "auburn hair and clear, blue eyes," whose melancholy renditions of "Sweet Hour of Prayer" lulled the camp to sleep every night, clung to hope in the midst of grinding despair. She prayed that somehow, somewhere, her wounded son had survived the three days of battle, even as the weeks began to inexorably add up.

With the local newspapers up and running again, Mrs. Hanness decided to try a new approach in finding her son. "As late as July 20th, the noble, heart-sore mother had not yet given up the quest of her son, as is shown by the following prominently displayed in the editorial column of one of the Gettysburg papers:

> INFORMATION WANTED.
>
> Mrs. Hanness, of New York State, is now among us searching for her son who was wounded in the first day's fight. She has visited all the hospitals, but he cannot be found. She thinks that he is lying in some private house; and

63. *Ibid.*, pp. 54, 43.
64. *Ibid.*

would be thankful and ever remember any person that would inform her of his whereabouts by leaving notice at the residence of Mr. David Warren, in Gettysburg. Her husband was wounded in the first day's fight and died soon after.[65]

So ran the advertisement in the editorial column of a Gettysburg newspaper on July 20, 1863. "Searching for her son . . . but he cannot be found."[66]

Early August would come, and, one by one, the patients would be stabilized and transported out of town or to the new Camp Letterman General Hospital out on the York Pike. The Second Corps Hospital would soon strike its tents, pack the remaining medical wagons and ambulances, and set out to rejoin the Army of the Potomac. "No trace of the boy was ever found. He probably sleeps amongst the one thousand unknown dead of the National Cemetery," was the opinion of local farmer and historian J. Howard Wert.[67]

"As the field hospitals were gradually closed there was no more work for the willing hands of Mrs. Hanness. She faded away from the field of slaughter, and I saw her nevermore." Wert often wondered what happened to the melancholy songstress from New York state. "But, wherever her lot was cast, it was a deep and silent grief that gentle, Christian lady bore with her, through the revolving years, until she sang for the last time:

'This robe of flesh I'll drop, and rise
To seize the everlasting prize;
And shout while passing through the air,
Farewell, farewell, sweet hour of prayer.'"[68]

Tuesday, July 21, 1863

Again the supply of comestibles was depleted; this time, dairy products were running dangerously low. "There was not an egg to be

---

65. Wert, "In the Hospitals of Gettysburg, July, 1863," no. II, *Harrisburg Telegraph*, July 25, 1907, p. 4. Gettysburg had three local papers—the Republican *Adams Sentinel*, the staunchly Democratic *Gettysburg Compiler*, and the Repubican *Gettysburg Star & Banner*. The *Compiler* brought out its first post-battle issue on July 13, with the *Sentinel* and the *Star and Banner* resuming operation around the same time.
66. *Ibid.*
67. *Ibid.*
68. *Ibid.*

had, and no butter, and *'butter'* is the perpetual petition of the poor soldiers, when a country vehicle all dusty stopped near our tents, and bread and biscuits, butter, lard and eggs, were handed out, with dried fruit in quantity."[69]

With only the most serious cases left at the hospital, pessimism tended to run high in some circles. "A surgeon said yesterday that 'two-thirds of all these amputated cases must die.'" While the doctor's prognosis was fueled by exhaustion and discouragement, it did address the continued mortality rate at the hospital. "We did not know that our hospital experiences were to prepare us for this work," added Emily Souder pensively.[70]

With every passing day, more and more patients were being rotated out to either a general hospital or to their own homes. "Some men were to be sent home, who had no pantaloons. Doctor Ward, from Wilmington, Del., came to me: 'Two men were going to Delaware in the morning; could I get pantaloons for them?' I found two white linen pairs joyfully, but Mr. Shinn said there were cloth pantaloons in one of his boxes; so we had it opened and found what was needed. Mr. Shinn told me he distributed thirty pairs yesterday morning."[71]

While Emily Bliss Souder struggled with pants and dairy supplies, Cornelia Hancock seemed to be having the time of her life. On July 21, she snatched a few moments away from her patients to write home. "MY DEAR MOTHER, It is with trouble that I can find time and quiet to enough write to anyone. I have been sick but one day since I have been here, and then I went into a tent and was waited upon like a princess. I like to be here very much, am perfectly used to the suffering and the work just suits me; it is more superintending than real work, still the work is constant. I like being in the open air, sleep well and eat well."[72]

News of the new General Hospital being organized over in Wolf Woods was beginning to circulate in all the corps hospitals. "The rumors about camp are that this hospital is to be moved down to Gettysburg. I hope it is not so but I suspect it is. The field hospital is a number of tents and nothing more; it is in first rate order now, and I am

69. Souder, *Leaves from the Battle-Field of Gettysburg*, p. 43.
70. *Ibid.*, p. 42.
71. *Ibid.*, p. 43.
72. Hancock, *South After Gettysburg*, pp. 15-16.

sorry it has to be moved. All the officers will be changed I suppose. The men are very polite to me, and I get on remarkably well, but quiet is impossible to obtain at camp."[73]

The camp, even two and a half weeks after the battle, was still changing. Some modifications were quite beneficial: "I have succeeded in getting a washerwoman today which is a great institution here indeed." Others were familiar complaints: "Old sheets and pads of every description are wanted in my hospital. Food we are scarce of sometimes but it is generally plenty."[74]

With preliminaries out of the way, the New Jersey nurse quickly got down to the heart of her letter—she was ecstatic over a recent award from the soldiers in her care. "I received a few days ago, a silver Medal worth twenty dollars. The inscription on one side is 'Miss Cornelia Hancock, presented by the wounded soldiers 3rd Division 2nd Army Corps.' On the other side is 'Testimonial of regard for ministrations of mercy to the wounded soldiers at Gettysburg, Pa.—July 1863.'"[75]

Not surprisingly, this special recognition caused no little stir in the camp, especially among the other women volunteers. "There have been in the Corps Hospital I suppose some thirty women, and it seems I am the favored one in the lot. Several, since they have seen mine, have started a subscription for two other ladies."[76] Cornelia brushed other opinions aside, and briskly lumped the majority of the volunteer nurses into one unflattering classification: "Most of the ladies are dead heads completely."[77]

Adequate clothing continued to be a problem for all the volunteer staff, both men and women. Most were still wearing the same outfit they had arrived in, and the effects of eating, sleeping, and tending bleeding men with oozing wounds were taking a toll on everyone's wardrobe. "The Steward of our Hospital is a funny fellow; he has gone to New York to take some wounded and says he is going to bring me a calico dress. I have no dress now except what is torn in threads. I sent to Belle to make me a new one and send it to me."[78]

---

73. *Ibid.*, p. 16.
74. *Ibid.*
75. *Ibid.*
76. Nurse Mary Lee would also receive a medal from her patients—this one was gold, handsomely engraved, and in the shape of a trefoil, the Second Corps insignia. One can only imagine Cornelia Hancock's reaction to this news. [Brockett and Vaughn, *Woman's Work in the Civil War*, p. 486.]
77. Hancock, *South After Gettysburg*, p. 16.
78. *Ibid.*

Lest her letter worry her mother in far-off Hancock's Bridge, New Jersey, the young Quakeress was quick to reassure the family of her safety as she closed: "You need not fear for me, I am all right. From thy daughter—C. HANCOCK"[79]

In a postscript, she continues: "I get letters from the soldiers that have left here, but do not get many letters from home. I wish you could see the hospital now; but I would never wish anyone to see a battlefield. I have succeeded in getting the men some beef steak for dinner, which I feel very thankful they are to have. The boys are going out on horse-back this afternoon to try to get some butter. I have written probably as much as is practical.

From thy daughter,

C. HANCOCK"[80]

One such letter received by Cornelia Hancock was signed merely "a Soldier":

> Camp Bradford, Baltimore, Md.
> July 21st, 1863.
>
> TO OUR SOLDIERS' FRIEND, MISS HANCOCK,
>
> You will please excuse a Soldier for writing a few lines to you to express our thankfulness for your kindness to our poor wounded comrades after the late battle. You little know the pleasure a Soldier feels in seeing a woman at camp. I only wish that we were able to express our gratitude in a different manner, but "Uncle Sam" happens to be in debt to us and until he "come down" with his greenbacks we are not able to do any more. You will never be forgotten by us for we often think of your kind acts and remember them with pleasure. Please excuse a Soldier for taking the liberty to write to you, for although we are Soldiers we know how to appreciate a kind act.
>
> Your sincere friend,
> A SOLDIER[81]

---

79. *Ibid.*
80. *Ibid.*, pp. 16-17.
81. *Ibid.*, p. 17.

Meanwhile, in spite of silver medals, admiring letters, and beef steak dinners, men still continued to unobtrusively die from their wounds in the Second Corps Hospital. Emily Bliss Souder noted, almost as an aside, in a letter to her brother: "A man named Crowley, who enlisted at St. Paul, was breathing his last, when we left the camp last evening [Tuesday, July 21]." For these men, the battle still raged, often in the quietness and loneliness of the night.[82]

For friends and loved ones, a new kind of sorrow had now begun. "We learn from one of our undertakers in town, that the number of coffins manufactured here for the transportation of the dead soldiers home by their friends amounts probably to 600 or 700 already," noted the *Adams Sentinel* on July 21, "and we presume this mournful business will be kept up for some time yet."[83]

Wednesday, July 22, 1863

Fatigue, pressure, and unsanitary conditions were beginning to take an inexorable toll on Emily Bliss Souder and her Philadelphia party.

> I remained in town to-day to rest, with the expectation of being able to return to labor in the field tomorrow with renewed strength. The duties here are undoubtedly arduous, and were it not for the special blessings of God, giving needful strength for the hour of necessity, we should have failed at the outset.
>
> Every lady of our party looked sadly worn yesterday, and I am sorry to say that I gave out totally. We purpose hereafter to remain in town alternately, to look after our affairs here, write letters, and visit sick soldiers who are quartered very near us, beside trying to obtain a little rest, which will be, we trust, a great benefit.[84]

Even the male portion of the delegation were suffering ill effects from the dangerous and polluted surroundings. "Mr. Bringhurst called last night to see us. He was sick, and going home. Few persons are able

---

82. Souder, *Leaves from the Battle-Field of Gettysburg*, p. 41. Minnesotan Frederick Crawley was tougher than Emily Bliss Souder imagined—he clung to life for another six days before succumbing to the effects of his wounds.
83. *Adams Sentinel*, July 21, 1863.
84. Souder, *Leaves from the Battle-Field of Gettysburg*, p. 42.

to remain here more than a week. The water has been very bad; the atmosphere shocking. I only wonder how we have borne it."[85]

Rumors floating around camp that the Second Corps Hospital was preparing to move the remaining patients to a location closer to Gettysburg proved to be absolutely correct, for a change.

By July 22, 11,425 wounded had been evacuated by rail from the festering environs of Gettysburg. Of those, 7,608 were Union, and 3,817 Confederate. An additional 4,000 battle casualties were dispatched to Baltimore from temporary hospital facilities in Westminster and Littletown. The remaining 1,995 Northern and 2,922 Southern wounded were still so fragile that it could be fatal to move them any great distance. The massive corps hospitals of a few weeks earlier were now caring for only a few hundred men each, yet every single one was critically wounded.[86]

Doctor Janes and his staff had been at work since July 15, clearing the Wolf Woods site, digging wells and latrines, and pitching hospital, embalming, "dead house," and cook tents. On July 22, the new facility—Camp Letterman General Hospital—was officially opened.

Both Sanitary and Christian Commissions were there on opening day, having set up separate supply facilities, complete with commissioners and delegates, "at the southeast angle" of the new hospital. The Sanitary Commission had "some six or eight" large tents pitched "beneath tall oaks and hickorys." One tent was a "Lodge" for up to thirty people, while the remainder served as "store-tents and offices." This was in addition to a kitchen, which specialized in light diet for the convalescent patients. The Christian Commission's presence was far more modest—"a store tent, a sleeping tent, and an eating tent, with some twelve delegates, formed the Christian Commission establishment at the general field hospital."[87]

With the general hospital now open, Doctor Janes immediately began consolidating the widely scattered hospital sites. It would be a complex operation, involving the methodical evacuation of the few

85. *Ibid.*, p. 44.
86. *OR*, vol. 27, pt. 1, p. 27.
87. Wormeley, *The United States Christian Commission*, p. 145; *The United States Christian Commission for the Army and Navy. For the Year 1863. Second Annual Report*, pp. 84, 85.

remaining Gettysburg hospitals, the Confederate hospitals west of town, and the sprawl of Union corps hospitals to the east.

On July 22, however, as the process was just beginning, all roads seemed to lead east to the Wolf Woods. "A line of stretchers a mile and a half in length . . . told us where lay our work," recalled one volunteer nurse.[88]

Meanwhile, at the Second Corps Hospital, it was business as usual for another day. Although the hospital was daily shrinking in size, it continued to be a mishmash of names, dialects, and hometowns. "Almost every State is represented here, but there are a great number of New York men, many Pennsylvanians, many Minnesotans, many from Maine and Ohio. Our soldiers manifest, almost without exception, a lofty courage and devotion to the cause of our country, which must excite our heartfelt sympathy and admiration."[89]

The tide of visitors had slowly begun to shift from those seeking the living wounded to those searching for burial sites. Family gravesites and burial plots, often many generations old, stood ready to receive many of the fallen soldiers back home, if only their immediate resting place could be discovered. "A constant procession of coffins meets the eye; groups of men, standing in the fields, searching for the name of some friend or brother. The town has been filled with people on these mournful errands."[90]

For those still clinging to life, fresh bandaging and clean clothing continued to be an ongoing need. "No one can estimate the value of pieces of old sheets, or indeed of the smallest rag, who has not been in such a place as this, and the poorest shirt, drawers, or pantaloons, is a real blessing."[91]

Thursday, July 23, 1863

It had been a pleasant interlude in the ceaseless round of agony, humiliation, and dying, but finally the "four gentlemen"—Mr. Souder,

88. Sophronia Bucklin, *In Hospital and Camp: A Woman's Record of Thrilling Incidents among the Wounded in the Late War.* (Philadelphia: John E. Potter and Co., 1869), p. 142.
89. Souder, *Leaves from the Battle-Field of Gettysburg*, p. 51.
90. *Ibid.*, pp. 52-53.
91. *Ibid.*, p. 53.

Mr. Claghorn, Mr. Campion, and Mr. Chaplain—packed their bags, and headed back home to Philadelphia. This freed the ladies to concentrate on the very serious business of moving the hospital. "On Thursday, after the gentlemen left, the camp was changed to another location, better known as 'the clover field,' a change which was very needful on every account."[92]

The move would take all the logistical skills of the entire team of doctors, nurses, aides, soldiers, and volunteers of the hospital. "The move was a very serious matter. It was necessary to carry every man on a stretcher, about a third of a mile. The tents were taken down and moved beforehand."[93]

Needful or not, the thought of actually being picked up and physically toted across uneven terrain to a man whose leg or arm stump could hemorrhage at the least jostle was terrifying. "It was pitiful to see the faces of many of these men, who feared and dreaded to be moved, and yet exhibited a degree of fortitude which was truly wonderful. A Massachusetts boy, with a mischief-loving eye, amused me by his remark, that 'he wished he had only lost a toe, so that he would not have to carry any more men over the run.' I told him we would call for Doctor Hayward directly (a Boston surgeon), and have it taken off."[94]

The move was carried off smoothly, with no reports of any patient suffering complications as the result. With everyone safely transferred to the new site, Emily Bliss Souder surveyed the new location. "The hospital is now located on a beautiful ridge, open to the sun and air, and forms a hollow square. The ladies' tents are in a little hollow, among the trees. It is a lovely spot. A bright stream flows close to the encampment, and the water is good. The former encampment was shaded with forest trees, which prevented the sun and wind from exerting their purifying influences."[95]

The necessity of moving the hospital had been a growing concern of the doctors and nursing staff for some time. "While the hospital remained in the *woods*, the number of deaths daily was very large; as soon as the removal to the clover-field was accomplished, where all were in the sun, the change for the better was very decided; the night after, only two deaths occurred."[96]

---

92. *Ibid.*, p. 56.
93. *Ibid.*
94. *Ibid.*, pp. 56-57.
95. *Ibid.*, p. 57.
96. Holstein, *Three Years in Field Hospitals*, p. 42.

With the hospital safely relocated, it was back to ministering to the wounded.

> A friend sent me a bottle, containing some preparation considered valuable for dressing a wound, directed to a member of the Seventy-third Reg., Third Division, Second Corps.[97] I went to a tent of the Third Division and inquired if any one in the tent belonged to that regiment.
>
> A pleasant-faced young man, lying on the front stretcher, promptly answered, "Yes."
>
> "What is his name?" said I.
>
> He gave me his own name, Joseph K-----, the very person I was looking for.[98]

The consolidation of patients at the new Camp Letterman General Hospital was now in full swing, under the keen eye of Surgeon Henry Janes. On July 23, Surgeon William F. Norris of the First Corps was ordered to move all of his patients from the Catholic Church and all other scattered locations to the new hospital grounds. By 7:00 p.m., Norris was pleased to report that all of his patients had made the move, many of them making the trip on hand-carried stretchers.[99]

Friday, July 24, 1863

It was becoming increasingly evident to some of the surgeons, now that there was sufficient time to reflect upon the events of the last several weeks, that the magnitude of what had been accomplished medically at the Second Corps Hospital had been a team effort, blending the surgical skills of the medical staff with the logistical acumen of many volunteer agencies. Surgeon Harry McAbee of the Third Division was particularly impressed with the efforts of the Christian Commission, and had written them a cordial note of thanks:

---

97. There is no 73rd Regiment in the Third Division, nor in the entire Second Corps.
98. Souder, *Leaves from the Battle-Field of Gettysburg*, pp. 57-58.
99. William F. Norris, "A Hospital at Gettysburg," *The General Magazine and Historical Chronicle*, vol. 45 (1942-43): 39-40.

Hospital, Third Division, Second Corps,
Near Gettysburg, Pa., July 15, 1863.
Messrs. Stillson, Adams, Fields, and Others of the Christian Commission.
Gentlemen:

Please allow me to say that the society which you represent more than earned a right to the title it has assumed, in the work it did at Gettysburg for the wounded of this Division. The supplies of food and clothing furnished were wisely selected, and generously and judiciously distributed, and the agents sent, by the manliness of their bearing, the unpretending devotion with which they gave themselves to the work, and the Christian-like deportment which characterized their conduct throughout, stamped them as being eminently fitted for the work of faith and labor of love to which they had been assigned.

Such laborers will always be welcome where large-hearted, true men are needed.

H. M. McAbee,
Surgeon in charge.[100]

Although Civil War relief agencies altruistically existed to provide benevolence and care to the men of the military, they drew their operational funds from the no-nonsense world of politics and commerce. One letter of commendation went a long way toward ensuring continued funding. However, the possibility of additional recommendations from the Second Corps Hospital must have certainly niggled at "Messrs. Stillson, Adams, Fields, and Others," for, a week later, a letter, on Christian Commission letterhead, arrived at the Second Corps Hospital:

Office U. S. Christian Commission,
Gettysburg, July 22d, 1863.
Dr. Dwinell,[101] Surgeon in charge 2d Corps Hosp.
Dear Sir,

It would be gratifying to the United States Christian Commission to have the testimony of yourself and your

---

100. *The United States Christian Commission for the Army and Navy. For the Year 1863. Second Annual Report*, p. 72.

101. Capital "D" written over "G" in misspelled "Gwinell."

associate Surgeons with reference to the work of the Commission in your Corps Hospital.

Thanking you most heartily in the name of the Commission for your many favours toward us in the work of relieving the wants of the soldiers, I remain

Very Respectfully yours,

F. E. Shearer,

Agent U.S.C.C.[102]

Surgeon Dwinelle was indeed willing to send off a testimonial from himself and his associates. Now that he was freed from the crushing weight of thousands of casualties waiting for treatment, the surgeon-in-charge promptly penned a reply:

Headquarters Second Corps Hospital

July 24, 1863.

F. E. Shearer,

Agent United States Christian Commission.

Sir: It affords us pleasure to bear testimony to the noble work of the United States Christian Commission in affording timely and substantial relief to the physical and religious wants of the wounded and dying soldiers of this corps since the battle of Gettysburg. A vast aggregate of suffering has been relieved, and no doubt many lives saved.

JUSTIN DWINELLE,

Surgeon in charge.

NATHAN HAYWARD,

Surgeon Twentieth Massachusetts Volunteers.

WM. J. BURN[*sic*],

Surgeon Forty-second Massachusetts Volunteers[*sic*][103]

F. F. BURMEISTER,

Surgeon Sixty-ninth Regiment Penna. Volunteers

---

102. Union Field Hospitals Vertical File, Gettysburg National Military Park Library.

103. William J. Burr was actually surgeon of the 42nd New York Volunteers.

E. DAY,
Surgeon Thirty-ninth Regiment N. Y. Volunteers,
in charge Third Division, Second Army Corps.

CHARLES T. KELSEY,
Surgeon in charge First Division, Second Army Corps.

A. STOKES JONES,
Asst. Surgeon Seventy-second Regiment Penna. Volunteers.

H. C. LEVENSALERS,
Assist. Surgeon Nineteenth Regiment Maine Volunteers.

T. O. CORNISH,
Assist. Surgeon Fifteenth Massachusetts Volunteers.[104]

"Capt. Nickerson is some better, and there is some hopes of his recovery."[105] So wrote Hospital Steward Charles Merrick before he set off for his regiment on July 15. But now, nine days later, while the remaining Second Corps surgeons were busy endorsing a letter of commendation to the Christian Commission with their signatures, Nickerson still lingered perilously close to death. "When I entered upon the third week of my enforced detention I began to have a great longing to be removed to my native State. The surgeons held a consultation and concluded that the change could not materially hasten or delay what appeared to them to be the inevitable. So they promised me that if, at the end of the next week, I was alive they would give their consent to my removal."[106]

With the death of his Indiana drinking companion, Nickerson clung to that slim medical promise like a drowning man to a life preserver. "The agents of the Christian Commission had hung upon the wall of the tent facing me a calendar, or scroll, underneath each date of which were inscribed in large type numbers of texts or passages of the Scriptures supposed to be suited to the reader, the time, and place.

104. *The United States Christian Commission for the Army and Navy. For the Year 1863. Second Annual Report*, p. 88.
105. Charles H. Merrick, Letter to his wife, Dr. Myra H. Merrick, July 15, 1863.
106. Nickerson, "Personal Recollections of Two Visits to Gettysburg," p. 25.

Immediately on the doctors giving me the above-mentioned promise, this calendar assumed an interest which no other calendar, before or since, has ever attained."[107]

The minutes of each day dragged by with agonizing sluggishness. Nickerson willed himself to survive each passing hour. The Ohio captain turned every ounce of his remaining stamina to one single goal: living through another day. Time hung particularly heavily as darkness finally settled over the camp. "From ten to twelve o'clock each night I do not think that five minutes were allowed to pass without my asking whoever was attending me, the hour; and before the words announcing the departure of the old day were fairly out of his mouth I begged him to 'please turn down that date.'"[108]

Saturday, July 25, 1863

Saturday was a busy day for Jane Boswell Moore and her mother. In a report to the Baltimore Christian Commission, Miss Moore outlined their day's activities in the rebel wards of the Second Corps Hospital.

"In the morning we rode to town in an ambulance to procure some stores, and on our return visited the thirteen tents entrusted to our care. These contain some sixty or seventy wounded rebels now in separate tents, for though we of course would have preferred ministering to our own men, still owing to this preference on the part of many, there was a certainty they would suffer, we were quite willing to attend to them."[109]

Nor could the two ladies have found a more appreciative group of men to attend to.

> And grateful suffering creatures we found them; many say that our kindness has done more to subjugate them than all the shells and balls that have been fired during the war,—they never expected such treatment, and have not the heart to raise a hand against us.
>
> Only a few days after the battle, one who had laid out in the storm told us that he would never forget our kindness; "and," said he, "if I only know how to keep from going into the army again, I would not go."

---

107. *Ibid.*
108. *Ibid.*
109. Moore, "Letter From Gettysburg," in the "Our Country" column, *Lutheran Observer*, August 21, 1863.

I answered that he could readily avoid it by taking the oath, and remaining within our lines. "But," said he, "then in sixty days I would be taken into your army, and seeing there is no escape, I might as well fight with my own people as not, though if I could, I would give up fighting altogether."

I told him that I was not aware of any such fact, nor did it exist, on which he and his neighbor were very much astonished, the one remarking, "You see, Jim, they tell us whatever suits their purpose."

A North Carolinian said, I would hardly believe him if he were to tell me all he had undergone. But with little to eat, he had to march hard and fight hard, tramp twenty to thirty miles, with no rations but a few crackers. Officers were so tyrannical, they would not even allow them to take a drink as they ran along.

I remarked, "Were they afraid you would desert?"

"Yes, I suppose so.—This was the worst whipping we ever got; Antietam was bad, but nothing like this. Plenty of us wanted to desert then as we were coming into Maryland, but they told us the bushes were full of Yankees who were waiting to shoot us, and would not show us a bit of mercy, but cut us right down."

"Did you not know that some of your companions got away?"

"Yes, we knew that a good many left us as we came over the mountain, but we never heard of them, and thought they had been shot."

Wishing to keep up their spirits, I remarked playfully to one, "How foolish it is in me to be feeding you and strengthening you to fight us again?"

"Well, if [we] do," rejoined one, "I'll do it on one leg."—Another said, "Don't blame us. War is not what it is cracked up to be. We did not want to come, but it wasn't for *us* to say whether we would stay or come."[110]

Anxious visitors continued to swarm through the camp, peering apprehensively into hospital tents, asking doctors, nurses, provost guard, and Commission agents, over and over again, the location of some soldier husband, son, or father. "Nearly every day wives,

110. *Ibid.*

mothers, sisters and friends visit the hospital for the purpose of finding the graves and bodies of their loved ones who have fallen in the strife, so that our sympathies are not only enlisted for the wounded and suffering, but also in behalf of their sorrowing friends. The other evening a lady came in search of her husband, but she was too late, as he was dead. 'OH,' she said, with tearful eyes, 'he talked so of me and his little lame girl.'"[111]

A second wave of relatives were now arriving, these from the farthest corners of the Union. Hindered by the vast distances to be covered, and by unexpected delays along the way, lone women and huddled family groups came from the timber country of Minnesota and the distant Wisconsin frontier. Others came from remote seacoast villages and rural hamlets of Rhode Island, New Hampshire, Vermont, and Maine. "A perfectly girlish woman came all the way from Maine on a three days' fruitless journey, the New York rioters having cut the telegraph wires, so that the second dispatch announcing his death did not reach her. And now, on her return, she was dreading to meet his aged, poor and feeble parents. His father was scarcely able, from rheumatism, to carry his food to his mouth, and his mother had never recovered from injuries received from being thrown from a wagon. She said the Maine women would be out to help with the soldiers but they were so far away, and the newspaper accounts were very different from reality.—In the little village where she lived they had raised since the battle eleven hundred dollars."[112]

Two days after helping the hospital to relocate, Jane Boswell Moore was well pleased with the new site, convinced that it was "much more healthy and pleasant. The tents extend round the edges of a beautiful clover field, a little below which, in a grove near a brook, are the tents of the Commission and numerous other parties. Just at present, as the cool air is surging delightfully through the trees, the view presented to our gaze is a very pretty one. In front is the waving clover still wet with last night's rain, and the white sun-lit tents relieving a background of dark gray clouds. In the distance looms the summit of Round Top, the frightful rocky position whose strength gained the day for our forces. Their graves are thickly strewn, but many an unburied form is stretched on the rocks and near the brook."[113]

---

111. *Ibid.*
112. *Ibid.*
113. *Ibid.*

Dr. Theodore Dimon had been hard at work, tirelessly trying to fulfill all the aspects of his difficult commission from the State of New York. Thankfully, he had secured some very powerful allies along the way: "Every possible aid was rendered by the United States Medical Inspector, Dr. Cuyler and Director Janes; by Dr. Brenton and quarter-master Rankin and others. The Sanitary and Christian Commission and Adams' Express honored all orders upon them for such articles as they had, and without them our labor would have availed little." On a more personal note: "I was greatly aided by the Rev. David Swope, from Livingston County New York, who was here doing Christian service, and also by the State Couriers, Messrs. Dunlevy, McMahon and McCluskey, who were very diligent and efficient in their attention to our soldiers, and who as soon as the arrangements were perfected for sending our soldiers to the New York City General Hospitals, accompanied them on the trains thither."[114]

Word of his inspection tour spread rapidly through each hospital he visited, and New Yorkers flocked to meet him. He and his team were impressed with "their patient and cheerful endurance of suffering as they lay wounded at our feet; even while the tide of life was rapidly ebbing, they would rise on their blankets, their countenances brightening with delight, when told that they were remembered at home, and their bravery appreciated by a grateful people."[115]

"New York had between 60 and 70 regiments at Gettysburg," according to Dimon's figures, not counting artillery outfits. The Second Corps alone had sixteen regiments and two battalions of New Yorkers, and Dimon was anxious to check on their condition. Although it is unclear as to when he reached the Second Corps Hospitals, his report seems to indicate that it was sometime shortly after the move to the clover field on Thursday, July 23.[116]

Dimon demonstrated an excellent understanding of the hospitals' history and movements. He related, in some detail, how the hospital had been shelled out of its Taneytown Road locations back to the lowlands along Rock Creek, and then the emergency move to the heights of the Schwartz property during the flooding.[117]

---

114. Dimon, *Report of the General Agent of the State of New York*, pp. 43, 56.
115. *Ibid.*, p. 44.
116. *Ibid.*, pp. 44, 53.
117. *Ibid.*, pp. 52-53.

The First and Second Divisions had been set up on a wooded hill, while the Third Division had established their hospital on "an open will [*sic*] half a mile further south." At the northern location, Dimon had found "a number of members of the Christian Commission encamped, as also a number of women engaged in cooking for, and nursing the wounded. Large quantities of stores from the Sanitary Commission, Adams' Express Company, hospital wagons laden with supplies, and every effort being made to alleviate the condition of the suffering soldiers."[118]

Despite high marks in supplies and nursing, Dimon was highly critical of where the First and Second Divisions had been encamped. "The location of this hospital was not the most desirable. The trees kept out the sun and obstructed the circulation of the air. The space was too small, rendering it necessary to crowd the tents and narrow the streets, and the ground continued wet after the rains. Eventually, from these causes, the wounds began to assume unpleasant appearances."[119]

Fortunately, Doctor Dwinelle and staff had been aware of the same concerns, and had already moved the two divisions to "an open grassy slope, and the three Divisions united on the three sides of this slope, with abundant space between the tents, the Confederate wounded being also removed to the same locality. Speedy and manifest improvement in the condition of the wounds took place after this removal."[120]

Dimon diligently met and questioned New York patients, and mingled with New York staff and volunteers; only after first-hand investigation was Doctor Dimon ready to give his official verdict of the quality of medical care being offered at the Second Corps Hospitals. "I cannot help expressing my commendation of Surgeon Dwinelle in charge of the wounded of this Corps. Though encountering embarrassments and difficulties, unusual even in the vast number of casualties falling upon all the Corps of this Army from the battle, yet he failed not to meet and remedy each difficulty as it arose, with untiring patience and determined perseverance, never resting with the excuse that 'he was doing the best he could,' while any thing better was possible. The large number of New Yorkers wounded in this Corps

---

118. *Ibid.*, p. 53.
119. *Ibid.*
120. *Ibid.*

were in good hands." High praise indeed from a government fact-finder.[121]

As the workload slackened at the hospital, Jane Boswell Moore and her mother had opportunity to finally visit the battlefield. What they saw there sickened and sobered them, especially along the Second Corps lines. "We walk along the low stone wall or breastwork, which stretches across a wide plain, and feel that we walk here in safety, only because our men stood their ground, even though the foe leaped the wall and seized their guns, *they stood their ground indeed.* But the hillock of graves—the little forest of head boards scattered everywhere, and there over that field, the piles of empty haversacks, the caps and blue coats everywhere, and the guns used by hands now cold in death, seem to tell with mute eloquence at what awful price Maryland and Pennsylvania were redeemed!"[122]

The heavy rains that had flooded the hospital out of the Rock Creek floodplain had eroded the shallow Confederate mass graves; now a phantom army was emerging by degrees from their unhappy resting places. "Two immense trenches filled with rebel dead, and surrounded with grey caps, attest the cost to them. The earth is scarcely thrown over them, and skulls with ghastly grinning teeth appear, now that the few spadefuls of earth are washed away. In these trenches one may plainly see the rise and swell of human bodies; and *oh* how awful to feel that these are brethren—deluded and erring, yet brethren. Surely, no punishment can be too great for those, whose mad ambition has filled these graves! Very respectfully yours, Jane Boswell Moore."[123]

Sunday, July 26, 1863

As the closing of the Second Corps Hospital approached, the supply situation took a turn for the worse. The belt-tightening measures of the Sanitary Commission to "take in sail," as per Doctor Agnew's July 16 dispatch, had taken over a week to filter down to the level of the field hospitals.

121. *Ibid.*, pp. 53-54.
122. Moore, "Letter From Gettysburg."
123. *Ibid.*

Cornelia Hancock was up early. After checking her patients, she sat herself down with paper and pen to organize her thoughts:

> MY DEAR MOTHER, Today is Sunday but there is no semblance of it here. It is now about five o'clock in the morning. Our hospital has been moved and our stores are given out. There is nothing to cook with, hence I have nothing to do, and therefore, have time to write. Such days will come here that we have to see our wounded men fed with dry bread and poor coffee; and I can tell you it is hard to witness some cursing for food, some praying for it.
>
> All the luxuries that the men get come through the Christian Commission, Sanitary, Ladies Aid, etc. I would give anything to have a barrel of butter, and some dried rusk that I have seen in our parlor. I wish you would get up something of the kind and have Mrs. Jones requested to forward it to me. I should think it would be as satisfactory for *me* to have them as for them to be sown broadcast on the land. I could make a report of everything received and write to the Society.[124]

But even though troubled by shortages of food and supplies, Cornelia could not contain her excitement about how *her* soldiers had honored her. Although she had described it in detail in her Tuesday letter, she carefully recounted the details to her mother once again. "I received a silver medal from the soldiers which cost twenty dollars. I know what thee will say—that the money could have been *better* laid out. It was very complimentary though. One of the soldiers has a sword that he found on the battlefield, which he is going to give to me before I come home. If they were only where they could buy I should be so loaded with baggage, I should never be able to get home."[125]

Even though somewhat giddy over the honor bestowed on her, she was all business when it came to the well-being of the wounded men entrusted to her care. "I shall not come home, unless I get sick, while this hospital lasts. I have two men detailed to wait on me, which suits of course. They are now fixing up nice little tables and all such things all around the tent. I have eight wall tents full of amputated men. The tents of the wounded I look right out on—it is a melancholy sight, but you

124. Hancock, *South After Gettysburg*, pp. 17-18.
125. *Ibid.*, p. 18.

have no idea how soon one gets used to it. Their screams of agony do not make as much impression on me now as the reading of this letter will on you."[126]

As visitors poured into the hospital compound, the staff faced the difficult challenge of balancing patient care with offering what limited amenities were at their disposal to each friend and relative that arrived. "The most painful task we have to perform here, is entertaining the friends who come from home and see their friends all mangled up. I do hate to see them. Soldiers take everything as it comes, but citizens are not inured."[127]

No doubt concerned about distorted or misleading reports filtering from the field and into hometown newspapers, Cornelia added a final reassurance of her welfare, although her mother probably drew scant encouragement from the candid details. "You will think it is a short time for me to get used to things, but it seems to me as if all my past life was a myth, and as if I had been away from home seventeen years. What I do here one would think would kill at home, but I am well and comfortable. When we get up early in the morning, our clothes are so wet we could wring them. On they go, and by noon they are dry. From thy affectionate daughter—C. Hancock"[128]

Monday, July 27, 1863

As the Second Corps Hospital continued to dwindle, and as the voracious draw on the supply depots of the Sanitary Commission and the Christian Commission slackened, the commissioners looked for other creative ways to encourage the wounded men in their slow recovery. One foursome developed a daily ritual that proved to be a camp favorite to both patients and staff alike.

"After the wounded were moved to the wheat field [July 23], four men of the Sanitary Commission went among the 600 men every night, singing their favorite hymns." Never one to be shy, Clarissa Fellows Jones joined in with these twilight serenades. "I always went with them and led the singing. My voice was clear and strong then," she would recall fifty years later, "and, beside, I was accustomed to leading my boys in school."[129]

---

126. *Ibid.*
127. *Ibid.*
128. *Ibid.*, pp. 18-19.
129. Jones, "Nursed the Confederates at Gettysburg," p. 4.

Every night was Request Night, and the wounded men reveled in having even the slightest bit of control over their surroundings. Invariably, the songs were not the bawdy ballads and patriotic rabble-rousers sung around regimental campfires, but instead the sweet modest melodies sung in churches and parlors back home. "For the Union men we sang 'Sweet Hour of Prayer.'"[130] Mrs. Hanness' evening serenades had certainly produced quite a following among the hardened Northerners.

"But the Confederates always wanted their old plantation hymn. Every night, when we asked 'What will it be tonight, boys?' the answer always was 'Oh, Sing to Me of Heaven.' It was a beautiful hymn and the first stanza began 'Oh, sing to me of Heaven, when I am called to die.' The chorus went:

There'll be no more sorrow there,
In Heaven above where all is love,
There'll be no more sorrow there.'"[131]

And as the sun slowly sank beyond the Round Tops, with the cicadas and crickets taking up the refrain, men who had given every ounce of energy to killing each other just a fortnight before now closed their eyes, and, if just for a moment, were safely home again with family and friends, and far from the sounds and smells of a corps hospital.

Tuesday, July 28, 1863

Emily Bliss Souder's health continued to deteriorate in the tainted air of Gettysburg.

> I have not been well enough for two or three days to go to the field. On Sunday, I was really sick all day and the greater part of yesterday.
>
> This morning I thought I would ride to the Seminary hospital and see what was wanted there, for our stores seem like the widow's cruse, always being replenished, and we all look much the worse for our experiences. I don't know what Sarah may decide to do, but our little company will probably depart Thursday.
>
> After leaving the Seminary, I paid a visit to the Sanitary Commission tent, near the railroad. I wanted some brandy for

130. *Ibid.*
131. *Ibid.*

an Ohio soldier, who was lying very near death, directly opposite our boardinghouse. It was given me in an oddly shaped bottle, which I intend to preserve as a memento. They gave me also a couple of cans of condensed milk, which was all I could manage. I had the most melancholy-looking vehicle and the most miserable horse that ever were seen in a civilized country, and the little boy who drove had hard work to get over the ground at all.[132]

The Christian Commission was beginning to phase out the Commission Stations at the corps hospitals, preparatory to downsizing their operation. "When the several field hospitals were finally merged in the general field hospital, the special field organization of the Christian Commission was broken up. . . . July 28th, about the time of our removal to the General Hospital, a district committee was chosen . . . to look after the interests of the Commission in Gettysburg and that vicinity, and to decide cases of difficulty which might arise."[133]

As to the downtown supply depot, "the two extensive stores of which we have before spoken, were occupied till the general Hospital was established, when we pitched our tents there, and removing the greater part of the Commission's property thither, made arrangements for religious services, and with the consent and approval of the surgeon in charge, continued to labor in our appropriate sphere, till the necessity for such labor no longer existed."[134]

Wednesday, July 29, 1863

The transfer of the wounded from the corps hospitals to Camp Letterman General Hospital was steadily gaining momentum. "The sick have been removed from several of the churches, and the process of purifying is going on very energetically. The Third and Fifth Corps are being brought into the General Hospital, which is near the railroad. The Twelfth Corps is entirely removed; the Eleventh nearly so." The

---

132. Souder, *Leaves from the Battle-Field of Gettysburg*, pp. 58, 59-60.

133. *The United States Christian Commission for the Army and Navy. For the Year 1863. Second Annual Report*, pp. 85, 80.

134. *Ibid.*, p. 80.

Second Corps Hospital, with its larger numbers and high proportion of grievously wounded men, was going to take a little longer.[135]

Everyone—from doctors to drivers to the horses—were working long and hard to get the patients moved as rapidly and as safely as possible. "The ambulances and litters are constantly passing through the town. This morning, the poor wearied horses attached to the ambulance refused to carry their burden up Cemetery Hill, and we alighted and walked quite a distance toward the camp."[136]

It was quite a walk from the corps hospitals, especially for those carrying the deadweight of a severely injured soldier. Only the most critically wounded were carried by stretcher; all others were sent by ambulance. Consequently, frequent rest stops were necessary for everyone concerned. "We passed several litters, the bearers and the wounded soldiers all resting a little by the way. Several of them offered us flowers that they had gathered in some demolished garden."

"As we received them I said, '*Your* garlands shall be green, and they shall last forever."

"One of the number responded with deep feeling, 'They ought to be, ma'am. We have worked hard enough for them.'"[137]

Another reason for the overworked condition of ambulances and their crews was discovered late in the day after the delegation from Philadelphia reached the Second Corps Hospital at the Schwartz Farm. "We learn this evening that the ambulances are all ordered to join the regiments to which they belong. At all events, the Second Corps is being moved to the General Hospital with all convenient dispatch."[138]

And even that was not all. "Dr. Duinelle [*sic*] said that the surgeons were wanted with their regiments, which made concentration necessary. One hundred men, he said, could not be moved for two weeks. I think Sarah will go to the General Hospital, and would like to see her settled there, with some one to aid her. We do not feel satisfied to leave her alone."[139]

And still the grieving women came, now mostly from the distant states. "We found today a kind woman from Minnesota, Mrs. Milliken, attending to several fellows from that State. I received a note from ----, this afternoon. Mrs. Waterman we have not yet seen, but will inquire for her to-morrow."

---

135. Souder, *Leaves from the Battle-Field of Gettysburg*, pp. 61-62.
136. *Ibid.*, p. 62.
137. *Ibid.*
138. *Ibid.*, p. 61.
139. *Ibid.*

"I have just returned from the hospital. . . . To-night, I have a telegram. 'All well at Cape May.'" Emily Bliss Souder's family had finally packed up on their own, and headed off to their seashore retreat.[140]

"I wrote you yesterday that we should be ready to go home to-morrow; but our visit to the battle-field has been postponed, and a heavy rain to-night, I am afraid, will prevent us to-morrow. . . . I hope to hear from home to-morrow. Good night. E.B.S."[141]

Thursday, July 30, 1863

Dr. Theodore Dimon had finished his exhaustive, and unusually exhausting, survey of the Union hospitals treatment of New Yorkers. He offered his final report to his superior, John F. Seymour, General Agent of the State of New York. "I am happy to state that, while acting as Special Agent of our State, I discovered no instance of neglect of our wounded by the medical officers in charge of them. On the contrary, any proper suggestion from me was met with ready assent on the part of these officers, with thanks for the assistance thus afforded them."[142]

But Doctor Dimon was still troubled by one thing: "I was constantly solicited for pecuniary aid in the expense attending the exhumation, disinfecting, coffining and transportation of our dead soldiers to their former homes." Pennsylvania was furnishing free transportation of her dead patriots, but it was exorbitantly expensive to ship bodies all the way to distant New York.[143]

Before packing his bags for the trip back east, Dimon came up with an novel idea to help save the cost and still give New Yorkers, and men from all loyal states, the honor that they so richly deserved. If the government could bring a general hospital to the battlefield, why not a national cemetery as well? "It occurred to me as practicable to have a piece of ground purchased for a burial place on or near the battlefield, to which the dead bodies of all our soldiers should be removed and there buried by regiments and states and their graves permanently marked. David Wills, Esq., the agent of Pennsylvania, heartily

140. *Ibid.*, p. 65.
141. *Ibid.*, pp. 61, 63.
142. Dimon, *Report of the General Agent of the State of New York*, pp. 56-57.
143. Dimon, *From Auburn to Antietam.*

approved the project and we both addressed the Governors of Pennsylvania and New York on the subject."[144]

Finally, with all the loose ends tied up, "our wounded having been reduced in numbers here by transportation to the Eastern general hospitals and a temporary general hospital having been established at Gettysburg to provide for the rest, there seemed to be no great need of my remaining longer and I accordingly returned to New York."[145]

Friday, July 31, 1863

July 31. Just another hazy, hot day for the few remaining patients and staff at the Second Corps Hospital. But to Capt. Azor Nickerson, given up for dead by the surgical staff, the end of July meant his promised release from the hospital, and a trip home. "Finally, on the last of the month, two attendants placed me on a stretcher, and while my father held an umbrella over me to keep off the rays of the mid-summer sun, they carried me to the village."[146]

The day was quite warm, and the hike of several miles, while carrying a loaded stretcher, began to tell on the men entrusted with gently transporting Captain Nickerson to the railroad station. "On entering the town we passed a large brick house that stood flush with the sidewalk, along which was a row of beautiful maples. Under the shade of the thick foliage the stretcher bearers set me down for a few minutes' rest."[147]

Amazingly, even after the mad inundation of wounded men had stretched Gettysburg and its residents to the maximum, the passage of one wounded man was still able to move the hearts of local residents. "The little procession attracted the attention of the occupants of the house, and a young lady, accosting my father from one of the upper windows, asked if I would not like a luncheon. The offer was made in such sympathetic tones that I felt a refusal would cause actual pain to the lady tendering the hospitality, so I accepted."[148]

With August just around the corner, the kitchen larders of Gettysburg were just beginning to be stocked, largely due to the

---

144. *Ibid.* Doctor Dimon would formally submit this idea in writing to Agent Seymour on August 1, 1863.

145. *Ibid.*

146. Nickerson, "Personal Recollections of Two Visits to Gettysburg," pp. 25-26.

147. *Ibid.*, p. 26.

148. *Ibid.*

largess of the many volunteer agencies funneling supplies into the shattered town, and the generosity of out-of-town friends. "While the dainty little spread was being prepared, the windows of the lower story, or parlor, were thrown open, another exceedingly attractive young lady appeared, and I had the first chat with a lady, in a real house, I had been privileged to enjoy for many a weary month."[149]

Even in the midst of mass devastation, social consciousness and mores still held sway. "When I had finished so much of the delicious repast as I was able to do, we exchanged visiting cards, and the young ladies presented me with an exquisite national flag about two inches in length by half an inch in width. I still retain this little emblem among the most cherished mementoes of my first visit to Gettysburg."[150]

Then the stretcher-bearers picked up the litter, and made their way down to the train station. It would be a long trip home for the Buckeye captain, still weak from his wounds. But by raw determination, a pictorial calendar, two bottles of wine, and a dying friend, Capt. Azor Nickerson had somehow managed to survive his first visit to Gettysburg, Pennsylvania.

Saturday, August 1—Saturday, August 8, 1863

The new general hospital, located within sight of Gettysburg, was now up and running full bore. Dr. Cyrus N. Chamberlain, the surgeon-in-charge of the new facility, christened Camp Letterman in honor of the Army of the Potomac Medical Director Jonathan Letterman.

The hospital quickly became a model of the best in clean, sanitary, and modern hospitals (by 1863 standards). Tents were pitched in double rows, about ten feet apart, each group of four tents in the rows designated as individual wards. The large hospital tents housed ten men each, and a Sibley camp stove kept the tents warm as the intense heat of summer slowly faded to the brisk evenings of autumn.

Dr. Henry Janes immediately found himself under intense pressure by local residents to move the few remaining patients out of public buildings—and the sooner, the better. The local school board wrote on August 4: "There is no building in the town whose use for this purpose could work as much public inconvenience. By its occupying, not only are all our teachers (most of whom are in dependent circumstances) thrown out of employment, but all the children of the borough,

149. *Ibid.*
150. *Ibid.*

numbering four hundred, are thrown upon the streets and deprived of school privileges."[151]

The Lutheran Seminary penned a similar letter, anxious to be able to paint and thoroughly clean the school building before the fall term began. When they discovered, however, that Janes planned to keep some of the most critically wounded out at the school, the irate seminary board fired off an incensed communiqué to the surgeon general's office.

The harried Gettysburg medical director received a harsh letter from Washington, D.C. by return mail: "It is reported that there is much sickness at the Seminary Hospital at Gettysburg owing to the proximity of bodies improperly buried. You will please report the facts of the case at once and take such action as may be most proper to remedy the evil, reporting your actions also." It was, in thinly disguised words, an eviction notice, brought about by the Lutheran Seminary board's continued pressure on the surgeon general's office.[152]

A compromise was finally reached between the feuding parties—Janes would have the grounds cleared of all wounded by August 30.[153]

The overwhelming desire to return to normalcy was evident elsewhere. The Fahnestock brothers wanted their store back—could the Sanitary Commission please vacate the premises as soon as possible? The Commission declined at first, but were eventually compelled to move their operations, ending up directly across the Diamond once again from the Christian Commission. Since the Christian Commission was in the midst of moving their entire operations out to Camp Letterman, downtown traffic snarled in the ensuing congestion as one Commission moved in while another moved out.

Even the army added ever-increasing pressure on Surgeon Janes to expedite the move of the wounded to Letterman General Hospital. They wanted their surgeons back. A month should have been sufficient for the medical mop-up around Gettysburg, reasoned the army brass.

The surgeons, assistant surgeons, and what few hospital stewards and chaplains remained, were also anxious to be on their way. Any mail

---

151. Henry Janes File, Medical Officers Files, Record Group 94, National Archives and Records Administration, Washington D.C.

152. J. R. Smith, Letter to Henry Janes, August 25, 1863, Office of the Surgeon General, Letters and Endorsements Sent to Medical Officers, Volume 4, Record Group 112, National Archives and Records Administration.

153. *Ibid.*

from home followed their regiment, rather than being shunted to the detached medical staff. A month was a long, lonely time without a mail call, or the companionship of regimental friends and messmates. A growing restiveness could be felt in the surgeons' quarters at the Second Corps hospitals each night.

Anna Holstein had made the move to Letterman Hospital; so had Cornelia Hancock, accompanying some of "her boys" from the Second Corps, Third Division Hospital. On August 6th, she sat down to update her sister on her new situation: "MY DEAR SISTER, We have all our men moved now to General Hospital. I am there, too, but the order in regard to women nurses has yet to be issued, and I do not know what my fate will be; I only know that the boys want me to stay very much."[154]

As to nursing assignment, Cornelia Hancock had fared quite well. "I have been assigned to ward E. It is a great deal nicer here except that I have but fourteen of my old boys which is very trying—it is just like parting with part of one's family. I go see the boys and some of them cry that I cannot stay. I have the first four tents abreast of the cook house, and the handiest tents in the whole hospital. I have Steward Olmstead for my *headquarter influence*, and we have an elderly doctor for our ward. I have a large hospital tent and sleep with three other ladies, so unless I struggle very hard to find it my friends need fear no harm for me. I am better than I am at home. I feel so good when I wake up in the morning."[155]

With the return to a more civilized lifestyle, her thoughts turned once again to the conventional amenities of society. "I do want my watch very much indeed; if you can get any show of a safe way of sending it—do so; I want my own gold one. I expect I shall be able to draw twelve dollars from the government now, but if thee can draw any money for hospital purposes or for me, send it along, for it is a poor place to be without money. If there should be an opportunity to send my purple dress, best bonnet and mantilla, I should like to have them; this hospital will not stay here more than three weeks and nobody

154. Hancock, *South After Gettysburg*, p. 19.
155. *Ibid.*

knows what I may want to do by that time. I may come home if there is no other battle."[156]

Her unstinting efforts at the Second Corps Hospital had not gone unnoticed. "Dr. Dwinelle gave me a splendid recommendation to Dr. Chamberlain, Surgeon in charge here. I am good friends with Sanitary, Christian, and all here, if it only lasts."[157]

Men still struggled with their wounds, and most were steadily improving. But the dying continued; slower, to be sure, than in the bloody aftermath of the battle, but still a constant possibility, even at the shiny new general hospital. "One of the boys died yesterday, and one had his leg amputated fresh.[158]

The Provost Guard at Letterman were a different breed than at the Second Corps Hospitals, and Cornelia quickly ran afoul of their soldierly discipline. "No citizens are allowed in Camp without a pass only after four o'clock. The militia go around after dark and pick up stragglers to take them out of camp. The other night they asked me if I was a detailed nurse. As it was before I was sworn in, I had to say 'No.' They said their orders were peremptory, so I would have to go, but Steward Olmstead appeared and told them that I was all right, so they went away. I expect I shall be in the guard house!—but that is only a part of soldiering if I am."[159]

The new setting posed a whole new set of relationships, and Cornelia was struggling to fit in, especially with other volunteer nurses. "I do not meddle or make up with anyone here but the ward master, doctor of our ward and Steward Olmstead. We have twenty women here about, some of them are excellent, but a more willful, determined set you never saw. Send this letter to mother for I hate to take the time to write often. C. Hancock"[160]

And still there were those too severely injured to be transferred, even by hand litter, from the corps hospitals.

---

156. *Ibid.* Camp Letterman did not actually disband until the week of November 17, some three months after Cornelia Hancock wrote this letter. All medical officers were officially relieved on November 20, 1863.
157. *Ibid.*, pp. 19-20.
158. *Ibid.*, p. 20.
159. *Ibid.*
160. *Ibid.*

> When all who could be had been removed to the general hospital, there were nearly four hundred left on the ground, severe cases of amputation, compound fractures, &c., of whom probably not more than one-third lived. Among these men, many of whom suffered excruciatingly, some of our delegates continued to labor till the last, through the surgeons and in connection with other commissions supplying their bodily wants, but seeking chiefly to direct them to the Great Physician for the healing of the soul.
>
> Many gave evidence of a renewed state. Especially was this true among the rebels. And as the delegates went through the tents you would hear the inmates invoke blessings upon their heads, and beg them to stop and pray and sing. A more glorious work was never engaged in. The blessings of philanthropy were not simply seen, but felt.[1561]

"All of our wounded that could bear transportation were forwarded, as rapidly as it could be done, to hospitals in Pennsylvania and Maryland," wrote Anna Holstein of those days of transition in all the corps hospitals. "By the 7th of August there still remained *three thousand*, who were moved into tents at the United States General Hospital on the York Turnpike; when our corps hospital was merged into this, we removed there; I remained as its matron until the close."[162]

The last week had been a hard one at the Second Corps Hospital, as the terminal cases had died, one by one. Litter crews gently carried the last few fragile wrecks of what had once been strong, young men off to the new general hospital. "On the eight[h] of August the last man was sent to the General Hospital at Gettysburg. The intervening time has been occupied in turning over the Hospital property to the proper authorities."[163]

---

161. *The United States Christian Commission for the Army and Navy. For the Year 1863. Second Annual Report*, pp. 71-72.
162. Holstein, *Three Years in Field Hospitals*, p. 43.
163. Dr. Justin Dwinelle, manuscript report of the Second Corps Hospital operations during the Battle of Gettysburg, MSC 129, National Library of Medicine, Bethesda, Maryland; copy in the Union Field Hospital Vertical File, Gettysburg National Military Park Library.

Now it all worked in reverse. One of Doctor Dwinelle's assistants supervised the breakdown of the camp. Down came the big hospital tents, to be aired, and folded, and packed away for next time. A tally was made of dispensary supplies—medicines, utensils, and stores — and all hospital instruments before carefully packing them away in the medical wagons. Kitchen supplies were gathered together, pots, pans, and kettles clattered together into a wagon, and foodstuffs secured for the bumpy trip.

The clerical assistant put the finishing touches on the mountains of paperwork generated by the hospital during its five-week stay. Complete patient records, surgical records for the three division hospitals, discharge records, transfer records, interment records, orders, dispatches, memos, passes—the paper trail seemed to go on forever.

Just enough time for one last look around. Not much to show for all that had taken place there: geometric squares of crushed straw, randomly stained and scuffed, where each tent had stood; trails and shortcuts worn into the farm fields between now-absent destinations; strange newly-turned plots of ground, inset into the verdant cropland, sprouting mismatched headboards instead of corn; latrines, heavily limed now and filled in; rich crops of corn and clover, generally trampled into a pulp and ruined.

Finally, with the physical camp packed up, and the paperwork either dispatched or safely filed away, it was time to go. Officers and doctors mounted up, teamsters cracked their whips, and the medical wagons and ambulances ponderously rumbled down the Schwartz farm lane, then out onto the Baltimore Pike. The war had moved on.

Part 4
Retrospective

Aye, this is the ground,
My blind eyes even as I speak behold it re-peopled from graves. . . .
Here we lay encamp'd, it was this time in summer also.
As I talk I remember all. . . .

The Centenarian's Story
Walt Whitman

POSTLUDE

1863-1913

". . . I was quite anxious to see again the old hospital. . . ."

Dr. Bushrod Washington James
Christian Commission

Throughout the next half century, Gettysburg would continue to irresistibly draw many who ministered at, or were treated at, the Second Corps Hospital. Everyone had been irrevocably altered during those days that they spent here. As the landscape of the battlefield began to heal and regained its bucolic atmosphere, more and more found the Pennsylvania town to be a lodestone, the magnetic north for their hearts.

It all began within a few short months of the battle, and would not ultimately end until the last patient, the last doctor and nurse, the very last volunteer had ultimately joined together in the final sleep of death.

Capt. Azor H. Nickerson, 8th Ohio Volunteers

Through dogged determination and constantly giving himself some reason, *any* reason, to live, Capt. Azor Nickerson had managed to survive his first visit to Gettysburg. It had been a long, hot, uncomfortable and painful journey back to Ohio. Now, after three and a half months of inactivity, the Ohio captain was itching to get back to his regiment.

"In November succeeding my first visit to Gettysburg, I was in the National capital, partly convalescent but still not permitted to rejoin my regiment. While awaiting a decision of the surgeons in my case, the ceremonies that were to take place on the occasion of the dedication of the proposed monument were announced, and I resolved to be present."[1]

On the way, Captain Nickerson encountered an old army friend, and they traveled on together to Gettysburg. The pair switched trains at Hanover Junction, which was once again just a sleepy rail junction without the bustle and activity associated with the Christian Commission's refreshment car. The car had been drawn up on a siding during the height of rail evacuations of the wounded from Gettysburg hospitals, but now only empty boxcars and flatcars filled the rail spur.

The two friends managed to board an official train bound for Gettysburg, filled to overflowing with an assortment of state delegations, politicians, and miscellaneous dignitaries and officials. Running into a former commanding officer, the now-retired general personally introduced Nickerson to Ohio governor David Tod. After being fully briefed on the captain's wounding and his hospital survival saga, Tod "told me that he would like to arrange it so that I could see and hear everything that transpired at the dedication ceremonies, and that he could best insure that if I and my friend were to accept the positions of aides-de-camp on his staff, which he then tendered. Of course we gratefully accepted the proferred honor."[2]

As the train huffed its way back to the battlefield, Captain Nickerson's thoughts turned once again to the gracious ladies who had served him lunch during his stretcher trip to the depot, now over three months past. Nickerson wanted to seek them out to express his sincerest appreciation for their hospitality to a gravely injured stranger.

> When we arrived at the station, though it was nearly eleven o'clock at night, I took McDowell and sought out the residence of my hosts of the previous July. Nearly everyone in the village was up, their houses illuminated and open in anticipation of their being called upon to entertain the immense crowds of incoming visitors.
>
> We found the house of my former hostesses open like the rest, and upon my making myself known (for it must be remembered that they had never seen me except for a few

---

1. Nickerson, "Personal Recollections of Two Visits to Gettysburg," p. 26. The "monument" Nickerson refers to is the National Cemetery at Gettysburg.
2. *Ibid.*

minutes, as I had laid upon the stretcher in front of their house) we were most cordially received.[3]

The ladies immediately threw open their home, lodging the two friends and several visiting newspaper editors for the night.

> At the dedication ceremonies on the following day, November 19, 1863, I had a seat on the platform within a few feet of the speakers, and could hear not only every word, but could mark every expression on the face of America's most polished orator, Edward Everett, as he delivered that masterly oration.
>
> When, therefore, Mr. Lincoln arose in obedience to the announcement that the President would now pronounce the dedication, everyone felt sorry for him. To say that Mr. Lincoln arose, can only be appreciated by those who have been near him when he got up to speak; but he had never before seemed to me to be so tall as he did on this occasion. He appeared to continue to arise as it were, until when he finally stood up I thought that he was the tallest and most awkward man I had ever seen.
>
> I thought then, and still think, it was the shortest, grandest speech, oration, sermon, or what you please to call it, to which I ever listened. It was the whole matter in a nutshell, delivered distinctly and impressively, so that all in that vast concourse could hear him. My own emotions may perhaps be imagined when it is remembered that he was facing the spot when only a short time before we had had our death-grapple with Pickett's men, and he was standing almost immediately over the place where I had lain and seen my comrades torn to fragments by the enemy's cannon-balls.[4]

Azor H. Nickerson eventually rose to the rank of major and went west to fight Apaches. But Gettysburg, in a very real way, lived on with Captain Nickerson for the rest of his life, and he mentally visited it many times during his stint out west. Thirty years later, he would vividly describe his two visits in an article in *Scribner's Magazine*, entitled "Personal Recollections of Two Visits to Gettysburg."

---

3. *Ibid.*, p. 27.
4. *Ibid.*, pp. 27-28.

Emily Bliss Souder, Volunteer Nurse from Philadelphia

Emily Bliss Souder was also back in Gettysburg on November 19, 1863. She had been forced to leave Gettysburg in late July because of the noxious atmosphere of rotting flesh, the greasy smoke of burning horses, and festering wounds, coupled with emotional and physical exhaustion. Nevertheless, illness or no illness, she was absolutely determined to return for the dedication of the new National Cemetery. "I had felt as if I *must* be in Gettysburg whenever the ceremonies did take place."[5]

She encountered a large number of people on her trip with the same goal—it seemed as if all of Pennsylvania was on the way to witness this solemn consecration ceremony. Rail and road travel were snarled, and accommodations were at a premium.

Finally arriving in town, she visited Camp Letterman Hospital, "now occupied as a camping ground for the soldiers who have come hither to take part in the ceremonies." Back in town, she found "the churches were lighted and warmed for the reception of those who could not find quarters elsewhere. The streets were filled with crowds of people."[6]

One of the chief attractions was the presence of President Abraham Lincoln. "A band played the national airs in front of the house where the Mr. Lincoln was staying, and eager calls were made for 'the President,' who finally stood a few minutes in the door-step, and in response to the wishes of the people, made a few characteristic remarks. . . . It was quite a new experience, you may be sure, and the whole time and circumstances were unlike anything we had known before."[7]

The next day, November 19, dawned gloomy and cloudy, but gradually cleared in time for the ceremonies.

> I gathered in the Cemetery many little sprays and green leaves, to send to friends at a distance, who might value such mementos of the day and hour.[8]
>
> At five in the afternoon, the citizens were introduced to the President, and we did ourselves the honor of paying our

---

5. Souder, *Leaves from the Battle-field of Gettysburg*, pp. 133-34.
6. *Ibid.*, pp. 137, 138.
7. *Ibid.*, p. 138.
8. Thus the significance of the title of her book: *Leaves from the Battle-field of Gettysburg.*

> respects to him and to the Governor. In the evening various meetings were held, and many speeches were made in the open air, some of which were greeted with hearty applause by citizens and soldiers. It seemed difficult to settle down to quietness.[9]

Moved by the unique experiences and impressions of her two visits to the Pennsylvania battlefield, Emily Souder also decided to write about her twin trips to Gettysburg. Instead of putting together a factual reminiscence decades later, as did Captain Nickerson, Mrs. Souder compiled her correspondence from the field, and added a collection of original patriotic poetry. Publishing in 1864, the slim folio bore the title *Leaves from the Battle-field of Gettysburg. A Series of Letters from a Field Hospital and National Poems.*

Maj. Gen. Winfield Scott Hancock, Commander, Second Corps

Maj. Gen. Winfield Scott Hancock would also find himself back again at Gettysburg. Not one to be outdone, he would return twice more to the battleground. However, there were still many months of difficult recovery and rehabilitation from his traumatic thigh wound to consider. And as July turned to August, the prognosis was looking decidedly grim.

It took until July 27 for General Hancock, commander of the Union Second Corps, to finally arrive home. First, he stopped to convalesce in Philadelphia, the City of Brotherly Love and Quaker hospitals. Upper level staff officers, however, did not recuperate in general hospitals with common soldiers, so Hancock was put up at the swanky LaPierre House on Broad Street, where he was personally attended to by Dr. D. Agnew.

A steady stream of famous physicians and noteworthy surgeons poked and probed for the elusive bullet in the general's upper thigh, with little success and much excruciating pain. Whether because of the oppressive heat or the agonizing attention of the local physicians, Hancock decided to set off for home in rural Norristown, Pennsylvania.[10]

---

9. Souder, *Leaves from the Battle-field of Gettysburg*, pp. 140, 142.
10. Letter of William G. Mitchell to Dr. L. W. Read, September 20, 1880 [transcribed copy in the General Winfield Scott Hancock Vertical File, Gettysburg National Military Park Library].

When it became known that Hancock was leaving town, a contingent of Philadelphia firemen turned out in full dress uniform to carry the Gettysburg hero to the depot. Through the crowded city streets they went, carefully avoiding stepping into any potholes or on any loose cobbles. At the train station, his stretcher was laid across several seats of the passenger coach for the eighteen mile trip.[11]

When the Philadelphia, Norristown, and Germantown train lurched to a halt at the Mill and Washington Street Station, it was immediately mobbed with a celebratory crowd of well-wishers. Fortunately, a contingent of the Invalid Corps, under the command of a Lieutenant Burns, was on hand to rescue the ailing general from his fans, and ferry him across town to his father's house on Swede Street. Although a grand gala had been prepared for the town's favorite son, Hancock's evident agony and exhaustion caused a postponement of the homecoming festivities.[12]

Despite a steady stream of get-well wishes and congratulatory telegrams, Hancock's condition continued to deteriorate. Now a fresh retinue of physicians arrived with probes and sounders, all in search of the missing Gettysburg bullet.

The turning point came when General Meade granted Dr. Louis Wernwag Read, a local Norristown doctor, a ten-day leave with specific instructions to attend to the failing general. Doctor Read had seen medical service under Czar Nicholas I in the Crimean War, and now served as medical director of the Pennsylvania Reserves and chief surgeon of the McKim United States Hospital in Baltimore. If anyone could find the lost bullet, it was Doctor Read.[13]

His first visit to Hancock was a sobering one.

> I found him much disheartened. He had grown thin, and looked pale and emaciated. He said he felt as if he was going to die, and that he had been probed and tortured to such an extent that death would be a relief. I endeavored to cheer him up, and as I was bidding him farewell he said, "Goodbye, Doctor. I may never see you again."

---

11. Hancock, *Reminiscences of Winfield Scott Hancock*, p. 99.
12. *Ibid.*; *Norristown Times Herald*, July 31, 1863; February 11, 1924.
13. *Philadelphia Times*, undated clipping, Historical Society of Montgomery County, Pennsylvania; Joseph T. Riemer, "General Hancock and Dr. Read," *The Bulletin of the Historical Society of Montgomery County, Pennsylvania*, vol. 18, no. 2 (Spring, 1972): 173-79.

> I had my hand on the door knob of the chamber, when he said: "See here, Doctor, why don't you try to get this ball out. I have had all the [doctors of] reputation in the country at it; now, let's have some of the practical."[14]

As Read examined Hancock from across the room, he noticed that "he was lying in the bed with his wounded limb actually flexed, and all the probing had been done with his leg at right angles. The ball had hit him just below the right groin, within an inch of the femoral artery, while he was sitting in the saddle with his legs distended." He had just discovered what all the other prominent doctors and their heavy-handed probings had not—the key to finding the minié ball.[15]

Doctor Read called several other physicians to assist him with the procedure. Helping Hancock into a chair "on top of the dining room table," Read used a "probe with a concealed blade" to examine the wound from the angle of the bullet's entry. Standing on the floor, "I inserted the probe and dropped fully eight inches into the channel and struck the ball, which was imbedded in the sharp bone which you sit upon." The next day, Saturday, August 22, Read surgically removed the ball "by cutting open the wound from the point in front at which . . . it . . . had entered the body." The ball was "located posterior to the femur." The general described the slug as weighing "one ounce and ninety grains."[16]

The turnabout in Hancock's condition was immediate. "In a week's time the General was out on crutches, and in two weeks more, the general even attended a Masonic gathering at Odd Fellows' Hall."[17]

---

14. *Philadelphia Times*, undated clipping; Riemer, "General Hancock and Dr. Read," p. 174; Letter of Winfield Scott Hancock to Maj. William G. Mitchell, August 24, 1863, Hartzell Collection; William G. Mitchell, Letter to Dr. L. W. Read, September 20, 1880; *Norristown Times Herald*, February 11, 1924.
15. *Philadelphia Times*, undated clipping; Riemer, "General Hancock and Dr. Read," p. 174; Letter of Winfield Scott Hancock to Maj. William G. Mitchell, August 24, 1863, Hartzell Collection; William G. Mitchell, Letter to Dr. L. W. Read, September 20, 1880; *Norristown Times Herald*, February 11, 1924.
16. *Philadelphia Times*, undated clipping; Riemer, "General Hancock and Dr. Read," p. 174; Letter of Winfield Scott Hancock to Maj. William G. Mitchell, August 24, 1863, Hartzell Collection; William G. Mitchell, Letter to Dr. L. W. Read, September 20, 1880; *Norristown Times Herald*, February 11, 1924.
17. *Norristown Republican*, August 28, 1863.

Hancock set himself an aggressive schedule as he convalesced. First, it was off to visit New York City and West Point Academy in mid-September. Then, he spent six weeks at his home in Longwood, near St. Louis, Missouri, devoting himself to tending trees and planting new saplings on his eleven acre property; when he became overtired, it was into the house to relax. "I threw aside my crutches a few days after my arrival," he wrote his father on October 12, "and now walk with a cane. I am improving but do not yet walk without a little 'roll.' My wound is still unhealed, though the doctors say it is closing rapidly. I find some uneasiness in sitting long in a chair, and cannot yet ride. The bone appears to be injured, and may give me trouble for a long time."[18]

Despite the fact that he could barely sit a chair, let alone a horse, optimism springs ever anew, especially in the resolute heart of General Winfield Scott Hancock. "I hope, however, I may be well enough in two weeks to join my Corps." With that in mind, he urged his physicians to regularly forward reports on his physical condition to the office of the adjutant general of the army.[19]

Hancock did return to the army—not in two weeks as he predicted, but five and a half months after his injury. In severe pain and extreme discomfort, Hancock resumed command of the Second Corps on December 27, 1863. It was painfully obvious to everyone involved, except perhaps to Hancock himself, that it was a premature return to duty; he was headed north again on January 8, 1864.

Frustrated with his inability to resume command, Hancock was determined to live up to his sobriquet as "the Superb." First it was off to Harrisburg on a recruiting drive to stimulate flagging enlistments. Then, throughout February, even with a superating wound, he staged a whirlwind tour of Philadelphia, New York, Albany, and Boston. On Washington's Birthday, Philadelphia threw a formal reception for the Gettysburg hero at Independence Hall, a very rare distinction indeed. The Union League of Philadelphia presented him with a handsome silver medal in recognition of his military achievements. Even the citizens of his hometown—Norristown, Pennsylvania—presented him with a nine-piece gold and silver service, each piece elegantly

18. Rev. C. W. Denison, *Winfield, the Lawyer's Son and How He Became a Major General* (Philadelphia, 1865), pp. 214-15; Hancock, *Reminiscences of Winfield Scott Hancock*, p. 101.

19. Rev. C. W. Denison, *Winfield, the Lawyer's Son and How He Became a Major General* (Philadelphia, 1865), pp. 214-15.

engraved with the Second Corps trefoil and commemorative inscriptions.[20]

Everywhere he went, he was hosted and feted as a conquering champion, wining and dining on only the choicest of rich and fatty foods. Forced into a life of inactivity by his injury, the general's weight ballooned, and he had put on an additional fifty pounds by June of 1864. The diabetes that ran in his family, and would eventually kill him, began to show up in fatigue, unusual thirst, and slowness of his wound to heal.

He returned to the army again on March 24, 1864, but his wound would haunt him throughout the rest of the war, and even force him to relinquish command on occasion. The pain and discomfort frequently led to fiery outbursts of anger. Despite all of his suffering, he still retained much of his old military chutzpah; he handled the Second Corps well at the Wilderness, and received his brevet to major general in the regular army when his corps smashed through the Confederate salient at Spotsylvania.

His mobility was severely curtailed by his injury, and Hancock fretted at his new limitations. "Through the Wilderness, and other fights following, he would leave the ambulance, mount his horse, and go through to the end without complaint," remembered his wife in later years. Yet he wrote her in frustration: "I suffer agony on these occasions, but must go into action on horseback or ask to be relieved. Can't you secure me a bandage of some sort in New York that will give me assistance?" But no such medical marvel could be found.[21]

Shortly after the Battle of Cold Harbor in June of 1864, the general was spotted, sitting along the Chickominy River with a canteen, pouring cold water over his reopened wound. In fact, so well known did his wound become that New Yorkers presented him with a barouche, so that he could ride when his wound was too painful to allow command from horseback. Even in his pain, Hancock was still extravagantly vain; he absolutely refused to direct an army corps from a carriage seat.[22]

---

20. Hancock, *Reminiscences of Winfield Scott Hancock*, pp. 100, 101-2.
21. Ibid., p. 101.
22. Paper read by Col. Theodore Lyman, January 9, 1882, *Papers of the Military Historical Society of Massachusetts*. (Boston: 1905), vol. 5, p. 19; Walker, *History of the Second Army Corps*, p. 539; *OR*, vol. 40, pt. 1, pp. 307, 318; *ibid.*, pt. 2, p. 122, 162; Meade, *The Life and Letters of George Gordon Meade*, 2:208-9; Willard Glazier, *Heroes of Three Wars* (Philadelphia: 1879), p. 351.

Things really started to unravel for Hancock in the final year of the war. In early June, a breakdown in the command structure failed to clearly communicate the goal of capturing Petersburg, and the general, pleading unfamiliarity with the battle plans, passed command (and a golden opportunity to end the war in mid-1864) to a subordinate officer. In all fairness, the Pennsylvania general was in intense agony, doggedly commanding his troops while forced by pain to sit on the ground, and traveling by ambulance as the corps moved. By June 18, fragments of bone were working their way out of the wound, and Hancock was forced to taken a ten day leave of absence, chafing at being laid up yet again.

Hancock returned, only to be totally mortified by the stunning defeat of the old Second Corps at Reams' Station. As his command began to disintegrate in the face of fierce Confederate resistance, he rode up to a battery and, turning to an officer, muttered: "Colonel, I do not care to die, but I pray God I may never leave this field."[23]

In November, the old campaigner was finally forced to face reality—he simply was no longer capable of the intensely active lifestyle required of a corps commander. With great sadness, he relinquished his field command; it was Thanksgiving Day, November 26, 1864, and he left without fanfare.

Out of active service, but unwilling to retire to private life, Hancock first turned his attention to recruiting the lst Veteran Volunteer Corps. When results were disappointing there, he was named commander of the Department of West Virginia and the Middle Military District on January 27, 1865. This appointment, which put him in overall charge of Washington, D.C., Maryland, West Virginia, and the Shenandoah Valley, integrally involved him in the trial of the Lincoln conspirators. He was able to slip away for a few days during the hectic summer months to give his eight year old daughter, Ada, a personal tour of the Gettysburg battlefield, carefully pointing out where her papa had done this or that.

He was finally mustered out of the volunteer service on July 26, 1866, the same day that he received the appointment of major general in the regular army. With war finally over, Hancock was assigned, in dizzying succession, to the Department of the Missouri (there to work with Sherman in dealing with hostile Plains Indians), the Fifth Military District (overseeing Louisiana and Texas), the Division of Atlanta, the

---

23. Francis A. Walker, *General Hancock* (New York: D. Appleton and Company, 1894), p. 275.

Department of the Dakotas (a military backwater covering Minnesota and the Dakotas), the Military Division of the Atlantic, and the Department of the South.

National politics, ever and always a sweet temptation for distinguished old soldiers, sounded its siren call to the general in 1868. The forty-four-year-old Hancock lost to Horatio Seymour at the Democratic Convention. He declined the nomination in 1872, and also turned down a chance to run for Governor of Pennsylvania, overcome with grief over the death of his beloved daughter from typhoid fever in 1875. But when he did run again, this time in the 1876 campaign, he was again edged out at the Democratic Convention by New York lawyer Samuel J. Tilden.

Undeterred, he bided his time in his various military postings, patiently waiting for the next campaign season (political, not military) to open again. Hoping to pull in the Southern voters with a familiar name, Hancock got the nod in 1880 at the Cincinnati Convention. But in a nail-biter of a presidential election, he was narrowly defeated by another old soldier, James A. Garfield.

That was finally the end, as far as Hancock was concerned. He had staged runs for the Oval Office on three occasions, and each one ended in a humiliating defeat. Hancock carefully packed up his political aspirations, and permanently locked them away in a remote corner of his heart. He devoted himself instead to being commander-in-chief, not of the army, but of the Military Order of the Loyal Legion, and tending to his duties at Governor's Island, in New York Harbor, where he now commanded the Department of the East. His office doors were always open to visits by veteran soldiers and aging friends from the glory days of the old Second Corps.

Ever a student of military affairs, he gladly assisted Francis Walker in compiling copious records, correspondence, articles, and references, forwarded with plenty of free advice, when his one-time aide set out to write a Civil War history of the Second Corps. He also collaborated with Alexander Webb, once a Second Corps division commander, but now president of City College of New York, when he wrote a book on the Peninsula Campaign. Hancock evidenced some of his old fire (and, no doubt, a good share of his old invective language) when Abner Doubleday published a history of the Battle of Gettysburg, rife with errors concerning the Second Corps (the gaffs were corrected when the second edition appeared).

Gettysburg continued large in Hancock's heart; he had never been better, more *right*, than he had been at that battle. Everything since had just been a postlude to that massive cantata of death and dismemberment in which the Pennsylvania general had shone so brightly. So, when a request came in 1885 from noted mapmaker and battlefield historian Col. John Bachelder, Hancock was soon on his way once again to the crossroads town.

Bachelder was facing a daunting task in his work with the Battlefield Association. Regimental survivors were returning in droves to the site of the battle, all intent on erecting heroic monuments honoring their achievements in the fierce fight. Each unit insisted that its monument must be just as close to the front as possible. Shouting matches, lawsuits, even fistfights, ensued when vitriolic veterans insisted that they most certainly *should* know where they fought, since they had been there. Bachelder desperately needed an impartial source to set the record straight.

Hancock was, by now, an imposing man, in reputation and in size. His weight had continued to skyrocket as his diabetes progressed. Dressed in a greatcoat against the chill November breezes, he towers over his companions in the photos of his visit. The aging general greatly relished being the star again. A cloud of old soldiers and junior officers followed him as he moved about town, obviously in awe, hanging on his every word.

Accompanied as well by his close personal friend Thomas B. Musgrave and his son Percy, Hancock walked back and forth over the field, pointing out positions of artillery, infantry movements, and enemy advances and retreats to Bachelder. Turning to his companion, Hancock intoned: "Your boy will remember what has been said when we have passed away."[24]

It was destined to be his last visit to the fields of Gettysburg, where the stars had shone so brightly on Winfield Scott Hancock. On February 9, 1886, he died at Governor's Island while still in command of the Department of the East. The old foe, diabetes melittus, finally caught up with him. Characteristic of his active life, he died in mid-sentence, muttering in his sleep to his beloved wife Almira: "Oh, Allie, Myra, good." He is buried in Montgomery Cemetery, Norristown, near the final resting place of General Zook, one of his brigade commanders, another casualty of Gettysburg.[25]

---

24. *Ibid.*, p. 312; Military Service Institute, *Letters and Addresses Contributed at a General Meeting of the Military Service institute at Governor's Island, New York Harbor, February 26, 1886, in Memory of Winfield Scott Hancock, etc.* (New York: Military Service Institute, 1886), p. 35.
25. *Norristown Times Herald*, February 11, 1924.

Cornelia Hancock, Independent New Jersey Nurse

For blonde, blue-eyed Cornelia Hancock, born to Thomas and Rachel Hancock in 1840, learning the ropes of nursing at Gettysburg proved to be but the beginning of a long and illustrious career in nursing, education, and social work, a circular career that would one day bring her back once again to Gettysburg.

When the Second Corps Hospital moved all its remaining wounded to Camp Letterman General Hospital, twenty-three-year-old Cornelia made the transition as well. On August 6, she wrote her sister: "We have all our men moved now to General Hospital. I am there, too, but the order in regard to women nurses has yet to be issued, and I do not know what my fate will be; I only know that the boys want me to stay very much, and I have been assigned to ward E." Ward E housed some of the most grievously wounded at Camp Letterman. Eleven days after arriving at her new home, Cornelia would write to her mother that "not one of the men under my care can get up yet! How patient they are though, never complain and lay still from day to day."[26]

September of 1863 found the young nurse in Philadelphia. She explained in a letter home: "The hospital got so full of women that one had to sit down while the others turned around, so I thought the most patriotic one was she who took her board off of Uncle Sam until there was a greater need of services."[27]

Loathe to return to the tedium of small town life, Miss Hancock moved on to Washington, D.C. On November 1, she "went to the Contraband Hospital on the northern outskirts of Washington and remained there until Feb. 15th, 1864." Following her stint at the refugee slave hospital, she moved on "to Brandy Sta[tion] to the 3rd Div. 2nd Corps Hospital, Dr. F. A. Dudley, 14th Conn Vol in charge."[28] Cornelia had met Dr. Frederick A. Dudley briefly at Gettysburg, where he had received a shoulder wound and was captured, and every one of Cornelia's letters until the end of the war would mention him.

When General Grant took command of the Union armies in 1864, the Second Corps' Third Division was broken up and divided between the other two divisions of the Corps. "All civilians were ordered to leave the Army. I returned to Philadelphia, but remained only a short time."

---

26. Hancock, *South After Gettysburg*, pp. 19, 23.
27. *Ibid.*, p. 27.
28. Cornelia Hancock, Pension Records, National Archives and Records Administration.

The Battle of the Wilderness produced a glut of wounded "almost as bad as Gettysburg," and Cornelia rushed to Fredericksburg to resume nursing.[29]

On May 31, 1864, a New York *Tribune* correspondent described Cornelia as she made the rounds in Fredericksburg: "Let me rise ever so early, she has already preceded me at work; and during many long hours of the day she never seemed to weary or flag. . . . She belonged to no association, and had no compensation. She commanded respect, for she was lady-like and well educated; so quiet and undemonstrative that her presence was scarcely noticed except by the smiling faces of the wounded as she passed."[30]

Cornelia Hancock and her nursing followed closely on the heels of the advancing army. From Fredericksburg, she moved on to Port Royal; soon she was off to White House where she treated the wounded from the heavy fighting at the North Anna River. On June 26, 1864, she arrived at City Point. "The dust here is just like ashes, 6 inches deep. . . . It is really awful here. The cannons boom along the line almost all the while, the heat is intense and the day of the explosion it seemed like what we read about hell. . . . I pray for health. I can stand all other hardships but sickness." She would remain at City Point until a month after General Lee surrendered.[31]

After two years of army nursing and social work with displaced blacks, Cornelia was still reluctant to return to the bucolic life of Hancock's Bridge, New Jersey, so she eagerly sought out other areas of endeavor. Convinced of the desperate need among the contrabands, she journeyed to South Carolina with a Miss Laura Towne under the auspices of the Philadelphia Society of Friends, intent on providing education and practical lifeskill training to the

---

29. Hancock, *South After Gettysburg*, pp. 89, 92.
30. Dr. Vanderpool, *New York Tribune*, May 31, 1864 (but compare Mr. John Vassar, "Miss Cornelia Hancock," in Brockett and Vaughn, *Woman's Work in the Civil War*, pp. 285, 286).
31. Hancock, *South After Gettysburg*, pp. 126-27. The "explosion" was the detonation of a large ordinance barge tied up at City Point supply depot wharf. As Anna Holstein described it: "There rose to a great height a dense cloud of smoke, spread out at top in the form of an umbrella, and from it fell a shower of death-dealing missiles; it literally *rained* muskets; shells flew in all directions; some passing over us, exploding beyond the hospital. The scene upon the bluff near the landing was sickening: dismembered bodies were strewn about the ground, the dead and dying side by side; the wounded were soon gathered up and brought to the hospital." [Holstein, *Three Years in Field Hospitals*, pp. 85-86.]

former slaves and their families. Miss Towne was so impressed by her audaciousness and natural adaptability that she promptly set her loose to start her own school. The result was the Laing School of Mount Pleasant, South Carolina, a highly successful educational facility that continued well into the twentieth century.[32]

After ten years in South Carolina, Miss Hancock returned to the North, and soon set sail with friends for Great Britain. There she expressed great concern over the vast number of poor and homeless she saw in the streets. Using her own social work experience, she was able to gain access to British social institutions, where she talked to members of their staffs and carefully studied their methods. When she returned to the United States, she brought with her many new ideas about how to help the poor and needy in American cities.[33]

The Philadelphia home of Dr. Henry Childs, the brother-in-law who had gained her access to the Gettysburg battlefield, was a well-known hotbed of social and humanitarian discussion. It was there that the Society for Organized Charity (later to become the Family Society of Philadelphia) was born in 1878. Cornelia was one of the first social workers employed by the fledgling relief agency. She operated on the personal concept, rooted in her experiences in the army and working with black schools in the South, that the social worker serves not only those needing assistance, but also the interests of those with the means and the desire to help.[34]

When the families of Philadelphia's Sixth Ward convinced Cornelia of the need for specialized aid to children, she campaigned tirelessly for the formation of a relief agency devoted specifically to their needs. In 1882, her dream came true with the founding of the Children's Aid Society and Bureau of Information (later known simply as the Children's Aid Society of Philadelphia). As secretary to the Board of Directors, her minutes of the proceedings reflect her deep-rooted philosophy: "We have been anxious not only to do something, but to do it well; to guard the child and to guard society: to help the suffering little one of today, and not, at the same time, to create a pauper for tomorrow. We cannot reconcile it to an enlightened conscientiousness in charity to act without inquiry, blindly trusting that the kind motive will ensure beneficent results."[35]

---

32. *Ibid.*, p. x.
33. *Ibid.*
34. *Ibid.*, pp. x-xi.
35. *Ibid.*, p. xi.

In 1884, she turned her attention to Wrightsville, Pennsylvania, a squalid slumtown suburb of Philadelphia. Serving as agent and associate to Edith Wright, she put into action an experimental housing program which went beyond mere sanitation, public utilities, and repairs; the school system was improved, a library was opened, a savings bank founded, and recreational activities instituted. By 1914, the former shantytown was a burgeoning community, with each resident a property owner.[36]

In 1913, she interrupted her work at Wrightsville to make the trip to Gettysburg to celebrate the fiftieth reunion with the remaining few of her "boys." After half a century, many of those old familiar faces that she remembered were sadly absent. Nonetheless, she was feted, celebrated, and warmly greeted by the old veterans, most of them strangers. For them, she served as a vivid reminder of the unstinting care and compassion that other Civil War nurses had lavished on them when they lay critically wounded in some primitive battlefield hospital.

While there, she was photographed with three other volunteer nurses, all seated in front of a giant American flag. Each is decked to various extents with reunion ribbons, souvenir buttons and commemorative medallions. Cornelia holds a smaller flag on her lap, and bears upon her breast the distinctive silver medal presented to her by "her boys" of the Second Corps. Even though half a century had come and gone, there is still something in the set of her jaw that harks back to that iron-willed, good-looking young woman who determined that "I, too, would go and serve my country" by helping the wounded on a distant battlefield.[37]

In later years, Cornelia, who never married, enjoyed regaling her nieces and younger cousins with thrilling anecdotes of her adventures. To Henrietta Stratton Jaquette, the granddaughter of one cousin, and a social worker herself, Cornelia bequeathed her yellowed collection of correspondence. "There is room, perhaps, for speculation over a bundle of letters which were left, at her death, 'to be burned without reading,'" says Mrs. Jaquette. "Her real interest in Dr. Frederick Dudley with whom she worked in the Hospital at Brandy Station is apparent, as is also his friendship for her."[38]

Cornelia Hancock died in Atlantic City in 1926 at age eighty-seven. Life had certainly been full for the Quaker girl from Hancock's Bridge,

---

36. *Ibid.*, pp. xi-xii.
37. *Ibid.*, p. 4.
38. *Ibid.*, p. xii.

New Jersey. She had literally seen the world, made a significant impact on the lives of many thousands of people, and come full circle to return home once again. She was laid to rest in Harmesville, New Jersey, just a few short miles from her rural home.[39]

In all of the return visits to Gettysburg of Second Corps Hospital doctors, nurses, patients and volunteers—whether for dedication of the National Cemetery, or for personal tours, or for reunions with returning comrades—no mention is ever made of desiring to see the old hospital grounds out at the Schwartz Farm, with one notable exception. In a battle where the contours of the land contributed so strongly to victory or defeat, only one participant ever expressed any interest in revisiting the actual ground where his previous labors made the difference between life and death for the men he treated.

Dr. Bushrod Washington James, Christian Commission September 19, 1895

With the battle now thirty-two years in the past, Dr. Bushrod Washington James made his way back to Pennsylvania, intent on seeking out the old Second Corps Hospital site. But first, a tour of the battlefield to refresh faded memories.

He carefully looked around him, deliberately noting each landmark, just another tourist taking in the pastoral scenery and crisp atmosphere of a typical early autumn day. It seemed scarcely conceivable that over three decades had come and gone since momentous events had swept down upon a relief doctor with the Christian Commission, and upon a small unknown village in Pennsylvania, making "Gettysburg" a household word all across America.

A third of a century past, the vista had been harsh and grisly—a mad muddle of bloated animal carcasses and putrefying bodies, fields gashed by projectiles, buildings with raw holes in the side or smoldering in ruins, bloated blowflies, and the scattered litter of discarded military equipment and bloody body parts everywhere. Now, "every point [was] laid out and marked by the Government, by

39. *Ibid.*; Conklin, *Women of Gettysburg*, p. 239.

individual States, or such military organizations as the 'Grand Army,' so that the entire area of twenty-five square miles or more, occupied in the great contest, spreads out before one in a grand panorama on a clear, bright, sun-lit day, is certainly a notable event in one's lifetime."[40]

No longer the brash young doctor of 1863, but now a well-seasoned middle-age physician, his hair shot with gray, Doctor James was doggedly determined to see all of the battlefield this time. Heading out by carriage, and accompanied by a battlefield guide, he went to the initial point of contact between the two hostile armies, moving purposefully and slowly, and pausing from time to time, as he scrupulously followed the course of the battle. The initial Confederate lines, the first Union stand out beyond Seminary Ridge, the bloody Railroad Cut, the rout back through Gettysburg, the obstinate Union stand down along Cemetery Ridge to the Round Tops—all were there to be seen, peopled once again by soldiers still young and bloody in the memory of Doctor James.[41]

However, where rank upon rank of seasoned veteran troops had once stood, and held, then fell bleeding or dead, now there were sprouting new legions—defenders of cold marble and granite, forged metal and chiseled stone, casting stony and defiant glares at the memory of an attack now long fought and repulsed. "At present it is as grand in its autumn loveliness as could well be imagined. This was the culmination of my experience after riding over that wide, extended area known as the 'Gettysburg Battle-Field.'"[42]

There was one site in particular, though, that drew Doctor James with its magnetic memories. "I was quite anxious to see again the old hospital along White Creek, where three thousand wounded Union and Confederate soldiers where [*sic*] lying on the side of the hill, many of them waiting there to be operated upon for the removal of limbs which had been shattered by the various missiles in the terrible conflict. I rode out on the Baltimore turnpike beyond Cemetery Hill, beyond Rock Creek, and on to a small run."[43]

Unfortunately, three decades of rebuilding ruined homesteads and the removal of war's detritus had served to largely obscure most recognizable landmarks of that troubled time.

---

40. James, *Echoes of Battle*, p. 107.
41. *Ibid.*, pp. 107-10.
42. *Ibid.*, p. 110.
43. *Ibid.*

> Not finding the locality, I was so much disappointed that I chided myself on having such a meagre [*sic*] "bump of locality," or cerebral convolutions, as mine just then appeared to be. . . . I asked my guide, Mr. Culp, if there was not some other stream of water in the immediate neighborhood, as this did not correspond at all with my recollections of the situation of the three hospitals which were located in close proximity, along the road, which I was then told was the Baltimore turnpike. I thought I had probably mistaken the situation, or possibly it was on the Taneytown road, or possibly the Emmittsburg [*sic*] road?
>
> He said, "Yes, there is another stream a mile further on, crossing the Baltimore pike, but it is away off from the battle-field." Ah, yes, said I, there is where the hospitals were placed, as far away from the noise of conflict as possible. Let us drive to that point and examine it, and should it not prove to be the exact spot, I should like to take the Emmittsburg [*sic*] road so as to be certain of finding the old place where I had labored so arduously thirty-two years before, and where my system broke down so completely that I was compelled to return home under the severe pressure of a violent cholera morbus.
>
> Driving to White Creek, and crossing the bridge, I immediately recognized the former location of the three hospitals, which were located within a quarter of a mile of each other, close to the stream. . . . Turning in along the stream, we drove off to the westward and crossed it again by fording, and continued up a farm lane to the crest of a hill.[44]

Even though the march of time had seen the destruction and rebuilding of a neighbor's barn, and the major deforestation of the area by lumbering, there could be no mistaking this steep ascent of the lane, cut into the hillside by generations of wagons; this weathered house and scattered outbuildings; the fields of grain climbing still higher up the ridge behind the structures—this was the Schwartz Farm, all right. The barn, smokehouse, and carriage house stood eerily silent now, save for the lowing of the cattle and the sighing of the wind. The porch was devoid of any sign of ripped and bleeding soldiers except for some faint rust-colored stains, almost obliterated by years of rain and

44. *Ibid.*, pp. 110, 111, 112.

drifting snow. The two wells stood alone in the barnyard, mute sentinels of other days, of people now only faintly recalled in the receding mists of memory.[45]

Doctor James stepped down from the carriage, walking slowly up the dirt lane that snaked left between the house and the farm buildings, familiar sensations of location battling with the unaccustomed serenity of the setting. "This was the place where our hospital tents and operating tables were situated," he mused, taking in the rolling curves of the fields to the left and right of the lane as he climbed to the top of Red Hill; "and where the three thousand wounded men lay."[46]

Despite the removal of all manmade signs of the hospital, it was the natural setting itself that gave away the former location of the Second Corps Hospital. "I went along the crest of the hill among the scattered trees and numerous stumps, and recognized the flat area on the top where the rows of tents had been placed, and some of the depressions which had been made for the tent poles and posts were still visible. The hay and straw which we had used in the tents had enriched a growth of grass the following year, and annually, this grass had gone on seeding, and springing up, and reproducing a crop from year to year, and the old tent lines and avenues are thus made visible or are marked out at the present day."[47]

What a host of memories there were. Even now, Doctor James remembered the names and faces of so many who had lived and died there—patients, doctors, members of relief organizations, and volunteer assistants. "I recognized also the position of the commissary and culinary departments, called to memory many friends I made, and the noble ladies who worked there in such a self-sacrificing manner, preparing meals and suitable dishes for the soldiers. I also recalled the hospital stewards and nurses who were constantly going and coming from this important culinary department to the hundreds of men under their nursing care, as I did, too, many of the wounded."[48]

Doctor James continued to wander over the green field and through the woodlots, recreating the scenes of horror and hope that had transpired there.

> My next object was to ascertain the situation of the operating tables where I spent so many wearisome and

---

45. *Ibid.*, p. 112.
46. *Ibid.*
47. *Ibid.*, pp. 112-13.
48. *Ibid.*, p. 113

fatiguing hours, with my sleeves rolled up, and with copious drops of perspiration covering my brow, in the sweltering days of that fearful July; and taking the markings of the rows of tents as my guide, I speedily ascertained the exact location; and the depression in the ground which we made for the blood and water to run into, was even visible, while some two or three little elevated, mound-like spots indicated the places where we buried the many limbs which we were obliged to remove. If they had been struck by a minie-ball, it shattered the bone completely for inches around, and in order to save the life of the soldier and prevent gangrene, the limbs had to come off. . . .

Satisfying myself with these identifications, I followed out the line of sod or grass to the present fence, and there I saw that the old road by which we had come in from the Baltimore pike in 1863 had been closed up and tilled over, but the cut-out at the pike well located its former position. I also recognized the former situation of the other hospital of tents alone, which had no building nearby.

This situation was quite near the Baltimore road, and it was here the surgeons told me they had 2,500 men under their care. Those of the barn hospital, across the turnpike had informed me that they had about 1,500, so that, with the 3,000 in the hospital in which I worked, in that small area alone there were about 7,000 wounded men, while off to the west and northeast were many hospitals which I had no time or disposition to visit.

As I came away I walked down along the side of the hill where so many of the wounded men were then lying under the shade of the trees awaiting operation; many of these were Confederates. All along the side of this hill for a long distance, from the operating tables down to the White Creek itself, there arose again in my memory the harrowing scenes which I encountered here among the suffering and dying, the moaning and the dead, for every hour or two several of those men passed into eternity.

Officers and men were lying there, pleading to be operated upon, and yet we were doing everything that humanity could do to reach and relieve them as rapidly as possible. Day after day as I walked along those lines of wounded men my heart was touched with sympathy, and I

> felt the injunction placed upon me when I entered the medical profession, of "cure the sick, relieve the suffering, wherever and whenever you can," come up forcibly to my mind so many times that I fully realized that to be a physician, with this strict requirement placed upon me at my graduation, made it a noble calling.... To see a hospital, after a battle, always mollifies one's human nature in behalf of each and every suffering individual, in the compassionate physician, throughout all his after-life.[49]

The visit to the old hospital site was drawing to a close. Doctor James turned to go, but not before looking about for some memento of this horribly vivid wedge of his past.

> I turned to see if I could not find some relic from this point to carry home, but nothing presented itself save a young hickory tree which had sprung up from the root of an older tree close to the site of the operating table. I said, "Truly, this hickory growth will amply repay me as a trophy when turned into a cane." I set about with my stout penknife, which was exceedingly dull, to whittle away the root itself on either side of the little hickory sapling, and it was only after half an hour's whittling, with the blistering of my right hand, that I succeeded in bringing away enough for the handle of a cane, which I resolved should be my Gettysburg relic from the White Creek hospital, where I spent so much energy and so much sympathy in our cause.[50]

With his amputated sapling in hand, Dr. Bushrod Washington James, late of the Second Corps Hospital, turned his back on the rushing sound of Rock Creek, and ambled through the verdant-green squares of long-gone hospital tents. He walked past the now-empty burial sites in Farmer Schwartz's corn patch, and in the field over toward the Bushman Farm, and behind the barn, and along the farm lane. Stiffly clambering up in the carriage, he urged his guide, Mr. Culp, to drive back to the battlefield.

Doctor James would never return to the Schwartz Farm.

---

49. *Ibid.*, pp. 113-16

50. *Ibid.*, p. 114.

Afterword

THE SECOND CORPS HOSPITAL TODAY

The Schwartz Farm is still there. Its distance from the uncoordinated sprawl of Gettysburg, plus being cut off, literally and figuratively, by the four-lane ribbon of Bypass 15, has served to protect the old farm from the developers: so far. But now a chic new golf course has sprung up across the road, slapdash housing allotments are shouldering their way ever closer, and the entire rural peacefulness of the area is changing to one of suburban bustle, replete with joggers, boomers, and car pools.

The old barn, too, is still there (the original), where, once upon a distant time, hundreds of Confederate wounded moaned, screamed under the knife and saw, and died in agony. There is an eerie quality to the place as it stands silent now, a repository for aged farm implements, and habitat for barn swallows and field mice. A ramshackled farmhouse (possibly the original) is off to the side, across the farmyard. One must still cross White Run on a feeble bridge and climb a centuries-old farm lane, cut deep into the bank, to reach the place.

Out back, rising beyond the buildings, wheat and corn still grow in the fields where the three division hospitals pitched their tents. The graves in Yards A, B, C, and D are empty now—the Southerners have been shipped to Richmond for burial in Hollywood Cemetery, the Northerners have migrated over to the National Cemetery in the Gettysburg National Military Park. Some Yankees and Rebels were moved home to rural or urban family burial plots by relatives and friends. Yet, one cannot help but wonder if, in some secluded spot, maybe under that stand of trees, or, perhaps, over on the slaty ridge where the plow never tills the rocky Pennsylvania soil, there does not still rest the remains of one or two of the men who died here.

The owner, Mr. H. R. Schaeffer, in retirement now from the frantic rat-race of Washington, D.C., sublets the property out to a local farmer. He often allows people on his property, whether electronic archaeologists with metal detectors, or medical historians who desire nothing more than to simply browse about the property and remember the vastness of the hospital that once visited this ground for five agonizing weeks. Please respect the fact that this is private property by contacting Mr. Schaeffer before visiting.

Mr. H. R. Schaeffer
P.O. Box 3112
Gettysburg, PA 17325
(717)334-3795

The idea of a moveable surgical hospital facility—capable of setting up, operating, packing up, falling back, and repeating the process as often as necessary—was a good one, but one that would need to see the passing of several more wars before achieving its full potential. Military medical care remained largely unchanged throughout the remainder of the nineteenth century. Most of the clashes were small enough, or remote enough, that the principles of Jonathan Letterman's mobile field hospital were largely set aside.

The universality of Letterman's hospital system, however, were demonstrated half a world away, and almost a half century distant, in the messy conflict optimistically christened the "Great War," the "War to End All Wars." Although the terminology is exotic, the wounds and what the wounded experienced are hauntingly familiar. The wounded (*blessés*) were taken by their comrades to a first aid station set up in the trenches. From there, stretchermen (*brancardiers*) would carry them through communication trenches to an advanced dressing station (*postes de secours*), ideally out of the line of direct fire in some bombproof structure, about a mile to the rear. There their immediate wounds were treated—cleaning, dressing, immobilizing fractures, and any emergency amputations.

Converted Ford jitneys and European touring car ambulances, driven by *ambulanciers*, would next transport the wounded capable of sitting up (*assis*), as well as those lying recumbent on stretchers (*couchés*), to a still more rearward triage hospital, where they were divided into three groups—those requiring immediate attention, those who were stable enough to be sent to rear-line hospitals, and those with mortal wounds to be relegated to the moribund ward. Transportation to more distant urban hospitals was then accomplished by train.[1]

While the advent of motorized ambulances in the First World War certainly revolutionized patient transportation, it was not until World War Two that the mobile field hospital concept was truly put to the test. There is arguably no finer example of its working than the 77th Evacuation Hospital. It was certainly highly mobile—England during the summer of 1942, Oran in November, Constantine in January of 1943, Tébessa in February, La Meskiana in March, back to Tébessa, Bône in April, Palermo in September, Licta in October, and finally returning to England to prepare for the June 6, 1944, D-Day Invasion.[2]

The armed incursion into Fortress Europe produced one of the greatest influxes of American battlefield casualties since the Battle of Gettysburg. The 77th Evacuation Hospital landed on Utah Beach on June 7, 1944, and was open for business at Ste. Mère-Eglise the next day. During its first twelve hours of operation, the 77th treated 1,450 patients at the rate of two per minute. Its first six days saw 6,304 patients go through triage; patients arrived at a round-the-clock rate of one per minute during the entire first week.

The line of ambulances pulling up to the 77th facility was nearly two hundred yards long at times, and ran three abreast. Six doctors were just barely able to keep up with the litter crews as they carried the wounded into the receiving tent. There was space for only one hundred litters in its cramped confines; the casualties were diagnosed, treated, and then carried out the back door. The walking wounded were clustered around the outside, swapping stories and war mementoes while they waited for a lull so that their injuries could be treated.

Record keeping was still a priority, as it had been at the Second Corps Hospitals. Patient tags revealed how much morphine the patient had received and each was closely questioned by doctors and nurses

1. Arlen J. Hansen, *Gentlemen Volunteers: The Story of the American Ambulance Drivers in the Great War, August, 1914—September, 1918* (New York: Arcade Publishing, 1996), pp. xiii-xvii.
2. Stephen E. Ambrose, *Citizen Soldiers: The U.S. Army from the Normandy Beaches to the Bulge to the Surrender of Germany, June 7, 1944 to May 7, 1945* (New York: Simon and Schuster, 1997), pp. 322-23.

about his injuries. The information was then dutifully entered in the patient's medical file.[3]

The nurses brought some sense of reality and normalcy to these men, just as they had at the Schwartz Farm. They checked vital signs, administered medication, and made notations on the patient's chart. With a smile, they straightened each sufferer's blanket. And then it was time to move on. It was the same old time crunch of the Civil War, only modernized and mechanized. The experience deeply touched the nurses; Lt. Aileen Hogan, expressing sentiments that Cornelia Hancock and Jane Boswell Moore would have deeply understood, remembered Normandy with these words: "I have never worked so hard in my life. I can't call it nursing. The boys get in, get emergency treatment, penicillin and sulfa, and are out again. It is beyond words."[4]

As the army moved, the 77th Evac. traveled in its shadow. After a month at Ste. Mere-Eglise, they moved forward to St.-Lô , then on to Le Mans, and then Chartes, Verviers, and so on. The 77th, true to its name, served as an evacuation hospital, moving the wounded to more secure hospitals further to the rear. They also served alternatively as a holding hospital (where wounded from multiple hospitals were gathered) and a triage hospital (a gruesome function sadly unchanged from the days of the Civil War, eighty years before).

It was not until the bitter "police action" in Korea that the concepts practiced in prototype by Doctor Dwinelle and his dedicated staff blossomed into full reality in the Mobile Army Surgical Hospital [MASH] model.

The average MASH was a well-equipped facility with approximately sixty beds, eleven doctors, and some one hundred personnel. It was the first place in the medical evacuation procedure where surgery could actually be performed. The system was remarkably similar to that experienced by the patients at the Second Corps Hospital ninety years before; the wounded in Korea were taken to a battalion aid post, where the bleeding was stopped and the patient stabilized, then rushed to a

3. Max Allen, *Medicine Under Canvas: A War Journal of the 77th Evacuation Hospital* (Kansas City: The Sosland Press, 1949), p. 118.
4. Judy Litoff and David Smith, "Today We Have Lived History: The D-Day Letters of U. S. Women," a paper given at the Eisenhower Center, May 16, 1994.

casualty clearing station. From there, they were evacuated by jeep or helicopter to a MASH unit. After the patient's wounds were treated, and he was well enough to travel, it was on to a rear line medical unit. If his injuries were serious enough, he was airlifted to a base hospital in Japan, and then home to the States.[5]

The experiences of the Norwegian MASH [NorMASH], of the Eighth Army, echo much of what the Second Corps Hospital experienced at Gettysburg; the NorMASH, however, was staffed with a wider range of specialists and newer procedures. During its three years of active existence, NorMASH had a cumulative staff of one-hundred and eleven female nurses, twenty-two male nurses, eighty doctors, five dentists, six pharmacists, seven chaplains, and three-hundred and ninety-two additional staff. The hospital treated both military and civilian casualties, often on an out-patient basis, providing food and coffee for transient patients whenever possible. Altogether, the unit treated over 90,000 patients (14,755 as in-patients) during its three-year existence. None of the Norwegian staff was killed in action, but two died in an accident.[6]

Dr. Odd Oyer remembers that "the unit for shock treatment, X-Ray, and the operating theatre with four operating tables, worked around the clock almost to the point of complete exhaustion. For example, at one time in 1953, 173 operations were performed in a 72-hour period. It was vital during such periods that some of the professional personnel be rested, so as to prevent all of us becoming exhausted at the same time. During such periods, non-medical personnel were put on to assist during operations and did a fine job."[7]

Blood transfusions helped save many that would have been lost during Doctor Dwinelle's day. "After an operation we usually kept patients for about three days but sometimes they stayed longer. The consumption of blood was enormous. The medical practice at the time was blood for blood lost. . . . Every bottle was tapped in [the] USA, transported to Japan and from there to Korea. 30 transfusions for one wounded man was not unusual."[8]

The wounds were no less terrible than in the Civil War, just different in location and scope. "Typical wounds were shrapnel and mine

---

5. "MASH," in George Forty, *At War in Korea* (London: Ian Allen Ltd., 1982; reprint, The Cassell Group, 1997), pp. 126-27.
6. *Ibid.*, pp. 127-28.
7. *Ibid.*, p. 128.
8. *Ibid.*

casualties, and the lower extremities suffered most. Legs crushed up to the knee was a tragic event. Because of splinters most casualties had multiple wounds. All central nervous system damage and eye injuries were taken by helicopter to specialized units further behind the front."[9]

The wars that America became involved in would continue with monotonous regularity, with Vietnam, Panama, Grenada, and the Persian Gulf being but a few. Muzzle velocities have increased, bombs have become smarter, technology more sophisticated and ruthless. But the principles and practices laid out by Doctor Letterman in the middle of the Civil War, and put into practice by the dedicated men and women of the Second Corps Hospital, would prove to be viable even in the world of evolving warfare and ever-changing medical technology, where new procedures continue to be implemented, new pharmaceutical discoveries speed recovery, and new equipment assists in the care and transport of the wounded.

Doctor Dwinelle and the staff of the Second Corps Hospital demonstrated the tremendous potential for a mobile, high-quality, military surgical facility; their dedicated care and professional treatments during a medical catastrophe of the greatest magnitude continue to serve as a example of what medicine has always aspired to be. We all reap the benefits of their pioneering work in the high quality of medical care that we now enjoy.

9. *Ibid.*

Appendix 1

ORDER OF BATTLE AND UNIT LOSSES, Union Second Corps

UNION SECOND CORPS

Maj. Gen. Winfield Scott Hancock

(wounded on July 3)

Brig. Gen. John Gibbon

General Headquarters Staff

6th New York Cavalry
Companies D and K
Second Corps Headquarters Escort

53rd Pennsylvania
Companies A, B, and K
Second Corps Provost Guard

FIRST DIVISION

Brig. Gen. John Curtis Caldwell

116th Pennsylvania, Company B — Provost Guard

FIRST BRIGADE

Col. Edward Everett Cross

(wounded on July 2)

Col. Henry Boyd McKeen

5th New Hampshire — Lt. Col. Charles Edward Hapgood

61st New York, "Clinton Guards" — Lt. Col. Knut Oscar Broady

81st Pennsylvania — Lt. Col. Amos Stroh

148th Pennsylvania — Col. Henry Boyd McKeen (moved to brigade command on July 2), Lt. Col. Robert McFarlane

SECOND BRIGADE

Col. Patrick Kelly

28th Massachusetts — Col. Richard Byrnes

63rd New York, "Third Regiment Irish Volunteers" (two companies) — Lt. Col. Richard Charles Bentley (wounded July 2), Capt. Thomas Touhy

69th New York, "First Regiment Irish Brigade" (two companies) — Capt. Richard Moroney (wounded July 2), Lt. James Joseph Smith

88th New York, "Fifth Regiment Irish Brigade" (two companies) — Capt. Denis Francis Burke

116th Pennsylvania (four companies) — Maj. St. Clair Augustin Mulholland

THIRD BRIGADE

Brig. Gen. Samuel K. Zook

(wounded on July 2)

Lt. Col. John Fraser

52nd New York, "German Rangers," "Sigel Rifles" — Lt. Col. Charles Godfrey Freudenberg (wounded July 2), Maj. Edward Venuti (killed July 2), Capt. William Scherrer

57th New York, "National Guard Rifles," "Clinton Rifles," "Zook's Voltiguers" — Lt. Col. Alford B. Chapman

66th New York, "Governor's Guard" — Col. Orlando Harriman Morris (wounded July 2), Lt. Col. John Sweeney Hammell (wounded July 2), Maj. Peter Adolph Nelson

140th Pennsylvania — Col. Richard Petit Roberts (killed July 2), Lt. Col. John Fraser (assumed brigade command after mortal wounding of General Zook)

FOURTH BRIGADE

Col. John R. Brooke

(wounded on July 2)

27th Connecticut (two companies) — Lt. Col. Henry Czar Merwin (killed July 2), Maj. James H. Coburn

2nd Delaware — Col. William P. Baily, Capt. Charles Henry Christman (commanded regiment on July 3)

64th New York, "First Cattaraugus Regiment" — Col. Daniel G. Bingham (wounded July 2), Maj. Leman W. Bradley

53rd Pennsylvania (three companies, Second Corps Provost Guard) — Lt. Col. Richards McMichael

145th Pennsylvania (seven companies) — Col. Hiram Loomis Brown (wounded July 2), Capt. John William Reynolds (wounded July 2), Capt. Moses Warren Oliver

SECOND DIVISION

Brig. Gen. John Gibbon

(wounded on July 3)

Brig. Gen. William Harrow

1st Minnesota, Company C -- Provost Guard

FIRST BRIGADE

Brig. Gen. William Harrow

Col. Francis Edward Heath

19th Maine — Col. Francis Edward Heath (wounded July 3, assumed brigade command when General Harrow took over division command), Lt. Col. Henry Whitman Cunningham

15th Massachusetts — Col. George Hull Ward (wounded July 2), Lt. Col. George Clesson Joslin

1st Minnesota (2nd Company Minnesota Sharpshooters attached) — Col. William Colvill (wounded July 2), Capt. Nathan Messick (killed July 3), Capt. Henry C. Coates

82nd New York, "Second New York State Militia" — Lt. Col. James Huston (killed July 2), Capt. John Darrow

SECOND BRIGADE

"The Philadelphia Brigade"

Brig. Gen. Alexander S. Webb

69th Pennsylvania, "Second California" — Col. Dennis O'Kane (wounded July 3), Capt. William Davis

71st Pennsylvania, "California Regiment" — Col. Richard Penn Smith, Jr.

72nd Pennsylvania, "Baxter's Philadelphia Fire Zouaves," "Third California" — Col. De Witt Clinton Baxter (wounded July 2), Lt. Col. Theodore Hesser

106th Pennsylvania "Fifth California" — Lt. Col. William Lovering Curry

THIRD BRIGADE

Col. Norman J. Hall

19th Massachusetts — Col. Arthur Forrester Devereux

20th Massachusetts — Col. Paul Joseph Revere (wounded July 2), Lt. Col. George Nelson Macy (wounded July 3), Capt. Henry Livermore Abbott

7th Michigan — Lt. Col. Amos Steele, Jr. (killed July 3), Maj. Sylvanus Wright Curtis

42nd New York, "Tammany Regiment" — Col. James E. Mallon

59th New York (four companies), "Union Guards" — Lt. Col. Max A. Thoman (wounded July 2), Capt. William McFadden

UNATTACHED

Massachusetts Sharpshooters — Capt. William Plumer (wounded June 1863, rode to Gettysburg in an ambulance), Lt. Emerson L. Bicknell

THIRD DIVISION

Brig. Gen. Alexander Hays

10th New York Battalion — Provost Guard

FIRST BRIGADE

Col. Samuel S. Carroll

14th Indiana — Col. John Coons
4th Ohio — Lt. Col. Leonard Willard Carpenter
8th Ohio — Lt. Col. Franklin Sawyer
7th West Virginia — Lt. Col. Jonathan Hopkins Lockwood

SECOND BRIGADE

Col. Thomas A Smyth

(wounded on July 3)

Maj. Theodore Grenville Ellis

Lt. Col. Francis Edwin Pierce

14th Connecticut — Maj. Theodore Grenville Ellis

1st Delaware — Lt. Col. Edward Paul Harris (arrested July 2, restored to command July 4), Capt. Thomas Bullock Hizar (wounded July 2), Lt. William Smith (killed July 3), Lt. John T. Dent

12th New Jersey — Maj. John T. Hill

10th New York Battalion, "National Zouaves" — Maj. George Faulkner Hopper

108th New York, "Rochester Regiment" — Lt. Col. Francis Edwin Pierce

THIRD BRIGADE

Col. George Willard

(killed on July 2)

Col. Eliakim Sherrill

(wounded on July 3)

Lt. Col. James M. Bull

39th New York (four companies), "Garibaldi Guards" — Maj. Hugo Hildebrandt

111th New York — Col. Clinton Dougald MacDougall (wounded July 3), Lt. Col. Isaac M. Lusk (wounded July 3), Capt. Aaron Platt Seeley

125th New York — Lt. Col. Levin Crandell

126th New York — Col. Eliakim Sherrill (wounded July 3), Lt. Col. James M. Bull

ARTILLERY BRIGADE

Capt. John G. Hazard

1st New York Light, Battery B, "Empire Battery," "Pettit's" — Capt. James McKay Rorty (killed July 3), Lt. Albert S. Shelden (wounded July 3), Lt. Robert Eugene Rogers[1]

1st Rhode Island Light, Battery A — Capt. William Albert Arnold

1st Rhode Island Light, Battery B — Lt. Thomas Frederic Brown (wounded July 2), Lt. William Smith Perrin

1st United States, Battery I, "Rickett's" — Lt. George Augustus Woodruff (wounded July 3), Lt. Tully McCrea

4th United States, Battery A — Lt. Alonzo Hereford Cushing (killed July 3), Sgt. William Frederick Fuger

UNIT STRENGTH, KILLED, WOUNDED, AND MISSING SECOND CORPS BY STATE

Units strengths and losses of the Union Second Corps, even with the mountains of paperwork connected with running the vast complexity of an army, are very difficult to determine with one hundred percent accuracy. Different writers present different perspectives, and often different numbers of strengths and losses. Even men present at the battle did not always agree on the numbers.

Consequently, these figures represent the best attempts of this writer to consider the horrible losses of Gettysburg. Whenever possible, they represent men "present for duty." Units on other assignments (detached, divisional duty, etc.) are so noted.

These figures are the result of analysis of numerous regimental histories, monographs, and the following resources on Gettysburg and the Civil War:

John W. Busey, *The Last Full Measure: Burials in the Soldiers' National Cemetery at Gettysburg* (Hightstown, New Jersey: Longstreet House, 1988).

1. Transferred from the Artillery Reserve on July 1, 14th New York Battery attached.

———, *These Honored Dead* (Hightstown, New Jersey: Longstreet House, 1988).
John W. Busey and David G. Martin, *Regimental Strengths at Gettysburg* (Baltimore, Maryland: Gateway Press, Inc., 1982).
William F. Fox, *Regimental Losses in the American Civil War, 1861-1865* (Albany, New York: Brandon Printing Company, 1898).
Thomas L. Livermore, *Numbers and Losses in the Civil War in America 1861-1865* (Boston: Houghton, Mifflin Company, 1901; reprint, Bloomington, Indiana: Periodicals Service Company, 1957).
The United States War Department, *War of the Rebellion: A Compilation of the Official Records of the Union and Confederate Armies*, 70 vols. in 128 parts (Wasington, D.C.: Government Printing Office, 1880-1901), series 1, vol. 27, pts. 1 and 3.

Regiment	Strength	Killed	Wounded	Missing	% Loss
14th Connecticut	200	10	52	4	33.0
27th Connecticut Companies D and F	160	10	23	4	23.1
1st Delaware	288	10	54	13	26.7
2nd Delaware	280	11	61	12	30.0
14th Indiana	236	6	25	0	13.1
19th Maine	543	29	170	4	37.4
Mass. Sharpshooters 1st Company	50	2	6	0	16.0
15th Massachusetts	304	23	97	28	48.7
19th Massachusetts	231	9	61	7	33.3
20th Massachusetts	301	30	94	3	42.2
28th Massachusetts	265	8	57	35	37.7

7th Michigan	165	21	44	0	39.4
1st Minnesota[2]	420	50	173	1	53.3[3]
	416[4]	80[5]	149	6	56.5[6]
(2nd Company Minnesota Sharpshooters, attached as Company L)					
5th New Hampshire	182	27	53	0	44.0
12th New Jersey	532	23	83	9	21.6
1st New York Light, Battery B (**14th New York Battery** Attached)	114	10	16	0	22.8
6th New York Cavalry Companies D and K Second Corps Headquarters Escort	—	1	3	0	—
10th New York Battalion Companies A, B, C, and D	98	2	4	0	6.1
39th New York Companies A, B, C, and D	322	15	80	0	28.6

2. This is the loss for the entire 1st Minnesota regiment. During their costly charge on July 2, however, Company L was serving as skirmishers, and fifty-six men from Company C were detached for divisional duties.
3. Edmund J. Raus, Jr., *A Generation on the March: The Union Army at Gettysburg* (Lynchburg, Virginia: H. E. Howard, 1987), p. 47.
4. There is still dispute over how many men were involved in the charge of the 1st Minnesota on July 2, even among those that were there. On June 30, the regiment was paid in Uniontown, Maryland. The roster shows 27 officers and 358 enlisted men as present for duty, a total of 385 men. Company L were members of Berdan's Sharpshooters, under the command of Captain Berger, with 3 officers and 28 men, bringing the total strength to 416. [Robert and William Haiber, *The First Minnesota Regiment at Gettysburg* (LaGrangeville, New York: Info Devels Press, 1991), Appendix A/B, A-1.]
5. Thirty-seven men died of their wounds, thus accounting partially for the discrepancy of these figures with the ones directly above. [John W. Busey, *These Honored Dead* (Hightstown, New Jersey: Longstreet House, 1988).
6. *Minnesota in the Civil and Indian Wars*, 2 vols. (St. Paul, Minnesota: Pioneer Press, 1890), vol. 2, pp. 373-76. Seventy percent of those actually engaged in fighting were casualties. [Richard Moe, *The Last Full Measure: the Life and Death of the First Minnesota Volunteers* (New York: Henry Holt and Company, 1993), pp. 295-96.]

42nd New York	197	15	55	4	37.6
52nd New York	134	2	26	10	28.4
57th New York	179	4	28	2	19.0
59th New York Companies A, B, C, and D	182	6	28	0	18.7
61st New York	148	6	56	0	41.9
63rd New York Companies A and B	112	5	10	8	20.5
64th New York	221	15	64	19	44.3
66th New York	176	5	29	10	25.0
69th New York Companies A and B	75	5	14	6	33.3
82nd New York	394	45	132	15	48.7
88th New York Companies A and B	126	7	17	4	22.2
108th New York	305	16	86	0	33.4
111th New York Companies A, D, E, F, G, H, J, and K	390	58	177	14	63.8
125th New York	500	26	104	9	27.8
126th New York	511	40	181	10	43.2
4th Ohio	229	9	17	5	13.5
8th Ohio	209	18	83	1	48.8

53rd Pennsylvania Companies A, B, and K Second Corps Provost Guard	136	7	67	6	58.8
69th Pennsylvania	329	40	80	17	41.6
71st Pennsylvania	331	21	58	19	29.6
72nd Pennsylvania	458	44	146	2	41.9
81st Pennsylvania	190	5	49	8	32.6
106th Pennsylvania	335	9	54	1	19.1
116th Pennsylvania Companies A, B, C, and D	123	2	11	9	17.9
140th Pennsylvania	590	37	144	60	40.8
145th Pennsylvania Seven Companies	228	11	69	10	39.5
148th Pennsylvania	468	19	101	5	26.7
1st Rhode Island Light, Battery A	139	3	28	1	23.0
1st Rhode Island Light, Battery B	103	7	19	2	27.2
1st United States, Battery I	113	1	24	0	21.2
4th United States, Battery A	129	6	32	0	29.5
7th West Virginia	319	5	41	1	14.7

Appendix 2

ARMY AND VOLUNTEER STAFF OF THE UNION SECOND CORPS HOSPITAL AT GETTYSBURG, JULY 2 THROUGH AUGUST 8, 1863

[**—Denotes person who wrote of his or her experience]
[?—Denotes uncertainty of person being in Gettysburg, or at the Union Second Corps Hospital]

Surgeons, Assistant Surgeons, Volunteer Surgeons, and Doctors

Second Corps Hospital Administration

Surg. Alexander N. Dougherty, medical director, Second Corps**
Surg. F. LeBaron Monroe, Second Division, First Brigade, 15th Massachusetts, assistant to Medical Director Dougherty
Surg. Justin Dwinelle, chief surgeon, Second Corps Hospital, 106th Pennsylvania**

Second Corps, First Division Administration

Medical Director Richard C. Stiles, First Division**
Surg. Charles T. Kelsey, First Division surgeon-in-charge, Fourth Brigade, 64th New York
Surg. William Warren Potter, First Division surgeon-in-charge (at the Taneytown Road facility), Third Brigade, 57th New York**
Surg. Dr. Charles Squire Wood, First Division chief operator, 66th New York

First Brigade

Surg. John W. Bucknam, 5th New Hampshire

Asst. Surg. William P. Bush, 61st New York

Surg. William Child, 5th New Hampshire**

Surg. Uriah Q. Davis, 148th Pennsylvania

Surg. Alfred Thornley Hamilton, primary aid station at the 148th Pennsylvania, Jacob Hummelbaugh Farm, attended General Barksdale**

Surg. John Houston, 81st Pennsylvania

Asst. Surg. Charles M. Trask, 5th New Hampsire?

Surg. Theodore C. Wallace, 61st New York?

Second Brigade

Asst. Surg. John C. Barrington, 28th Massachusetts

Asst. Surg. A. H. Crosby, 69th New York?

Surg. Patrick Aloysius O'Connell, 28th Massachusetts

Asst. Surg. John Eleazer Parsons, M.D., 28th Massachusetts

Asst. Surg. Richard Powell, Licentiate Royal College of Surgeons, Ireland, 88th New York

Surg. Francis Reynolds, Fellow Royal College of Surgeons, Ireland, 88th New York

Surg. Laurence Reynolds, 63rd New York

Asst. Surg. Dr. Charles Smart, Licentiate College of Surgeons, Aberdeen, Scotland, 63rd New York

Third Brigade

Asst. Surg. G. A. Bingel, 52nd New York?

Asst. Surg. Robert Corry, 57th New York?

Surg. Moritz Frolick, 52nd New York?

Asst. Surg. Benjamin F. Hill, 140th Pennsylvania

Asst. Surg. Gustavus Jacobi, 52nd New York?

Asst. Surg. Nelson Neeley, 57th New York

Surg. Julius C. Rappold, 52nd New York?

Asst. Surg. Griffin Reno, 66th New York?

Asst. Surg. W. W. Sharp, 140th Pennsylvania

Surg. Albert Vander Veer, 66th New York**

Surg. Ernst Weiler, 52nd New York?

Surg. John W. Wishart, 140th Pennsylvania

Fourth Brigade

Asst. Surg. John C. Claypoole, 2nd Delaware
Surg. David H. Houston, 2nd Delaware?
Surg. Dana E. Kelsey, 64th New York?
Asst. Surg. Philip M. Plunkett, 2nd Delaware?
Surg. George L. Potter, 145th Pennsylvania
Asst. Surg. D. W. Richards, 145th Pennsylvania
Asst. Surg. J. S. Whildin, 145th Pennsylvania

Second Corps, Second Division Administration

Medical Director J. Franklin Dyer (surgeon-in-charge of division after Surgeon Dwinelle took charge of corps), Third Brigade, 19th Massachusetts

Justin Dwinelle, Second Division surgeon-in-charge, (later surgeon-in-charge of the Second Corps Hospital), Third Brigade, 106th Pennsylvania**

Surg. Nathan Hayward, Second Division chief operator, Third Brigade, 20th Massachusetts

First Brigade

Surg. A. J. Billings, 19th Maine?
Asst. Surg. Wallace Bolan, 19th Maine?
Asst. Surg. Theodore O. Cornish, 15th Massachusetts
Asst. Surg. William R. Fitch, 82nd New York?
Asst. Surg. Peter Gabrielson, 1st Minnesota?
Asst. Surg. Henry C. Levensaller, 19th Maine
Asst. Surg. Morgan L. Lewis, 82nd New York?
Asst. Surg. J. R. McCullough, 82nd New York
Asst. Surg. Fred G. Parker, 19th Maine?
Surg. S. Hiram Plumb, 82nd New York
Asst. Surg. E. G. Pugsley, 1st Minnesota
Asst. Surg. Henry Rockwood, M.D., 15th Massachusetts

Second Brigade

Dr. John Aiken [Akin], 71st Pennsylvania
Surg. Frederick F. Burmeister, 69th Pennsylvania
Asst. Surg. Erasmus D. Gates, 106th Pennsylvania
Asst. Surg. A. Stokes Jones, 72nd Pennsylvania
Asst. Surg. C. P. Marshall, 71st Pennsylvania
Asst. Surg. Henry D. McLean, 106th Pennsylvania

Asst. Surg. B. A. McNeill, 69th Pennsylvania
Surg. Martin Rizer, 72nd Pennsylvania
Asst. Surg. G. R. B. Robi[n]son, 71st Pennsylvania

Third Brigade

Asst. Surg. Marvin A. Allen, 7th Michigan?
Surg. William J. Burr, 42nd New York
Surg. Gilbert Chaddock, 7th Michigan?
Asst. Surg. George Dougherty, 59th New York
Asst. Surg. James W. Hughes, 59th New York?
Asst. Surg. William Dickson Knapp, M.D., 19th Massachusetts
Asst. Surg. Henry B. Landon, 7th Michigan?
Surg. S. Hiram Plumb, 59th New York?
Asst. Surg. P. R. H. Sawyer, 42nd New York?
Surg. Elisha Mann White, 20th Massachusetts?

Second Corps, Third Division Adminitration

Surg. Isaac Scott, Third Division medical director, First Brigade, 7th West Virginia
Surg. Ebenezer Day, Third Division surgeon-in-charge, Third Brigade, 39th New York
Dr. Harry McKindree McAbee, Third Division chief operator, primary aid station at the Catherine Guinn Farm, First Brigade, 4th Ohio**

First Brigade

Surg. Joseph L. Brenton, 8th Ohio?
Asst. Surg. Barzilla Gray, 4th Ohio?
Asst. Surg. W. T. Hicks, 7th West Virginia?
Surg. George W. McCune, 14th Indiana?
Asst. Surg. Francis William Morrison, 4th Ohio
Asst. Surg. Timothy W. Ross, 7th West Virginia?
Asst. Surg. Elias H. Sabin, 14th Indiana?

Second Brigade

Surg. Frederick A. Dudley, 14th Connecticut
Surg. Brower Gesner, 10th New York Battalion?
Asst. Surg. Uriah Gilman, 12th New Jersey
Asst. Surg. Levi Jewett, 14th Connecticut?
Surg. David W. Maull, 1st Delaware?
Asst. Surg. J. W. McCullough, 1st Delaware

Surg. Owen Munson, 108th New York?
Asst. Surg. Fred J. Owens, 1st Delaware?
Surg. Alvin P. Satterthwait [Satterwaite], 12th New Jersey
Asst. Surg. Francis M. Wafer, primary aid station at the Peter Frey Farm, 108th New York Volunteer**

Third Brigade

Asst. Surg. Washington Aiken, 125th New York?
Asst. Surg. James D. Benton, 111th New York
Surg. William S. Cooper, 125th New York?
Asst. Surg. Charles M. Frisbee, 111th New York?
Asst. Surg. W. W. Goodwin, 39th New York?
Surg. Fletcher M. Hammond, 126th New York
Asst. Surg. D. S. Hopkins, 111th New York
Surg. Charles S. Hoyt, 126th New York?
Surg. Pierre D. Peltier, 126th New York**
Asst. Surg. Emil Steiger, 39th New York
Surg. William B. Vasburgh, 111th New York?
Surg. Frederick Wolf, 39th New York

Surgical help from outside the Second Corps

Asst. Surg. William A. Barry, Eleventh Corps, 75th Pennsylvania
Dr. John H. Brinton, President, Army Medical Examining Board, Army Medical Museum**
Dr. H. B. Buck, Granite Schoolhouse hospital
Dr. John M. Cuyler, United States Army Medical Inspector, Georgia, Surgical care of the Confederates in the barn**
Bushrod W. James, civilian physician, Christian Commission, Philadelphia, Pennsylvania**
Asst. Surg. S. L. Morris, 5th Michigan Cavalry (probable identity of army surgeon only mentioned as "Morris" in Justin Dwinelle's report and Emily Bliss Souder's July 16 letter)
Asst. Surg. Louis E. Norris, Third Corps, First Division, Third Brigade, 17th Maine (probable identity of Army surgeon only mentioned as "Norris" in Justin Dwinelle's report)
Asst. Surg. E. J. Walker, Sixth Corps, First Division, Second Brigade, 121st New York (probable identity of Army surgeon only mentioned as "Walker" in Justin Dwinelle's report)
Doctor Ward, Wilmington, Delaware

Detailed Men From Various Units, Volunteer Nurses, Nursing Assistants, and Hospital Stewards

Nathaniel Beerly, Drummer, Company B, 148th Pennsylvania**
Hospital Steward Billy Berry, First Division, First Brigade, 148th Pennsylvania
Hospital Steward David T. Branch, Third Division, First Brigade, 4th Ohio
"Bridget," a soldier detailed to wash dishes
Hospital Steward Stephen Britton, Third Division, First Brigade, 14th Indiana?
Mrs. Campion & R. Campion (her son), Philadelphia, Pennsylvania**
Principal Musician Robert A. Cassidy, 148th Pennsylvania**
Mrs. Chaplain, Philadelphia, Pennsylvania?
Mrs. James L. Claghorn, Philadelphia, Pennsylvania
Hospital Steward Ralph B. Clarke, 106th Pennsylvania
Pvt. Elbert Corbin, Battery B, 1st New York Light Artillery
Mrs. Curtis, Gettysburg, Pennsylvania?
Hospital Steward Hugh Dinnin, Second Division, Third Brigade, 42nd New York?
Miss Eliza Farnham, Philadelphia, Pennsylvania**
Mary Cadwell Fisher, York, Pennsylvania**
John Y. Foster, Philadelphia, Pennsylvania**
Miss Cornelia Hancock, Third Division, Hancock Bridge, New Jersey**
Mrs. Hanness, central New York
Ellen Orbison Harris, First Division, Philadelphia, Pennsylvania**
J. B. Holloway, Drummer, Company D, 148th Pennsylvania**
Maj. William H. & Mrs. Anna Holstein, Merion, Pennsylvania**
Mrs. Hughes, Michigan
Mary Morris Husband (cared for Confederates in barn), Philadelphia, Pennsylvania**
Miss Clarissa Fellows Jones, Philadelphia, Pennsylvania**
Hospital Steward James Kirkman, 1st Minnesota?
Mary W. Lee, Philadelphia, Pennsylvania**
Hospital Steward G. F. Marble, 1st Minnesota?
Acting Hospital Steward William H. Mayer, 148th Pennsylvania**
Hospital Steward David McIlhattan, Hummelbaugh aid station, First Division, First Brigade, 148th Pennsylvania

Charlotte Elizabeth Johnson McKay, South Reading, Massachusetts**
Hospital Steward Charles W. Merrick, Third Division, First Brigade, 8th Ohio**
Sgt. Thomas P. Meyer, Company A, 148th Pennsylvania**
Charles Minard, Battery B, 1st New York Light Artillery**
Miss Jane Boswell Moore, Baltimore, Maryland**
Mrs. Moore, (Jane's mother), Baltimore, Maryland
Lewis Morgan, Company I, 4th Ohio, Delaware, Ohio
Miss Anna Raymond (Mrs. Claghorn's sister), Philadelphia, Pennsylvania
Mrs. Reynolds, Philadelphia, Pennsylvania
Sarah ———
Mrs. Emily Bliss Souder, Philadelphia, Pennsylvania**
Hospital Steward Charles H. Spear, 1st Minnesota?
Lt. John S. Sullivan, Third Division Ambulance Corps
Capt. Benjamin W. Thompson, 111th New York**
Mrs. Turley, Philadelphia, Pennsylvania?
Hospital Steward Charles A. Weideman, Third Division, Second Brigade, 12th New Jersey?
Mrs. Adam (Catherine "Aunt Katy") Wert, Gettysburg, Pennsylvania
J. Howard Wert, son of Katherine Wert, Gettysburg, Pennsylvania**

Chaplains, Clergy, and Commission Representatives

Rev. Jonathan E. Adams, co-captain of Third Division Christian Commission Station, New Sharon, Maine**
Rev. Mr. George Bringhurst, Christian Commission delegate Philadelphia, Pennsylvania (superintended the Station at the Fifth Corps after Rev. R. J. Parvin)**
Rev. ——— Chapin, New Stanton, Maine**
Chaplain F. A. Conwell, 1st Minnesota?
Chaplain Rev. William Corby, First Division, Second Brigade, 88th New York**
Rev. Dr. Cyrus Cort, Christian Commission delegate, Altoona, Pennsylvania**
Rev. Andrew Boyd Cross, Baltimore, Maryland**
Rev. R. C. Matlack, captain of First and Second Division Christian Commission Station, Philadelphia, Pennsylvania**

Chaplain Rev. Edward McKee, 116th Pennsylvania

Rev. Isaac W. Monfort, Indiana Military Agent, Indianapolis, Indiana**

Rev. B. W. Morris, Germantown, Pennsylvania

Chaplain Thomas G. Murphey, 1st Delaware**

Rev. R. J. Parvin, Christian Commission delegate, Philadelphia, Pennsylvania (also superintended the Station at the Fifth Corps)**

Rev. J. B. Poerner, Baltimore, Maryland**

Rev. Shinn, Rector of the Church of our Saviour, Philadelphia, Pennsylvania

Chaplain Henry S. Stevens, 14th Connecticut**

Chaplain William Henry Stevens, 148th Pennsylvania**

J. B. Stillson, co-captain of Third Division Christian Commission Station, Rochester, New York**

Chaplain Daniel G. Strong, Third Division, First Brigade, 4th Ohio

Chaplain Rev. Thomas Willet, S. J., First Division, Second Brigade, 69th New York

Chaplain ———, 2nd, 5th, or 8th Florida

Chaplain ———, 64th New York

Appendix 3

BIOGRAPHICAL SKETCHES OF SECOND CORPS NURSING STAFF

Pioneering social worker. Diplomatic consort. Author. Innovative nutritionist. Educator. Historical preservationist. Chair of a governmental agency. Visionary administrator. Journalist. Poet. Founder of a graduate school. Certainly sounds like the empowered women of our generation, on the fast track to success.

Surprisingly, the roles just mentioned were filled, not by women of our generation, but by those who volunteered their time and efforts to sustain the wounded and dying men at the Second Corps Hospital in Gettysburg. These were extraordinary women in every sense of the word—resourceful, tenacious, strong and compassionate—pioneers whose leadership set a standard of excellence in their chosen fields of endeavor.

Cornelia Hancock
Independent New Jersey Nurse
see Chapter 18

Ellen Orbison Harris
Secretary of the Philadelphia Ladies Aid Society and Correspondent

As Secretary of the Philadelphia Ladies Aid Society, Ellen Orbison Harris found herself traveling to some of the bloodiest battlefields of the Civil War, and living in some of the most primitive conditions imaginable. The fifth of twelve children of William and Eleanor Elliott Osborne, she was born on July 19, 1816, in Huntington County, Pennsylvania. In 1837, she married widower Dr. John Harris.

Mrs. Harris was far from a likely candidate for the job. By 1860, the forty-eight-year-old Ellen found herself comfortably married to a seventy-year-old Philadelphia physician/pharmacist, with no children. She was certainly not a robust crusader; instead, one acquaintance described her as "a pale, quiet, delicate woman, often an invalid for months."[1] Another thought her to be "one of those delicate, fragile, and feeble-looking ladies who are apparently condemned to lives of patient suffering and inactivity by constitutional defect of physical vigor."[2]

However, the secretariat of the Ladies Aid Society seemed to imbue her with a new stamina and endurance far beyond her abilities. She traveled extensively in the Eastern theater of war through 1863, visiting the devastated fields of Antietam, Fredericksburg, Chancellorsville, and Gettysburg. She then turned her attention to Western battlefields.

From time to time, she would make a swing through Philadelphia, to report to the Society in person, and to snatch a few days of rest at home. Inevitably, her strong sense of duty and personal responsibility for the Society's relief ministry drove her back out to care for the Northern soldiers. "I felt impelled to leave Philadelphia before I was restored, feeling anxious about our stores and the soldiers. We found all our co-workers gone, and no one knew what had to be done with our stores, many of which I knew could not have been distributed *judiciously*."[3] "[I] often wish for longer days and more strength, there are so many ways of doing good, and bearing the burdens of our poor soldiers."[4]

Mrs. Harris' overriding concern throughout all of her medical relief was proper nutrition for the wounded. "Everywhere we see the want of good cooks. The diet after all is the main thing—better be without surgeons than without good nurses and cooks."[5] She was a firm advocate of the healthful benefits of fresh foods and preserves, especially pickles. After distributing pickles, bread, and oranges on

---

1. Brockett and Vaughn, *Woman's Work in the Civil War*, p. 149.
2. Moore, *Women of the War*, p. 176.
3. *Third Semi-Annual Report of the Ladies Aid Society of Philadelphia with Letters and Copious Extracts of Letters from the Secretary of the Society* (Philadelphia: C. Sherman & Son, 1862), p. 43.
4. *Fourth Semi-Annual Report of the Ladies Aid Society of Philadelphia with Letters and Copious Extracts of Letters from the Secretary of the Society* (Philadelphia: C. Sherman & Son, 1863), pp. 17-18.
5. Rev. D. K. Turner, *History of Neshaminy Presbyterian Church of Warwick* (Philadelphia: Culbertson & Bache, 1876), pp. 352-53.

one hospital transport, "at least twenty of them told us the next day that the pickles had done them more good than all the medicine they had taken. So much for the pickle treatment."[6]

Always a powerful writer, her letters became more and more succinct as the war progressed. A deeply devout woman, her faith gave her an anchor even when the war drove her to the very edge of despair. "Meet with so many difficulties here in the prosecution of my work; would have given up in utter despair, had it not been for an unwillingness to quit a field where so few are found to testify for Christ. Not a bright spot appears in our heavens."[7] However, the sight of over one thousand sick and wounded exposed to the elements in severe winter weather caused even her to question God: "Are not the hairs on our heads numbered? Does He not see every throe of anguish, hear every sigh, count every groan, and know every pain? and yet he permits them all, giving a loose rein to His creatures, that they may in their madness destroy themselves. . . . Why hath He dealt so with us, is too often in my head."[8]

When the war finally played itself out in 1865, she returned to Philadelphia much the worse for her efforts, "her health feebler than before, suffering constantly from the effects of a sunstroke, received while laboring on the field at Savage Station."[9] In 1870, her husband was appointed U.S. Consul to Italy. "The consular residence in Venice was the meeting place of many of the most distinguished persons. Robert Browning, Whistler, and other men of the arts and letters were entertained by Dr. Harris and his wife."[10]

Doctor Harris died February 21, 1881, while spending some time in Venice. Following the death of her husband, Ellen "removed to Florence, where she has resided ever since, her health having been as such to make the voyage to the states too dangerous for her to undertake."[11]

Her untiring exertions to relieve the suffering of wounded and sick soldiers had finally caught up with her. The proposed voyage to the

---

6. *Third Semi-Annual Report of the Ladies Aid Society*, p. 23.
7. *Fourth Semi-Annual Report of the Ladies Aid Society*, p. 16.
8. *Ibid.*, pp. 16, 23.
9. Moore, *Women of the War*, p. 212.
10. William Meroni, *Harris (or Herris), Miller, and Dunlop* (Privately published, 1920), p. 94.
11. Obituary of Ellen Orbison Harris, *Democratic Watchman*, Bellfonte, Pennsylvania, December 12, 1902.

States never took place. Ellen Orbison Harris, Secretary Emeritus of the Ladies Aid Society of Philadelphia, died in 1902 in Florence, where she is buried.[12]

William and Anna Holstein
Independent Volunteer Nursing Attendant and Dietary Specialist

Only one married couple figured prominently in the care of the Second Corps wounded—William and Anna Morris Holstein from Upper Merion, Pennsylvania. "People of considerable wealth, and unexceptionable social position, beloved and honored by all who know them," forty-six-year-old William started visiting battlefield hospitals in 1862, leaving Anna, nine years younger, to collect and publish his hospital stories for use by aid societies.

However, when William returned with tales of grave need from the general hospitals around Antietam and Frederick, Maryland, Anna gave up her editing and society rounds to actively pursue nursing. They soon became familiar figures around the Second Corps hospitals near Falmouth, Virginia, following the Battle of Fredericksburg in December of 1862, and near Potomac Creek following the clash at Chancellorsville in May of 1863.[13]

William frequently suffered recurring episodes of malarial fever, and they returned home due to William's health just a week before the clash at Chancellorsville. But William was sufficiently recuperated to leave for Gettysburg within a week of the battle, and they immediately sought out the Second Corps Hospital. Like Ellen Orbison Harris, Anna Holstein was deeply concerned with proper diet for the weakened men in the hospital, and worked with the Second Corps special "diet kitchen."[14]

"By the 7th of August there still remained *three thousand* [wounded throughout Gettysburg], who were moved into tents of the United States General Hospital on the York turnpike; when our corps hospital was merged into this, we removed there; I remained as its matron until the close."[15] The Holsteins made quite an impression on Surgeon Henry May of the 145th New York: "In August of 1863, while

---

12. Conklin, *Women at Gettysburg*, p. 198.
13. Brockett and Vaughn, *Woman's Work in the Civil War*, p. 251; Conklin, *Women at Gettysburg*, p. 255; Holstein, *Three Years in Field Hospitals*, pp. 37-38.
14. Holstein, *Three Years in Field Hospitals*, pp. 38-39.
15. *Ibid.*, p. 49.

on duty at Camp Letterman General Hospital at Gettysburg, Pa., I met Mr. and Mrs. Holstein . . . who were devoting their whole time gratuitously to the cause of the sick and wounded soldier. Mrs. Holstein was placed in charge of the 'Lowdiet Kitchen' of that large Hospital and from its organization to its close in November 1863, she did most faithful, efficient, and acceptable service. Her work extended from the early hours of each day to its close; and a host of grateful men were ever loud in her praise for the many kind words and offices rendered aside from that of preparing their food."[16]

The men were deeply moved by the culinary kindness of Mrs. Holstein. "Mrs. H. had full charge of the diet kitchen and all the many delicacies we received were from her hands, and in addition to this she constantly visited the wounded to ascertain what would be good for them and to encourage them, and give them motherly care," wrote Capt. John Hilton of the 145th Pennsylvania. "The lives of badly wounded men depend more from nourishing food than medicine. Having been one of the doubtful cases, I know had it not been for such care I received from Mrs. Holstein, I never could have recovered."[17]

When Letterman Hospital was finally closed in November, Anna Holstein spent the remainder of 1863 giving a lecture series for the Sanitary Commission across the State of Pennsylvania. Even though it was time well spent, being away from the wounded galled her: "The inaction and feeling of doing nothing for the wounded was unbearable, and a constant source of anxiety and trouble."[18]

The Holsteins returned to the army in May of 1864; after leaving Belle Plain, she followed Cornelia Hancock's footsteps to Port Royal, White House, and City Point. "Nothing before us all day but wounded; wounded men at every step you take." Like Cornelia, she found the dust ever-present and aggravating: "Clouds of dust fill the air; and though the hospital is some distance from the traveled road to the front, yet by four o'clock the rows of tents which stand but a few yards from us are obscured."[19]

When William's health began to once again deteriorate in the torrid Virginia weather, the Holsteins headed for the cool hills of Upper

---

16. Holstein Pension Records, letter from Dr. Henry May, Private Act #141, 52nd Congress, National Archives and Records Administration.
17. Holstein Pension Records. For the account of Captain Hilton's wounding and care at the Second Corps Hospital, see Chapter 5.
18. Holstein, *Three Years in Field Hospitals*, p. 58.
19. *Ibid.*, pp. 76-77.

Merion, never to return to their soldier friends. Anna turned her attention to a rigorous schedule of speaking tours and working with newly-returned prisoners of war at Annapolis, Maryland.

With the end of the war, Anna sat down to record their Civil War adventures, entitling the 1867 book *Three Years in Field Hospitals of the Army of the Potomac*. Despite occasional lapses in dates and geography, and her harshly anti-Southern views, Anna Holstein's book is a lively and emotional account of life in Civil War Hospitals. For her unflagging relief service, she was awarded a $12 monthly pension in 1892 by a special act of Congress, her claim buoyed by numerous letters from other nurses, surgeons, patients, and even former Pennsylvania governor Andrew Curtin.

Without the war or a book to occupy her time, Anna turned her attentions to historical preservation, desiring "to arouse public sentiment and appreciation for the great historical importance of the hills of Valley Forge, where Washington's army was encamped during the terrible winter of 1777-1778. She was made regent of the Valley Forge Centennial and Memorial Association at its organization and held this office until her death. She labored untiringly that the association might purchase Washington's headquarters at Valley Forge and restore it 'as a memorial for all time to come.'"[20] One can almost imagine Brig. Gen. Samuel Zook smiling down on her efforts to preserve his old playground.

Anna Morris Holstein died on December 31, 1900, at her lifelong home and refuge in Upper Merion, Pennsylvania. She was buried beside her husband at Swedes Church Cemetery in Swedesburg, Pennsylvania, her modest headstone bearing, like so much of what she did, her inscribed and distinctive signature.[21]

Clarissa Fellows Jones
School Teacher and Independent Pennsylvania Nurse

Clarissa Fellows Jones was just twenty-eight when war invaded her peaceful world. It was a quiet and domestic existence, with Clarissa teaching at the Rittenhouse Grammar School in Germantown, Pennsylvania, which served to support her and her widowed mother. Clarissa simply expanded her life to include nursing whenever time

20. Gertrude Bosler Biddle and Sarah Dickinson [Dickson] Lowrie, *Notable Women of Pennsylvania* (Philadelphia: University of Pennsylvania Press, 1942), pp. 166-67.

21. Conklin, *Women at Gettysburg*, p. 264.

allowed, mostly during summer breaks and school holidays. "I did not register as a nurse, because being the breadwinner of the family I could not give my entire time to Hospital work. From the beginning to the close of the war I gave my best energies to the service of my country. . . . I never received pay in any form for services rendered thru [*sic*] the war."

"In 1861 I was a member of a class of women receiving instruction from a Professor who was coaching Students for their exam, as doctors. The Professor agreed to extend to a class of women who desired to become nurses a like benefit, so I was better fitted to go to the field than most women." Working around her teaching schedule, she served in 1861 as a volunteer in the hospitals scattered throughout the greater Philadelphia area; in December, she visited Camp Pierrepont hospital in Washington D.C. She sent ahead supplies to the surgeon-in-charge, and then spent her time there "distributing stores, instructing soldier nurses in the care of the sick, preparing food for them and finding the actual needs of the Camp Hospital."[22]

In early 1862, with school again in session, she continued volunteering in nearby hospitals. During July, however, she landed a berth on the hospital steamer *State of Maine*, which transported exchanged prisoners of war, as well as sick and wounded troops, to Northern hospitals. Surgeon-in-Charge H. L. W. Burrett wrote: "Miss Clarissa F. Jones has been acting as volunteer nurse on board our steamer for the last month and I am happy to say has satisfied me in every respect of eminent capacity for that position. Miss Jones is a lady of cultivated mind and refined deportment as well as great force of character. Her tender care and humanity toward the sick and suffering and her constant attention to them is remembered by all and will not soon be forgotten."[23]

In August, it was back to Philadelphia to secure supplies, then off to the surgeon general's office to pick up a pass to Alexandria, Virginia. Since Dorothea Dix had been appointed to oversee military nursing, Clarissa was sent to see her. Dix told her frankly that she had no use for her, since she could only work at limited times. Miss Jones was certainly not about to be put off by Dix; she simply did an end-run around the touchy superintendent of nurses. A visit to the War Department produced a pass for her, due to her impeccable credentials

22. Pension Submission File, Letter dated February 5, 1917, Commissioner of Pensions files, National Archives and Records Administration.
23. *Ibid.*

(including a letter from the mayor of Philadelphia). Planning ahead, Clarissa had obtained temporary leave from her teaching position, and remained in Alexandria nursing the victims of Second Bull Run until November, 1862.

The following summer, she did local nursing in Germantown until the crisis came at Gettysburg. "After Gettysburg, Mrs. Moore, her daughter and I went to Baltimore and Washington to replenish our stock, then commenced the hardest task of getting a Pass to the front. This I achieved and we went to Rappahannock Station where our army is resting. We remained there until Sept. 1 when my school duties called me home."[24]

During winter break, it was off again to the army's winter quarters at Rappahannock Station, as well as a visit to Brandy Station, bringing "barrels and boxes" of medical supplies. "My journey to and from was an eventful one. I was entirely alone, walking miles to find the Camps. The night of my arrival the mud was so deep that I could hardly pull my feet out of the mud which was nearly ankle deep. I wore high boots. The next morning everything was frozen. I was awakened by hearing the noise of chopping ice from around the mules whose legs were imbedded in solid ice. After leaving the stores and xmas cheer there I returned to Rappahannock Station and distributed the rest."[25]

Clarissa Fellows Jones' nursing trips came to an abrupt and unexpected halt: "My sister, dying in 1864, my trips to the front were discontinued, as she left me her family of three small children whose welfare prevented me from leaving home."[26] Now, in addition to supporting a widowed mother, Clarissa was responsible for eight-year-old Lydia, seven-year-old Elizabeth, and her namesake Clarissa J., aged three years. Nevertheless, she was deterrmined to maintain her relief efforts, and "continued collecting and forwarding hospital stores till the close of the war."[27]

Clarissa continued on as a school teacher after the end of the war. In December of 1872, she became Mrs. John H. Dye. Dye, a widower who had served a stint as lieutenant of Company G, 33rd Pennsylvania Volunteers, brought four children of his own to the marriage.

---

24. *Ibid.*
25. *Ibid.*
26. Clarissa's sister, thirty-five-year-old Elizabeth Logan, died of marasmus (a nineteenth-century term for wasting away). Her husband Daniel was serving time in the Philadelphia County Prison (as of 1860) for larceny.
27. Pension Submission File, Letter dated February 5, 1917, Commissioner of Pensions files, National Archives and Records Administration.

Even with seven inherited children, Clarissa continued to have a persistent heart for nursing. She became Chairman of the Pension Committee for the Association of Army Nurses of the Civil War. Oddly enough, despite her several applications for a nurse's pension, she was turned down each time.

In 1913, she was interviewed by an enterprising reporter from the Philadelphia *North American* about her memories of serving as an Army Nurse, now that the veterans were gathering for a fiftieth reunion at the old battlefield. Clarissa gave a lucid and candid account of her journey and the time there, spent mostly in caring for wounded Rebel prisoners. Her story appeared in a special section of the June 29, 1913 edition.

Clarissa Fellows Jones Dye, full-time teacher, unexpected mother, and part-time nurse with a full-time heart, died somewhere around 1920. Her burial site is presently unknown.[28]

Mary W. Lee
72nd Pennsylvania Volunteer Nurse

There was only one Mary Lee. She had a vision; a vision of being able to minister to every soldier that passed through Philadelphia—every single one.

"It had started in this way: Back in 1861, on April 23, Sherman's battery of eight howitzers, manned by eighty very hungry and thirsty men, passed through Philadelphia on its way to Washington. As the troops appeared on the water front, in a shabby working-class district, women came running out bringing the plates off their own tables, and the saucepans and frying pans off their own stoves full of their own family dinners. Others came rushing with bottles from the pantry shelves, and loaves out of the bread box. Loiterers on the street, seeing this, hastily bought up all the stocks of the pushcart men, who sold apples and oranges and peanuts, and added them to the food the women were assembling for the soldiers. A man passed around his hat and took up a collection which he spent buying out the nearest tobacco shop. The soldiers departing, replete with food, drink, and

---

28. *Ibid.*; Conklin, *Women at Gettysburg*, p. 302. Little is known of Clarissa Fellows Jones Dye, apart from the June 29, 1913, article in the *Philadelphia North American*, and her extensive pension application file, which contains many letters and "proofs" of her Civil War experience.

smoke, gave nine cheers, for the Union, the Constitution, and the ladies of Philadelphia."[29] At least, that's how the story goes.

Inspired by the impromptu feast, Mary put up a stove and coffeepot in an old boathouse, and hung a sign over the door: "Union Refreshment Saloon." She contacted all the housewives in the area to organize refreshments; whenever soldiers were arriving, whether day or night, by boat or by train, a signal gun would sound, and groups of volunteers would converge, food in hand, to man the "Saloon." These were largely the poorest folk of town, many crippled, but delighted nonetheless to be able to help in the war effort.

Word soon spread through the military community that there was always food and amenities to be found when passing through Philadelphia. Funds and donations began to flow in from all over the city. "Men of larger means and equally earnest sympathies" were attracted to this homegrown enterprise, and one, Samuel B. Fales, poured extensive funding and many hours of volunteer work into the Saloon. Over $100,000, besides enormous amounts of supplies, was funneled into the local relief agency during the four and a half years of its existence.[30]

Soon the "Union Refreshment Saloon" outgrew the boathouse, and building after adjoining building were annexed in the expanding enterprise. Bathing facilities were added when soldiers complained that they hadn't had a chance to clean up in days; when troops arrived dog-tired, they found dormitories ready for their use. Even sick and wounded men soon found a Saloon Hospital waiting to care for their needs—nearly 15,000 patients were treated there. It is estimated that, from 1861 to 1865, between 800,000 and 900,000 men found a home away from home at the pre-USO "Union Refreshment Saloon."[31]

Mary had had a lot of help along the way, but the Saloon was uniquely hers in the minds of most of the troops who walked through the door. But all that changed in August of 1862. Mary's son William had enlisted in Company B, 72nd Pennsylvania in August of 1861. After a year of separation, Mary decided to relocate her services to the front. When the hospital transport *Spaulding* set sail after dropping wounded troops off at Philadelphia, Mary was on board. Arriving at

---

29. Marjorie Barstow Greenbie, *Lincoln's Daughters of Mercy* (New York: G. P. Putnam's Sons, 1944), pp. 134-35.
30. Brockett and Vaughn, *Woman's Work in the Civil War*, pp. 733-34.
31. Greenbie, *Lincoln's Daughters of Mercy*, pp. 134-35.

Harrison's Landing, she was a welcome sight to the many wounded from the costly Peninsula Campaign.

Arriving at Antietam on the evening of September 16 via forage wagon, she set up along Sharpsburg Road, supplying bread and water to the wounded throughout the battle. "Mrs. Lee was probably nearer the front than any other woman on the day of the battle, and certainly much nearer than the commander in chief himself," noted one commentator with some acerbity.[32]

It was at Antietam that Mrs. Lee became legendary among the wounded of the Army of the Potomac. "At one of the field hospitals where Mrs. Lee was doing the best she could for the crowd of sufferers, there was nothing found in the way of commissary supplies but a barrel of flour, a barrel of apples, and a keg of lard. To a practical housekeeper, as she is, this combination seemed to point to apple dumplings as the dish in which they could all be employed to the best advantage; and the good-natured astonishment of the poor fellows, who looked for nothing but black coffee and hardtack, was merged in admiration for the accomplished cook who could there, almost on the battlefield, serve them with hot dumplings."[33]

By evening, Mary was cooking for the wounded at Sedgwick's division hospital. After a few days, she even scoured the battlefield with another nurse, searching for overlooked wounded.[34] Mary moved on to Hoffman's Farm Hospital, then on to the Second Corps' Smoketown General Hospital, remaining there for three months. She hurriedly left there when news came that a powder explosion in Harpers Ferry had killed and wounded many men from the 72nd Pennsylvania. Her son, however, was safe and sound.

After nursing the casualties from Fredericksburg in December of 1862, she accompanied her sick son home to Philadelphia, working at the Refreshment Saloon while he recovered. By March, 1863, she was back with the Second Corps Hospital at Potomac Creek Hospital and the Lacy House Hospital at Chancellorsville, accompanied now by her daughter and talented aide, Amanda.

Exactly when the Lees arrived at Gettysburg is unclear. Once again, she searched out the Second Corps Hospital. "For her services in this hospital she received from the officers and men a gold medal—a trefoil,

---

32. Moore, *Women of the War*, pp. 150-51.
33. *Ibid.*
34. They found two wounded soldiers in an old cabin, who had survived for days on a few crackers and some water.

beautifully engraved, and with an appropriate inscription."[35] When the corps hospital consolidated with Camp Letterman, Mrs. Lee stayed on for almost two months with her son, who had been detailed there as a nurse.

The wear and tear of campaigning were beginning to tell on Mary, and she headed home in late 1863. "Her health was impaired by her excessive labors at Gettysburg and previously in Virginia, and she remained at home for a longer time than usual . . . but early in February, 1864, she established herself in a new hospital of the second Division, Second Corps at Brandy Station, Virginia."[36] Again her daughter joined her, and she was soon back in the routine of army life again: "Mother has a small stove," wrote Amanda Lee; "the top is about half a yard square. On this she is now boiling potatoes, stewing some chicken-broth, heating a kettle of water, and has a large bread-pudding inside. She has made milk-punch, lemonade, beef-tea, stewed cranberries, and I cannot think what else since breakfast."[37] Cornelia Hancock confided that "I wish I was more like Mrs. Lee, did not think about anything but my biscuit, yeast, etc. She is delighted to have my division to cook for, the more work she has to do the better she feels."[38]

With Cornelia Hancock, she traveled through a progression of hospital sites—Belle Plain, Fredericksburg, White House, and City Point. By June of 1864, her tireless culinary exertions were taking a severe toll. "She is here but I think played out," noted Cornelia Hancock; "she has worked harder than any galley slave I ever saw." Miss Hancock thought in July that "Mrs. Lee will come home soon."[39]

After regaining her strength at home, Mary Lee attempted to return to the front in March of 1865. However, it was not as easy to secure a pass now as in the past, so she had to content herself with working in a hospital in Fredericksburg. She was there when the war ended, and stayed on through May in hospitals around Petersburg and Richmond. Returning to Philadelphia, she worked the final days of the Union Refreshment Saloon. The "bouncing little Scotch-Irish woman . . . homely and sweet as one of her famous apple dumplings," was forty-five when she returned from war, with both son and daughter intact.[40]

---

35. Brockett and Vaughn, *Woman's Work in the Civil War*, p. 486.
36. *Ibid.*
37. *Ibid.*
38. Hancock, *South After Gettysburg*, p. 82.
39. *Ibid.*, pp. 125, 136.
40. Greenbie, *Lincoln's Daughters of Mercy*, p. 133.

Her death on August 6, 1893, was as spectacular as she was herself. A public notice in the *Public Ledger* openly invited all of the friends, relatives, workers from the Union Refreshment Saloon, veterans, and the Ladies Aid Society of the 72nd Pennsylvania to attend. She was buried in the Ebenezer Methodist Episcopal Church Cemetery. In 1903, the church was abandoned, and part of the land sold to the city; numerous coffins and remains were moved to Arlington Cemetery, Delaware County. It is believed that Mary W. Lee was reburied there in 1905 in the Silverbrook Section, Lot #163, Grave #2. Sadly, this is a mass grave of eight individuals, with no headstone.[41] Selfless Mary Lee probably would have liked the idea of sharing her grave with others.

Charlotte Elizabeth Johnson McKay
Independent Massachusetts Nurse

Death had come to the McKay house, not once, but twice in five years. Charlotte McKay sat devastated and destitute in what had once been a happy family home.

Born Charlotte Elizabeth Johnson on August 2, 1818, she was one of seven children born to Dr. Abner and Julia Sargent Johnson of Waterford, Maine. The family moved about the state during her childhood—Waterford, Sullivan, Cherryfield, Brewer, Presque Isle. Her father, Dr. Johnson, was something of a pharmacist, and "was the originator and manufacturer of a popular liniment called 'Johnson's Anodyne Liniment' which he compounded in a small building in Sullivan Harbor [in 1834]."[42]

Charlotte became a teacher in a small private high school. On August 16, 1854, she married William P. McKay of South Reading, Massachusetts. Little Julia Sargent McKay, named for her grandmother, came along on May 14, 1855. The small family's joy was short-lived—William died in April of 1856. Charlotte raised little Julia alone until the child, too, died on February 1, 1861.

But Charlotte was not one to sit at home and mourn. "Her heart worn with grief, sought relief, where it was most likely to find it, in ministering to the sufferings of others." Some thought that she "sought oblivion, and at the same time usefulness, in the army of the Potomac." For Charlotte, the prospect was not pleasant: "The contemplated journey

---

41. Conklin, *Women at Gettysburg*, p. 205.
42. *The History of Waterford, Oxford County, Maine: A Compilation of Addresses, Records and Proceedings, published at the direction of the Town* (Portland, Maine: Hoyt, Fogg, and Donham, 1879), p. 264.

offered nothing inviting to my anticipations. I was leaving behind me all that I held pleasant in social life. . . . The rushing rail-car, the creaking, flying steamboat would bear me swiftly to scenes where all was strange and terrible to my apprehension."[43]

Charlotte first went to the Camden Hospital in Baltimore. Baltimore already had a glut of volunteer nurses, so, when a call came from Frederick, Maryland, she proceeded there. She would serve in the "Hessian Barracks" Hospital, two large grim stone buildings built to house Revolutionary War German prisoners-of-war. When the Confederates swept through Frederick on their first invasion of the North, the hospital (and Charlotte) surrendered. Promised protection, she nursed wounded Confederates during the occupation: "So ragged were they, so filthy and squalid in appearance . . . yet . . . many of them I found to be good, intelligent, thoughtful men, having implicit faith in their cause, in God as their especial leader, and next to Him in Stonewall Jackson."[44]

The hospital changed hands again as the Southern army fell back, and Charlotte ministered to many of the casualties of Antietam. Working in a number of hospitals in Washington (some even situated in governmental offices) during the winter following the Battle of Fredericksburg, she finally requested and received permission on January 12, 1863, to take supplies to the front. This was gratifying to Charlotte, since she had a brother, Lt. Dudley Johnson, camped along the Rappahannock River near Falmouth in winter quarters.

"In the spring the army was re-organized, camps were changed, and our division, with its hospital, was removed to Potomac Creek, four or five miles from Falmouth." When the Battle of Chancellorsville began on May 3, 1863, Charlotte headed for the front. "Just before we reached the river was a small house, that had been taken for an hospital. Horses were picketed around it in all directions; quartermaster's wagons, with their tents near by; a throng of soldiers coming and going. Finding many wounded men lying in and around the house, I immediately commenced the distribution of stimulants and nourishment." It was there that she learned that her brother had been shot and killed in the action. Death had again come to call on Charlotte McKay.[45]

---

43. Brockett and Vaughn, *Woman's Work in the Civil War*, p. 514; Moore, *Women of the War*, p. 279; McKay, *Stories of Hospital and Camp*, pp. 159-60.
44. McKay, *Stories of Hospital and Camp*, pp. 22-23.
45. *Ibid.*, pp. 33-39. Lt. Dudley Johnson left a widow and an eight-month-old daughter.

As the army fell back, so did Charlotte, stopping frequently to minister to the wounded along the road. Back at Fredericksburg, her hospital was again swamped with the casualties of the battle. Here she would stay until the hospital was finally disbanded as the army moved toward Gettysburg in pursuit of Lee.

Following her time at the Second Corps Hospital in Gettysburg, Charlotte followed the army as it moved in September. She ministered in Sulphur Springs, Virginia, then on to Rappahannock Station. After shunting between the capital and the front, Charlotte finally settled in to winter with the army at Brandy Station, where she nursed the sick. Ordered back to Washington when Grant cleared women out of the army encampment, she returned to Fredericksburg in time for the Battle of the Wilderness in May of 1864. She followed the army as it progressed, serving at Port Royal, then White House Landing, and finally ending at the Cavalry Corps Hospital at City Point.

With the capitulation of the South, Charlotte made her way into Petersburg to see the sights. She took over the special diet kitchen at Petersburg, but "my strength gave out, and I was obliged, with great regret, to relinquish the work, and leave the men who need the care I would gladly have continued to give."[46] As a token of their appreciation, the men from the hospital presented her with a gold medal and chain.

At loose ends after the war, Charlotte stayed in Virginia for the winter, distributing supplies from the North to freed slaves in Poplar Springs and Petersburg. Beyond this, little is known of her work with freedmen.

She sat down to write of her wartime experiences in 1876, at her home in Wakefield, Massachusetts, and, as Mrs. C. E. McKay, published a slender volume called *Stories of Hospital and Camp.* In 1893, at age seventy-five, she swore out a deposition for an increase of pension to her brother Dudley's widow. She, however, never bothered to file for a nursing pension for herself.

Charlotte died in San Diego, California, on April 10, 1894, thirty-eight years to the very day of her husband's death. She is buried in Section F, Division 3, Lot 2, Space 4 of the Olivewood Cemetery in Riverside, California.[47]

---

46. *Ibid.*, p. 142.
47. Conklin, *Women at Gettysburg*, p. 254.

Jane Boswell Moore

Independent Maryland Nurse and Newspaper Columnist

Jane Boswell Moore and her mother comprised a highly effective mother/daughter team at Gettysburg, but one that is almost totally lost to history. Even her mother's first name is unknown. They exist only in the observations of others, and in a scant number of printed sources. Even most of the newspaper articles written by Miss Moore have been lost.

Jane began her war experience by publishing a series of scathing responses to secession in the loyal newspapers of her hometown, Baltimore. In no uncertain terms, she labeled secession as high treason.

Once she became interested in the field of nursing, her mother became her inseparable companion. As she wrote of the war, Jane chose to relate poignant vignettes of nursing experiences rather than a dry recitation or a timeline of events. The duo worked in some of the most challenging spots of the war, and Jane painted vivid word pictures that spanned the years of war, caught by her sharp journalistic eye:

> By the light of a dimly-rising moon we rode over the burial trenches of Antietam to Smoketown Hospital, through whose scattered grove of trees the roaring of the December wind sounded like the notes of some great funeral organ.
>
> A picture of desolate grandeur was Harper's Ferry, with its rude hospitals, its dead on the hill-side, whose march was over, and its tens of thousands of the living thronging every winding path on their way to Fredericksburg, Martinsburg, and Cumberland. . . .
>
> Cumberland, in whose old mill, on a wild March evening, we watched the failing breath of Dutton, a New York soldier. . . .
>
> The old ruined town of Winchester, by whose desolate churches so many of our dead are sleeping, and our little room in Taylor Hospital then . . . crowded with fever patients.
>
> [At Chancellorsville] we had sad music—the bands on the hill-side with their mournful "dead march," by open graves, and the plaintive cry of the whippoorwill, when our busy day was done.
>
> . . . Gettysburg with all its horrors, among those dead and dying we passed a month. . . .

Visiting his [General Franz Sigel's] forces just before they left Winchester, with stationary, pickles, &c., and hurried back over deserted roads, with our precious mail-bags bearing thirteen hundred letters, many of them the last messages to friends. . . .

A deserted cabin formed our next quarters at Point of Rocks, close to the swamps of the Appomattox, where we saw the opening bombardment of Petersburg. The New Hampshire youth, Leonard Wiggins, fell asleep here as the guns were firing. . . . How distinctly memory recalls the night of his death—the doors, windows, and walls of our rude dwelling shook and rattled so under every gun, that we willingly left it, and stood at the stile in the light of a full moon, watching the exploding shells. We then made Leonard the lemonade he had enjoyed so much, for the *last* time.

Amid the booming of guns from the neighboring battlefield of Cedar Creek, on an October morning, we entered our little room on Braddock Street, Winchester. How many times were the barrels and boxes of that crowded spot replenished by the Sanitary and Christian Commissions during the six long, busy months of labor among the regimental hospitals, as well as in the snowy tents of Sheridan, covering so many suffering and dying souls.

O, the sad heart-rending letters written nightly to kindred far away, by the blazing fire of Virginia rails.

. . . We passed under Fort Drewry's now silent guns, with our stores, into Richmond, for ten weeks' labor among worn-out troops. This seems the hardest of our campaigns; but the end was near. . . .

[Throughout the war,] we drew liberal supplies from both the Sanitary and Christian Commissions, as well as largely from individuals, but have ourselves belonged to no association, and received no compensation from any quarter. None of our expenses were defrayed, except in the matter of government passes. As southern women who had no relatives to give to the cause, we have endeavored to be behind none in our devotion.[48]

---

48. Moore, *Women of the War*, pp. 556-59, 569-70.

Frank Moore noted in his book *Women of the War*: "[Major] General [William] Emory says of her and her mother, 'The names of Miss and Mrs. Moore are on the lips of thousands to whom they have ministered in camp and hospital.' General Grant also testifies to their remarkable usefulness."[49]

Jane Boswell Moore and her devoted mother certainly succeeded in their goal "to be behind none in our devotion." Absolutely nothing more is known of their lives, beyond the final disturbing note that "the health of Miss Moore has been seriously impaired by the hardships she has suffered, and by the agitations of those four years of unremitting military service." Devoted women, indeed.[50]

Emily Bliss Souder
Independent Pennsylvania Nurse and Poet

Just for the briefest moment did Emily Bliss Souder step onto the pages of public history. When the crisis came at Gettysburg, Emily decided to forego the annual family vacation, "our cot beside the sea" at Cape May, for a visit instead to the battlefield as a volunteer nurse.[51] Emily had a large and active family still living at home in Philadelphia—Emily (twenty-two), Stephen (twenty), Sarah (eighteen), Edward (eleven), Fanny (eight), Mary (four), and Sallie (one).[52] Her sudden trip must have put an unexpected strain on the family's routine.

Arriving in Gettysburg on July 14, she stayed just a little over two weeks, and ministered to the wounded at the Second Corps Hospital. Her departure was just as precipitate: her last letter from the field is dated July 29, and her dispatches of the final week chronicle her failing health in the noxious surrounds of Gettysburg.

Undaunted by her illness, she was determined to return for the dedication of the new National Cemetery. "I had felt as if I *must* be in Gettysburg whenever the ceremonies did take place."[53]

Moved by the unique experiences and impressions of her two visits to the Pennsylvania battlefield, Emily Souder compiled her

---

49. *Ibid.*
50. *Ibid.*
51. Souder, *Leaves from the Battle-field of Gettysburg*, p. 54.
52. Pennsylvania 1860 Census Records. Capt. Stephen Souder, age twenty, enlisted June 18 in a three month Philadelphia unit to face the "existing emergency" posed by the Confederate invasion. He mustered out August 1, 1863. This may well have been Emily's eldest son.
53. Souder, *Leaves from the Battle-field of Gettysburg*, p. 133.

correspondence from the field, and added a collection of original patriotic poetry. Publishing in 1864, the slim folio bore the title *Leaves from the Battle-field of Gettysburg. A Series of Letters from a Field Hospital and National Poems.*

And then she was gone. Until her death on December 22, 1886, at age seventy-two, very little is known of her life. She was buried in Philadelphia's Woodlands Cemetery, Section F, Grave 348-349. Although once marked by both headstone and footstone, her grave today is missing both. Her final resting place, like much of her life, is lost to history. But the lasting impression she made in the lives of men she touched during two terrible weeks in Gettysburg lives on in the history of the Second Corps Hospital.[54]

Jane Eliza Newton Woolsey and George Anna Muirson Woolsey Sanitary Commission "Lodge" Transit Hospital

The three-week-long visit to Gettysburg as representatives of the Sanitary Commission was coming to an end for Georgeanna Muirson Woolsey and her mother, Jane Eliza Newton Woolsey. Georgeanna was the third of eight children born to Charles and Jane Elizabeth Newton Woolsey through the years. It was a lopsided mix of siblings—seven girls (Abby, Jane, George Anna, Mary, Eliza, Harriet, and Caroline) and one boy (Charles). A wealthy and highly influential Boston family, the Woolseys migrated to New York City following Charles Sr.'s death in 1840. Once established in New York, Georgy had been instrumental in the formation of the "Women's Central Association of Relief," which in turn led directly to the formation of the United States Sanitary Commission.[55]

At first, all of the Woolsey ladies had contented themselves with sewing clothes, making lint, and collecting supplies. "We women regretfully 'sit at home at ease' and only appease ourselves by doing the little we can with sewing machines and patent bandage-rollers." Georgy, however, was not content to merely be a spectator to the war; she pursued nursing, gradually drawing along the rest of the family in her wake. Georgy and sister Eliza set off to joust with Dorothea Dix; once they had passed her strict scrutiny, they were attached to a tent hospital in Alexandria.[56]

---

54. Conklin, *Women at Gettysburg*, p. 313.
55. Woolsey Bacon, *Letters of a Family During the War for the Union*, p. 62.
56. *Ibid.*, p. 532; Moore, *Women of the War*, p. 146.

Now two years and numerous nursing assignments later, the mother/daughter team had hurried off to Gettysburg, worried that Charles Jr., on the staff of General Meade, had been killed or seriously wounded in the bloody, three-day battle. Charley was shaken, but intact, so the two ladies immediately took over the day to day affairs of the Sanitary Commission "Lodge" Transit Hospital by the railroad tracks, making use the large shipment of Commission supplies which they had accompanied to the field.

As things were being packed up for the trip home, a Baltimore fireman (whom they had met during their relief efforts) stopped by to give them an unforgetable going-away present. The enterprising firefighter "secured two bands before we came away and marched them down to camp to serenade us, which they did standing at the mouth of the long tent and refreshed themselves afterwards with gingerbread and punch." Their guests enjoyed the refreshments mightily, never knowing that the Canadaigua, New York Sanitary Commission delegation, already having enjoyed the snack, and with hands covered with sugary gingerbread, had quickly rinsed off their fingers in the punchbowl when the bands had unexpectedly arrived! "Our work was over, our tents were struck, and we came away, after a flourish of trumpets from two military bands, who filed down to our door, and gave us a farewell,—'Red, white, and blue.'"[57]

Boarding the train, they headed back home to New York City. The Sanitary Commission immediately urged Georgy to record their experiences as a fund-raiser publication for the Commission, to "fire the hearts" of sewing circles and aid societies throughout the north. Georgeanna dashed off a pamphlet entitled "Three Weeks at Gettysburg," then left to nurse the wounded at the Point Lookout Hospital, in Maryland. The Commission had already ordered 10,000 copies, so Abby, Georgy's oldest sister, was entrusted with overseeing the printing and distribution of the brochure.[58]

---

57. *Ibid.*
58. Woolsey Bacon, *Letters of a Family During the War for the Union*, p. 534. The promotional pamphlet would serve to annoy the entire family for the remainder of the war. In May, 1864, sister Caroline wrote to Georgy: "Miss E. M. wants to know if I wrote those everlasting Three Weeks in Gettysburg. Having read them, she cannot stay at home, and would like a little information as to what was needed for a nurse . . . she is the second anxious inquirer this morning. . . . We think of adding 'Army Gen'l Directory' to our door-plate, so many people of all sorts come to us for information." [*Ibid.*, pp. 597, 600.]

Soon after their return from Gettysburg, Georgeanna and Jane were contacted about a return visit. "The authorities want us to go back again, and look after the special diet in the new and fine General Hospital for 3000 men, too sick to be moved," wrote Georgy. "We can't do so, though, as Jane and I have promised to spend the winter at Point Lookout in the Hammond Hospital." For her part, mother Jane Eliza Newton Woolsey very much wanted to go back to Gettysburg. Beside a notebook filled with names and information on the many men she had met there, "she has many a minento [*sic*] of that strange battle—one, of a rebel lieutenant who died in her care, and a score of palmetto buttons from rebel coats—dirty but grateful, poor wretches."[59] Mother Woolsey made do with visiting a military hospital in Brattleboro, Vermont, during a family getaway. The widespread impact of the Pennsylvania battle was apparent when she immediately encountered a former Gettysburg patient as she walked in the door: "One man was almost convulsed at seeing Mother, and, with tears, would hardly let her hand go. 'I knew you, ma'am, the minute you came in. You were at Gettysburg, and were the first one that dressed my arm.' And there the poor arm still lay, useless and swollen, and constant streams of cold water necessary to keep down inflammation."[60]

Georgy and Jane were soon on the move again, this time to the Fairfax Theological Seminary Hospital in Virginia. It was there that the sisters had the opportunity to nurse their only brother back to health. Since Gettysburg, Charley had joined the 164th New York and been a command level staff officer in the Army of the Potomac. Young Woolsey was felled, not by Rebel fire, but by the development of inflammatory rheumatism. After convalescing at home, he was soon in the field again, and remained there for the remainder of the war.

Like Cornelia Hancock and Ellen Orbison Harris, Georgy was called to Fredericksburg in May of 1864. May 15 she wrote: "Fredericksburg-town full of wounded." In late May, however, the tragic news came that sister Mary Woolsey had died. Georgy and Jane rushed home to be with the family. After a period of mourning, Georgy accepted her final nursing assignment in Beverly, New Jersey. It was, by far, the most frustrating experience of her career: "The Beverly Hospital was perhaps the worst one claiming to be a Regular Army establishment

59. *Ibid.*, pp. 531-32, 535. For the story of the lieutenant and the Confederate buttons, see Chapter 14.
60. *Ibid.*, pp. 545-46.

that I ever went into, and the conditions exasperating, because it was in the midst of a land of plenty."[61]

Following the end of the war, the Woolseys visited the subjugated city of Richmond, then traveled on to Washington for the Grand Review. The rigors of wartime finally caught up with Georgy, who fell ill from an unspecified sickness. "I think the last four years is the matter with her," wrote one of her siblings. "It would not be human that she could endure, without some ill effects, the constant exposure and trials of that time."[62]

The numerous members of the Woolsey clan went on to distinguish themselves in numerous philanthropic and social arenas. Georgy married longtime acquaintance and correspondent Dr. Francis Bacon, professor of surgery at Yale Medical School, on June 7, 1866. Together, they would found the Connecticut Training School for Nurses, for which Georgy wrote the landmark text *Hand Book of Nursing for Family and General Use* in 1879. She spent the rest of her life using her medical skills in ministering to the underprivileged and social outcasts of her day—children, the mentally handicapped, and prisoners. She died in 1906, and was buried, full of honors, in the Grove Street Cemetery in New Haven.

The other half of the dynamic mother/daughter Gettysburg team, mother Jane Eliza Newton Woolsey, died in 1874, and is almost certainly interred in the family plot at Dsorios near Glen Grove, Long Island, New York.[63]

---

61. *Ibid.*, pp. 588, 622.
62. *Ibid.*, p. 714.
63. Conklin, *Women at Gettysburg*, p. 295.

Appendix 4

BIOGRAPHICAL SKETCHES OF 2ND CORPS SURGICAL STAFF[1]

The pernicious rumor still lives on, decade after decade, that the surgeons and assistant surgeons of the Civil War were a bunch of hacks and butchers, unskilled in medical acumen, and uncaring in their bedside manner.

True, there certainly are verifiable stories and anecdotes of ineptitude in professional skills, drunkenness while on duty, callousness toward patients, cowardice in the face of the enemy, and outright chauvinism and dogmatism toward volunteer nurses. These are a matter of record. As in every age and vocation, there were horrid examples in the Civil War of the very worst that the medical profession could produce.

Care must be taken, however, not to judge the whole by the sins of the few. Many of the medical men of the Civil War, and many within the Union Second Corps, were men of great reputation, trained in state-of-the-art technology, innovative, intelligent, and teachable. Records of the examinations that these surgeons and assistant surgeons underwent before being appointed to their regiments still survive. These tests included, as one would likely expect, detailed sections on anatomy, biology, and comparative physiology. Surprisingly, they also contained extensive questions on ancient history, government,

1. Unless otherwise noted, all information on Second Corps surgeons (however fragmentary) is based on *Roster of Regimental Surgeons and Assistant Surgeons in the U. S. Army Medical Department During the Civil War* (n.p., 1882; reprint, Gaithersburg, Maryland: Olde Soldier Books, Inc., 1989).

and literature. Contrary to our current concept of the medical profession, the army was looking not only for doctors, but for gentlemen as well.

The following biographical sketches demonstrate the level of ability evidenced by many of the men of the Second Corps Medical Department. While some left behind little or no record of their passing, others have left a legacy which is, in a very real sense, up to the very highest standards prescribed by the Hippocratic Oath, truly "physicians" and "healers."

[Note: "To" and "from" indicate service dates with various regiments. "?" preceding a name indicates uncertainty of this doctor's presence at Gettysburg]

Aiken, Surgeon Dr. John, 71st Pennsylvania

From April 1863?

Leave of absence from duty due to bronchitis with general debility —September, 1864

Contracted with the Army of the Potomac as acting assistant surgeon—August 19, 1864 to June 5, 1865

Contract ended—June 5, 1865[2]

Aiken, Assistant Surgeon Washington, 125th New York

Troy, New York

From August 1862

"Each regiment was entitled to two assistant surgeons, who were none too many in active service. The One Hundred and Twenty-fifth had several such connected with it. . . . But the one who started from home and returned with the regiment was Dr. Washington Akin [*sic*]."

"Dr. Akin was born at Johnsville, Rennsalaer County, New York, on the 22nd of August, 1835. He was graduated from the Cambridge Academy in 1855. He then pursued a course in medicine and surgery at the Albany Medical college, from which he was graduated December 31st, 1858. He became established in his profession in Troy, practicing here until his connection with the One Hundred and Twenty-fifth at its organization."

---

2. Record Group 94, Adjutant General's Office, Personal Papers of Medical Officers and Physicians, Box No. 5, National Archives and Records Administration. [Hereinafter cited as Record Group 94 with the appropriate box number.]

"From Gettysburg onward the writer noted in Dr. Akin the qualifications of a good surgeon. He was quick to decide and bold to act when the use of the knife was demanded. he was manifestly a born surgeon. . . . Dr. Akin faithfully performed his duty, and has earned the success which has attended his practice in Troy since the close of the war."[3]

Barrington, Assistant Surgeon John C., 28th Massachusetts
"mustered out with the regiment"[4]
To June 1864
Also 2nd Heavy Artillery

Benton, Assistant Surgeon James D., 111th New York
Syracuse, New York
To 98th New York in March 1865

Billings, Surgeon Adoniram J., 19th Maine
Freedom, Maine
Mustered in: June, 1862

"It appears from records that Dr. A. J. Billings was Surgeon of the 19th Me. Vols. from Aug. 5, 1862 to Jany 11, 1864, and was on duty with his regt 2d Div, 2 A. C. at the place specific to his affidavit during the months of June & July, 1863." Pension Commission Office

"June 63—Present with Regt. entire month. Camp near Falmouth, Va., & on the march—2d Div. July 63—Present with Regt entire month, 2d Div—In march from Gettysburg to the Rappahannock." Pension Evidence

Resigned: January 11, 1864[5]

Bingel, Assistant Surgeon Gustavus A., 52nd New York
96 Ten Eyck St., Brooklyn, New York
To March 1864[6]

?Bolan, Assistant Surgeon Wallace, 19th Maine
Augusta and New Sharon, Maine
Resigned—March 22,1864[7]

---

3. Simon, *One Hundred and Twenty-fifth New York*, pp. 293-94.
4. D. P. Conyngham, *The Irish Brigade and Its Campaigns* (New York: William McSorley and Co., 1867; reprint, Gaitherburg, Maryland: Olde Soldier Books, 1988), p. 589.
5. Smith, *The History of the Nineteenth Regiment*, p. 318; Record Group 94, Box No. 53.
6. Record Group 94, Box No. 53.
7. Smith, *The History of the Nineteenth Regiment*, p. 318.

Brenton, Surgeon Joseph L., 8th Ohio
Beloit, Wisconsin, or North Georgetown, Ohio
From March, 1863

Buck, Dr. H. B., U.S. Volunteers
Granite Schoolhouse Hospital

Bucknam, Surgeon John H., 5th New Hampshire

"John W. Bucknam was a noble, self-sacrificing, patriotic, genial man. He was born in Lancaster, N. H., December 4, 1833, of excellent New England stock. His ancestors served in the Revolution. He was educated in the common schools and the academy in his native town. He was a good scholar, a keen observer of nature, and of men and things. He began the study of medicine and surgery in 1856 and received his diploma at the Dartmouth Medical College in 1859 and at once began practice in his native town. He was called upon the staff of Colonel Cross as assistant-surgeon and was finally promoted to surgeon. He was with the Fifth in every battle while he was in the service, and at Gettysburg saw his beloved commander die, and with tender care folded his arms, which should never draw sword again, and closed those eyes which should never again flash in the din of battle. On the 12th of June, 1861, he married Miss Celia A. Buckland of Warehouse Point, Conn."

"Soon after his discharge Doctor Bucknam began practice at Great Falls, N. H. Here he soon gained a good name, fame, a large practice, a fair income, and made many friends. He died suddenly on the 18th day of December, 1870, mourned by his acquaintances, respected by his professional brethren, loved by his comrades and sadly missed by his family and friends. Only eight days after his death his wife, who had been an object of tender care, followed him to rest. A daughter, Anna Weeks, is the only survivor of the family of that gallant man, devoted friend and worthy citizen."

"In the service Doctor Bucknam was a most excellent surgeon, an officer of fine personal bearing; when mounted upon his fine, black horse he attracted much attention. He was modest yet brave, reticent yet affable, unassuming yet earnest and skillful, always at his post of duty and assiduous in his labors."[8]

---

8. Child, *A History of the Fifth Regiment*, pp. 324-25.

Burmeister, Surgeon Frederick F., 69th Pennsylvania
1942 Frankford Avenue, Philadelphia, Pennsylvania
With 73rd Pennsylvania until December 1862
With 69th Pennsylvania from December 1862
Dr. Justin Dwinelle found Doctor Burmeister to be a quality surgeon, and commented favorably on him and his work in his letters and correspondence.

Burr, Surgeon William J., 42nd New York
Newark Valley, New York
Assistant surgeon of the 59th New York, transferred to 42nd New York May 1863
Surgeon of 42nd New York from May 1863

Bush, Assistant Surgeon W. P., 61st New York

Chaddock, Surgeon Gilbert, 7th Michigan
Muskegon, Michigan
To January 1865[9]

Child, Surgeon William, 5th New Hampshire
Bath, New Hampshire (mustered out June 28, 1865)
From November 1862
Also U.S. Examining Surgeon for Pension Office

"William Child was born February 4, 1834, in Bath, N. H. His father was Dwight P. Child, a direct descendant of a sister of the Dwights of educational fame, and his mother, Nancy Morse Child, was a near relative of Morse, the telegraph inventor. The great-grandmother of the doctor and the mother of Morse were sisters. Thus in his veins meet two strains of most excellent families."

"William Child was born upon a magnificent farm, from which could be seen Mount Washington, the Presidential, Franconia and Moosilauke ranges, and the beautiful valley of the Connecticut for many miles. The views from the old homestead are the grandest and most beautiful in New England. Amid these surroundings young Child grew to be a lad of fifteen years, rarely leaving the farm for a day. He received the usual education in the modest school near his home. From the age of sixteen to twenty years he attended the Bath Academy, under the instruction of Rev. Edward Cleaveland, Nathan Lord, Jr., and Hon. A. P. Carpenter. During all those years he walked six miles each school day. Here he prepared for an advanced standing in college, but he

9. Record Group 94, Box No. 105.

entered the Dartmouth Medical School in 1854, graduating in 1857. During these years he was under the tuition of Professors Peaslee, Phelps, the Crosbys and in the hospitals of Boston and in the Demilt Dispensary of New York. After graduation and riding six months with the celebrated Dr. McNab, of Wells River, Vt., he began practice in his native town, living in the residence of the then well-known Dr. John French, which he bought and now owns. Here he met the most able physicians, as competitors, in Northern New Hampshire, such as McNab, Tuttle, Boynton, Spaulding, Leonard, Watkins, Moody and Carbee."

"In August, 1862, he was commissioned as second assistant-surgeon of the Fifth Regiment, and was finally promoted to be surgeon of the same regiment. He served almost three years, until the ending of the war. During his service he was often absent on detail. He served in the Antietam hospital, had charge of the hospital in the prisoners-of-war camp at Point Lookout, Md., where he often had the supervision of 1,500 sick, with six to eight Confederate surgeons as assistants; was detailed to examine prisoners of war who enlisted into the Union army, to fill vacancies in other regiments, and to accompany difficult and dangerous expeditions. He was present at every battle from South Mountain and Antietam to Deep Bottom and Reams' Station. At the close of the war he was division surgeon, and was discharged with the regiment."

"After the war, he at once resumed his medical and surgical practice, and entered upon a quiet and uneventful citizenship. He never sought public office, but was twice elected as representative from his native town, and was elected anniversary chairman and president of the New Hampshire State Medical Society. He has the credit of having read more papers before the society than any other member, and of having promulgated more original, and perhaps absurd and untenable ideas, though he has ever been ready to present good, if not sufficient, reasons therefor. He has been married twice; first to Caroline B. Lang, second to Luvia Lang, daughters of Sherburn Lang, Esq., of Bath. He is a Mason, Odd Fellow and Patron of Husbandry. He was Medical Director, Department of New Hampshire, Grand Army of the Republic, in 1870."[10]

---

10. Child, *A History of the Fifth Regiment*, pp. 327-29.

?Claypoole, Assistant Surgeon John C., 2nd Delaware

Twenty-two in 1861, graduate of Philadelphia College of Pharmacy "considerable experience in dressing wounds, &c"—Claypoole's August 12, 1861 application letter to the surgeon general.

To March 1865[11]

Cooper, Surgeon William S., 125th New York

Troy, New York

From August 1862

". . . A word is demanded on behalf of the surgeons, and the name of Surgeon Cooper must here have place. The men of the One Hundred and Twenty-fifth had reason to be grateful for the one who served as surgeon to the regiment from the beginning to the close of its history. The carefulness, kindness and skill of Surgeon Wm. S. Cooper uniformly impressed the writer, who, making his way to [the] field hospital after each battle, had abundant opportunity to observe those whose duty it was to care for the wounded. Great pains was always taken to spare men, so far as possible, the loss of limbs. The writer has known Surgeon Cooper to save a man one finger of a shattered hand, holding that one finger—the "little" finger—might be of some service. It is possible that the amputating knife was at times applied when, amid circumstances more favorable, long and close care might have rendered the loss of leg or arm unnecessary. But, at the front, with armies moving, amputation was sometimes a more merciful act. Still this record is here made, that of the many men who passed under the surgeons' hands, the writer never saw a needless case of the use of the knife. He did have occasion at times to persuade men, who plead with him to see to it that arm or leg should not be cut off, that the decision with them was, "limb or life."

"Surgeon William S. Cooper was born July 11th, 1819, in Stane, a village adjacent to Shott's Iron Works, Lanarkshire, Scotland. He studied medicine in the city of Glasgow from 1836 to 1840. He then went to sea as a surgeon of a whaling vessel. During the voyage in the Arctic regions . . . the ship in which Surgeon Cooper was serving was wrecked amid the ice in a severe storm on the 3d of May, 1840, in about 75 degrees north latitude. After three days he and his companions were picked up and taken to Scotland. In the following year, undaunted by his former perils, he shipped on a second voyage."

11. Record Group 94, Box No. 114.

"July 26th, 1842, he sailed for America, and was wrecked on Hempstead Beach, Long Island, about the 3d of September. Rescued and making his way to Albany, New York, he renewed his medical studies at the Medical College in that city, choosing in this way to take a double course. He was graduated at Albany, and entered upon practice of his profession at the Troy Iron Works, where he continued for twenty years, and until the War Committee of Rensselaer County waited upon him and requested him to take the position of surgeon in the One Hundred and Twenty-fifth."

"More fitting choice could not well have been made. Dr. Cooper proved himself not only skillful in his professional duties, but was regarded as a gentleman of strong convictions, and a man of careful culture. He returned with the regiment to Troy, where he has up to the present [1888] followed successfully his profession. A man who could face the dangers which Surgeon Cooper met in his earlier days was qualified by valor, as he was by undoubted ability, to serve even on battlefield. He was, at the close of the war, very justly brevetted Colonel."[12]

Cornish, Assistant Surgeon Theodore O., 15th Massachusetts
404 4th St., Boston, Massachusetts
Mustered in August 11, 1862
Mustered out July 29, 1864

Corry, Assistant Surgeon Robert, 57th New York
Commissioned—May 16, 1863
On duty with the regiment until July 23, 1863
Admitted to hospital for hemorrhage of lungs—July 27, 1863
Returned to duty—August 7, 1863
Medical discharged—September 5, 1863[13]

Davis, Surgeon Uriah Q., 148th Pennsylvania
Milton, Pennsylvania
Appointed assistant surgeon September 12, 1862
Promoted surgeon December 8, 1862
Mustered out with regiment June, 1865
Killed in railroad accident at Milton, Pennsylvania[14]

Day, Surgeon Ebenezer, 39th New York
Third Division surgeon-in-charge
Grand Tower, Illinois

---

12. Simon, *One Hundred and Twenty-fifth New York*, pp. 290-93.
13. Record Group 94, Box No. 130.
14. Muffly, *The Story of Our Regiment*, p. 923.

To 78th New York as assistant surgeon September 1863
With 78th New York from July 1863 to June 1864
78th New York consolidated with 102nd New York June 29, 1864

Dougherty, Surgeon Alexander N., Medical Director, Second Corps, U.S. Volunteers

Medical Director, New Jersey Brigade. Serving in this position proved something of a problem to Dougherty, as the following letter attests:

Office of Brigade Surgeon, Hd. Qrs. N. J. Brigade,
February 2nd, 1862

Capt. Jas. M. Wilson, A. A. G.,

Sir, I respectfully apply through you to be relieved from further service, as Surgeon of this Brigade.

I am impelled to take this step, by the fact, that I have not, apparently, though with my best endeavors, succeeded in pleasing the General; and further, that I have been subjected to the imputation, of officious intermeddling, in the concerns of a Department, with which I had nothing to do; said imputation, being contained in an official note, dictated by the General, under a misapprehension of the facts; and which, though I humbly think, completely refuted, by my answer thereto, still remains unwithdrawn, and even unexplained, and unmodified. After this, it is obvious, that my position here is irksome.

I am therefore, under the necessity of making this application; and I sincerely hope, and respectfully solicit, that the General, will do me the favor, to endorse, and forward it, at his earliest convenience.

I am, Your Obt. Servt.,
Alexr N. Dougherty, M. D.,
Brigade Surgeon, New Jersey Brigade[15]

Medical Director Charles S. Tripler of the Army of the Potomac, Maj. Gen. George McClellan commanding, recommended reassignment of Dougherty to brigade surgeon of Grosvenor's brigade, Stone's division, and Surgeon Henry Bryant to replace Dougherty—February 10, 1862

Becomes Medical Director, Second Corps—1862

---

15. Record Group 94, Box No. 165.

"In the aftermath of the Battle of Antietam, Dougherty, as medical director of the Second Corps, was singled out for special praise by Dr. Jonathan Letterman, the newly-minted medical director of the Army of the Potomac, in his official report: "The medical directors of corps, especially Surgeons Dougherty and McNulty, were untiring in their exertions and unceasing in their labors, and were ably assisted by the staff under their commands. Very few delinquencies occurred, and these were swallowed up in the devotion exhibited by the rest of the medical staff during and long after the battle."[16]

Relieved of duty as medical director of the Second Corps to become medical director of the Right Grand Division—December 5, 1862

Returned as Second Corps medical director—1863

"The doctor was a very fat man, and the picture of good-nature. His uniform, which was never, or very seldom, renewed, did not serve to lengthen his short and broad figure, and he rode a very fat and sturdy black horse as phlegmatic and good-natured as he. . . . Dr. Dougherty was . . . learned in medicine and literature, and an inveterate punster. His wife was his great admiration, and he showed us her picture, which proved her a very good-looking lady, and used to read us choice passages from her letters, which he lauded as the production of an extraordinary woman. He . . . smoked a meerschaum pipe, which he filled often. His face was fair and much covered with a full light-brown beard, and his blue eyes would twinkle with humor. . . . The doctor . . . was not one of those members of the medical profession who so rigidly sheltered their bodies by the privilege of being non-combatants as never to visit the field in time of battle, but was noted for his frequent presence under fire, where he encountered danger rather with the equanimity of a philosopher than the martial spirit of the professed fighting man."[17]

Wrote February 28, 1867, from the New Jersey Home for Disabled Soldiers, endeavoring to secure a promotion.[18]

Dougherty, Assistant Surgeon George, 59th New York

George Dougherty caught up with the Second Corps on June 20, while it was on the march north. He asked to resign on August

---

16. *OR*, vol. 19, pt. 1, p. 113.
17. Livermore, *Days and Events*, pp. 259-60, 309.
18. Record Group 94, Box No. 165.

5, 1863, in a letter addressed to Surgeon General Hammond. Dougherty was to replace Assistant Surgeon Henry C. Duane of the 59th New York, who officially served with that regiment until July 1, 1863. Duane had already left the 59th, but his official papers had still not cleared the army bureaucracy, with the confusion following the battle of Gettysburg.

Dougherty was serving without pay, and, as he writes: "My family is depending upon me for support, and if there is no possibility of receiving compensation for my services, and my expenses, for outfit, &c., I shall be compelled for the sake of my family, if for no other reason, to return to Brooklyn and resume my practice." He was released from service in August, 1863.[19]

Dudley, Surgeon Frederick A., 14th Connecticut

Pre-war—New Haven, Connecticut
Post-war—Kings Ferry, New York
Enlisted—August 11, 1862
Mustered in as assistant surgeon—August 23, 1862
Promoted—April 2, 1863
Wounded and captured at Gettysburg—July 3, 1863
Paroled—January 14, 1865
Mustered out with regiment—May 31, 1865[20]

Dwinelle, Jr., Surgeon Justin, 106th Pennsylvania

Mustered in at Fort Schuyler, New York, June 28th, 1861, as an assistant surgeon of the 1st California [71st Pennsylvania]
Promoted September 1, 1861, to surgeon of the 5th California [106th Pennsylvania]
Surgeon-in-charge, Second Division, Second Corps
Chief surgeon, Second Corps Hospital
Mustered out with regiment—September 10, 1864

Justin Dwinelle, Jr. was born on January 22, 1822, into a well-to-do family living in Cazenovia, New York. He was the third child of Justin Dwinelle, Sr. and Louisa Whipple Dwinelle. Justin grew up in the midst of a precocious and colorful group of people.

Justin Sr. had blazed a long political career in Madison County, serving as state assemblyman, United States Congressman, county court judge, and district attorney.

19. *Ibid.*
20. Page, *History of the Fourteenth Regiment*, pp. 374-75.

Louisa Whipple, his mother, was a relative of William Whipple, one of the signers of the *Declaration of Independence* for New Hampshire

His oldest brother, John Whipple Dwinelle (1816-1881), practiced law for ten years before joining the gold rush of '49—not as a miner, but as a lawyer. Opening an office in San Francisco, he quickly worked his way from attorney, to mayor of Oakland, and up to state assemblyman. In this position he was highly influential in planning the founding of the University of California. Mark Twain, writing for the *Territorial Enterprise* in 1868, was scathing in his assessment of John, feeling that "Dwinelle's [resolutions] are not the things that made the Californian name a synonym for liberality and generosity." He also served from time to time as something of a high-priced hired legal gun for several of the nineteenth century "Robber Barons."

John had gone to California with his younger brother, Samuel Hull Dwinelle, who became a prominent judge in San Francisco.

Justin's second oldest brother, Dr. William Henry Dwinelle (1819-1896), M.D., D.D., was one of the great pioneers of modern dentistry. Practicing by age nineteen, he made tools that he could not find, or invented ones that simply did not yet exist. He eventually opened a lucrative practice in New York City, where he was widely recognized as a sculptor, artist, avid art collector, and speaker. He was well-known as an authority on dentristry on both sides of the Atlantic, and his many innovations include dental bridgework and taking impressions of teeth.

Justin's youngest brother, Dr. James E. Dwinelle, was a prominent surgeon practicing in Baltimore, Maryland.

Little is known of Justin Jr.'s pursuit of medicine. However, his brother William Henry studied under Doctor Warner, a local Cazenovia physician, so it is quite likely that young Justin followed in his older brother's footsteps. Justin eventually went into practice in Syracuse and Tully, New York.

It was in Tully that Justin fell in love with Mary Viall King, daughter of local postmaster and businessman Henry Fidelio King. They married on May 25, 1847, and the family soon expanded to include four children—Mary, William Henry, Isabella, and little Julia. Julia was born just one month before Justin volunteered his services to the United States in May of 1861.

At the somewhat advanced age of thirty-nine, Justin enlisted in the 1st California Regiment. Its commander, Col. Edward Baker, a United States Senator from Oregon, and close personal friend of Abraham Lincoln, persuaded the president to allow him to raise this regiment under the name of the recently-added State of California. After the colonel's death at the ill-conceived Battle of Ball's Bluff, the regiment was renamed the 71st Pennsylvania, since most of its men were from Philadelphia. It would go on to be part of the hard-fighting "Philadelphia Brigade."

Justin had been giving considerable thought to the medical vacuum that his departure would create in the community. Before leaving to join his regiment, he wrote a practical medical "do-it-yourself" guide, with the inconceivably ponderous title of: *Domestic Practice Of Medicine: An Entirely New And Original Work, Containing A Minute And Faithful Description Of The Causes, Symptoms, And Treatment Of Diseases, And Designed For The Especial Use Of Heads Of Families, Planters, Emigrants, Sailors, And All Others, Who Are Deprived Of The Immediate Services Of A Physician.*" In a further gesture of public goodwill, it was published at the author's expense.

Justin was mustered in at Fort Schuyler, New York on June 28, 1861, to rank as an assistant surgeon. On September 1, 1861, he was promoted to surgeon of the 5th California, under the command of Col. Turner Moorehead. The 5th California, like its sister regiment, suffered something of an identity crisis, and was eventually renamed the 106th Pennsylvania. It, too, would fight its way into the history books as part of the "Philadelphia Brigade."

Justin served three years and three months in Federal service. During that time, he was present at every major action of the Army of the Potomac, from Ball's Bluff to the slaughter of Cold Harbor. His high sense of professionalism is evident in his appointment to surgeon-in-charge of the Second Corps Hospital, until that position was finally eliminated in April 1864. He then became surgeon-in-charge of the Second Division, Second Corps Hospital, eventually rising to surgeon-in-charge of the Post Hospital at City Point, Virginia. Doctor Dwinelle mustered out of service with his regiment in Philadelphia in September 1864, at age forty-two.

A long, quiet life as a small-town doctor was not to be his, however. During a cranial surgery at winter quarters in Brandy Station, Virginia, in 1864, the doctor, always a careful operator, somehow managed to nick himself during the delicate operation. In this pre-antiseptic era, erysipelas soon developed.

Although he battled the infection for years, it would eventually claim his life on December 9, 1871. "His brother, Dr. James E. Dwinelle of Baltimore was attending physician, and Dr. Nathan Smith of Baltimore was consulting physician. The official cause of death was a long exposure to camp life with the Army, Typhoid and Malarial fever, and the wound to his hand, received at Brandy Station, Va. In short he wore himself out." He died just short of his fiftieth birthday.[21]

Dyer, Surgeon J. Franklin, 19th Massachusetts

Second Division surgeon-in-charge (surgeon-in-charge of division after Surgeon Justin Dwinelle took charge of corps)

Fitch, Assistant Surgeon William R., 82nd New York

To October 1863[22]

Frisbee, Assistant Surgeon Charles M., 111th New York

Friendship, New York

Reported for duty—February 2, 1863

Served with regiment—from April 1863[23]

?Frolick, Surgeon Moritz, 52nd New York

Gabrielson, Assistant Surgeon Peter, 1st Minnesota

St. Paul, Minnesota

Mustered in—February 17, 1863

Mustered out—May 4, 1864

Assistant surgeon 11th Infantry—from September 1864[24]

Gates, Assistant Surgeon Erasmus D., 106th Pennsylvania

Fairview, Pennsylvania

106th Pennsylvania from September 13, 1862

---

21. "John Whipple Dwinelle" inscription in the foyer of Dwinelle Hall, University of California, Berkeley; *Territorial Enterprise*, March 2, 1868, Number XI, "Mark Twain's Letters From Washington: The Mining School"; William Dwinelle obituary, courtesy of Scott Michael Dwinelle and Margaret Ladd, town historian, Cazenovia, New York; Scott Michael Dwinelle, *Healer and Comforter: The Civil War Surgeon. A Collection of Orders and Letters belonging to Surgeon J. Dwinelle, 106th Penn. Inf.* (n. p., 1989), copy in the Civil War Hospitals and Medicine Vertical File, Gettysburg National Military Park Library, p. 1; Scott Michael Dwinelle letter to the author, February 27, 1999.
22. Record Group 94, Box No. 192.
23. *Ibid.*, Box No. 203.
24. John Quinn Imholte, *The First Volunteers: History of the First Minnesota Volunteer Regiment 1861-1865* (Minneapolis: Ross & Haines, Inc., 1963), pp. 134-35.

Transferred to 106th Battalion
Discontinued—June 15, 1865

Gesner, Surgeon Brower, 10th New York Battalion
Contracted as private physician to serve with the army
Assistant surgeon 38th New York—until November 1862
Reported to the 10th New York Battalion—April 13, 1863
To February 1865[25]

Gilman, Assistant Surgeon Uriah, 12th New Jersey
Woodstown, N. J.
To June 1865

?Goodwin, Assistant Surgeon Willis W., 39th New York
Born in Brownsville, New York, July 30, 1825
Studied medicine with Doctor Clayton of Clayton, New York
Attended University Medical College, New York, graduated—March, 1854
Enlisted in the 2nd New York Artillery in 1861
Applied repeatedly to become a medical cadet—May, August, November, 1862
Signed as contract physician—October 28, 1862
Requested reexamination as surgeon for a colored regiment—June 9, 1863
Worked at Clay General Hospital, Louisville, Kentucky, and Jeffersonville General, Jeffersonville, Indiana—1863-1864
To July 31, 1865
Died—July 25, 1887[26]

Hamilton, Surgeon Alfred Thornley, 148th Pennsylvania
Primary aid station at the Jacob Hummelbaugh Farm, attended General Barksdale
Lewistown, Pennsylvania
Appointed February 4, 1863
Mustered out with regiment June, 1865[27]

Hammond, Surgeon Fletcher M., 126th New York
Penn Yan, New York
Appointed and awaiting muster into U.S. service

"SURGEON FLETCHER M. HAMMOND was born in Pleasant Valley, at the head of Crooked Lake (since called Hammondsport), in March, 1815. He was reared on a farm, and worked at farm labor

---

25. Record Group 94, Box No. 212.
26. *Ibid.*, Box No. 224.
27. Muffly, *The Story of Our Regiment*, p. 923.

until manhood, when he commenced the study of medicine with E. D. PULLING, M.D., of Bath, Steuben county, New York, in 1840. In 1841 he went to Albany, and prosecuted his studies in the office of J. P. Boyd, M.D., and at the Albany Medical College, until the year 1844, when he graduated and commenced the practice of his profession in Penn Yan, Yates county, New York. He continued in the practice of medicine at that place until he was appointed Surgeon of the 126th Regiment, New York Volunteers, in July, 1862, when he entered upon his duties in the organization of the Regiment, and was commissioned and mustered its Surgeon, with rank from July 15th, 1862. He accompanied the Regiment to the field, and to Maryland Heights in the engagement there."

"He continued on duty with the Regiment till after its exchange and return to the field again; but in January, 1863, he was assigned to duty on the staff of General HAYS, as Surgeon-in-Chief of the Brigade, and established a hospital at Union Mills, Va., and when in the spring of 1863 the headquarters were removed to Centreville, the hospital was moved thither also."

"When the Brigade was assigned to the Army of the Potomac as the 3d Brigade 3d Division 2d Corps, Doctor HAMMOND continued Surgeon-in-Chief of the Brigade through the Gettysburg campaign, and the battles of Auburn, Bristow, Mine Run, and Morton's Ford; and when the army was consolidated, and the Brigade increased by other Regiments, and assigned to the 1st Division of the 2d Corps as the 3d Brigade of that Division, Surgeon HAMMOND was still continued Surgeon-in-Chief, and was attached to the field hospital of the 1st Division of the 2d Corps during the campaign from the Rapidan to Petersburg."

"In the latter part of June, 1864, he was ordered to City Point to organize and establish the Base Hospital, of the 1st Division, 2d Corps, after accomplishing which, he was ordered to organize, establish, and take charge of the hospital for the colored troops of the army of the Potomac, at City Point. This he did, and remained in charge of this hospital from September to the 20th of the following December, when he was ordered on detached duty as Medical Inspector for the Western Division of the State of New York; with headquarters at Elmira. While on this duty he made three tours of inspection of the Provost-Marshall's Head-quarters, and of the recruits at the following places, including the rebel prison in Elmira: Elmira, Utica, Syracuse, Sackett's Harbor, Auburn,

Canandaigua, Rochester, Lockport, Buffalo, Dunkirk and Binghamton."

"He returned to the field on the 20th day of the following March, and was assigned to duty on the staff of Major-General MILES, as Surgeon-in-Chief of the 1st Division, 2d Corps, and served in that capacity during the closing campaigns of the war, and was mustered out with his Regiment, June 2d, 1865. He then returned to Penn Yan and resumed the practice of his profession."

"Surgeon HAMMOND was a man who could be fully appreciated only by those who knew him well. Within his large and manly breast beat a warm and sympathetic heart, ever ready to do good and to alleviate suffering. It was his nature not to make loud professions of sympathy, tickling the ears with smooth words, but rather with skill and indefatigable perseverance, to contribute to the comfort of the sick and the wounded in the hospital or on the field, and if possible to restore them to health; taking neither thought or care that his efforts for their good should ever be known by those for whom he labored."[28]

Hawes, Surgeon J. Q. A., 19th Maine
Hallowell, Maine
To November 1864

Hayward, Surgeon Nathan, 20th Massachusetts
Second Division chief operator
M.D. 1855
Assistant surgeon 20th Massachusetts July 1, 1861
Surgeon 20th Massachusetts September 10, 1861
Prisoner at Sharpsburg, Maryland, while taking care of his wounded lieutenant colonel (Palfrey, 1851)
Mustered out September 19, 1864
Brevet lieutenant colonel U.S. Volunteers March 13, 1865
Brevet colonel U.S. Volunteers March 13, 1865
In practice of medicine at St. Louis, Missouri
Died at St. Louis, Missouri, August 17, 1866[29]

Hicks, Assistant Surgeon W. T., 7th West Virginia
On duty with the regiment—March, 1863

---

28. Willson, *Disaster, Struggle, Triumph*, pp. 358-60.
29. Francis H. Brown, *A Record of Services Rendered in the Army and Navy of the United States by the Graduates and Students of Harvard College and the Professional Schools* (Boston: Cupples, Upham, and Company, 1886), p. 47.

To January 1865
Died November 9, 1867[30]

Hill, Assistant Surgeon Benjamin F., 140th Pennsylvania
Candor, Pennsylvania
From November 1862

?Hopkins, Assistant Surgeon D. S., 111th New York[31]

Houston, Surgeon David H., 2nd Delaware
Lewes, Delaware
With 2nd Delaware from October 1861
"July 63—On duty with Regt"[32]

Houston, Surgeon John, 81st Pennsylvania
Marietta, Pennsylvania
July, 1863—On duty with the regiment
To September 1864[33]

Hoyt, Surgeon Charles S., 126th New York
Canadaigua, New York
To 39th New York May 1864

"Surgeon CHARLES S. HOYT was born in Ridgefield, Fairfield county, Ct., June 8th, 1822. He commenced the study of medicine in 1843, and engaged in the practice of his profession, in Potter, Yates county, New York, in the spring of 1847. When the war broke out he took an active part in recruiting in Yates county, and in sustaining the loyal feeling first awakened; and when the call for three hundred thousand volunteers was made, in July, 1862, he was appointed by Governor MORGAN one of the War Committee of the twenty-sixth senatorial district."

"He immediately entered upon the duty of recruiting, and identified himself with the 126th Regiment, and, having assisted with the examination of the men, was commissioned and mustered Assistant Surgeon of the Regiment, with rank from August 11th, 1862. He accompanied the Regiment to Harper's Ferry, and was ordered on duty at the post hospital there September 1st, 1862, and was continued on duty there after the surrender of that post until the 11th of October following, when the sick and wounded were transferred to Annapolis, Md., and he joined his Regiment at Chicago, Ill., arriving there October 29th."

---

30. Record Group 94, Box No. 266.
31. *Ibid.*, Box No. 276.
32. *Ibid.*, Box No. 279.
33. *Ibid.*

"Surgeon HAMMOND having been detailed Brigade Surgeon, December 12th, 1862, Assistant Surgeon HOYT became Acting Surgeon of the Regiment, and, excepting absence, on account of sickness, from September 22nd, 1863, to November 13th, 1863, he retained that charge until the 20th of May, 1864, when he was promoted to be Surgeon of the 39th New York Volunteers. On the 10th of June following, he was detached as executive officer of the 1st Division, 2d Corps hospital, by Special Order No. 441, Headquarters 1st Division, 2d army Corps, and continued on that duty until January 12th, 1865, when he was detailed Surgeon in charge of the hospital during the absence of Surgeon J. A. WISHART, 140th Pennsylvania Volunteers. On the 28th of March following he returned to his former duty of executive officer, and on the 25th of May, 1865, he again became Surgeon in charge of the hospital, and continued on that duty until his discharge on the muster out of his Regiment, on the 1st of July, 1865, when he returned to his home, in Yates county, and resumed the practice of medicine."

"Surgeon HOYT was on duty with the army in all the battles in which the 126th Regiment New York Volunteers was engaged, except Auburn Ford and Bristow Station, and being with the Regiment a large portion of the time he became more generally acquainted with the officers and enlisted men of the Regiment than any other officer."

"Surgeon Hoyt was assiduous in his attentions to his charge and devoted to his duty, ever providing and improvising as necessities required, comforts, and accommodations for the sick and wounded. Having been detailed to accompany the sick to Washington just before the movement on Gettysburg in 1863, he rejoined the Regiment at Frederick City, Maryland, and being without a horse, he marched on foot to Gettysburg, was on duty as field Surgeon, attending to the wounded at times even on the line of battle. When the army left Gettysburg, he procured the body of the lamented [Col. Eliakim] SHERRILL [of the 126th New York] and accompanied it to Baltimore, Maryland, where sorrowing friends from Geneva, New York, relieved him of the sacred trust. He immediately rejoined the army and marched on foot with the men to Elk Run, attending to his arduous duties, and, by his example, encouraging many a weary and faint soldier to eke out his strength till rest and refreshment came to his relief."

"While executive officer of the Division hospital he brought everything into order and system so that all parts worked smoothly together without delays or jars. With the musicians of the Division, organized into a Company under an officer—a strict disciplinarian—who had charge of erecting, taking down and removing hospital tents and accommodations; bringing in and carrying out the wounded and such as had died; with a corps of nurses to attend to the sick and wounded, and cooks to provide them nourishment and food, and in fine with a complete system of labor and duty, everything was done with such dispatch that the Hospital accommodations seemed ever to accompany the Division, and however rapid the movements of the army, or suddenly the enemy was engaged, the wounded found well appointed hospital arrangements in the rear, where were in attendance, nurses in waiting, cooks to prepare food, and added to all the Sanitary and Christian Commissions to shower with a lavish hand, unexpected but much needed and tempting delicacies and comforts."

"For the position of executive officer of the hospital, Surgeon HOYT was peculiarly adapted, as many thousand maimed and crippled soldiers who came under his charge can now testify, with grateful feelings for the uniform kindness and attention upon all occasions received at his hands."[34]

Hughes, Assistant Surgeon James W., 59th New York

Recommended by Rev. Henry Bowen to serve with the 59th New York—May, 1863

Applied to serve as assistant surgeon in a colored regiment—August, 1863

Transferred to 152nd New York as surgeon in April 1865

"Dr. Hughes has recently been examined & pronounced insane and sent to the Asylum at Binghamtom, N. Y. for treatment." Deposition to Surgeon General's Office, received April 4, 1893. Signed, Dr. William J. Burr, late surgeon, 42nd New York [see "Burr, William J." above][35]

Jacobi, Assistant Surgeon Gustavus, 52nd New York

To September 1863—returned to Germany[36]

Jewett, Assistant Surgeon Levi, 14th Connecticut

Pre-war—Windsor Locks, Connecticut

Post-war—357 W. 14th St., New York, New York

---

34. Willson, *Disaster, Struggle, Triumph*, pp. 360-62.
35. Record Group 94, Box No. 283.
36. *Ibid.*, Box No. 292.

Enlisted: July 14, 1862

Commissioned assistant surgeon of the 14th Connecticut Volunteers—August 11, 1862

Mustered in: August 23, 1862

Wounded in the head: August 25, 1864, at Reams' Station

Discharged due to disability: January 4, 1865

Contracted to serve at New York as acting assistant surgeon with Surg. William J. Sloan at West's Buildings Hospital from March 18, 1865 to May 25, 1865[37]

Jones, Assistant Surgeon A. Stokes, 72nd Pennsylvania

Ottsville, Pennsylvania

With 72nd Pennsylvania from August 1862

With 200th Pennsylvania from September 1864

Kelsey, Surgeon Charles T., 64th New York

First Division surgeon-in-charge

Mecklenburgh, New York

To January 1865

Kelsey, Surgeon Dana E., 64th New York

Joined 64th New York as a replacement for George W. Barr, April 22, 1863

With 64th New York to December 1864[38]

Knapp, Assistant Surgeon William Dickson, M. D., 19th Massachusetts

Assistant surgeon 19th Massachusetts March 19, 1863

Battles: Second Fredericksburg, Virginia; Gettysburg, Pennsylvania; Bristoe Station, where he was slightly wounded.

Dismissed December 2, 1863[39]

Laird, Assistant Surgeon John B., 4th Ohio

Assistant surgeon February 13, 1863

Resigned: July 11, 1864[40]

Landon, Assistant Surgeon Henry B., 7th Michigan

Bay City, Michigan

To April 1864[41]

Le Blond, Surgeon John B., 1st Minnesota

Sioux Falls, Dakota Territory or Brownsville, Minnesota

---

37. Page, *History of the Fourteenth Regiment*, pp. 374-75; Record Group 94, Box No. 297.
38. Record Group 94, Box No. 308.
39. Brown, *A Record of Services Rendered*, p. 279.
40. Kepler, *History of the Three Months' and Three Years' Service*, p. 243.
41. Record Group 94, Box No. 330.

To May 1864
Recommissioned—May 17, 1865[42]
Personally helped remove Color Cpl. John Densmore and Maj. Mark Downie from the battlefield.

Levensaller, Assistant Surgeon Henry C., 19th Maine
Thomaston, Maine
Discharged August 17, 1863
Surgeon 8th Maine from September 1863[43]

Lewis, Assistant Surgeon Morgan L., 82nd New York
Resigned October 29, 1863 due to disability
Died about 1882[44]

McAbee, Surgeon Harry McKindree, 4th Ohio
Third Division chief operator
Primary aid station at the Catherine Guinn Farm

"H. M. McAbee, M. D., son of Rev. I. M. McAbee, was born May 12th, 1827, in Westmoreland county, Pennsylvania; graduated from the Cleveland, Ohio, Medical College in 1851; several years after he entered the ministry and at the outbreak of the rebellion he was pastor of the First Methodist Episcopal Church in Beaver, Pennsylvania; was among the first that offered his services to the Governor of Ohio—for years his adopted State—was appointed Surgeon of the Fourth Ohio May 1st, 1861, resigned September 16th, 1863, and was killed soon after in a railroad accident near Painesville, Ohio. His reputation as a man, surgeon and physician had preceded him, on which account he was on detached duty the greater part of the time, acting as Surgeon in Chief of the Department of West Virginia under Generals [Benjamin F.] Kelley and [Frederick W.] Lander; had charge of Camp Ohio until March, 1863, and of over a thousand wounded men after the battle of Gettysburg, having been for some time Surgeon in Chief on the Staff of General Reynolds."

"He was possessed of an intensely affectionate yet highly sensitive nature. He was a hard worker, and a good organizer. His many plans for the welfare of the sick and wounded, his reports to his superiors from subordinates, of examinations into a large number of cases, his letters to and from friends of the sick and wounded that had been under his care and treatment, convince

---

42. *Ibid.*, Box No. 338.
43. Smith, *History of the Nineteenth Regiment*, p. 318.
44. Record Group 94, Box No. 339.

one that Surgeon McAbee was most assiduous in his attentions to the needs of those in his charge. He expected well men to be men, and had a supreme contempt for the man who tried to play off sick. For the truly sick, in his intense desire to do his whole duty, he ofttimes gave his eyes but little sleep or his weary body the needed rest. He cared for his wounded even though he had to go inside of the enemy's lines, and hazarded a conflict with his superiors for the sake of the comfort of his sick."

"His letters are characteristic of one who had noble purposes, firm resolves, high ideals, and lofty conceptions of Christian duty. The following is a specimen from his letter of resignation, written to Secretary Stanton:

> 'After the battle of Gettysburg, with but three assistants, I was left in charge of a thousand badly wounded men, not a few of whom, I fear, absolutely died for want of appropriate and good professional care. And it is my deliberate opinion that the failure to furnish a sufficient number of medical officers on that occasion has cost the country more good men than did the charge of any rebel brigade on that severely contested field. I have no candidates to urge for places, and have nothing to ask for myself. I have been in the field since May 1st, 1861, and although I believe now, as I did then, that a place in the army in times like these is the most honorable to which a citizen can aspire, yet I have so entirely despaired of seeing the medical staff of the army made what the country and age have a right to expect, that I shall accept it as a personal favor to be allowed honorably to retire to the quiet of private life.'"[45]

To September 1863

McAbee was killed in a railway accident near Cleveland, Ohio, early in 1864, and is buried in Canton, Ohio.

The following is from the pen of Sgt. Frank B. Nickerson, 8th Ohio.

"On the afternoon of July 2d, 1863, at Gettysburg, I was carried back badly wounded, to the hospital of the Second Corps, near Round Top, and placed with hundreds of desperately wounded.

---

45. Kepler, *History of the Three Months' and Three Years' Service*, pp. 192-93.

Surgeon McAbee was constantly at work, and it was midnight before he reached me; having asked a few questions and promised to specially care for me at daybreak, he turned to a mere boy on my left—a Confederate—not more than seventeen years old; death's pallor was on his brow and the blood flowed from his mouth; he was moaning pitifully, in striking contrast to the silent way so many were suffering and dying all around. Dr. McAbee seemed touched with his youthful appearance and disquietude of mind, and said to him, 'My poor fellow, you cannot be helped; you can live but a little time.' The boy broke out in a despairing cry, 'My poor mother, what will she do? I cannot die, I cannot die. She will never know what became of me. I was shot on the skirmish line and no one knows it.' The Surgeon wrote in his notebook his name as a member of a Georgia regiment, and his mother's address, and promised, if possible, to write to his mother, and then knelt down by his side, holding the lantern in his blood-stained hand; with the other he took a pocket Bible from his pocket and read the first fourteen verses of the Fourteenth of St. John, and then offered up a prayer for the soul that was passing away, in such simple, earnest language that helped the faith of all. Twenty-two years have passed and I still have a tender memory of the heartfelt ministrations of that man that night. Last summer, in visiting the battle-field, I rode to that barn, noticed the blood stains upon its sills, and asked the owner if any Confederates were brought here. He replied, 'Yes, one boy—and I buried him across that little rolling by the fence. I miss the place when I plow. He is there.'"[46]

McCullough, Assistant Surgeon J. R., 82nd New York
Dismissed—February 1864

McCullough, Assistant Surgeon J. W., 1st Delaware
Died—March 1881

McCune, Surgeon George W., 14th Indiana
From January 1863
Died in Montezuma, Indiana—1891[47]

McLean, Assistant Surgeon Henry D., 106th Pennsylvania
1531 Pine St., Philadelphia, Pennsylvania
November 5, 1862 to December 5, 1863

McNeill, Assistant Surgeon B. A., 69th Pennsylvania
To August 1864

---

46. *Ibid.*, pp. 193-94.
47. Record Group 94, Box No. 359.

Marshall, Assistant Surgeon C. P., 71st Pennsylvania
To April 1864
Maull, Surgeon D. W., 1st Delaware
Wilmington, Delaware
Recommended for service—1853
Surgeon in Chief Isaac Scott requests that Second Corps Medical Director Dougherty appoint Doctor Maull to act as temporary surgeon in chief during Doctor Scott's short absence—August 8, 1863
To April 1865
U.S. examining surgeon[48]
Monroe, Surgeon F. LeBaron, 15th Massachusetts
Assistant to Medical Director Dougherty
101 Fulton St., Brooklyn, New York
First lieutenant assistant surgeon
1st Battery Light Artillery, May 18, 1861
Mustered out August 2, 1861
Appointed assistant surgeon 1st Massachusetts—September 3, 1861
With regiment near Fort Worth, Virginia—September 30, 1862
With that regiment in the Army of the Potomac and Department of Virginia until promoted surgeon, 15th Massachusetts, December 29, 1862
To 15th Massachusetts—January 25, 1863
During months of August and September, 1863, served as acting medical inspector of the Second Corps
Medical Inspector General Second Corps, July 23, 1863
With regiment near Stevensburg, Virginia—April 30, 1864
With regiment near Petersburg, Virginia—June 30, 1864
With that regiment in the Second Army Corps, Army of the Potomac until mustered out with regiment, July 24, 1864
Mustered out of 15th Massachusetts July 29, 1864
Acting assistant surgeon at Galloups Island, Boston Harbor from September 12, 1864 to April 30, 1866
Acting assistant surgeon at Fort Preble, Maine—April 1, 1867 to October, 1867
Post surgeon in the Colorado and Wyoming Territories, and at Raleigh, North Carolina until September, 1875

48. *Ibid.*, Box No. 387.

Failing to be promoted to surgeon in the Regular Army, he resigned effective December 31, 1875

At age fifty-four, applied to the surgeon general to be reinstated as an assistant surgeon, April 17, 1890, in response to newspaper advertisements for army surgeons—his application was declined by a standard form letter from the surgeon general's office

Address: 3500 Cottage Grove Avenue, Chicago, Illinois as of 1890[49]

Morrison, Surgeon Francis W., 4th Ohio

Delaware, Ohio

From November 1863 (as surgeon)

"After a long illness, Dr. Francis W. Morrison died March 16th, 1886, at his residence on East Central Avenue, Delaware, Ohio."

"Francis W. Morrison, M.D., of Delaware, was born near Mansfield, Ohio, July 13th, 1831, and is the son of James and Ruth (Billings) Morrison. He entered college at Delaware in the spring of 1853, and graduated in June, 1856. Being without means, he earned what he could by manual labor and teaching school, both to carry him through college and while in pursuit of his medical education. He graduated at the medical schools of Cincinnati in the spring of 1860, when he commenced the practice of his profession with his former preceptor, Dr. Blymyer. In the spring of 1861 he enlisted as a private in Company I of the Fourth Ohio Volunteers, in the three months' service. He again, July 7th, 1861, enlisted for three years in the Eleventh Ohio Volunteer Infantry as Hospital Steward, and continued with the command in West Virginia until August, 1862, when he was commissioned Assistant Surgeon of the Fourth Ohio Volunteer Infantry, and was ordered east to join his new command, with which he was ever present on active service. In November, 1863, the doctor was commissioned Surgeon of the regiment, in which capacity he served until his regiment was mustered out of service in June, 1864. He then married Miss Elizabeth Willey, of Delaware, Ohio, June 29th, 1864, and on the10th of July following entered the contract service as Surgeon at Camp Dennison, Ohio, where he continued until September 20th, when he was commissioned Surgeon of the Seventy-fourth Ohio Volunteer Infantry, and in this position he

49. *Ibid.*, Box No. 405.

faithfully served until January, 1865, when he was detailed as Brigade Surgeon, on the Staff of General Minor T. Thomas, where he continued until ordered home to be mustered out with his regiment in July, 1865, at the close of the war. Since then he has continued to reside in Delaware, except four years of residence in his native place."

"Dr. Morrison was a member of the Delaware County Medical Association, was twice annually chosen its Secretary and finally President. He was independent and self-reliant; like many others made his own fortune unaided, and was thus in a position to comprehend the obstacles and inconveniences which beset the pathway of the youth who would obtain an education and a competency in life. He left a family of three children and a wife to mourn his loss."[50]

?Munson, Surgeon Owen, 108th New York

Served October, 1862 to April, 1864 as contract surgeon

Constantly in and out of the hospital due to ill health[51]

Neeley, Assistant Surgeon Nelson, 57th New York

To June 1864

O'Connell, Surgeon Patrick Aloysius, 28th Massachusetts

Moved to surgeon U.S. Volunteers—June 1863

Mustered out—June 30, 1865

M.D. 1860

Assistant surgeon 9th Massachusetts May 13, 1861

Mustered into service June 11, and a new commission issued of that date; on duty at Arlington Heights, Virginia, until September 29, and then took part in forward movement of the army.

Surgeon 28th Massachusetts October 25, 1861

On duty in South Carolina, Virginia, and Maryland; battles of James Island, South Carolina; Second Bull Run, Virginia; Fredericksburg; Antietam, Maryland; surgeon in chief of brigade in First Division, 9th Corps, September, 1862; and soon after surgeon in chief of the division; medical director of the 9th Corps, October, serving in Maryland, Virginia, and Kentucky

Surgeon U.S. Volunteers June 13, 1863

Battles: Gettysburg, Pennsylvania; medical inspector district of Indiana and Michigan, July; medical director of left wing of

50. Kepler, *History of the Three Months' and Three Years' Service*, pp. 195-96.
51. Record Group 94, Box No. 416.

forces in East Tennessee, September; rejoined 9th Corps as medical director, January, 1864; medical inspector of corps, April; in charge of U.S. General Hospital Lexington Avenue, New York, March 14, 1865

Brevet lieutenant colonel U.S. Volunteers June 1, 1865

Mustered out August, 1865

Died at Santa Barbara, California, January 6, 1874.[52]

Owens, Assistant Surgeon Fred J., 1st Delaware

Vernon, Delaware

To August, 1864

"Having been connected with the 1st Reg of Del. Vol., attached to the Army of the Potomac, as Assist. Surg., and finding Active service to [*sic*] Arduous, I should be pleased if I could procure a situation as a contract Surgeon, in your Department. Fred J. Owens, Late Asst. Surg., 1st Del. Reg., Sept. 5th, 1864"[53]

Contracted as private physician with the Army—September 22, 1864—October 26, 1865—served at Carlisle, Pennsylvania, Phillipsburg, Pennsylvania, and Harrisburg, Pennsylvania[54]

Parker, Assistant Surgeon Fred G., 19th Maine

Presque Isle and Stetson, Maine

Discharged—March 5, 1864

Died—November 11, 1883[55]

Parsons, Assistant Surgeon John Eleazer, M. D., 28th Massachusetts

Ayer, Massachusetts

To July 1863

Assistant surgeon 28th Massachusetts March 18, 1863

Battles Chancellorsville, Virginia; Gettysburg, Pennsylvania

Discharged for disability July 30, 1863.

Acting assistant surgeon U.S. Navy October 10, 1863

Acting passed assistant surgeon U. S. Navy March 24, 1866

Resigned: December 10, 1866.[56]

Peltier, Assistant Surgeon Pierre D., 126th New York

Hartford, Connecticut

To November 1863

---

52. Brown, *A Record of Services Rendered*, p. 104.
53. Record Group 94, Box No. 437.
54. *Ibid.*
55. Smith, *History of the Nineteenth Regiment*, p. 318; Record Group 94, Box No. 441.
56. Brown, *A Record of Services Rendered*, p. 281.

"ASSISTANT SURGEON PIERRE D. PELTIER was born at Fort Gratiot, Michigan, on the 15th of November, 1835. He was reared and educated in the State of New York, and, after a regular course in the study of medicine, he entered upon its practice in Ontario county, New York; and while the 126th New York Volunteers was being recruited, he was appointed Assistant Surgeon of the Regiment, and was commissioned and mustered as such, with rank from August 11th, 1862. He served with his Regiment until the latter part of August, 1863, when he was attacked with camp fever, induced by the arduous duties performed during the Gettysburg campaign, and exposures in the field, and on account of continued ill health he was discharged from the service while in the field, on the 3d day of November, 1863, by Special Order No. 285, Headquarters Army of the Potomac. In the spring of 1864 he re-entered the service, and was appointed Acting Post Surgeon at Martinsburg, West Virginia, but at the close of the summer campaign of 1864 he again retired from the service, and engaged in the practice of his profession, at Clifton Springs, New York. Surgeon PELTIER, while with the Regiment, won the full confidence of the officers and men under his charge, as well as of his medical associates, by his skill and success as a Physician and Surgeon, and endeared himself to all by his uniform kindness, his genial and social qualities as a gentleman, and by his unfailing fund of pleasant wit and humor, that never required a victim."[57]

?Plumb, Surgeon S. Hiram, 59th New York
Red Creek, New York
Died—August 13, 1880[58]

?Plunkett, Assistant Surgeon Philip M., 2nd Delaware
Willington, Delaware
Appointed and awaiting muster into the U.S. service[59]

Potter, Surgeon George L., 145th Pennsylvania
Bellfonte, Pennsylvania
Appointed and waiting muster into U.S. service

Potter, Surgeon William W., 57th New York
Surgeon-in-charge, First Division

"William Warren Potter was born in Strykersville, Genesee (now Wyoming) county, N. Y., December 31, 1837. . . ." Potter came

57. Willson, *Disaster, Struggle, Triumph*, pp. 362-63.
58. Record Group 94, Box No. 458.
59. *Ibid.*, Box No. 459.

from a very medical family, with father, grandfather, and uncle all practicing physicians. "The early life of William W. Potter was passed in the vicinity of his birth, and his lay education was received in the private schools, at Arcade Seminary, and at Genesee Seminary and College at Lima, N.Y. He came to Buffalo in 1854, received his medical education at Buffalo Medical College, where he graduated February 23, 1859. Soon after graduating he was offered a partnership in the practice of medicine, by his uncle, Dr. M. E. Potter, of Cowlesville, N.Y., where he located in the spring of 1859. Upon the breaking out of the civil war he made haste to offer his services in a professional capacity to the Government, and passed the examination of the Army Medical Examining Board at Albany, N.Y., April 25, 1861. He became interested in the organization of the Second Buffalo Regiment (the Forty-ninth New York Volunteers) in the summer of 1861, and was commissioned by Governor Morgan its Assistant Surgeon, September 16, 1861, at the insistance of the Union Defense Committee. . . ."

"Dr. Potter served as its junior medical officer during all of its earlier career, from the date of its organization; was with it when it joined the Army of the Potomac; followed its fortunes during the peninsular campaign; then when it was temporarily under Pope; again when it was under McClellan during the Maryland campaign; and finally when under Burnside in the Fredericksburgh [*sic*] disaster. He was left with the wounded of Smith's division on the night of the 29th of June, 1862, by order of General Franklin, commanding the Sixth Corps, when the army was retreating by the flank to Harrison's Landing, and next morning fell into the hands of the enemy, when he had an interesting interview with redoubtable 'Stonewall' Jackson. In a few days he was removed to Richmond and given quarters in Libby prison, then under command of the celebrated Lieutenant Turner. He was released among the first exchanges under the cartel arranged between the hostile powers, and delivered to the hospital steamship *Louisiana*, July 18, 1862, and immediately thereafter rejoined his regiment at Harrison's Landing, Va. On December 16, 1862, just after the battle at Fredericksburgh [*sic*], he was promoted surgeon of the Fifty-seventh Regiment New York Volunteers, in Hancock's division of the Second Corps. He served with his regiment during the Chancellorsville and Gettysburg campaigns; and, in August, 1863, was assigned to the charge of the First Division Hospital,

Second Corps, continuing upon that duty until his muster-out of service with his regiment near the close of the war. He was breveted Lieutenant-Colonel United States Volunteers for faithful and meritorious service, by the President of the United States, and of New York Volunteers by the Governor of the State of New York, for like reasons."

"After the war he performed services for the Government in connection with the Pension Office as General Examining Surgeon, and was appointed Coroner of the District of Columbia. He resigned the latter office to return to the more congenial field of private practice, and located temporarily in Mount Morris, Livingston county. For several years he resided in Batavia, Genesee county, where he was a physician to the New York State Institution for the Blind; he was a member of the Genesee County Medical Society. . . . Finally he returned to Buffalo in 1881, where he has since resided pursuing the practice of his profession."

Potter was member in a number of local and national medical associations and societies, and a frequent contributor to medical journals and publications. Over time, he became known as a specialist in the gynecological diseases, and a prominent surgeon.

He married a direct descendant of Ethan Allen, and had three children: Frank, Helen, and Alice. Dr. Frank H. Potter followed his father into the medical field, and became clinical assistant (by 1888) to the chair of surgery in the medical department of Niagara University.[60]

Doctor Potter died at age seventy-two in Buffalo, on March 14, 1911.[61]

Powell, Surgeon Richard, 88th New York

"Licentiate Royal College of Surgeons, Ireland, is a native of county Clare, Ireland. Came out with the regiment as assistant-surgeon; continued as such until August, 1863, when he was appointed surgeon, Dr. Reynolds having mustered out. His three years' term of service having expired in November, 1864, he was mustered out. Dr. Powell was highly respected in the Brigade both for his professional skill and gentlemanly demeanor."[62]

Died—May, 1872

---

60. Potter, *Three Years with the Army of the Potomac*, p. 0—Prefatory Remarks.
61. *Buffalo Enquirer*, March 14, 1911.
62. Conyngham, *The Irish Brigade*, p. 559.

Pugsley, Assistant Surgeon E. G., 1st Minnesota
Contracted with the army—July 2, 1846
Served at Fort Smith, Arkansas—July 22, 1846 to April 14, 1847
Mustered in—April 29, 1862
Mustered out—August 15, 1863
Cashiered
Assistant surgeon 9th Minnesota from October 1864, acting surgeon Pioneer Corps, First Division
Appointed to act as divisional purveyor in addition to surgical duties with the 9th Minnesota January 16, 1865[63]

Rappold, Surgeon Julius C., 52nd New York
750 Flushing Ave., New York, New York
To November 1863[64]

Reno, Assistant Surgeon Griffin, 66th New York
To October 1863[65]

Reynolds, Surgeon Francis, 88th New York

"Fellow Royal College of Surgeons, Ireland, came out with the regiment as surgeon. He was a native of County Kilkenny, Ireland, and served on the British Medical Staff during the Crimean War. As a professional man he had no superior in the Army of the Potomac, particularly in operative surgery. He was during the time he remained in the west, one of the operating surgeons of the division; was a most cultivated gentleman and a jovial companion. He remained with the regiment till August, 1863, when he was mustered out of service to accept a commission from the President as assistant-surgeon, U.S.V., which he retained till the organization of the First Corps by General Hancock, when he was appointed surgeon of the Second Regiment in that corps."[66]

Care of the adjutant general, U.S.A. to August 1863
2nd U.S. Veteran Volunteer Infantry Retired from March 1865 to March 1866

Reynolds, Surgeon Lawrence, 63rd New York

"A native of Waterford, a highly educated and refined gentleman, and a very experienced surgeon, a true Irish gentleman and patriot, served with honor as surgeon of the regiment from its first organization; although advanced in years is still young in vigor. He has written several beautiful and touching poems on his

63. Imholte, *The First Volunteers*, pp. 134-35; Record Group 94, Box No. 469.
64. Record Group 94, Box No. 475.
65. *Ibid.*, Box No. 482.
66. Conyngham, *The Irish Brigade*, p. 559.

unfortunate native land, and is endowed with wit and humor to a great degree, also a remarkable memory. He was a distinguished Chartist in England, and was also amongst those of his countrymen who had to fly from Ireland in '48, his only crime being that he loved his country dearly."[67]

Reynolds had served a stint as surgeon in the British army. His Irish roots ran deep, however, and he eventually joined the Fenian Brotherhood, a secret militant organization committed to securing independence for Ireland. Reynolds rose to head the "Potomac Circle," the official Fenian group within the Army of the Potomac.

"Surgeon Lawrence Reynolds, late of the 63rd New York reg (Irish Brigade) served under my command from the battle of Antietam until near the close of the war, when I left the Second Corps. He was distinguished for attention to his duties. . . ."
General Winfield Hancock, personal affidavit

Oswego, New York

Assistant surgeon 24th New York to January 1862

Surgeon 63rd New York from February 1863

Signed contract as acting assistant surgeon with army—June 5, 1867[68]

Richards, Assistant Surgeon D. W., 145th Pennsylvania

Assisted Chaplain Stuckenberg in retrieving the wounded left on the field during the night of July 2-3

Applebachsville, Pennsylvania

To November 1864

Rizer, Surgeon Martin, 72nd Pennsylvania

Philadelphia, Pennsylvania

From August 1861

Robison [Robinson], Assistant Surgeon G. R. B., 71st Pennsylvania

Sharpsburgh, Pennsylvania

From May 1863

Rockwood, Assistant Surgeon Henry, M. D., 15th Massachusetts

South Weymouth, Massachusetts

Mustered in August 7, 1862

Assistant surgeon 15th Massachusetts August 7, 1862—September 14, 1863

Dismissed September 14, 1863[69]

---

67. *Ibid.*, p. 567.

68. Record Group 94, Box No. 484.

69. Brown, *A Record of Services Rendered*, p. 246.

Ross, Assistant Surgeon Timothy W., 7th West Virginia
Waynesburgh, Pennsylvania
To August, 1863[70]

Sabin, Assistant Surgeon Elias H., 14th Indiana
To October 1863
Moved to San Antonio, Texas[71]

Satterthwait [Satterwaite], Surgeon Alvin P., 12th New Jersey
Assistant surgeon, 7th New Jersey
To 12th New Jersey as surgeon—July 19, 1862
Surgeon, 12th New Jersey to June 1865

?Sawyer, Assistant Surgeon P. R. H., 42nd New York
Bedford, New York
From July 1863[72]

Scott, Surgeon Isaac, 7th West Virginia
Third Division medical director
Parkersburgh, West Virginia
To December, 1864 U.S. examining surgeon

Sharp, Assistant Surgeon W. W., 140th Pennsylvania
Amity, Pennsylvania
To 18th Pennsylvania Cavalry January 1864

Smart, Assistant Surgeon Dr. Charles, 63rd New York

"A Scotchman by birth, and a licentiate of the College of Surgeons, Aberdeen, joined the Sixty-third as assistant surgeon; was afterwards promoted to be medical inspector of the corps. He underwent a very creditable examination for the regular service, in which he is at present (1867) serving. Dr. Smart was a refined scholar, a good surgeon, and a young man of the most amiable disposition, taking second place out of a large list of competitors. He also possessed very high qualifications as a poet, producing pieces that might rate favorably with Burns."[73]

Care of adjutant general, U.S.A.
To assistant surgeon U.S.A.—March 1864

Steiger, Assistant Surgeon Emil, 39th New York
Prairie du Chien, Wisconsin
To February 1864[74]

---

70. Record Group 94, Box No. 498.
71. *Ibid.*, Box No. 503.
72. *Ibid.*, Box No. 508.
73. Conyngham, *The Irish Brigade*, pp. 568-69.
74. Record Group 94, Box No. 548.

Stiles, Surgeon Richard C., First Division, U.S. Volunteers
Sturgis, Assistant Surgeon Benjamin Franklin, 19th Maine
Auburn and North Gloucester, Maine
U.S. examining surgeon
Auburn, Maine to October 1864
Assistant surgeon 19th Maine April 23, 1864
Battles: Wilderness, Virginia; Spottsylvania; North Anna; Cold Harbor; in front of Petersburg; Weldon R.R.; Reams' Station
Discharged on account of disability October 22, 1864."[75]
Trask, Assistant Surgeon Charles M., 5th New Hampshire
No. 21 Pleasant St., Boston, Massachusetts
To Oct. 1864

"Dr. Trask joined the regiment from Stewartstown, and was hospital steward until promoted to assistant-surgeon, June 1, 1863. He was mustered out December 27, 1864. Dr. Trask was a faithful, noble man, who performed every duty without a murmur. Probably no man in the Fifth did his duty more fully without any desire for promotion, notorious attention and display, than did Dr. Trask. He was honest, able, kind, attentive and cheerful under all circumstances. As a physician he possessed all those qualities that commanded the respect and love of officers and men. After the war he practiced his profession at Wells River, Vt. He then, on account of bad health, entered the drug business in Boston, and later followed the same business at White River Junction, Vt. He died in the very prime of life from disease contracted in his army service."[76]

Van Devere [Vander Veer], Surgeon Albert, 66th New York
Albany, New York
?Vasburgh, Surgeon William, 111th New York[77]
Wafer, Assistant Surgeon Francis M., 108th New York
Primary aid station, at the Peter Frey Farm
Kingston, Canada
Wallace, Surgeon Theodore C., 61st New York
Cambridge, New York

75. Smith, *History of the Nineteenth Regiment*, p. 318; Brown, *A Record of Services Rendered*, p. 283.
76. Child, *A History of the Fifth Regiment*, p. 331; Record Group 94, Box No. 590.
77. Record Group 94, Box No. 603.

93rd New York assistant surgeon until March 1863
Resigned—March 5, 1864[78]

Weiler, Surgeon Ernst, 52nd New York
Dismissed—March 1865[79]

Whildin, Assistant Surgeon J. S., 145th Pennsylvania
Philadelphia, Pennsylvania
Moved to 208th Pennsylvania—February, 1865

White, Surgeon Elisha Mann, 20th Massachusetts
99 Court St., Boston
Assistant surgeon 37th Massachusetts March 29, 1864[80]
Serving as surgeon 37th Massachusetts—December 21, 1864
Appointed surgeon 37th Massachusetts from January 1865 to June 1865

Wishart, Surgeon J. W., 140th Pennsylvania
30 6th Ave., Pittsburgh, Pennsylvania
From October 1862
U.S. examining surgeon

Wolf, Surgeon Frederick, 39th New York
St. Louis, Missouri
To April 1864

Wood, Surgeon Charles Squire, 66th New York
First Division chief operator
171 W. 47th St., New York, New York
Moved to surgeon U.S. Volunteers, September 1863

---

78. *Ibid.*, Box No. 611.
79. *Ibid.*, Box No. 620.
80. Brown, *A Record of Services Rendered*, p. 283.

Appendix 5
SECOND CORPS HOSPITAL WOUNDED AND PATIENTS

Their names are evocative of a bygone century in their multisyllabic grandeur—Artemus, Phineas, Erastus, Hiram, Archibald, Chauncey, Horatio, Ambrose, Romulus, Octavius. Some ring with Biblical fervor—Nimrod, Abraham, Isaac, Jacob, Eli, Elijah, Elisha, Nehemiah, Jabez, Amos, Jona; others are redolent of distant cultures and far-off lands—Ignatz Heimbucher, Ludwig Kreisel, Frederick Rambmeier, and Patrick O'Brien. Musicians, generals, pioneers, cavalrymen, captured Confederates, artillerymen, and common soldiers—each have their place on the roll of this institution.

The one thing that unites them all is what each experienced during the hot, tedious summer of 1863, in an army care facility outside a small, festering town in Pennsylvania. As much as is possible, with some records incomplete or simply absent, this is a list of the men who lived, and died, while under the care of the Union Second Corps Hospital at Gettysburg.

FATALLY WOUNDED / DEAD ON ARRIVALS PROCESSED AT A SECOND CORPS HOSPITAL FACILITY, BUT NOT INCLUDED IN PATIENT COUNT

The following parameters were used in compiling this roster of mortally wounded or dead on arrival patients processed by some portion of the Second Corps Hospital (usually at the aid station level):

—Soldiers killed outright are not included in this listing, unless their body was processed by some aspect of the Second Corps medical system. This was done quite frequently for officers at the regimental, brigade, or divisional command levels. Staff aides of dead officers used the Second Corps facilities (especially within the triangle prescribed by the Bryan, Peter Frey, and Hummelbaugh Farms) as a temporary morgue until funeral arrangements could be made following the end of the battle.

—Fatally wounded who died in transit to, or immediately upon arrival at, the Second Corps Hospital are included. Many were not even registered at the hospital, and so may not appear in this roster.

—# preceding a name indicates a Second Corps soldier buried on the G. Herling Farm, a location which has yet to be determined.

Pvt. Joseph Ashley, Company C, 16th Vermont [First Corps] [KILLED July 3, buried on the Jacob Hummelbaugh Farm near the Second Corps aid station, reinterred in A-2 in the Vermont Plot]

Pvt. John E. Bailey, Company I, 111th New York, wounded in the head [KILLED July 3, buried on the south side of the Catherine Guinn Farm near the 111th New York aid station of the Second Corps, reinterred in E-63 in the New York Plot, age 30]

First Sgt. Henry C. Ball, Company F, 15th Massachusetts, shot in the left chest [KILLED July 2, buried near the Second Corps aid station in the Peter Frey Farm field, age 28]

Sgt. John K. Barclay, Company C, 8th Ohio [KILLED July 2, buried on the south side of the Catherine Guinn house adjacent to the 8th Ohio, Second Corps aid station, reinterred in A-20 in the Ohio Plot, age 20]

Pvt. Edward Barry, Company G, 20th Massachusetts [KILLED July 2, buried on the ridge between the A. Bryan Farm and the Peter Frey Farm, enroute to the Second Corps aid station at the Peter Frey Farm, reinterred in A-11 in the Massachusetts Plot, age 23]

Pvt. Dayton D. Bartholomew, Company E, 111th New York, wounded in the head [KILLED July 3, buried near the Second Corps aid station in the Peter Frey Farm field, age 37]

Pvt. Edwin Beebe, Company E, 7th Michigan [KILLED July 2, buried on the ridge between the A. Bryan Farm and the Peter Frey Farm, enroute to the Second Corps aid station at the Peter Frey Farm, reinterred in A-21 in the Michigan Plot, age 18]

Pvt. George W. Bemis, Company K, 111th New York, wounded by a shell in the head [KILLED July 3, buried near the Second Corps aid station in the Peter Frey Farm field, reinterred in B-37 in the New York Plot, age 25]

Sgt. Ira Z. Bennett, Battery B, 1st Rhode Island Light Artillery (detailed from Company B, 19th Maine) [KILLED July 3, buried to the right between the A. Bryan and the Peter Frey farms, reinterred in A-1 in the Rhode Island Plot, age 32]

#Pvt. Adin W. Biles, Company I, 71st Pennsylvania, wounded in the head [KILLED July 3, buried on the G. Herling Farm]

Sgt. William S. Booth, Company E, 71st Pennsylvania, wounded in the left side [KILLED July 3, buried in the Peter Frey Farm field near the Second Corps aid station]

Cpl. William S. Boothwell, Company I, 111th New York, wounded in the head [KILLED July 3, buried near the Second Corps aid station in the Peter Frey Farm field, age 25]

Pvt. Thomas J. Boyd, Company H, 82nd New York [KILLED July 2, buried near the Peter Frey stone house adjacent to the Second Corps aid station, reinterred in B-53 in the New York Plot, age 35]

#Sgt. Jeremiah W. Boyle, Company H, 69th Pennsylvania [KILLED July 3, buried on the G. Herling Farm, reinterred in D-8 in the Pennsylvania Plot]

John Brodie, Massachusetts [KILLED, buried at the Peter Frey Farm pump adjacent to the Second Corps aid station, reinterred in C-12 in the Massachusetts Plot; *however, the only Massachusetts man with this name was discharged in 1862—this could have been Pvt. John Brodie, Company D, 126th New York (missing July 3, no further record, probably killed), or Sgt. John Broudy, Company H, 82nd New York*]

Pvt. William Brown, Company B, 8th Ohio [KILLED July 3, buried on the east side of the Catherine Guinn house adjacent to the 8th Ohio, Second Corps aid station, reinterred in A-19 in the Ohio Plot, age 18]

#Pvt. William Brown, Company D, 71st Pennsylvania, wounded in the forehead [KILLED July 3, buried on the G. Herling Farm, reinterred in C-22 in the Pennsylvania Plot]

Pvt. Hiram Burch, Company K, 111th New York, wounded in the head [KILLED July 3, buried near the Second Corps aid station in the Peter Frey Farm field, reinterred in A-48 in the New York Plot, age 21]

Cpl. William G. Burred, Company E, 111th New York, wounded by a shell in the back [KILLED July 3, buried near the Second Corps aid station in the Peter Frey Farm field, age 23]

Pvt. Henry C. Burrill, Company I, 20th Massachusetts [KILLED July 3, buried on the ridge between the A. Bryan and the Peter Frey farms, reinterred in A-5 in the Massachusetts Plot, *no one by this name is listed in Company H of the 20th Massachusetts—this could have been Horace P. Burrill of Company H (killed July 3)*]

Pvt. Abraham C. Cadmus, Company I, 126th New York [KILLED July 3, buried near the Second Corps aid station by the side of the Peter Frey Farm house, reinterred in G-78 in the New York Plot, age 20]

Pvt. William P. Camray, Company K, 82nd New York [KILLED July 2, buried near the Peter Frey stone house adjacent to the Second Corps aid station, reinterred in C-34 in the New York Plot, age 21]

First Sgt. George F. Cate, Company A, 20th Massachusetts, wounded in the body by a shell [KILLED July 3, buried near the Second Corps aid station at the Peter Frey Farm near the fortifications, reinterred in A-18 in the Massachusetts Plot, age 18]

Cpl. James P. Cheney, Company C, 15th Massachusetts, shot in the head [KILLED July 2, buried in the lot near the Second Corps aid station on the Peter Frey Farm, age 19]

Sgt. Edwin B. Cilley, Company C, 5th New Hampshire [KILLED July 3, buried west of the William Patterson Farm near a cedar tree near the Second Corps Hospital, his body was removed from the field prior to disinterment to the National Cemetery, age 30]

Pvt. William W. Clark, Company A, 72nd Pennsylvania [KILLED July 3, buried on the Peter Frey Farm near the Second Corps aid station, reinterred in C-21 in the Pennsylvania Plot]

Pvt. James Clay, Company G, 69th Pennsylvania, wounded in the brain by a shell [KILLED July 3, buried in the Peter Frey Farm lot near the Second Corps aid station, reinterred in A-34 in the Pennsylvania Plot]

Pvt. Martin J. Cook, Company D, 16th Vermont [First Corps] [KILLED July 3, buried between the A. Bryan and Peter Frey farms under the trees, reinterred in A-8 in the Vermont Plot]

Pvt. Isaac H. Copeland, Company E, 12th New Jersey [KILLED, buried near the Peter Frey stone house in the orchard near the Second Corps aid station, reinterred in A-6 in the New Jersey Plot]

Pvt. James Coyle, Company G, 69th Pennsylvania, wounded in the brain by a shell [KILLED July 3, buried in the Peter Frey Farm lot near the Second Corps aid station, reinterred in A-35 in the Pennsylvania Plot]

Pvt. Alexander Creighton, Company F, 148th Pennsylvania [KILLED July 3, buried on the Jacob Hummelbaugh Farm near the Second Corps aid station, reinterred in A-4 in the Pennsylvania Plot]

Pvt. John Cripps, Company E, 111th New York, wounded in the head [KILLED July 3, buried near the Second Corps aid station in the Peter Frey Farm field (or in the Neinstadt Farm field), reinterred in C-29 in the New York plot, age 28]

Pvt. James Cullen, Company F, 42nd New York [KILLED July 3, buried near the Peter Frey stone house adjacent to the Second Corps aid station, reinterred in C-17 in the New York Plot, age 21]

Pvt. Alden Cunningham, Company D, 19th Maine [KILLED July 3, buried at the Second Division, Second Corps Hospital, age 21, single]

First Sgt. James P. Cush, Company C, 59th New York [KILLED July 2, buried near the Peter Frey stone house adjacent to the Second Corps aid station, reinterred in D-11 in the New York Plot, age 21]

Lt. Alonzo Hereford Cushing, 4th United States, Battery A [KILLED July 3] His body was carried by his men past the Second Corps hospitals and laid out under a tarpaulin at the artillery bivouac.

#Pvt. Thomas C. Diver, Company I, 69th Pennsylvania [KILLED July 3, buried on the G. Herling Farm, reinterred in Evergreen Cemetery]

First Lt. Herman Donath, Company C, 19th Massachusetts [KILLED July 3, buried in the lot near the Second Corps aid station at the Peter Frey Farm, later removed to Evergreen Cemetery, age 21]

Cpl. William Donavan, Company A, 69th Pennsylvania, shot in the lungs [KILLED July 3, buried in the Peter Frey Farm lot near the Second Corps aid station]

Pvt. Thomas Downey, Company E, 20th Massachusetts [KILLED July 3, buried on the ridge between the A. Bryan Farm and the Peter Frey Farm, enroute to the Second Corps aid station at the Peter Frey Farm, reinterred in A-14 in the Massachusetts Plot, age 35]

Pvt. George Dukinfield, Company I, 72nd Pennsylvania [KILLED July 2, buried on the Peter Frey Farm near the Second Corps aid station, reinterred in C-18 in the Pennsylvania Plot]

Pvt. August Duttling, Company C, 20th Massachusetts [KILLED July 3, buried on the ridge between the A. Bryan Farm and the Peter Frey Farm, enroute to the Second Corps aid station at the Peter Frey Farm, reinterred in A-17 in the Massachusetts Plot, age 20]

Pvt. Ira Emery, Company A, 16th Vermont [First Corps] [KILLED July 3, buried on the A. Bryan lot under a walnut tree, reinterred in A-18 in the Vermont Plot, apparently his remains were subsequently removed]

Sgt. Mark Englert, Company I, 108th New York [KILLED July 3, buried near the Peter Frey stone house or in the orchard adjacent to the Second Corps aid station, reinterred in A-46 in the New York Plot, age 26]

Pvt. John Enosens, Company A, 59th New York [KILLED July 3, buried on the Peter Frey Farm near the Second Corps aid station, reinterred in C-20 in the New York Plot, age 21]

#Pvt. William Evans, Company I, 71st Pennsylvania, wounded in the head [KILLED July 3, buried on the G. Herling Farm, reinterred in C-19 in the Pennsylvania Plot]

Pvt. John Finlen, 15th New York Light Battery [KILLED July 2, buried near the Second Corps aid station in the Peter Frey Farm orchard, reinterred in D-73 in the New York Plot, age 26]

Sgt. William Finnecy, Company H, 72nd Pennsylvania [KILLED July 3, buried in the Peter Frey Farm lot near the Second Corps aid station]

Pvt. Edgar H. Fiske, Company E, 13th Vermont [First Corps] [KILLED July 3, buried near the Peter Frey Farm pump adjacent to the Second Corps aid station *(name noted as "Weybridge"), reported killed in unit casualty reports, but state Adjutant Gen. Office records show him mustered out of the regiment July 30, 1863*]

Pvt. Michael Flynn, Battery B, 1st Rhode Island Light Artillery (detailed from Company E, 15th Massachusetts) [KILLED July 3, buried on the side of the A. Bryan Farm, reinterred in D-3 in the Massachusetts Plot, age 20]

Sgt. Frank B. Fox, Company G, 72nd Pennsylvania [KILLED July 3, buried in the Peter Frey Farm lot near the Second Corps aid station]

Pvt. James Gallagher, Company H, 71st Pennsylvania, wounded in the head [KILLED July 3, buried on the Peter Frey Farm near the Second Corps aid station, reinterred in D-11 in the Pennsylvania Plot]

Pvt. Timothy Gallagher, Company B, 69th Pennsylvania, wounded in the brain [KILLED July 2, buried on the Peter Frey Farm near the Second Corps aid station (also recorded as being buried in the Catholic Cemetery), reinterred in C-45 in the Pennsylvania Plot]

Pvt. Samuel R. Garvin, Company E, 72nd Pennsylvania [KILLED July 3, buried on the Peter Frey Farm near the Second Corps aid station, reinterred in B-19 in the Pennsylvania Plot]

Capt. Peter Generous, Company B, 5th Michigan [Third Corps] [KILLED July 2, buried near the Second Corps aid station on the Jacob Hummelbaugh Farm, reinterred in G-9 in the Michigan Plot, age 22]

Pvt. E. Gilbert, Company A?, 64th New York? [KILLED July 2 or 3?, buried near the Peter Frey Farm, *not listed in the state Adjutant General Office records*]

Sgt. Nicholas Goshy, Company E, 7th Michigan [KILLED July 3, buried on the ridge between the A. Bryan Farm and the Peter Frey Farm, enroute to the Second Corps aid station at the Peter Frey Farm, reinterred in A-20 in the Michigan Plot, age 21]

Pvt. John Grady, Company I, 15th Massachusetts [KILLED July 3, buried near the Second Division, Second Corps Hospital at its original position on the Sarah Patterson Farm, reinterred in D-12 of the Massachusetts Plot, age 19]

Second Lt. Erastus M. Granger, Company D, 111th New York, wounded in the chest [KILLED July 3, buried near the Second Corps aid station on the east side of the Peter Frey Farm house]

Pvt. James A. Gray, 1st New York Light Battery [Sixth Corps], shot in the head [KILLED July 3, buried near the Second Corps aid station in the field of the Peter Frey Farm, reinterred in C-116 in the New York plot, age 19]

Pvt. William E. Green, Company G, 13th Vermont [First Corps] [KILLED July 3, buried on the Jacob Hummelbaugh Farm near the Second Corps aid station, reinterred in A-10 in the Vermont Plot]

Pvt. Edgar Grinnell, Company K, 111th New York, wounded in the lungs [KILLED July 2, buried near the Third Division, Second Corps aid station in back of the Jacob Swisher farmhouse, reinterred in Evergreen Cemetery, age 19]

Pvt. James H. Griswold, Company E, 111th New York, wounded by a shell in the abdomen [KILLED July 3, buried near the Second Corps aid station in the lot of the Peter Frey Farm, reinterred in D-21 in the New York Plot, age 18]

Pvt. Thomas R. Gulwin, Company F, 20th Massachusetts [KILLED July 3, buried on the ridge between the A. Bryan Farm and the Peter Frey Farm, enroute to the Second Corps aid station at the Peter Frey Farm, reinterred in A-9 in the Massachusetts Plot, age 35]

#Sgt. James Hand, Company D, 69th Pennsylvania, wounded in the lungs [KILLED July 3, buried on the G. Herling Farm]

Pvt. Simeon Harmon, Company E, 111th New York, wounded by a shell in the side [KILLED July 3, buried near the 111th New York, Second Corps aid station opposite the Catherine Guinn Farm house, age 19]

Pvt. John Harrington, Company K, 69th Pennsylvania, wounded in the brain [KILLED July 2, buried in the Peter Frey Farm field near the Second Corps aid station, reinterred in B-69 in the Pennsylvania Plot]

Pvt. Sidney G. Harris, Company D, 7th Michigan [KILLED July 2, buried in the lot of the Peter Frey Farm near the Second Corps aid station, reinterred in G-3 in the Michigan Plot, age 18]

Pvt. John Harvey, Jr., Company A, 69th Pennsylvania, wounded in the brain by a shell [KILLED July 3, buried on the east side of the Peter Frey Farm house adjacent to the Second Corps aid station, reinterred in D-72 in the Pennsylvania Plot]

Pvt. Thomas D. Hawkins, Company E, 111th New York, shot in the head [KILLED July 3, buried near the Second Corps aid station in the lot of the Peter Frey Farm, reinterred in C-25 of the New York Plot, age 33]

Cpl. Samuel Hayburn, Company B, 106th Pennsylvania, wounded in the left eye [KILLED July 2, buried in the Peter Frey Farm field near the Second Corps aid station, reinterred in B-18 in the Pennsylvania Plot]

First Lt. Elijah Hayden, Company H, 8th Ohio [KILLED, buried on the Catherine Guinn Farm adjacent to the 8th Ohio, Second Corps aid station, age 32]

Sgt. Joseph H. Hervey, Company C, 19th Massachusetts [KILLED July 3, buried near the Jacob Hummelbaugh House on the ridge coming from the A. Bryan Farm, enroute to the Second Corps aid station at the Jacob Hummelbaugh Farm, age 20]

Pvt. Daniel Holland, Company D, 19th Massachusetts [KILLED July 3, buried in the lot near the Second Corps aid station on the Peter Frey Farm, reinterred in D-32 in the Massachusetts Plot, age 22]

Second Lt. Rufus P. Holmes, Company G, 126th New York [KILLED July 3, buried near the Second Corps aid station on the Peter Frey Farm, reinterred in B-34 in the New York Plot, age 30]

#Pvt. John Hurley, Company H, 69th Pennsylvania, wounded in the lungs [KILLED July 3, buried on the G. Herling Farm, reinterred in C-17 in the Pennsylvania Plot]

Lt. Col. James Huston, 82nd New York [KILLED July 2]

Pvt. William Inch, Company D, 20th Massachusetts [KILLED July 3, buried on the ridge between the A. Bryan Farm and the Peter Frey Farm, enroute to the Second Corps aid station at the Peter Frey Farm, reinterred in A-16 in the Massachusetts Plot, age 32]

First Sgt. Matthew G. Isett, Company C, 53rd Pennsylvania [KILLED July 2, buried in the orchard of the Peter Frey Farm near the Second Corps aid station, reinterred in C-64 in the Pennsylvania Plot]

Sgt. Maj. Irving P. Jaques, 111th New York, shot in the head [KILLED July 2, buried near the Second Corps aid station in the lot of the Peter Frey Farm, body removed before reinterment in the National Cemetery, age 18]

First Sgt. George Joeckel, Company B, 20th Massachusetts [KILLED July 3, buried on the ridge between the A. Bryan Farm and the Peter Frey Farm, enroute to the Second Corps aid station at the Peter Frey Farm, reinterred in A-12 in the Massachusetts Plot, age 25]

Pvt. Peter Keefe, Company F, 20th Massachusetts [KILLED July 3, buried on the ridge between the A. Bryan Farm and the Peter Frey Farm, enroute to the Second Corps aid station at the Peter Frey Farm, reinterred in A-13 in the Massachusetts Plot, age 20]

Pvt. Thomas Kelley, Company A, 20th Massachusetts [KILLED July 3, buried on the ridge between the A. Bryan Farm and the Peter Frey Farm, enroute to the Second Corps aid station at the Peter Frey Farm, reinterred in A-6 in the Massachusetts Plot, age 22]

Pvt. Michael Kelly, Company E, 106th Pennsylvania (apparently temporarily attached to the 2nd United States Cavalry) [KILLED July 3 (apparently as a member of the 106th Pennsylvania), buried in the Peter Frey Farm field near the Second Corps aid station, reinterred in B-67 in the Pennsylvania Plot]

Pvt. William Kiker, Company K, 72nd Pennsylvania [KILLED July 3, buried in the Peter Frey Farm field near the Second Corps aid station, reinterred in A-37 in the Pennsylvania Plot]

Pvt. John King, Company K, 82nd New York [KILLED July 2, buried near the Peter Frey stone house adjacent to the Second Corps aid station, reinterred in B-54 in the New York Plot, age 41]

Pvt. Alois Kraft, Company C, 20th Massachusetts [KILLED July 3, buried on the ridge between the A. Bryan Farm and the Peter Frey Farm, enroute to the Second Corps aid station at the Peter Frey Farm, reinterred in A-8 in the Massachusetts Plot, age 30]

Pvt. Ludwig Kreisel, Battery A, 1st Artillery [KILLED July 3, buried near the Peter Frey stone house adjacent to the Second Corps aid station, reinterred in A-4 in the New Jersey Plot]

Pvt. George Kutter, Battery A, 1st Artillery [KILLED July 3, buried near the Peter Frey stone house adjacent to the Second Corps aid station, reinterred in A-5 in the New Jersey Plot]

Pvt. James Lane, Company F, 20th Massachusetts [KILLED July 3, buried on the ridge between the A. Bryan Farm and the Peter Frey Farm, enroute to the Second Corps aid station at the Peter Frey Farm, reinterred in A-30 in the Massachusetts Plot, age 45]

Pvt. George Larsons, Company D, 20th Massachusetts [KILLED July 2 or 3, buried on the ridge between the A. Bryan and the Peter Frey Farms (*not listed on the unit casualty report or in the state Adjutant General Office reports)*]

Capt. Dorastus B. Logan, Company H, 11th New Jersey [Third Corps] [KILLED July 2, buried near the Peter Frey pump adjacent to the Second Corps aid station]

#Pvt. Michael Logan, Company I, 69th Pennsylvania [KILLED July 2, buried on the G. Herling Farm]

Pvt. Alexander Lord, Company C, 15th Massachusetts [KILLED July 3, buried in the lot near the Second Corps aid station on the Peter Frey Farm, age 45]

Cpl. Archibald G. McAfee, Company A, 111th New York, shot in the head [KILLED July 3, buried near the Second Corps aid station on the Peter Frey Farm, reinterred in C-31 in the New York Plot, age 28]

#Cpl. James McCann, Company D, 69th Pennsylvania [KILLED July 3, buried on the G. Herling Farm, reinterred in D-10 in the Pennsylvania Plot]

Pvt. James McEntyre, Company G, 69th Pennsylvania [KILLED July 3, buried in the Peter Frey Farm field near the Second Corps aid station, reinterred in A-33 in the Pennsylvania Plot]

Pvt. David McGill, Company A, 10th New York [KILLED, buried near the Peter Frey Farm near the Second Corps aid station, reinterred in C-32 in the New York Plot, age 22]

Pvt. Alexander McGillora, Company G, 111th New York, shot in the chest [KILLED July 2, buried near the Second Corps aid station in the lot of the Peter Frey Farm, reinterred in B-36 in the New York Plot, age 39]

Pvt. John McHugh, Company K, 72nd Pennsylvania [KILLED July 3, buried in the Peter Frey Farm field near the Second Corps aid station, reinterred in B-20 in the Pennsylvania Plot]

Pvt. Jeremiah McNulty, Company F, 7th New Jersey [Third Corps] [KILLED July 2, buried near the Second Corps aid station on the Peter Frey Farm, reinterred in D-11 in the New Jersey plot]

Sgt. James McShea, Company B, 69th Pennsylvania [KILLED July 2, buried in the Peter Frey farm field near the Second Corps aid station, reinterred in C-44 in the Pennsylvania Plot]

#Pvt. John McWilliams, Company D, 69th Pennsylvania [KILLED July 3, buried on the G. Herling farm]

Pvt. John Marsh, Company B, 15th Massachusetts, wounded in the head [KILLED July 3, buried on the ridge midway between the A. Bryan and the Peter Frey Farm, enroute to the Second Corps aid station at the Peter Frey Farm, reinterred to D-2 of the Massachusetts Plot, age 26]

Pvt. George H. Martin, Company A, 12th New Jersey [KILLED July 3, buried in the Peter Frey orchard near the Second Corps aid station, reinterred in A-9 in the New Jersey Plot]

Pvt. Joseph M. Martin, Company D, 16th Vermont [First Corps] [KILLED July 3, buried on the A. Bryan Farm under a walnut tree, reinterred in A-9 in the Vermont Plot]

Capt. Luther Martin, Company D, 11th New Jersey [Third Corps] [KILLED July 2, buried near the Peter Frey pump adjacent to the Second Corps aid station]

Pvt. James Matz, Company K, 72nd Pennsylvania [KILLED July 3, buried in the Peter Frey Farm field near the Second Corps aid station]

Cpl. Charles E. Mead, Company G, 14th Vermont [First Corps] [KILLED July 3, buried on the Jacob Hummelbaugh Farm near the Second Corps aid station, reinterred in A-4 in the Vermont Plot]

Lt. Col. Henry Czar Merwin, 27th Connecticut [KILLED July 2]

Pvt. George Mickle, Company C, 72nd Pennsylvania [KILLED July 3, buried in the Peter Frey Farm field near the Second Corps aid station, reinterred subsequently in Evergreen Cemetery, reinterred again in F-63 in the Pennsylvania Plot]

Pvt. Andrew Moore, Company F, 1st Massachusetts [Third Corps] [KILLED July 2, buried near the Second Corps aid station on the Jacob Hummelbaugh Farm; age 43]

Pvt. Ozro Moore, Company I, 8th Ohio [KILLED July 3, buried on the south side of the Catherine Guinn House adjacent to the 8th Ohio, Second Corps aid station, reinterred in A-18 in the Ohio Plot]

Pvt. Robert Morrison, Company A, 69th Pennsylvania [KILLED July 3, buried in the Peter Frey Farm field near the Second Corps aid station (possibly recorded as having been interred on the east side of Evergreen Cemetery), reinterred in B-17 in the Pennsylvania Plot]

Cpl. Charles Morse, Jr., Company A, 16th Vermont [First Corps] [KILLED July 3, buried on the A. Bryan Farm under a walnut tree, reinterred in A-16 in the Vermont Plot]

Pvt. Charles Murphy, Company B, 72nd Pennsylvania [KILLED July 3, buried in the Peter Frey Farm field near the Second Corps aid station]

Pvt. Amos Myers, Company G, 148th Pennsylvania [KILLED July 3, buried in the William Patterson orchard adjacent to the Second Corps Division Hospital]

Pvt. Patrick O'Brien, Company A, 69th Pennsylvania, wounded in the brain [KILLED July 3, buried in the farm field of Peter Frey near the Second Corps aid station, reinterred in C-16 in the Pennsylvania Plot]

Sgt. John O'Connor, Company G, 69th Pennsylvania, wounded in the brain [KILLED July 3, buried on the Jacob Hummelbaugh Farm near the Second Corps aid station, reinterred in B-68 in the Pennsylvania Plot]

Pvt. Patrick O'Neal, 15th New York Light Battery [KILLED July 2, buried near the Second Corps aid station in the Peter Frey Farm orchard, age 21]

Pvt. James O'Neil, Company B, 69th Pennsylvania, wounded in the brain [KILLED July 2, buried in the Peter Frey Farm field near the Second Corps aid station, reinterred in C-41 in the Pennsylvania Plot]

Pvt. Danford Parker, Company K, 8th Ohio [KILLED July 3, buried on the south side of the Catherine Guinn house adjacent to the 8th Ohio, Second Corps aid station, reinterred in A-22 in the Ohio Plot, age 36]

Pvt. Edward Peto, 1st New York Light Battery [Sixth Corps], wounded by a shell in the abdomen [KILLED July 3, buried near the Second

Corps aid station in the field of the Peter Frey Farm, reinterred in C-117 in the New York Plot, age 28]

Pvt. John K. Phillips, Company F, 126th New York [KILLED July 3, buried near the Second Corps aid station near the Peter Frey farm house, reinterred in A-45 in the New York Plot, age 27]

Pvt. George L. Plant, Company A, 20th Massachusetts [KILLED July 3, buried in the lot of the Peter Frey Farm near the Second Corps aid station, reinterred in A-21 in the Massachusetts Plot, age 37]

First Lt. Augustus W. Proseus, Company E, 111th New York, shot in the head [KILLED July 2, buried near the Second Corps aid station in the lot of the Peter Frey Farm, age 26]

Pvt. Patrick Quinlan, Company F, 20th Massachusetts [KILLED July 3, buried near the stone house on the Peter Frey Farm near the Second Corps aid station, reinterred in A-20 in the Massachusetts Plot, age 28]

Pvt. Charles A. Reed, Company H, 15th Massachusetts, wounded in the left chest [KILLED July 3, buried in the lot near the Second Corps aid station on the Peter Frey Farm, reinterred in E-17 in the Massachusetts Plot, age 19]

Pvt. James Rice, Company G, 69th Pennsylvania [KILLED July 3, buried in the Peter Frey Farm field near the Second Corps aid station, reinterred in A-36 in the Pennsylvania Plot]

Pvt. Henry W. Roberts, Company E, 111th New York, shot in the lungs [KILLED July 3, buried near the Second Corps aid station in the field of the Peter Frey Farm, reinterred in C-26 in the New York Plot, age 18]

Col. Richard Petit Roberts, 140th Pennsylvania [KILLED July 2]

Second Lt. Sherman S. Robinson, Company A, 19th Massachusetts [KILLED July 3, buried in the lot near the Second Corps aid station on the Peter Frey Farm, reinterred in E-29 in the Massachusetts Plot, age 21]

Pvt. Edmond Roche, Company E, 19th Massachusetts [KILLED July 3, buried near the Second Corps aid station by the stone house on the Peter Frey Farm, reinterred in C-30 in the Massachusetts Plot, age 30]

Cpl. Dyer Rogers, Company D, 13th Vermont [First Corps] [KILLED July 3, buried on the Jacob Hummelbaugh Farm near the Second Corps aid station, reinterred in A-13 in the Vermont Plot]

Sgt. Edward B. Rollins, Company A, 15th Massachusetts, shot in the left chest on [KILLED July 2, buried near the Second Corps aid station on the Peter Frey Farm near the stone house, reinterred to D-11 in the Massachusetts Plot, age 33]

First Lt. Henry Ropes, Company K, 20th Massachusetts, wounded by the premature explosion of a shell from a Union cannon firing over his position, while he sat reading a Dickens novel during the cannonade [KILLED July 3, age 23 (body was almost certainly returned to the Second Corps Hospital awaiting shipment to his family in Massachusetts)]

Capt. James McKay Rorty, Battery B, 1st New York Light, [KILLED July 3]

Pvt. Garrett L. Roseboom, Company D, 13th Vermont [First Corps] [KILLED July 3, buried on the Jacob Hummelbaugh Farm near the Second Corps aid station, reinterred in A-17 in the Vermont Plot]

Pvt. Charles W. Ross, Company G, 13 Vermont [First Corps] [KILLED July 3, buried on the Jacob Hummelbaugh Farm near the Second Corps aid station, reinterred in A-3 in the Vermont Plot]

Pvt. Thomas J. Rudrow, Company G, 12th New Jersey [KILLED July 3, buried in the Peter Frey orchard near the Second Corps aid station, reinterred in A-15 in the New Jersey Plot]

Cpl. Henry C. Russell, Company F, 13th Vermont [First Corps] [KILLED July 3, buried by the Peter Frey stone house adjacent to the Second Corps aid station]

Pvt. George S. Sawtell, Company K, 20th Massachusetts [KILLED July 3, buried in the lot of the Peter Frey Farm near the Second Corps aid station, age 21]

Cpl. Patrick Scannel, Company H, 19th Massachusetts [KILLED July 3, buried on the ridge between the A. Bryan Farm and the Peter Frey Farm, enroute to the Second Corps aid station at the Peter Frey Farm, reinterred in D-24 in the Massachusetts Plot, age 21]

Cpl. Frank Shaffer, Company D, 8th Ohio [KILLED July 3, buried on the south side of the Catherine Guinn House adjacent to the 8th Ohio, Second Corps aid station, reinterred in A-21 in the Ohio Plot, age 32]

Pvt. Jacob Sheak, Company I, 4th Ohio (on duty with the Third Division, Second Corps provost guard), wounded by a shell in the chest on July 2 or 3 [KILLED, buried in the Peter Frey Farm orchard near the Second Corps aid station, reinterred in A-19 in the New Jersey Plot, age 21]

Cpl. John B. Sheetz, Company D, 1st Delaware [KILLED, buried on the Schwartz Farm, reinterred in A-4 in the Delaware Plot]

Pvt. Frederick Shoner, Company E, 72nd Pennsylvania [KILLED July 3, buried in the Peter Frey Farm field near the Second Corps aid station, reinterred in D-7 in the Pennsylvania Plot]

Second Lt. Albert Slafter, Company E, 7th Michigan [KILLED, buried in the lot of the Peter Frey lot near the Second Corps aid station, reinterred in G-13 in the Michigan Plot, age 28]

Sgt. Maj. Henry H. Smith, 13th Vermont [First Corps] [KILLED July 3, buried by the Peter Frey Farm pump adjacent to the Second Corps aid station, reinterred in A-25 in the Vermont Plot]

First Lt. William Smith, Company A, 1st Delaware [KILLED July 3]

Second Lt. William H. Smith, Company B, 106th Pennsylvania [KILLED July 2, buried in the Peter Frey Farm field near the Second Corps aid station, reinterred in C-42 in the Pennsylvania Plot]

Cpl. James C. Somerville, Company E, 20th Massachusetts [KILLED July 3, buried on the ridge between the A. Bryan Farm and the Peter Frey Farm, enroute to the Second Corps aid station at the Peter Frey Farm, reinterred in A-15 in the Massachusetts Plot, age 18]

Cpl. Joseph B. Spachius, Company B, 12th New Jersey [KILLED July 3, buried in the Peter Frey orchard near the Second Corps aid station, reinterred in A-8 in the New Jersey Plot]

Pvt. William H. Spencer, Company B, 12th New Jersey [KILLED July 3, buried in the Peter Frey orchard near the Second Corps aid station, reinterred in A-16 in the New Jersey Plot]

Pvt. David Stainrock, Company E, 72nd Pennsylvania [KILLED July 3, buried in the Peter Frey Farm field near the Second Corps aid station, reinterred in C-20 in the Pennsylvania Plot]

Lt. Col. Amos E. Steele, 7th Michigan [KILLED July 3, buried in the lot of the Peter Frey Farm near the Second Corps aid station]

Cpl. Theodore Streyline, Company C, 72nd Pennsylvania [KILLED July 3, buried in the Peter Frey Farm field near the Second Corps aid station, reinterred in A-2 in the Pennsylvania Plot]

Cpl. George Stuart, Company G, 72nd Pennsylvania [KILLED July 3, buried in the Peter Frey Farm field near the Second Corps aid station, reinterred in the east side of Evergreen Cemetery]

Cpl. Wesley C. Sturdevant, Company E, 13th Vermont [First Corps] [KILLED July 3, buried near the Peter Frey Farm pump adjacent to the Second Corps aid station]

Pvt. Peter Tees, Jr., Company C, 72nd Pennsylvania [KILLED July 3, buried in the Peter Frey Farm lot near the Second Corps aid station, reinterred in Evergreen Cemetery]

Pvt. James H. Todd, Company H, 69th Pennsylvania, wounded in the lungs [KILLED July 2, buried in the Peter Frey Farm field near the Second Corps aid station]

Lt. Col. Martin Tschudy, 69th Pennsylvania, wounded July 2, wounded in the bladder on July 3 [KILLED July 3, buried on the east side of the Peter Frey Farm house adjacent to the Second Corps aid station]

Sgt. Sylvester Vanderpool, Company I, 125th New York [KILLED July 3, buried on the Catherine Guinn Farm near the 125th New York, Second Corps aid station, reinterred in E-66 in the New York Plot, age 23]

Cpl. Ambrose L. Van Valkenburgh, Company E, 111th New York, shot in the head [KILLED July 3, buried near the Second Corps aid station in the field of the Peter Frey Farm, reinterred in E-57 in the New York Plot, age 19]

Pvt. Benjamin Van Wort, Company K, 111th New York, shot in the abdomen [KILLED July 3, buried near the Second Corps aid station in the field of the Peter Frey Farm, reinterred in Evergreen Cemetery, age 23]

Sgt. John Vaughan, Company C, 13th Vermont [First Corps] [KILLED July 3, buried on the Jacob Hummelbaugh Farm near the Second Corps aid station]

Maj. Edward Venuti, 52nd New York [KILLED July 2]

Pvt. Charles J. Walker, Company B, 16th Massachusetts [Third Corps] [KILLED July 2, buried near the original location of one division of the Second Corps Hospital on the west side of the William Patterson Farm, near the fortifications, age 22]

Pvt. Orville A. Warren, Company K, 8th Ohio [KILLED July 3, buried on the south side of the Catherine Guinn House adjacent to the 8th Ohio, Second Corps aid station, reinterred in A-17 in the Ohio Plot, age 23]

Pvt. Charles Webster, Company C, 26th Pennsylvania [Third Corps] [KILLED July 3, buried near the Second Corps aid station on the Jacob Hummelbaugh Farm, reinterred in B-80 in the Pennsylvania Plot]

Pvt. Martin V. Westbrook, Company E, 111th New York, shot in the head [KILLED July 3, buried near the Second Corps aid station in the field of the Peter Frey Farm, age 22]

Pvt. William E. Whitmore, Company E, 111th New York, shot in the head [KILLED July 3, buried near the Second Corps aid station in the field of the Peter Frey Farm, reinterred in C-28 in the New York Plot, age 18]

Sgt. John B. Wilson, Company C, 82nd New York [KILLED July 3, buried near the Peter Frey house adjacent to the Second Corps aid station, reinterred in A-74 in the New York Plot, age 32]

Sgt. Nathan W. Wilson, Company F, 11th Massachusetts [Third Corps] [KILLED July 2 or 3, buried near the Second Corps aid station on the Jacob Hummelbaugh Farm, aged 25]

Sgt. John Wogan, Company G, 69th Pennsylvania, wounded in the stomach [KILLED July 3, buried in the Peter Frey Farm field near the Second Corps aid station, reinterred in A-32 in the Pennsylvania Plot]

Sgt. Esty E. Wood, Company G, 111th New York, shot in the head [KILLED July 2, buried near the Second Corps aid station in the field of the Peter Frey Farm, body removed prior to reinterment in the National Cemetery, age 18]

WOUNDED DOCUMENTED AS TREATED AT A SECOND CORPS HOSPITAL FACILITY

(PROCESSED BY SECOND CORPS STAFF, AND INCLUDED IN THE PATIENT COUNT)

The following parameters were used in compiling this roster of wounded treated at the Second Corps Hospital:

—Soldiers sustaining "flesh wounds" are not included here. The average soldier's extreme aversion to hospital care meant that he might (or just as likely might not) retire to the rear if he were merely nicked, grazed, contused, or even slightly wounded. Some minor injuries were simply bound up and ignored, since "the enlisted men were exceedingly accurate judges of the probable result which would ensue from any wound they saw." [Frank Wilkeson, *Recollections of a Private Soldier in the Army of the Potomac* (New York: G. P. Putnam's Sons, 1886; reprinted as *Turned Inside Out: Recollections of a Private Soldier in the Army of the Potomac* (Lincoln: University of Nebraska Press, 1997), pp. 206-7.]

One year later, on the road to Petersburg, Second Corps "wounded soldiers, it mattered not how slight the wounds, generally hastened away from the battle lines. A wound entitled a man to go to the rear and to a hospital." But there were still "many exceptions to this rule, as there would necessarily be in battles where twenty thousand to thirty thousand men were wounded." [Wilkeson, *Recollections of a Private*, p. 201.]

—Only soldiers known to have been wounded are listed here. Men listed in records as "supposed wounded" are not included here.

—Only Confederates known to have been captured in assaults against the Union lines, or those left behind in Gettysburg and known to be treated at the Second Corps Hospital, are included in this roster.

—*** denotes that the soldier who was treated at the Second Corps Hospital wrote of his experience.

—? precedes names of patients presumed to be treated at the Second Corp Hospital.

—Wounded from the Army of Northern Virginia are listed in "**bold print**," while patients from the Army of the Potomac are printed in "non-bold print."

As the Confederate wounded, especially from the July 3 fighting, were collected, assorted ambulance crews from various Union corps hospitals picked them up and transported them to their own individual hospitals. Consequently, members of the same Confederate unit were often treated by as many as three or four different Union hospitals. This was especially true of the First, Second, Third, and Twelfth Corps Hospitals, as they worked together in the desperate days immediately following the end of the Battle of Gettysburg.

After being treated at the Second Corps Hospital, Confederate casualties were transferred to four major hospital complexes for further care—DeCamp General Hospital, New York; West's Buildings Hospital, Baltimore; U.S. General Hospital, Chester, Pennsylvania; and Camp Letterman General Hospital, Gettysburg. When sufficiently recuperated, they were either paroled, or transferred again to a more secure prisoner-of-war camp, such as Johnson's Island, off Sandusky, Ohio (if officers), or Fort Henry, in Baltimore, or David's Island, New York.

Pvt. Daniel B. Abbott, Company H, 19th Maine, wounded in the side and arm.

Pvt. Henry Abbott, Company I, 1st Minnesota, wounded in the leg on July 2, age 20

Cpl. Marion Abbott, Company F, 1st Minnesota, wounded in the right arm on July 2, discharged due to disability on November 1, 1863

Lt. Col. Charles Powell Adams, 1st Minnesota, struck six times in the chest and hip on July 2, the last ball passing through the chest, lungs and back, treated at Second Division Hospital in Sarah Patterson's stone barn, survived to command the 1st Minnesota

Pvt. John B. Adams, Company C, 19th Maine, wounded in the hip and shoulder

Second Lt. Edwin Thomas Adams, Company D, 8th Virginia, battlefield fracture of the left leg on July 3, captured, treated at the Second Division Hospital [DIED July 18, buried in Yard D, Row 1 in Schwartz's cornfield by Rock Creek, disinterred to Richmond on June 13, 1872, with 110 others in ten large boxes marked "S"]

Pvt. George M. Adams, Company E, 1st Minnesota, wounded in the shoulder on July 2

***Capt. John "Jack" G. B. Adams, 19th Massachusetts, shot in the groin and right hip on July 2, carried on the back of Private Collopee to a Third Corps aid station, moved late July 3 to the Second Corps, but abandoned along the Taneytown Road at an ambulance collection point; evacuated under shellfire on July 3 to the Second Corps Rock Creek facility, diagnosed as mortally wounded; eventually hired a wagon with some friends to transport them after a week to Littlestown, where his wounds were treated, and he was finally evacuated by railroad.

Pvt. Lucius A. Adams, Company A, 1st Minnesota, wounded in the hand on July 2, age 29

?Pvt. William H. Agnew, Company G, 11th Virginia, age 30, teacher, battlefield fracture of both superior and inferior maxilla (jaws), no further record, probably died at either the Second or Twelfth Corps hospitals

Pvt. Elisha Allen, Company A, 59th New York, wounded by a shell in the right shoulder on July 2 [DIED July 15, buried in the Schwartz cornfield near Rock Creek, reinterred in D-30 in the New York plot, age 22]

Pvt. Erastus A. Allen, Company I, 145th Pennsylvania, wounded July 2 [DIED July 4, buried on the Schwartz Farm near "Red Rock," reinterred in B-41 in the Pennsylvania Plot]

Pvt. William R. Allen, Company D, 1st Minnesota, shot in the lower abdomen on July 2 [DIED July 18]

Pvt. David A. Ammerman, Company B, 148th Pennsylvania, wounded July 2 [DIED July 4, 5, or 6, buried in the Schwartz cornfield near a walnut tree, reinterred in B-33 in the Pennsylvania Plot]

Pvt. John Thompson Ammerman, Company B, 148th Pennsylvania, wounded July 2

Pvt. Adam Areman, Company G, 1st Minnesota, wounded in the shoulder on July 2

?Pvt. Richard C. Archer, Company B, 14th Vermont [First Corps], wounded July 3 [DIED July 14, recorded (possibly incorrectly) as having been buried on the Jacob Hummelbaugh Farm, reinterred in B-11 in the Vermont Plot]

Pvt. Benjamin Archer, Company G, 68th Pennsylvania [Third Corps], wounded in the stomach on July 2 [DIED July 3, buried on the Schwartz Farm opposite White Run]

Pvt. George Arnold, Company B, 1st Minnesota, wounded in the shoulder and leg on July 2, celebrated his twenty-sixth birthday in the hospital on July 3

Pvt. Dawson W. Arnold, 5th Florida, age 18, shot in the upper third of the left femur on July 3, captured, leg amputated at the Second Corps Hospital, transferred on August 5 to the Letterman General Hospital [DIED September 15 of exhaustion and chronic diarrhea, buried there]

Pvt. Edwin R. Ash, Company F, 72nd Pennsylvania, wounded July 2 [DIED July 3 at the Second Division Hospital]

Pvt. Minor Atherton, Company C, 1st Minnesota, wounded in the legs and thigh on July 3, transferred to the Invalid Corps on December 13, 1863, age 19

Pvt. John R. Atwood, Company E, 19th Maine, wounded in the leg

Pvt. William H. Aucker, Company B, 1st Minnesota, wounded in the right hip and through the intestines on July 2, never returned to duty, age 23

Pvt. John W. Austin, Company H, 18th Virginia, age 42, farmer, shot in the arm on July 3, captured, treated at First Division Hospital, exchanged September 23, 1863, from Chester Hospital

Pvt. James F. Bachelor, Company F, 1st Minnesota, wounded in the foot on July 2, age 24

Cpl. Assner Baker, Company A, 19th Maine, wounded in the chest [DIED August 6 at Summit House Hospital, Philadelphia]

Pvt. Harry S. Baker, Company H, 72nd Pennsylvania, mortally wounded [DIED, buried in the Schwartz cornfield near a walnut tree]

Pvt. Ozias P. Baker, Company L, 1st Minnesota, wounded on July 3

Pvt. Horatio N. Barber, Company F, 1st Minnesota, wounded in the back on July 3

Brig. Gen. William Barksdale, 13th Mississippi, gunshot wounds in the chest and legs on July 2, captured [DIED July 3 at the Second Corps aid station at the Hummelbaugh Farm, buried there near the Second Corps aid station]

Pvt. John Barmoy, Company F, 148th Pennsylvania, wounded July 2, transferred to the Veterans Reserve Corps

Cpl. Josiah D. Barnes, Company I, 120th New York [Third Corps], mortally wounded July 2 [DIED July 2, buried on the Schwartz Farm, reinterred in D-52 in the New York Plot, age 20]

Pvt. James Barry, Company I, 20th Massachusetts, wounded

Cpl. George W. Barter, Company I, 19th Maine, wounded

Pvt. George W. Bartlett, Company D, 1st Minnesota, wounded in the thigh on July 2

Pvt. Dana S. Barton, Company G, 1st Minnesota, wounded in the chest and arm on July 2

Pvt. George L. Bass, Company B, 15th Massachusetts, wounded in the hip by a shell on July 2 [DIED July 5, buried on the Schwartz Farm on Rock Creek opposite the George Bushman Farm, reinterred in D-10 of the Massachusetts Plot, age 19]

Pvt. Oliver S. Bates, Company A, 20th Massachusetts, wounded

Col. Dewitt Clinton Baxter, 72nd Pennsylvania, wounded on July 2

Second Lt. John A. Bayard, Company H, 148th Pennsylvania, wounded July 2 [DIED July 3]

Pvt. George W. Bayne, Company K, 8th Virginia, age 25, farmer, gunshot flesh wound in the right leg on July 3, captured, treated at the Second Division Hospital, exchanged March 6, 1864

Pvt. Bradford W. Beale, Company A, 20th Massachusetts, wounded

Pvt. James E. Beales, Company H, 148th Pennsylvania, wounded July 2 [DIED August 8, buried in C-85 of the Pennsylvania Plot]

Pvt. Benjamin F. Beans, Company G, 148th Pennsylvania, wounded July 3

Pvt. James Bear, Company E, 148th Pennsylvania, wounded July 2

Pvt. Charles Behr, Company K, 1st Minnesota, wounded in the chest, treated at the Second Corps Hospitals

***George Washington Beidelman, 71st Pennsylvania, wounded at "The Angle" on July 3, a minié ball cut across both legs above the knees, just bruising the left, and cutting a gash in the right about the depth of a finger, treated at the Second Corps Hospital, transferred July 7 to Chestnut Hill General Hospital, Philadelphia

Pvt. George W. Bellomy, Company H, 57th Virginia, gunshot fracture of the thigh on July 3, captured [DIED July 10 at the Second Corps Hospital, buried there in Yard C west of the Schwartz farm house in the woods on the red hill above the creek; disinterred June 13, 1872, to Richmond with 110 others in 10 large boxes marked "S"]

Lt. Col. Richard Charles Bentley, 63rd New York, wounded July 2

Pvt. Amos O. Berry, Company E, 1st Minnesota, wounded in the leg on July 2

Pvt. Charles A. Berry, Company E, 1st Minnesota, wounded in the leg on July 2, age 21

Cpl. Joshua Besse, Company A, 20th Massachusetts, wounded

Cpl. Gardiner W. Bigelow, Company A, 19th Maine, wounded in the arm on July 2

Cpl. Jeremiah Bigelow, Company K, 111th New York, wounded by a shell in the stomach on July 3 [DIED July 4 at the Third Division Hospital, buried on Michael Trostle's "Walnut Row," reinterred in Evergreen Cemetery, age 28]

Col. Daniel G. Bingham, 64th New York, wounded on July 2, died a year later from his wounds

Second Lt. Jeremiah Birtcil, Company F, 145th Pennsylvania Volunteers, wounded in the right arm on July 2

Capt. William Rombough Bissell, Company A, 8th Virginia, shot in the head and shaft of the upper arm on July 3, captured, treated at the Second Division, Second Corps Hospital, arm amputated at the shoulder by Surgeon Charles Squire Wood of the 66th New York [DIED July 16, buried at the Presbyterian Graveyard, Gettysburg, Pennsylvania]

Pvt. Gorham L. Black, Company I, 19th Maine, wounded

Pvt. Richard M. Blaisdell, Company K, 19th Maine, wounded in the leg

Pvt. Edwin Blake, Company K, 19th Maine, wounded in the hand

Sgt. Thomas Blake, Company A, 13th Vermont [First Corps], wounded July 3 [DIED July 4, buried on the Sarah Patterson Farm near the original position of the Second Division Hospital, reinterred in A-28 in the Vermont Plot]

Pvt. Rufus Gair Blanchard, Company B, 1st Minnesota, wounded in the side on July 3, transferred to Letterman Hospital, still absent on disability when regiment mustered out on May 5, 1864

Pvt. James L. Blethen, Company C, 19th Maine, wounded in the hand and arm

Capt. John J. T. Blinn, Assistant Adjutant General, First Brigade, Second Division, Second Corps, hip shattered on July 3, treated at the Second Division Hospital [DIED July 14 or 18, age 23]

Color Cpl. William S. [or L.] Bodwell, Company C, 27th Connecticut, shot in the lung on July 2 [DIED July 5, buried at Schwartz's "Red Rock"]

Pvt. Cyrus S. Bondurant, Company G, 1st Minnesota, wounded in the right thigh and hip on July 2, treated at the Second Corps Hospitals

Pvt. Casper Bonnet, Company C, 66th New York, gunshot fracture of the femur at the left knee [DIED July 18, buried in the Schwartz cornfield near Rock Creek, reinterred in D-29 in the New York plot, age 35]

Pvt. James P. Boss, Company H, 8th Virginia, gunshot fracture of the femur on July 3, captured, treated at the First Division Hospital [DIED]

First Sgt. John L. C. Boswell, Company E, 57th Virginia, gunshot fracture of the hip and thigh on July 3, captured [DIED July 14, buried in Yard D in the Schwartz cornfield, disinterred June 13, 1872, to Richmond with 110 others in 10 large boxes marked "S"]

Lt. George Boyd, Company I, 1st Minnesota, wounded in the leg and thigh on July 2

Color Sgt. Jacob Boyd, Company I, 2nd Delaware, shot in the forearm, amputated [DIED July 6, buried in Yard D, in the Schwartz cornfield, reinterred in B-4 in the Delaware Plot]

Pvt. Adam Boyer, Company A, 148th Pennsylvania, wounded July 3, transferred to the Veteran Reserve Corps

Pvt. Philip Boyer, Company I, 148th Pennsylvania, wounded July 2, transferred to the Veteran Reserve Corps

Pvt. George W. Bradbury, Company H, 1st Minnesota, wounded in the shoulder on July 3

Cpl. Henry C. Bradley, Company E, 1st Minnesota, wounded in the ankle on July 2

Capt. Joseph R. Bradley, Company F, 27th Connecticut, wounded

Pvt. Thomas J. Brainard, Company F, 14th Connecticut, shot in the right shoulder [DIED July 3 at Third Division Hospital]

Pvt. Clark Brandt, Company A, 1st Minnesota, wounded in the knee on July 2 [DIED July 21]

Pvt. John Brant, Company D, 39th New York, wounded July 2 or 3 [DIED July 3 at the Third Division Hospital of a wound to the genitals, *Brant is not listed in the unit casualty list, nor in the state Adjutant General Office records*]

First Lt. William Harvie Bray, Company E, 53rd Virginia, VMI Class of 1861, wounded in the thigh on July 3, captured, leg amputated [DIED July 14, buried in Yard D in the Jacob Schwartz cornfield; disinterred June 13, 1872, to Richmond with 110 others in 10 large boxes labeled "S"]

Cpl. George E. Briggs, Company G, 72nd Pennsylvania, shot in the back on July 3 [DIED July 18, buried in the Schwartz cornfield]

Cpl. William Briggs, Company B, 19th Maine, wounded in the ankle

Pvt. Ira L. Brigham, Company H, 8th Ohio, wounded July 2 [DIED July 4, buried on the Jacob Swisher Farm near the Third Division, Second Corps aid station, reinterred in D-21 in the Ohio Plot, age 34]

Pvt. Brice D. Brisbin, Company G, 148th Pennsylvania, wounded July 3

Pvt. Dwight T. Brockett, Company D, 27th Connecticut, wounded

Pvt. Thomas Broinham, Company K, 20th Massachusetts, wounded

Col. John R. Brooke, Second Corps, First Division, Fourth Brigade commander, debilitating ankle wound on July 2

Pvt. James R. Brower, Company B, 148th Pennsylvania, wounded July 2

Pvt. Bartlett Brown, Company E, 111th New York, shot in the lung on July 3 [DIED July 3 or 4, buried behind the Jacob Swisher house near the Third Division aid station location, reinterred in C-15 in the New Hampshire Plot, age 33]

Capt. Benjamin Brown Jr., Company H, 19th Virginia, age 19, farmer, VMI class of 1864, wounded in the right foot on July 3, captured, treated at the Second Division Hospital, paroled for exchanged on February 24, 1865

Lt. Thomas Frederic Brown, Battery B, 1st Rhode Island Light, wounded July 2

Sgt. Henry O. Brown, Company I, 11th Massachusetts [Third Corps], wounded in the abdomen on July 2 [DIED July 2, buried on the Schwartz Farm on Rock Creek, opposite White Run, age 20]

Col. Hiram Loomis Brown, 145th Pennsylvania, wounded in the right arm above the elbow on July 2

Pvt. James C. Brown, Company D, 19th Maine, wounded in the leg

Pvt. John Brown, Company D, 20th Massachusetts, wounded

Pvt. Michael A. Brown, Company B, 148th Pennsylvania, wounded July 2, transferred to the Veteran Reserve Corps

Sgt. William Brown, Company I, 145th Pennsylvania [apparently DIED at Second Corps Hospital]

Pvt. William W. Brown, Company G, 1st Minnesota, wounded in the right leg on July 2

Cpl. James Bryant, Company D, 1st Minnesota, wounded in the thight on July 2

Pvt. John Buckley, Company A, 108th Pennsylvania, shot in the abdomen July 2 or 3 [DIED July 4 at the Third Division Hospital, *not listed on the state Adjutant General Office records*]

Pvt. Timothy Buckley, Company F, 20th Massachusetts, wounded

Second Lt. Samuel E. Bucknam, Company K, 19th Maine, wounded in the leg

Pvt. Charles Buesco, Company D, 6th New York Cavalry (Second Corps Headquarters escort), wounded in the chest and shoulder by a shell on July 2 [DIED July 4 at the Third Division Hospital, buried in the back of the Jacob Swisher house adjacent to the aid station location, age 30]

Pvt. William F. Buker, Company A, 19th Maine, wounded in the hands

Pvt. Daniel Bumgardner, Company A, 141st Pennsylvania [Third Corps], shot in the right thigh and left knee [DIED July 23, buried on the Schwartz Farm lane near White Run, reinterred in C-24 in the Pennsylvania Plot]

Pvt. James M. Burchett, Company K, 8th Virginia, wounded in the lower third of the left leg, shoulder dislocated on July 3, captured, leg amputated, exchanged November 17, 1863, from West's Buildings Hospital [nephew of Andrew Johnson, Governor of Tennessee, strongly disliked by his comrades for strongly expressed Union sentiments]

Pvt. Henry Burgetorf, Company F, 1st Minnesota, wounded in the back on July 3, age 20

Pvt. John Burns, Company A, 59th New York, wounded by a shell which fractured his skull on July 2 [DIED July 13, buried in the Schwartz cornfield, reinterred in B-43 in the New York Plot, age 43]

Cpl. John Q. Burrill, Company F, 1st Massachusetts [Third Corps], wounded July 2 [DIED July 4, buried on the Schwartz Farm on Rock Creek opposite White Run; age 20]

Junior Second Lt. Walter Butts, Company F, 9th Virginia, age 20, shot in the lung on July 3, captured, treated at the First Division Hospital [DIED July 11, buried there in Yard D, Row 1 of the Jacob Schwartz cornfield by Rock Creek; disinterred June 13,

1872, to Richmond with 110 others in 10 large boxes marked "S"]

Pvt. John S. Buzzard, Company I, 148th Pennsylvania, wounded July 2, transferred to the Veteran Reserve Corps

Pvt. Charles F. Buzzell, Company E, 12th New Hampshire [Third Corps] [DIED July 14 of typhoid fever, buried in the Schwartz cornfield on Rock Creek, reinterred in A-5 in the New Hampshire Plot, age 21]

Pvt. Henry D. Byard, Company D, 19th Maine, wounded in the leg on July 2

Pvt. Mathew Byrnes, Company C, 82nd New York, wounded July 2 [DIED July 5, buried in the Schwartz field opposite White Run, reinterred in D-55 in the New York Plot, age 19]

Pvt. Frederick S. Call, Company C, 19th Maine, mortally wounded [DIED August 25]

Pvt. Albert Caplazi, Company B, 1st Minnesota, wounded in the thigh and foot on July 2

Pvt. Bartholomew Carmody, Company A, 125th New York, mortally wounded July 3 [DIED July 3, buried on the Schwartz Farm, reinterred in B-71? in the New York Plot, age 18]

Pvt. James H. Carney, Company G, 1st Minnesota, wounded in the thigh on July 2

***Sgt. Alfred P. Carpenter, Company K, 1st Minnesota, wounded in the foot on July 2

Sgt. Charles F. Carpenter, Company F, 20th Massachusetts, wounded

***Pvt. Austin A. Carr, Company F, 82nd New York, treated for a glancing shell wound of the collarbone, and hemorrhoids

Pvt. Rinaldo A. Carr, Company H, 19th Maine, wounded in the thigh

Pvt. Bartholomew Carriegiet, Company B, 1st Minnesota, wounded in the thigh on July 2, still recovering as of February 23, 1864

Pvt. Charles J. Carroll, Company G, 19th Maine, wounded July 3 [DIED July 7]

First Sgt. William H. Carroll, Company E, 20th Massachusetts, wounded

Capt. Edward Carter, Company K, 8th Virginia, VMI class of 1864, shot in both legs on July 3, captured, treated at the Second Division Hospital, paroled December 15, 1864

Pvt. Jacob L. Carter, Company C, 148th Pennsylvania, wounded July 2

Pvt. William G. Cason, Company H, 57th Virginia, wounded and captured on July 3 [DIED July 17, 1863, buried there in Yard D,

Row 3 in the Schwartz cornfield; disinterred June 13, 1872, to Richmond with 110 others in 10 large boxes marked "S"]

Pvt. John Caswell, Company G, 28th Massachusetts, shot in both thighs on July 2 [DIED July 29, buried on the Schwartz Farm, reinterred in D-18 in the Massachusetts Plot, age 33]

Musician Lauriston Chamberlain, Company F, 19th Maine, wounded in the back

Pvt. Benjamin F. Charles, Company A, 19th Maine, wounded in the leg on July 3

Pvt. Daniel B. Chase, Company I, 20th Massachusetts, wounded

Pvt. Samuel O. Cheatham, Company D, 14th Virginia, shot in both legs on July 3, captured [DIED July 17, buried there in Yard D, Row 1; disinterred June 13, 1872, to Richmond with 110 others in 10 large boxes labeled "S"]

Pvt. George F. Chapman, Company B, 19th Maine, wounded in the arm and side

Sgt. Almond M. Chesbro, Company G, 53rd Pennsylvania, wounded in both legs on July 2 [DIED July 10, buried in the Schwartz cornfield east of a walnut tree, reinterred in B-39 in the Pennsylvania Plot]

Pvt. John C. Chiles, Company C, 14th Virginia, age 19, shot in the head on July 3, captured, treated at the Second Division Hospital [DIED August 9, 1863, at Chester Hospital, buried there in Grave #128]

Pvt. Samuel Christian, Company I, 20th Massachusetts, wounded

Pvt. John P. Church, Company A, 19th Maine, wounded in the arm

Pvt. Daniel Clancy, Company C, 1st Minnesota, wounded in the shoulder on July 3

Pvt. Hiram Clapp, Company I, 19th Maine, wounded

Cpl. Henry W. Clark, Company F, 27th Connecticut, wounded

Pvt. Luther Clark, Company I, 19th Maine, wounded

Pvt. John Clausen, Company H, 1st Minnesota, wounded in the chest on July 2

Pvt. Charles H. Clements, Company D, 19th Maine, wounded July 2

Pvt. William G. Coen, Company G, 1st Minnesota, wounded in the left foot on July 2

Pvt. Frank Coffin, Company B, 19th Maine, wounded in the thigh on July 3, leg amputated at middle third of the thigh [DIED July 14, buried in Yard D, in the Schwartz cornfield, reinterred to B-2 in the Maine Plot, age 18, single]

Sgt. Gorham Coffin, Company A, 19th Massachusetts, wounded July 3 [DIED July 3, buried on the Schwartz Farm, reinterred in C-28 in the Massachusetts Plot, age 26]

Sgt. Charles H. Colburn, Company A, 19th Maine, wounded in the leg on July 3

***Jacob H. Cole, 57th New York, shot in the arm and wounded by shrapnel in the right leg on July 2, stranded behind Confederate lines, retrieved by ambulance on July 5, and treated at the Rock Creek facility

Pvt. Franklin Cole, Company G, 61st New York, shot in the leg on July 2, leg amputated [DIED July 12, buried in the Schwartz cornfield, reinterred in B-39 in the New York Plot, age 26]

Pvt. William C. Coleman, Company L, 1st Minnesota, wounded on July 3

Pvt. William J. Colsin, Company E, 19th Maine, wounded in the leg

***Col. William Colvill III, 1st Minnesota, shot through the upper chest and foot on July 2, treated at the Second Division Hospital in Sarah Patterson's stone barn, moved to the Rock Creek facility, removed to the Schwartz Farm location, left partially disabled for the rest of his life due to his wounds

Pvt. John Conley, Company G, 12th New Jersey, shot in the abdomen on July 2 [DIED July 4 at the Third Division Hospital]

Pvt. William Conlin, Company H, 140th Pennsylvania, shot in the thigh on July 2, leg amputated at the upper third of the thigh [DIED July 15, buried south of the Schwartz buildings under an apple tree, reinterred in A-42 in the Pennsylvania Plot]

Cpl. Orrin T. Conway, Company I, 19th Maine, mortally wounded in the leg [DIED September 1 in Baltimore]

Sgt. William Coogan, Company C, 69th Pennsylvania, shot in the hip on July 3 [DIED July 21]

Pvt. Joseph G. Cookson, Company E, 19th Maine, wounded in the hand

Pvt. Martin Coon, Company A, 20th Massachusetts, wounded

Second Lt. Giles H. Cooper, Company D, 24th Virginia, wounded in the left leg on July 3, captured, leg amputated at the lower third of the left thigh [DIED July 27, buried in Yard B on the hill between the Schwartz and Bushman farms under a walnut tree, disinterred to Richmond on June 13, 1872, in Box #202]

Pvt. Michael Corcoran, Company G, 82nd New York, shot in the leg on July 2 [DIED July 17, buried in the Schwartz cornfield, reinterred in A-56 in the New York plot, age 38]

Pvt. Joseph Coro, Company H, 19th Maine, wounded in the arm and side

Cpl. Patrick Coughlin, Company G, 20th Massachusetts, wounded

Second Lt. Charles Cowgill, Company G, 20th Massachusetts, wounded

Pvt. Chauncey J. Crandall, Company K, 125th New York, wounded July 3 [DIED July 9, buried on Michael Trostle's Farm near a sycamore tree opposite "Walnut Row," reinterred in A-90 in the New York Plot, age 18]

Pvt. Albert L. Cranston, Company E, 72nd Pennsylvania, gunshot fracture of the lower third of the left leg on July 3 [DIED July 6 at the Second Division Hospital]

Cpl. Frederick Crawley, Company A, 1st Minnesota, wounded on July 2 [DIED July 27]

Sgt. Frederick Crome, Company B, 1st Minnesota, wounded in the arm on July 2

Pvt. Samuel S. Cronkhite, Company H, 1st Minnesota, wounded in the head on July 3

Sgt. Benjamin S. Crooker, Company B, 19th Maine, wounded in the head

Pvt. Abijah Crosby, Company C, 19th Maine, wounded in the left leg on July 2 or 3, amputated at the middle third of the thigh [DIED July 8 (regimental history) or July 12 (Busey—corroborated by Ellen Orbison Harris), buried in the clearing of the Jacob Swisher Farm temporary aid station on the Taneytown Road, reinterred to G-3 in the Maine Plot; age 37, single]

Pvt. Nimrod Cross, Company I, 8th Virginia, (present in arrest for being AWOL), shot in the left groin on July 3, captured, treated at the Second Division Hospital, joined U. S. service on February 9, 1864

Col. Edward E. Cross, Second Corps, First Division, First Brigade commander, mortally wounded in the abdomen July 2 [DIED at a aid station early July 3, age 31]

Maj. Richard E. Cross, 5th New Hampshire (brother of Col. Edward E. Cross), wounded

Pvt. William Cross, Company G, 61st New York, shot in the right leg on July 2, leg amputated at the middle third [DIED July 13, buried in the Schwartz cornfield, reinterred in C-33 in the New York Plot, age 34]

Pvt. Orson E. Crummett, Company B, 19th Maine, wounded in the head

Color Sgt. Michael Cuddy, Company I, 42nd New York, wounded by a shell in the right arm and right lung on July 3 [DIED July 5 at the Second Division Hospital, buried on the Schwartz Farm in back of Rock Creek opposite the George Bushman Farm, reinterred in A-69 in the New York Plot, age 22]

First Lt. Edward R. Cunningham, Company D, 19th Maine, wounded in the chest

Pvt. John Curry, Company E, 1st Minnesota, wounded in the shoulder on July 2

Capt. Charles J. Curtis, Company D, 20th Massachusetts, wounded

Pvt. Watson Curtis, Company B, 19th Maine, wounded in the head

Pvt. William H. Curtis, Company B, 19th Maine, wounded in the side

Cpl. George Dalgleish, Company K, 82nd New York, gunshot fracture of the thigh on July 2 or 3 [DIED July 10, buried in the Schwartz cornfield at the edge of the woods near a walnut tree, reinterred in A-60 in the New York Plot (state Adjutant General Office records show him as mustering out of the regiment on May 21, 1864)]

First Sgt. ____ Damon, 19th Massachusetts, wounded in the leg on July 2, shattering the bone, transported with Capt. John "Jack" G. B. Adams to the Rock Creek facility, leg amputated

Pvt. Sylvester O. Dare, Company F, 71st Pennsylvania, wounded July 3 [DIED July 5, buried in the Schwartz cornfield on Rock Creek opposite White Run, reinterred in D-13 in the Pennsylvania Plot]

Pvt. Almaron Davis, Company F, 1st Minnesota, wounded in the shoulder on July 3, age 19

Pvt. Asa O. Davis, Company G, 4th Ohio, shot in the left side on July 2 [DIED July at the Third Division Hospital, reinterred in E-13 in the Ohio Plot, age 19]

Pvt. Joseph Davis, Company E, 8th Virginia, battlefield fracture of the right tibia on July 3, captured, right leg amputated at the Second Division Hospital [DIED July 11, buried in Yard D, Row 2 of the Schwartz cornfield by Rock Creek, disinterred to Richmond on June 13, 1872, with 110 others in ten large boxes marked "S"]

Pvt. Philip Davis, Company I, 14th Virginia, age 23, carpenter, battlefield wound fracture of the thigh on July 3, captured [DIED July 24, buried behind the Schwartz barn]

Lt. Samuel Boyer Davis, staff of Confederate general Isaac Trimble

Pvt. Leroy T. Dawson, Company C, 24th Virginia, wounded on July 3, captured, treated at the Third Division Hospital [DIED July 21, buried in Yard B, Row 2 on the hill between the Schwartz and

Bushman farms under a walnut tree, disinterred to Richmond on June13, 1872, in Box #10]

Pvt. Horace Dean, Company D, 19th Maine, wounded

Pvt. Leonard Dearborn, Company E, 19th Maine, wounded in the hand

Pvt. Artemus Decker, Company F, 1st Minnesota, wounded in the knee on July 3

Color Cpl. John W. Dehn, Company A, 1st Minnesota, wounded in the arm on July 3, arm amputated, discharged due to disability in November 1863

Pvt. George Deisroth, Company F, 147th Pennsylvania [Twelfth Corps], mortally wounded in the head on July 3 [DIED July 3, buried in the Schwartz cornfield near the creek, reinterred in A-30 in the Pennsylvania Plot]

Second Lt. David B. Demerest, 1st Minnesota, wounded in the hip on July 2 [DIED July 30]

Color Cpl. John Densmore, Company B, 1st Minnesota, severely wounded in the jaw, chest, leg, and thumb on July 2, removed from the field by Surgeon LeBlond to a Second Corps aid station, eventually removed to a hospital in Harrisburg, where he was still recuperating as of February 23, 1864

Pvt. Michael Devlin, Company A, 1st Minnesota, wounded on July 3

Pvt. Peter De Vos, Company E, 111th New York, wounded in the leg on July 2, leg amputated above the knee [DIED July 12 at the Third Division Hospital, reinterred in B-70 in the New York Plot, age 21]

Pvt. Alfred H. Dibble, Company G, 14th Connecticut, shot in right shoulder on July 3 [DIED July 5 at Third Division Hospital, reinterred B-1 in the Connecticut Plot]

Sgt. Frederick Diehr, Company H, 1st Minnesota, shot in the right lung and wounded by a shell fragment in the side on July 2, remained delirious until his death [DIED July 23, reinterred B-4 in the Minnesota Plot]

Pvt. Robert E. Dignum, Company H, 1st Virginia, age 19, coach trimmer, shot in the head on July 3, captured, treated at the Second Division Hospital, exchanged

Pvt. Lewis Dilly, Company D, 140th Pennsylvania, shot in the elbow joint, scrotum, penis, and thigh on July 2, arm amputated [DIED July 19, buried in the Schwartz cornfield near the creek, reinterred in B-44 in the Pennsylvania Plot]

Cpl. John Dippolt, Company B, 20th Massachusetts, wounded July 2 or 3 [DIED July 12 or 14, buried on the Schwartz Farm near Rock

Creek under a walnut tree, reinterred in A-25 in Massachusetts Plot, age 24]

Pvt. John H. Docken, Company H, 1st Minnesota, wounded in the arm on July 3

Pvt. Adrian C. Dodge, Company I, 19th Maine, wounded in the cheek

Pvt. Martin V. B. Dodge, Company H, 19th Maine, wounded in the arm and side

Pvt. William Doenecke, Company B, 39th New York, wounded July 2 [DIED July 15, buried on the Schwartz Farm near "Red Rock," reinterred in D-59 in the New York Plot, age 28]

Pvt. Jeremiah Donevan, Company I, 1st Minnesota, wounded in the wrist on July 2

Pvt. Thomas Donovan, Company H, 20th Massachusetts, wounded

***First Lt. John E. Dooley, Company C, 1st Virginia, shot through both thighs on July 3, captured, paroled for exchange February 20, 1865**

Sgt. William A. H. Dooley, Company A, 1st Minnesota, wounded in the wrist on July 3

Pvt. Isaac E. Dorman, Company A, 145th Pennsylvania, shot in the shoulder on July 2 [DIED July 11 or 25, buried in the Schwartz cornfield near a walnut tree, reinterred in A-44 in the Pennsylvania Plot]

Sgt. Jesse A. Dorman, Company H, 19th Maine, mortally wounded [DIED July 6]

Pvt. William G. Dorsey, Company D, 1st Delaware [listed as KILLED, but recorded as buried on the Schwartz Farm, reinterred A-3 Delaware Plot]

Pvt. John Dougherty, Company I, 145th Pennsylvania, gunshot fracture of the skull on July 2 [DIED July 8 at the First Division Hospital, buried in the Schwartz cornfield near a walnut tree]

Pvt. James H. Dowdy, Company E, 18th Virginia, shot in the head on July 3, captured [DIED July 16, buried in Row 3, Yard D in the Jacob Schwartz cornfield, disinterred June 13, 1872, with 110 others to Richmond in 10 large boxes marked "S"]

Maj. Mark Downie, 1st Minnesota, severely wounded in the chest, foot, and twice in the right arm on July 2, removed from the field by Surgeon LeBlond and sent to the Second Corps Hospitals, hospitalized for three months

Cpl. Nahum Downs, Company E, 19th Maine, wounded in the leg [DIED July 10]

Pvt. Charles S. Drake, Company A, 1st Minnesota, wounded in the arm on July 3

Pvt. Hiram Drake, Company E, 1st Minnesota, wounded in the foot on July 2

Pvt. Kellian Drondt, Company H, 1st Minnesota, wounded in the head on July 2

Capt. Cornelius J. DuBois, Company D, 27th Connecticut, wounded

Sgt. George Dunbary, Company C, 19th Maine, wounded in the elbow

Pvt. Richard Duncum, Company E, 14th Virginia, wounded and captured on July 3, treated at the First Division, Second Corps Hospital [DIED December 1, 1863, of smallpox at Point Lookout]

Cpl. Phineas L. Dunham, Company G, 1st Minnesota, battlefield fracture of the thigh on July 2, leg amputated [DIED July 15]

Pvt. Edwin L. Dunnell, Company F, 19th Maine, wounded

Pvt. John J. Dunning, Company D, 111th New York, wounded in the head July 2 or 3 [DIED July 10 or 11 at the Third Division Hospital, buried on Michael Trostle's "Walnut Row," reinterred in B-68 in the New York Plot, age 18]

Pvt. Ezekiel L. Dunton, Company K, 19th Maine, wounded in the leg

Pvt. Chester H. Durfee, Company K, 1st Minnesota, wounded in the leg on July 2 and 3, age 17

Pvt. Israel Durr, Company K, 1st Minnesota, shot in the side and lung on July 2 [DIED July 4]

Pvt. John Durst, Company D, 148th Pennsylvania, wounded July 3 [DIED October 6 in Harrisburg, Pennsylvania]

Pvt. Alden W. Dyer, Company I, 19th Maine, wounded in the shoulder

Pvt. Joseph S. Eaton, Company K, 1st Minnesota, wounded in the thigh, "a long flesh wound along the entire leg," on July 2, age 21

Pvt. Frederick B. Easley, Company E, 14th Virginia, age 25, clerk, wounded and captured on July 3 [DIED, buried by the Jacob Schwartz farm lane, near the creek, under a walnut tree]

Pvt. Moritz Ehardt, Company B, 1st Minnesota, wounded in the ankle on July 2

Cpl. John Einfeldt, Company K, 1st Minnesota, wounded in the shoulder on July 2

Capt. Martin W. B. Ellegood, Company E, 1st Delaware, shot in the stomach on the skirmish line on July 2 [DIED July 4 at the Third Division Hospital]

Pvt. August Ellenberger, Company B, 59th New York, gunshot fracture of the elbow joint on July 3 [DIED August 1, buried on the Schwartz Farm, reinterred in C-41 in the New York Plot, age 18]

Second Cpl. Lemuel O. Ellett, Company I, 1st Virginia, shot in the head on July 3 and captured, [DIED July 12, buried in Yard D, disinterred June 13, 1872, with 110 others to Richmond in 10 large boxes marked "S"]

Pvt. Samuel H. Elliott, Company G, 11th Virginia, age 19, trader, shot in the foot and/or the right knee on July 3, captured, treated at the Second Division Hospital, exchanged on September 8, 1863, from DeCamp Hospital

Cpl. Alvin H. Ellis, Company B, 19th Maine, wounded in the thigh

First Lt. Elisha W. Ellis, Company B, 19th Maine, wounded in the side

Pvt. John E. Ellsworth, Company C, 1st Minnesota, leg fractured on July 2, leg amputated [DIED July 20]

Pvt. Charles Ely, Company K, 1st Minnesota, wounded in the abdomen on July 2

Pvt. Henry Emery, Company C, 19th Maine, wounded in the foot

Sgt. William H. Emery, Company C, 19th Maine, wounded in the head

Cpl. Amos Erhard, Company A, 148th Pennsylvania, wounded July 3, "a nasty hole through the thigh just grazing the femoral artery," treated at the Rock Creek facility, transferred to the Veteran Reserve Corps

Pvt. Anthony W. Ernst, Company G, 1st Minnesota, wounded in the shoulder on July 3 [DIED August 5 at Fort Schuyler, New York, of purulent inflammation of the lungs, left side, due to the bullet which broke his clavicle and two ribs and lodged in his chest, age 24]

Cpl. Christopher Erskine, Company C, 19th Maine, mortally wounded on July 3 [DIED July 5]

Pvt. Redford M. Estes, Company H, 19th Maine, wounded in the leg

Pvt. Peter Everson, Company B, 1st Minnesota, wounded in the jaw on July 2

Sgt. Charles H. Farnsworth, Company G, 126th New York, shot July 2 or 3 [DIED July 9 at the Third Division Hospital, buried in the Schwartz cornfield opposite White Run, reinterred in D-56 in the New York Plot, age 32]

Pvt. Jerome Farnsworth, Company G, 1st Minnesota, wounded in the thigh on July 2, leg amputated [DIED July 27 at the Jarvis Hospital in Baltimore, interred in Jordan Park Cemetery]

Pvt. Daniel H. Farquhar, Company A, 1st Minnesota, compound fracture of the left tibia on July 2

Pvt. John Farquhar, Company A, 1st Minnesota, wounded in the thigh on July 3

Capt. Wilson B. Farrell, Company C, 1st Minnesota, shot in the right shoulder and left side on July 3 [DIED July 5 at the Second Division Hospital, age 31]

First Sgt. Patrick Farrington, Company G, 82nd New York, shot in the legs on July 2, legs amputated [DIED July 10, buried in the Schwartz cornfield near a walnut tree, reinterred in D-24 in the New York Plot, age 19]

Pvt. George M. Feary, Company B, 108th New York, shot in the thigh on July 3, severing the femoral artery, leg amputated, secondary hemorrhaging occurred July 13 or 14 [DIED July 25 at the Artillery Reserve Hospital, buried on the Schwartz Farm, age 22]

Pvt. Patrick Fee, Company F, 20th Massachusetts, wounded

Pvt. Benjamin Fenton, Company E, 1st Minnesota, wounded in the hand on July 3

Second Lt. George H. Finch, Company E, 145th Pennsylvania, wounded in the left thigh and right ankle on July 2 [DIED July 6, buried in the Schwartz cornfield, reinterred in A-43 in the Pennsylvania Plot]

Pvt. Elijah C. Fink, Company A, 28th Virginia, age 26, carpenter, shot in the right foot on July 3, captured, treated at the First Division Hospital, exchanged August 28, 1863, from West's Buildings Hospital; deserted September 14, 1863, from Farmville, Virginia Hospital

Pvt. Henry I. Fisher, Company E, 1st Minnesota, wounded in the left heel on July 2, returned to active duty on October 31, 1863

Pvt. Jabez B. Fisk, Company K, 86th New York [Third Corps], shot in the left lung on July 2 [DIED July 4, buried on the Schwartz Farm opposite White Run, reinterred in D-54 in theNew York plot, age 18]

Pvt. Job P. Flagg, Company B, 19th Maine, wounded in the chest [DIED December 2, in York, Pennsylvania]

Pvt. James Fletcher, Company G, 7th New Jersey [Third Corps], wounded in the buttocks on July 2 [DIED July 8, buried in the Schwartz cornfield, reinterred in B-6 in the New Jersey Plot]

First Sgt. William Flynn, Company H, 42nd New York, wounded in the spine and left lung on July 3 [DIED July 12, buried on the Schwartz Farm, age 22]

Pvt. Daniel Foley, Company H, 20th Massachusetts, wounded

Pvt. Frank M. Forbes, Company I, 145th Pennsylvania, wounded through the right lung on July 2, treated at the First Division Hospital on July 3

Cpl. Gilbert A. W. Ford, Company C, 27th Connecticut, wounded

Second Lt. Francis H. Foss, Company C, 19th Maine, wounded in the neck

Pvt. Horace H. Foster, Company G, 18th Virginia, wounded July 3, captured [DIED July 17, buried in Row 1, Yard "D" in the Schwartz cornfield on Rock Creek; disinterred on June 13, 1872, to Richmond with 110 other remains in 10 large boxes marked "S"]

Pvt. Edward B. Fowler, Company F, 27th Connecticut, wounded

Pvt. Jacob F. Freeze, Company I, 1st Minnesota, wounded in the hand and foot on July 2 [DIED August 2]

Lt. Col. Charles Godfrey Freudenberg, 52nd New York, wounded on July 2

Pvt. Frederick Frey, Company F, 108th New York, end of his nose shot off on July 3

Col. Birkett D. Fry, 13th Alabama, shot through the thigh on July 3, captured, leg amputated, moved to Fort McHenry as a prisoner of war, transferred from prison to prison before finally being returned South by a special prisoner exchange in March of 1864.

***Second Lt. Charles A. Fuller, 61st New York, shot in the shoulder and left leg on July 2, transported to the First Division Hospital on Granite Schoolhouse Road, evacuated south to the Jacob Weikert house when the hospital was shelled, removed at 10:00 p.m., July 3 to the new Rock Creek facility, leg amputated

Cpl. Francis P. Furber, Company H, 19th Maine, wounded in the mouth

Pvt. Moses H. Gale, Company E, 20th Massacusetts, wounded

Pvt. Thomas Galvin, Company H, 1st Minnesota, wounded in the arm on July 3

Pvt. Thomas Gannon, Company D, 6th New York Cavalry (Second Corps Headquarters escort), wounded in the leg on July 2 or 3 [DIED, buried in the Jacob Swisher field near the woods, reinterred in A-104 in the New York Plot, age 26]

Pvt. Alfred G. Gardner, Battery B, 1st Rhode Island Light, Second Corps Artillery Brigade, mortally wounded on July 3 when a shell almost completely tore off one arm [DIED July 3, buried at the

Michael Fiscel Farm (just south of the Jacob Schwartz Farm), just east of the house]

Pvt. Tom Gardner, Company H, 14th Connecticut, shot in the head on July 3, bullet deeply grazed his skull

Sgt. Charles P. Garland, Company H, 19th Maine, wounded in the leg

Second Lt. Franklin G. Garland, Company A, 61st New York, shot in the lung on July 2 [DIED July 4, buried on the J. Bair Farm at the foot of a tree, reinterred in C-35 in the New York Plot, age 21]

Third Sgt. Calvin Garner, Company H, 14th Virginia, age 22, overseer, shot in the right leg on July 3, captured, treated at the First Division Hospital, exchanged March 6, 1864

Pvt. Malachi Garrity, Company E, 20th Massachusetts, wounded

Pvt. John Gatze, Company G, 1st Minnesota, wounded in the right thigh on July 2

First Sgt. Leonidas J. Gee, Company B, 56th Virginia, gunshot fracture of arm and middle third of the thigh, captured, leg amputated at the Third Division Hospital [DIED there on July 17, 1863, buried in Yard D, Row 2 of the Schwartz cornfield by Rock Creek; disinterred June 13, 1872, to Richmond with 110 others in 10 large boxes labeled "S"]

Pvt. Charles W. Geer, Company D, 1st Minnesota, wounded in the shoulder on July 2

Pvt. Lewis B. Geer, Company D, 1st Minnesota, wounded in the chest and hand on July 2

Pvt. William F. Gerald, Company H, 19th Maine, wounded in the thigh

***Brig. Gen. John Gibbon, commander Second Division, Second Corps, gunshot wound in the shoulder, treated at the Rock Creek facility, evacuated by ambulance to Westminster on July 4, then by train to Baltimore

***__Col. William Gibson, 48th Georgia, severely wounded at the Codori Farm on July 2, entire regiment surrendered in order to obtain Union medical treatment for the colonel, transported by ambulance to the Second Division Hospital, personally treated there by Dr. Justin Dwinelle, attempted to escape from the hospital, recaptured__

Pvt. George W. Gilbert, Company G, 148th Pennsylvania, wounded July 3

Cpl. Manassas Gilbert, Company A, 148 Pennsylvania, shot in the shoulder on July 2, treated at the Rock Creek facility

Sgt. Maj. James C. Gill, 18th Virginia, age 17, student, shot in the side at the stone wall on July 3, captured [DIED at the Second

Division Hospital, buried there in Row 2, Yard D in the Schwartz cornfield, disinterred June 13, 1872, with 110 others to Richmond in 10 large boxes marked "S"]

Pvt. Frederick Gillhousen, Company I, 148th Pennsylvania, wounded July 2 [DIED July 17]

Pvt. James Gilman, Company C, 1st Minnesota, wounded on July 3

Pvt. Lorenzo D. Gilman, Company C, 19th Maine, wounded in the knee

Pvt. Frederick Giser, Company A, 1st Minnesota, wounded on July 2

Pvt. Thomas Glacken, Company G, 20th Massachusetts, wounded

Pvt. James S. Glassell, Company I, 11th Virginia, age 34, clerk, battlefield fracture of the cranium on July 3, captured, [DIED July 5, buried there at an unknown location]

Pvt. Frederick Glave, Company A, 1st Minnesota, wounded in the knee on July 2, leg amputated [DIED July 10]

Pvt. Michael Gleason, Company A, 20th Massachusetts, wounded

First Sgt. Vincent C. Goad, Company B, 14th Virginia, shot in the thigh on July 3, captured, treated at the First Division Hospital, exchanged September 23, 1863, from Chester Hospital

Pvt. Charles E. Goddard, Company K, 1st Minnesota, wounded in the shoulder and leg on July 2, age 17, wounds never completely healed, died at age 23

Pvt. Merrill Godfrey, Company H, 111th New York, wounded in the face on July 2 [DIED July 3 at the Third Division Hospital, age 21]

First Sgt. Russel B. Godfrey, Company B, 7th Michigan, wounded July 3 [DIED July 5, buried on the Schwartz Farm opposite White Run, reinterred in D-18 in the Michigan Plot, age 23]

First Sgt. David H. Goff, Company A, 126th New York, shot in the chest and lungs on July 2 [DIED July 3 at the Third Division Hospital, age 29]

Pvt. Michael Goff, Company G, 11th New Jersey [Third Corps], shot in the left shoulder July 2 or 3 [DIED July 9, buried in the Schwartz cornfield, reinterred in B-7 in the New Jersey Plot]

Sgt. Thomas Gomm, Company C, 108th New York, shot in the knee joint on July 3 [DIED July 28 at the Third Division Hospital, age 21]

Pvt. Jona Goodrich, Company G, 1st Minnesota, wounded in the leg on July 2

Pvt. Drew Goodridge, Company H, 19th Maine, wounded in the leg

Sgt. Matthew Goodson, 52nd North Carolina, shot through both lungs (the bullet exiting through the left side of the chest cavity) on July 3, captured [DIED July 12 at the Second Corps Hospital, buried there in Yard D, Row 2 in the Schwartz cornfield; reinterred

January 29, 1866, in Lot #169, Section E, of the Evergreen Cemetery by Gettysburg resident Hiram Warren; in August, 1867, the Evergreen Cemetery Board ordered all Confederate dead removed from the cemetery to a "more secluded place"; in the process, all records of Goodson's remains were lost; present burial site unknown]

Capt. Goodwin, 5th New Hampshire

Pvt. August A. Goppinger, Company D, 1st Minnesota, wounded in the foot and hand on July 2

Cpl. Patrick Gorman, Company E, 20th Massachusetts, wounded

First Sgt. James T. Goulding, Company C, 20th Massachusetts, wounded

Pvt. Charles H. Gove, Company B, 1st Minnesota, shot in the chest and spine on July 2 [DIED July 30 at the Second Division, Second Corps Hospital, reinterred in A-6 of the Minnesota Plot, age 22]

Pvt. Thomas Graham, Company H, 1st Minnesota, wounded on July 3

Pvt. George Grandy, Company D, 1st Minnesota, wounded in the chest on July 2 [DIED July 4]

Sgt. George L. Grant, Company K, 19th Maine, wounded July 3 [DIED November 5]

?Capt. G. A. Graues, 22nd North Carolina, wounded and captured

Pvt. John Green, Company H, 148th Pennsylvania, wounded July 2 [DIED August 2, buried in the National Cemetery, Loudon Park, Baltimore, Maryland]

Pvt. John Greene, Battery B, 1st Rhode Island Light Artillery, shot in the thigh on July 3, leg amputated [DIED July 16, buried in the Schwartz cornfield on Rock Creek, reinterred in A-5 in the Rhode Island Plot]

Pvt. Alvin L. Greenlee, Company F, 140th Pennsylvania, battlefield fracture of the thigh on July 2, transferred to Letterman General Hospital, leg amputated there [DIED August 3]

Quartermaster Sgt. Aaron Greenwald, Company C, 1st Minnesota, wounded on July 2 [DIED July 7]

Pvt. John Griffin, Company G, 27th Connecticut, wounded

Capt. George G. Griswold, Company I, 145th Pennsylvania Volunteers, slightly wounded in the hand on July 2, transferred to Philadelphia [DIED after contracting erysipelas in the wound]

Pvt. George Groft, Company E, 148th Pennsylvania, wounded July 2

Pvt. Alfred Grover, Company F, 19th Maine, wounded in the thigh

Pvt. Joseph Groves, Company E, 72nd Pennsylvania, wounded July 2 or 3 [DIED July 4, buried on the William Patterson Farm near the Second Corps Division Hospital]

Pvt. Henry Grum, Company A, 28th Pennsylvania [Twelfth Corps], mortally wounded July 3 [DIED July 3, buried in the Schwartz cornfield

Pvt. Matthias Guiser, Company A, 148th Pennsylvania, wounded July 2

Pvt. John T. Hagerman, Company K, 18th Virginia, age 19, clerk, gunshot fracture of left knee, captured, left thigh amputated at the middle third at the Second Division Hospital, exchanged November 17, 1863, from West's Buildings Hospital

Pvt. Roswell Haire, Company D, 19th Maine, shot in the right portion of the chest on July 3 [DIED July 4 at the Second Division Hospital; age 39, married]

Pvt. Edward P. Hale, Company I, 1st Minnesota, wounded in the hip and leg on July 2, leg amputated [DIED September 12]

Cpl. George P. Hall, Company B, 148th Pennsylvania, wounded July 3

Pvt. Charles R. Hamilton, Company D, 19th Maine, wounded in the arm and face

Pvt. James R. Hamilton, Company A, 20th Massachusetts, wounded

?Second Lt. William H. Hamilton, Company I, 13th Vermont [First Corps], wounded July 3 [DIED July 6, buried on Michael Trostle's "Walnut Row" west of the creek, reinterred in B-1 in the Vermont Plot]

Pvt. Charles L. Hamlen, Company H, 19th Maine, wounded in the leg

First Lt. James H. Hamlin, Company I, 145th Pennsylvania, wounded in the heel on July 2

Pvt. Charles Hamman, Company B, 1st Minnesota, wounded in the head and hand on July 2

Lt. Col. John Sweeney Hammell, 66th New York, wounded July 2

Pvt. Benjamin F. Hanaford, Company F, 20th Massachusetts, wounded

***Maj. Gen. Winfield Scott Hancock, Second Corps commander, severe wound in the upper thigh, treated at the Rock Creek facility, evacuated by ambulance to Westminster on July 4, then by train to Philadelphia

Pvt. Willard R. Hardy, Company B, 19th Maine, wounded in both hands

Pvt. William S. Harker, Company H, 12th New Jersey, shot in the head on July 2 [DIED July 2 in the Third Division Hospital, reinterred in

B-17 in the New Jersey Plot (but also recorded as buried in Woodstown, New Jersey)]

Pvt. Lewis Hanson, Company K, 1st Minnesota, wounded in the left calf on July 2

Pvt. James W. Harl, Company A, 4th Ohio, wounded July 2 [DIED July 9 at the Third Division Hospital, buried on Michael Trostle's "Walnut Row," reinterred in B-18 in the Ohio Plot, age 20]

***Second Lt. William Harmon, 1st Minnesota, wounded on July 3

***Capt. John H. Harpster, Company G, 148th Pennsylvania, wounded July 3

Pvt. Charles E. Harriman, Company E, 19th Maine, mortally wounded in both legs on July 3, left leg amputated [DIED July 10, reinterred to D-6 in the Maine Plot, age 18, single]

Pvt. Leonard Harrington, Company A, 20th Massachusetts, wounded

Cpl. Delos W. Harris, Company C, 7th Michigan, wounded in the left side by a shell which exposed the entire left lung on July 3 [DIED July 8 at the Second Division Hospital, buried in the Schwartz cornfield under a walnut tree, reinterred in D-12 in the Michigan Plot, age 21]

Lt. Col. Edward A. Harris, 1st Delaware, wounded on July 2, placed under arrest by General Hancock for pulling back a skirmish line without orders

Pvt. James L. Harris, Company F, 56th Virginia, shot in the left leg on July 3, captured, leg amputated [DIED July 16, buried in Row 3, Yard D in the Jacob Schwartz cornfield by Rock Creek; disinterred on June 13, 1872, to Richmond with 110 others in ten large boxes marked "S"]

Pvt. Henry H. Hartshorn, Company D, 19th Maine, wounded July 3

Pvt. Michael Harty, Company A, 20th Massachusetts, wounded

?Third Lt. Edward B. Harvey, Company H. 18th Virginia, age 35, laborer, shot in the right thigh July 3, captured [DIED August 6 at Camp Letterman Hospital of prostration fever and a secondary hemorrhage, buried in Section 3, Grave #13 of the Hospital Cemetery, disinterred on June 13, 1872, to Richmond in Box #45]

***Lt. Frank Haskell, staff aide to Union general John Gibbon, severe bullet bruise to the thigh

Pvt. Joseph E. Haskell, Company C, 19th Maine, wounded in the leg

First Lt. Daniel G. Hatcher, Company I, 24th Virginia, gunshot flesh wound in the upper third of the left thigh on July 3, captured,

treated at the Second Division Hospital, exchanged March 22, 1865

Sgt. Charles F. Hausdorf, Company A, 1st Minnesota, wounded in the leg on July 2

Pvt. Christ C. Havener, Company F, 148th Pennsylvania, wounded July 2

Pvt. James Hawkins, Company I, 12th New Hampshire [Third Corps], shot in the abdomen July 2 [DIED July 3, buried on the Schwartz Farm opposite White Run, reinterred in A-14 in the New Hampshire Plot, age 21]

Pvt. Newton A. E. Hawley, Company I, 28th Virginia, age 21, farmer, shot in the neck and flesh wounds in right side and neck on July 3, captured, treated at the Second Division Hospital, exchanged February 20 or 21, 1865

Pvt. Alonzo C. Hayden, Company D, 1st Minnesota, wounded on July 2 [DIED July 3]

Cpl. Anson R. Hayden, Company I, 1st Minnesota, wounded in the hand on July 2

Pvt. Patrick Hayes, Company D, 81st Pennsylvania, shot July 2 [DIED July 4 or 5, buried in the Schwartz cornfield east of a walnut tree, reinterred in B-29 in the Pennsylvania Plot]

Pvt. Faxon Hayford, Company C, 1st Minnesota, wounded in the right leg on July 3

Pvt. James T. Heal, Company K, 19th Maine, shot in the head on July 3 [DIED July 8 or 9, buried in Yard D, in the Schwartz cornfield above Rock Creek, reinterred to B-3 in the Maine Plot, age 31, single]

Cpl. Payson T. Heard, Company A, 19th Maine, wounded in the arm [DIED August 5 at Summit House Hospital, Philadelphia]

Col. Francis Edward Heath, 19th Maine, wounded in the shoulder July 3

First Lt. Christofer Heffelfinger, 1st Minnesota, wounded in the chest on July 2, survived wound to found a shoe company back home

Pvt. Ignatz Heimbucher, Company B, 39th New York, mortally wounded in the chest on July 3 [DIED July 3, buried on Michael Trostle's "Walnut Row" [at the Sixth Corps Hospital], reinterred in A-43 in the New York Plot, age 35]

Pvt. Frederick Heinzen, Company A, 39th New York, wounded by a shell in the chest and /or abdomen on July 3 [DIED July 4 at the Third Division Hospital, reinterred in F-13 in the New York plot, age 33]

Pvt. Charles H. Henderson, Company E, 27th Connecticut, wounded

Pvt. Martin J. Henry, Company B, 1st Minnesota, wounded in the back on July 2

Pvt. N. B. Herring, Company I, 7th Virginia, wounded in the left leg on July 3, captured, leg amputated, [DIED July 27, buried in Grave #6 behind the Schwartz barn]

Pvt. Greenhalt Hess, Company H, 1st Minnesota, wounded in the thigh on July 2

Second Lt. Lansing E. Hibbard, Company A, 20th Massachusetts, wounded

Sgt. Edward H. Hicks, Company G, 19th Maine, wounded in the arm and groin

Pvt. Jonas R. Hill, Company E, 1st Minnesota, wounded in both legs on July 2

Pvt. Isaac Hills, Company B, 19th Maine, wounded in the thigh

***Capt. John C. Hilton, 145th Pennsylvania, thigh shattered during the Confederate attack on July 3, leg amputated at the upper thigh, transferred to Camp Letterman General Hospital, returned to active service with an artificial limb

***Sgt. Benjamin Hirst, Company D, 14th Connecticut, wounded three times on July 3, one being a severely bruised right shoulder by a piece of flying stone

Capt. Thomas Bullock Hizar, 1st Delaware, wounded July 2

Pvt. George E. Hodgdon, Company C, 19th Maine, wounded July 2 [DIED August 24]

Pvt. Lorenzo W. Hoffses, Company D, 19th Maine, wounded in the legs

Cpl. Bernard Hogan, Company D, 17th Maine [Third Corps], shot in the hip on July 2 [DIED July 23, buried beside the Schwartz Farm lane, near the creek, under a walnut tree, reinterred in C-8 in the Maine Plot]

Pvt. John Hogan, Company D, 27th Connecticut, wounded

Pvt. William W. Holden, Company E, 1st Minnesota, wounded in the leg on July 2

Second Sgt. Robert C. Holland, Company I, 28th Virginia, shot in the right elbow joint on July 3, captured, treated at the First Division Hospital, exchanged October 28, 1863, from DeCamp Hospital

Cpl. George E. Holmes, Company I, 19th Maine, wounded in the head

Pvt. George J. Hopkins, Company G, 1st Minnesota, severely wounded in the right wrist and left hip on July 2, moved to a general hospital where he remained until December 31, 1863, transferred to the 134th Company, 2nd Battalion, Veteran Reserve Corps

Pvt. Henry Horner, Company E, 148th Pennsylvania, wounded July 2, transferred to the Veteran Reserve Corps

Capt. Charles K. Horsefall, Company E, 12th New Jersey, shot in the head on July 2 [DIED July 3 at the Third Division Hospital]

Pvt. Archibald Howe, Company D, 1st Minnesota, wounded in the hip on July 2

Pvt. Hiram V. Howard, Company D, 20th Massachusetts, gunshot fracture of leg on July 2 or 3 [DIED July 8 or 9, buried on the Schwartz Farm near Rock Creek, opposite the George Bushman Farm, age 23]

Pvt. William D. Howell, Company I, 1st Minnesota, wounded in the left hand on July 2

Sgt. John L. Hoyt, Company D, 19th Massachusetts, wounded July 3 [DIED July 6, buried on the Schwartz Farm by Rock Creek under a walnut tree, age 24]

First Cpl. Alexander Hubbard, Company C, 28th Virginia, age 31, farmer, wounded and captured on July 3, treated at the First Division Hospital [DIED either July 9 or July 19]

Pvt. William Hubbard, Company B, 19th Maine, wounded in the head

Pvt. Charles L. Hubbs, Company F, 1st Minnesota, wounded in the wrist on July 3

Pvt. Charles E. Hubles, Company F, 1st Minnesota, wounded on July 3

Cpl. Arthur Hughes, Company F, 20th Massachusetts, wounded

Cpl. Adam Huhn, Company A, 1st Delaware, wounded [DIED July 8, buried on M. Trostle's "Walnut Row," reinterred B-5 in the Delaware Plot]

Pvt. Franz Huhn, Company C, 20th Massachusetts, wounded

Sgt. Patrich Huite, Company C, 20th Massachusetts, wounded

Lt. Albert Hunter, Company H, 19th Maine, wounded in the throat on July 2

Pvt. George A. Hussey, Company G, 19th Maine, wounded in the hip

Sgt. George R. Huston, Company B, 148th Pennsylvania, wounded July 2, transferred to the Veteran Reserve Corps

Pvt. Daniel Hutchins, Company I, 1st Minnesota, wounded on July 2

Capt. George H. Ince, Company A, 66th New York, wounded in the chest on July 2 [DIED July 6, buried on Michael Trostle's "Walnut Row," age 37]

Pvt. O. L. Ivey, Company G, 11th Virginia, shot in the left hip on July 3, captured, treated at Second Division Hospital, exchanged on August 17, 1863, from Chester Hospital

Pvt. William H. Jackman, Company G, 19th Maine, wounded in the side

Pvt. Benjamin Jackson, Company I, 1st Minnesota, wounded in the leg on July 2

Pvt. Benjamin F. Jackson, Company B, 11th New Jersey [Third Corps], shot in the hip on July 2 [DIED July 7, buried in the Schwartz cornfield, reinterred in B-4 in the New Jersey Plot]

Pvt. Edwin S. Jacobs, Company I, 19th Maine, wounded in the head

Pvt. Romulus E. Jacobs, Company F, 1st Minnesota, wounded in the back and shoulder on July 3

Pvt. Josephus James, Company H, 19th Maine, wounded in the right leg, leg amputated

Pvt. Ernest Jefferson, Company E, 1st Minnesota, wounded in the left leg and foot on July 2, moved to Jarvis Hospital in Baltimore where his leg was amputated just below the hip, discharged due to disability on December 9, 1863

Pvt. Alvah Jellison, Company K, 19th Maine, wounded in the thigh

Second Sgt. James Jennings, Company I, 18th Virginia, age 28, farmer, wounded on July 3, captured [DIED July 16, buried in cemetery behind the barn]

Sgt. William S. Jinkins, 7th North Carolina, age 34, shot through the body on July 3, captured, treated at the aid station at the Peter Frey Farm [DIED July 4, buried in the Frey orchard, just south of the stone house; presumed disinterred to the South in 1872, final resting place unknown]

Cpl. Arthur Johnson, Company E, 20th Massachusetts, wounded

Pvt. David Johnson, Company B, 1st Minnesota, wounded in the knee on July 2

Pvt. Joseph Johnson, Company F, 82nd New York, wounded July 2 [DIED July 9, buried in the Schwartz cornfield near a walnut tree, age 24]

Pvt. James F. Joloph, Company G, 66th New York, gunshot fracture of the right femur at the hip on July 2 [DIED July 17, buried in the Schwartz cornfield, reinterred in A-55 in the New York Plot, age 21]

Pvt. Amos Jones, Company G, 19th Maine, wounded in the arm

Capt. Andrew J. Jones, Company I, 11th Virginia, age 30, farmer, gunshot flesh wound of the right foot during the July 3 advance, captured, wound was dressed with a simple dressing at the First Division Hospital, exchanged March 22, 1865

Pvt. Anthony Jones, Company G, 1st Minnesota, wounded in the head on July 3

Pvt. Benjamin Jones, Company K, 20th Massachusetts, wounded

Pvt. Charles W. Jones, Company C, 19th Maine, wounded in the head

Pvt. Edward P. Jones, Company H, 148th Pennsylvania, wounded July 3

Cpl. George W. Jones, Company B, 17th Maine [Third Corps], shot in the left thigh on July 2 [DIED July 23, buried beside the Schwartz Farm lane, near the creek, under a walnut tree, reinterred to C-3 in the Maine plot]

Pvt. John O. Jones, Company I, 11th Virginia, gunshot flesh wound of left knee and right femur on July 3, captured, treated with a simple dressing at the First Division Hospital, [DIED July 15, buried in Yard D in the Schwartz cornfield, disinterred to Richmond on June 13, 1872, with 110 others in ten large boxes marked "S"]

Pvt. Nathan E. K. Jones, Company I, 9th Virginia, farmer, age 18, farmer, shot in the hip on July 3, captured, treated at the First Division Hospital, exchanged September 8, 1863 from DeCamp Hospital

Pvt. John F. Julian, Company D, 14th Connecticut, battlefield compound fracture of the head [DIED July 6 or 8]

Pvt. John Jungunst, Company C, 39th New York, wounded July 2 [DIED July 10, buried in the Michael Trostle field near "Red Rock," age 30]

Pvt. John D. Kearney, Company G, 106th Pennsylvania, both legs crushed by a solid shot on July 2, both legs amputated [DIED July 5 at the Second Division Hospital]

Pvt. Calvin B. Keen, Company F, 19th Maine, wounded

Pvt. John F. Keene, Company E, 19th Maine, wounded in the arm

Cpl. Timothy Keiley, Company K, 1st Minnesota, wounded in the thigh and calf on July 2

Pvt. Jacob Keirsh, Battery F, Pennsylvania Independent Light Artillery [Artillery Reserve], wounded [DIED July 4, buried on the William Patterson Farm adjacent to the Second Corps Division Hospital, reinterred in D-28 in the Pennsylvania Plot]

Pvt. Edward Kelley, Company K, 28th Virginia, age 18, shot in the left foot on July 3, captured, treated at the Second Division Hospital, exchanged August 17, 1863, from Chester Hospital

Second Lt. John Kelliher, Company F, 20th Massachusetts, wounded

Pvt. George F. Kelly, Company D, 8th Virginia, gunshot flesh wound of the right thigh on July 3, captured, treated at the First Division

Hospital, exchanged on September 8, 1863, from Chester Hospital

Sgt. Hugh Kelly, Company G, 69th Pennsylvania, wounded July 3 [DIED July 20]

Pvt. James Kelly, 8th Ohio, leg badly shattered [DIED July 7, buried at the Second Corps Hospital]

Pvt. Lawrence H. Kelly, Company H, 1st Massachusetts [Third Corps], mortally wounded on July 2 [DIED July 2, buried on the Schwartz Farm on Rock Creek opposite White Run, age 20]

Pvt. Peter Kennan, Company K, 20th Massachusetts, wounded

Pvt. Andrew Kennison, Company A, 19th Maine, wounded in the leg on July 2, leg amputated

Pvt. Adolph Kernberger, Company C, 20th Massachusetts, wounded

Pvt. John W. Kessler, Company D, 70th New York [Third Corps], wounded July 2 [DIED July 8, buried near the Schwartz House, reinterred in D-42 in the New York Plot, age 24]

Pvt. Edward Kestin, Company D, 20th Massachusetts, wounded

Pvt. Joseph Khyle, Company G, 53rd Pennsylvania, wounded July 2 [DIED July 5, buried in the Schwartz cornfield, reinterred in B-40 in the Pennsylvania Plot]

Pvt. Thomas M. Kilcullen, Company D, 27th Connecticut, wounded

Pvt. George A. Kimball, Company K, 19th Maine, wounded in the foot

?Capt. J. A. Kincain, 52nd North Carolina, wounded and captured

Pvt. George C. King, Company C, 126th New York, wounded July 3 [DIED July 5, buried on Michael Trostle's "Walnut Row," (other sources report him as having died at the Seminary Hospital on July 5), age 20]

Pvt. Levi King, Company F, 1st Minnesota, wounded in the jaw on July 2

Pvt. Thomas A. King, Company F, 20th Massachusetts, wounded

Pvt. William H. Kinyon, Company K, 1st Minnesota, wounded in the knee on July 2

First Sgt. John C. Kipka, Company A, 8th Ohio, shot in the abdomen on July 3 [DIED July 4 at the Third Division Hospital, buried in Evergreen Cemetery, reinterred in F-2 in the Ohio Plot, age 29]

First Sgt. Oliver M. Knight, Company I, 1st Minnesota, wounded in the arm by artillery fire on July 2

Cpl. Jacob W. Kouts, Company D, 1st Minnesota, wounded in the arm and elbow on July 2

Pvt. William Kreiss, Company I, 52nd New York, shot in the chest on July 2 [DIED July 15, buried in the Schwartz cornfield, reinterred in D-28 in the New York Plot, age 40]

Pvt. David Kreps, Company C, 148th Pennsylvania, wounded July 2

Sgt. Andrew J. Kreuger, Company C, 1st Minnesota, wounded in the left thigh on July 3

Pvt. John Kunkle, Company E, 148th Pennsylvania, wounded July 2 [DIED July 2]

Cpl. Daniel G. Lamb, Company I, 19th Maine, wounded

Pvt. Levi Lamson, Company A, 20th Massachusetts, wounded

Sgt. Patrick Lanergan, Company I, 20th Massachusetts, wounded

Capt. James E. Larkin, Company A, 5th New Hampshire, wounded

Sgt. John Larkin, Company K, 82nd New York, shot in the chest on July 3 [DIED July 31, buried on the Schwartz Farm, reinterred in C-42 in the New York Plot, age 20]

Pvt. Mose Larrabee, Jr., Company B, 19th Maine, wounded in the thigh

Pvt. John W. Lattimer, Company G, 9th Virginia, age 25, clerk, married, battlefield wound fracture of the left leg on July 3, captured, leg amputated at the First Division Hospital [DIED September 18, 1863, at Camp Letterman Hospital of gangrene, buried there in Section 8, Grave #9]

Pvt. Irving Lawrence, Company D, 1st Minnesota, shot in the head on July 2 [DIED July 5 at the Second Division Hospital, reinterred in D-7 in the Minnesota Plot, age 21]

Cpl. Herman Lawson, Company I, 1st Minnesota, wounded in the thumb and hip on July 2 and 3

Pvt. George Lawton, Company H, 16th Massachusetts [Third Corps], wounded July 2 [DIED July 2, buried on the Schwartz Farm by Rock Creek, opposite White Run, reinterred in D-34 in the Massachusetts Plot, age 20]

Pvt. Peter T. Leach, Company K, 8th Virginia, compound gunshot fracture of the right arm and wounded in the shoulder on July 3, captured, treated at the Second Division Hospital, present at Point Lookout as of October 4, 1863, no further record

Pvt. Benjamin O. Lear, Company D, 19th Maine, wounded in the arm on July 2

Pvt. Samuel Leavitt, Company A, 19th Maine, wounded in the shoulder on July 3

Pvt. Richard H. Lee, Company I, 57th Virginia, gunshot fracture of the knee on July 3, captured [DIED July 15, buried in Yard D,

Row 3 in the Schwartz cornfield; disinterred June 13, 1872, to Richmond with 110 others in 10 large boxes marked "S"]

Pvt. William Lee, Company D, 27th Connecticut, wounded

Pvt. Hampton W. Leighton, Company G, 19th Maine, wounded in the arm

Sgt. George W. Leitzell, Company A, 148th Pennsylvania, wounded July 2, transferred to the Veteran Reserve Corps

Pvt. James Lenfest, Company D, 19th Maine, wounded in the leg on July 3

Pvt. Chester A. Leonard, Company K, 20th Massachusetts, wounded

Cpl. David Leonard, Company F, 20th Massachusetts, wounded

Pvt. Maurice F. Leonard, Company C, 1st Minnesota, wounded on July 3, treated for wound and scurvy

Pvt. William Leonard, Company H, 19th Maine, wounded in the leg

Pvt. John B. Leuthe, Company D, 41st New York [Eleventh Corps], shot July 2 [DIED July 9 at the Third Division Hospital, age 38]

First Lt. Horatio F. Lewis, Company D, 145th Pennsylvania, shot in the leg on July 2, leg amputated [DIED July 6]

Junior Second Lt. John T. Lewis, Company E, 14th Virginia, age 20, farmer, shot in the finger and hips on July 3, captured, treated at the First Division Hospital, released June 12, 1865, from Fort Delaware

Pvt. Jonathan Lewis, Company C, 19th Maine, wounded in the elbow

First Sgt. Richard B. Lewis, Company E, 14th Virginia, shot in the hips on July 3, captured, treated at the First Division Hospital, exchanged August 1, 1863

Pvt. Charles H. Libby, Company H, 19th Maine, wounded in the leg

Pvt. Samuel Lilly, Company G, 1st Minnesota, wounded in the back by a bullet which was slowed first by hitting his canteen on July 2

Cpl. Frederick Limbert, Company A, 148th Pennsylvania, wounded July 2

Capt. Willard Lincoln, Company H, 19th Maine, wounded in the head

Pvt. Washington Lininger, Company B, 145th Pennsylvania, gunshot fracture of the leg on July 2 [DIED July 10 or 18at the Second Corps Hospital, buried in the Schwartz cornfield, reinterred in A-41 in the Pennsylvania Plot]

Pvt. Thomas Little, Company I, 19th Maine, wounded in the leg on July 2

Pvt. David F. Lockhart, Company E, 148th Pennsylvania, wounded July 2

Pvt. Thomas R. Lockhart, Company E, 148th Pennsylvania, wounded July 2, transferred to the Veteran Reserve Corps

Pvt. Harrison Long, Company I, 148th Pennsylvania, wounded July 2 [DIED August 17, buried in A-56 in the Pennsylvania Plot]

Pvt. Marcus J. Long, Company D, 20th Massachusetts, wounded

Pvt. Stephen Longfellow, Company H, 20th Massachusetts, wounded

Pvt. Jack Looman, Company E, 82nd New York, wounded July 2 or 3 [DIED, buried on the Schwartz Farm on Rock Creek opposite the George Bushman Farm, *not listed in the state Adjutant General Office records*]

First Sgt. David Lord, Company B, 1st Minnesota, wounded in the shoulder on July 2

Pvt. William H. Losee, Company E, 1st Minnesota, wounded in the chest on July 2

Pvt. James Henry Love, Company G, 111th New York, shot in the thigh on July 2 or 3 [DIED August 3, buried on the Schwartz Farm, age 21]

Cpl. William B. Low, Company I, 20th Massachusetts, wounded

Pvt. Charles M. Lowe, Company K, 19th Maine, shot in the groin, head and arm [DIED July 12, buried in Yard D, in the Schwartz cornfield near Rock Creek, age 20, single]

Pvt. John D. Lucas, Company F, 148th Pennsylvania, wounded July 2

Lt. Col. Isaac M. Lusk, 111th New York, wounded July 3

Pvt. James H. Lynn, Company G, 140th Pennsylvania, wounded July 2 [DIED July 6 or 13, buried in the Schwartz cornfield east of a walnut tree, reinterred in B-34 in the Pennsylvania Plot]

Pvt. Harrison Lyons, Company A, 1st Minnesota, younger brother of Steven Lyons, wounded in the leg on July 3

Cpl. Steven Lyons, Company A, 1st Minnesota, wounded in the leg on July 2

Pvt. Daniel McAdams, Company I, 20th Massachusetts, wounded

Pvt. Charles McCarty, Company K, 72nd Pennsylvania, shot in the shoulder on July 3, arm amputated [DIED July 12, buried in the Schwartz cornfield east of a walnut tree, reinterred in B-30 in the Pennsylvania Plot]

Cpl. Collins McCarty, Jr., Company E, 19th Maine, wounded in the arm, arm amputated

Pvt. John McCauslan, Company D, 72nd Pennsylvania, right arm wounded by a shell on July 3, arm amputated at the shoulder

[DIED July 27 at the Second Division Hospital, reinterred in A-55 in the Pennsylvania Plot]

Pvt. John McCillip, Company C, 8th Ohio, shot in the hip on July 2 [DIED July 10 at the Third Division Hospital, buried on Michael Trostle's "Walnut Row," reinterred in B-20 in the Ohio Plot, age 31]

Cpl. Charles McConnell, Company K, 11th Pennsylvania [First Corps], wounded July 3 [DIED July 4, buried on the William Patterson Farm adjacent to the Second Corps Division Hospital, reinterred in D-25 in the Pennsylvania Plot]

Pvt. John McCormick, Company H, 38th Virginia, battlefield wound fracture of the hip on July 3, captured [DIED July 23, buried in Yard B, Row 2 on the hill between the Schwartz and Bushman farms; disinterred on June 13, 1872, to Richmond in Box #211]

Pvt. John T. McCormick, Company D, 10th New York, shot in the abdomen July 3 [DIED July 4 at the Third Division Hospital, buried on Michael Trostle's "Walnut Row," reinterred in C-61 in the New York plot, age 20]

Cpl. Thomas McCullough, Company I, 148th Pennsylvania, wounded July 2 [DIED August 17, buried in A-59 in the Pennsylvania Plot]

First Lt. John H. McDonald, Company E, 82nd New York, mortally wounded on July 3 [DIED July 3, buried on Michael Trostle's "Walnut Row," age 33]

Cpl. Patrick McDonnel, Company H, 82nd New York, shot in the stomach on July 2 [DIED July 19, buried in the Schwartz cornfield, reinterred in D-27 in the New York Plot, age 21]

Col. Clinton Dougald MacDougall, 111th New York, wounded July 3, treated at the Second Corps Hospitals

Pvt. Thomas McElwee, Company E, 148th Pennsylvania, wounded July 2

Pvt. Edward McGinty, Company E, 68th Pennsylvania [Third Corps], shot in the left knee on July 2, leg amputated at the thigh [DIED July 23, buried near the Schwartz lane under a walnut tree]

Pvt. Edward McGrath, Company F, 20th Massachusetts, wounded

Cpl. Bernard McGuire, Company B, 8th Ohio, wounded July 3 [DIED July 10 at the Third Division Hospital, buried on Michael Trostle's "Walnut Row," reinterred in B-19 in the Ohio Plot, age 25]

Cpl. Philip McGuire, Company E, 20th Massachusetts, wounded

Sgt. John McIvors, Company B, 5th New Jersey [Third Corps], shot in the back of the shoulder on July 2 [DIED July 16, buried in the

Schwartz cornfield near a walnut tree, reinterred in B-2 in the New Jersey Plot]

Cpl. Stephen P. McKenney, Company G, 19th Maine, wounded in the hands

Pvt. William McKenney, Company K, 19th Maine, wounded in the chest

Cpl. John McKenzie, Company E, 1st Minnesota, wounded in the right femur on July 2 [DIED August 7]

Pvt. Jeremiah McKinley, Company F, 148th Pennsylvania, wounded July 2

Pvt. John McKinstry, Company G, 1st Minnesota, wounded on July 2 [DIED August 22]

Cpl. Eugene McLaughlin, Company F, 20th Massachusetts, shot in the chest July 2 or 3 [DIED July 6 or 10, buried on the Schwartz Farm near Rock Creek, opposite the George Bushman Farm, reinterred in A-27 in the Massachusetts Plot, age 44]

Pvt. John McLean, Company F, 20th Massachusetts, gunshot fracture of the thigh on July 2 or 3, leg amputated at the lower third of the thigh [DIED July 20 of pyemia, buried on the Schwartz Farm near Rock Creek under a walnut tree, reinterred in A-24 in the Massachusetts Plot, age 23]

D. McRae, Company A, 13th Mississippi, wounded and captured on July 2

Lt. Col. George Nelson Macy, 20th Massachusetts, wounded on July 3, left hand amputated

Pvt. Joseph G. Maddox, Company I, 19th Maine, wounded in the arm

Pvt. George Magee, Company G, 1st Minnesota, wounded in the chest on July 2

First Sgt. Gustave Magnitsky, Company G, 20th Massachusetts, wounded

Col. John Bowie Magruder, 57th Virginia, age 24, shot in the chest and upper right arm on July 3, captured, treated at the Second Corps Hospital (Harrison and Busey contend it was at the Twelfth Corps Hospital) [DIED July 5, buried at the Schwartz Farm, disinterred October, 1863, by an Epsilon Alpha fraternity brother who placed the remains in a metallic coffin, transported to Richmond for final interment]

Pvt. Daniel Mahoney, Company B, 69th New York, wounded July 2 [DIED July 4, buried near "Red Rock" on the Schwartz Farm, reinterred in B-42 in the New York Plot, age 21]

First Sgt. Francis Malin, Company C, 116th Pennsylvania, wounded July 2 [DIED July 4 at the First Division, Second Corps Hospital]

Cpl. Horace Mann, Company I, 145th Pennsylvania, wounded in the thigh, recovered from his wound

Pvt. Patrick Manning, Company D, 20th Massachusetts, shot in both wrists on July 2 or 3, both radii resected [DIED July 12 or 13 of pyemia, buried on the Schwartz Farm near Rock Creek under a walnut tree, reinterred in A-23 in the Massachusetts Plot, age 24]

Cpl. Peter Marks, Company A, 1st Minnesota, wounded on July 2, leg amputated [DIED July 24]

Pvt. William Marlott, Company C, 39th New York, shot in the right chest on July 2 [DIED July 10 at the Third Division Hospital, buried in Michael Trostle's field near "Red Rock," reinterred in D-57 in New York Plot, age 27]

Pvt. Charles H. Marshal, Company E, 11th Virginia, gunshot fracture of the femur, captured, leg amputated at the Second Division Hospital, exchanged November 17, 1863, from West's Buildings Hospital

Pvt. George W. Marshall, Company G, 64th New York, gunshot fracture of the thigh on July 2, leg amputated at the lower third of the thigh [DIED July 16, buried in the Schwartz cornfield, age 27]

Pvt. George H. Martin, Company G, 4th Ohio, shot in the abdomen on July 2 [DIED July 4 or 6 at the Third Division Hospital, buried on Michael Trostle's "Walnut Row," reinterred in B-21 in the Ohio Plot, age 21]

Sgt. James M. Martin, Company B, 59th New York, skull fractured by a shell on July 3 [DIED July 4, buried by the Peter Frey stone house adjacent to the Second Corps aid station, reinterred in A-75 in the New York plot, age 32]

Pvt. Patrick Martin, Company H, 61st New York, wounded July 2 [DIED July 2, buried in the J. Bair cornfield, reinterred in A-58 in the New York Plot, age 34]

Lt. Col. Rawley White Martin, 53rd Virginia, age 27, physician, attended University of Virginia, graduated University of New York, wound at the Angle fractured the upper third of the right thigh, wound in the left thigh, shell wound of left foot, and flesh wound of the left leg, all on July 3, captured, treated at the Second Division Hospital, exchanged April 30, 1864, from Point Lookout, retired as lieutenant colonel October 22, 1864

Pvt. Reuben D. Martin, Company H, 19th Maine, wounded in the hip

Pvt. Adam Marty, Company B, 1st Minnesota, wounded in the thigh on July 2, spent eight months recuperating from his injuries

Pvt. Fridolin Marty, Company B, 1st Minnesota, severely wounded in the hand on July 2, still recuperating in a Philadelphia hospital as of February 23, 1864

Philip Martyler, 30th or 39th New York, wounded July 2 or 3? [DIED, buried on the Schwartz Farm, reinterred in D-39 in the New York Plot, *no record of this man in any other source material*]

***Sgt. Mathew Marvin, Company K, 1st Minnesota, wounded in the foot on July 2

Pvt. Charles F. Mason, Company I, 1st Minnesota, wounded in the leg on July 2

Second Lt. Charles H. Mason, Company K, 1st Minnesota, shot on July 3 [DIED August 18 of his wounds]

Capt. Herbert C. Mason, Company H, 20th Massachusetts, wounded

Pvt. John W. Massie, Company I, 19th Virginia, shot in the leg on July 3, captured, treated at the First Division Hospital [DIED July 10]

Pvt. Andrew J. Matthews, Company C, 28th Virginia, age 19, blacksmith, shot in the leg on July 3, captured, treated at the First Division Hospital [DIED July 23, buried there in Yard B, Row 2 on the hill between the Schwartz and Bushman farms under a walnut tree; disinterred June 13, 1872, to Richmond in Box #15]

Pvt. Richard T. Mattocks, Company C, 8th Virginia, shot in the left foot on July 3, captured, treated at the Second Division Hospital, exchanged March 20, 1864

Pvt. Sullivan A. Maxim, Company C, 19th Maine, wounded in the leg

Second Lt. William M. May, Company B, 1st Minnesota, wounded in the leg on July 2

Pvt. Robert D. Mays, Company G, 19th Virginia, age 20, farmer, shot through both thighs on July 3, captured, treated at the First Division Hospital, exchanged September 16, 1863, from DeCamp Hospital

Pvt. John Merriam, Company D, 19th Maine, mortally wounded [DIED August 25]

Pvt. Martin Merrill, Company G, 27th Connecticut, wounded

Pvt. Frederick Meyer, Battery I, 1st Ohio Light Artillery [Eleventh Corps], shot in the shoulder on July 2 [DIED July 18, buried in the Schwartz cornfield on Rock Creek, reinterred in A-25 in the Ohio Plot, age 36]

Pvt. Vincent Middlestadt, Company E, 1st Minnesota, wounded in the left foot, on July 2

Pvt. Daniel Miles, Company H, 69th Pennsylvania, mortally wounded July 3 [DIED July 3, buried in the Schwartz cornfield east of a walnut tree]

Pvt. Marcus T. C. Miles, Company K, 20th Massachusetts, wounded

First Sgt. James E. Millam, Company G, 53rd Virginia, shot in the arm on July 3, captured, treated at the First Division Hospital [DIED August 6, 1863 at Chester Hospital of pneumonia, buried there in Grave #123]

Pvt. David Miller, Company G, 148th Pennsylvania, wounded July 3

Color Cpl. Enoch K. Miller, Company F, 108th New York, mortally wounded during the July 3 Confederate attack [DIED, date uncertain]

Cpl. Ernst L. F. Miller, Company I, 1st Minnesota, wounded in the thigh and right eye on July 2

Pvt. George Miller, Company E, 148th Pennsylvania, wounded July 2

Col. Hugh Reid Miller, 42nd Mississippi, age 51, shot in the left chest and right knee on July 3, captured, treated at the Rock Creek facility, transferred to a private home in Gettysburg [DIED there on July 19, body was accompanied south by Thomas D. Witherspoon (regimental chaplain) and Edwin Miller (the colonel's son) under flag of truce, temporarily detained and interred in Baltimore, final reinterment in Richmond on July 29]

Sgt. Luke Miller, Company G, 20th Massachusetts, wounded

Cpl. George A. Milliken, Company I, 1st Minnesota, wounded in the left leg on July 2, leg amputated, discharged due to disability on December 15, 1863

Pvt. Alexander Mills, Company E, 72nd Pennsylvania, shot in the left portion of the chest on July 3 [DIED July 9, buried in the Schwartz cornfield east of a walnut tree, reinterred in B-32 in the Pennsylvania Plot]

Pvt. James P. Mills, Company I, 19th Maine, wounded in the leg

Lt. Joseph A. Milne, Battery B, 1st Rhode Island Artillery, serving with Battery A, 4th U.S. Artillery, shot in the abdomen on July 3 [DIED July 9]

Sgt. Elias Mingle, Company A, 148th Pennsylvania, wounded July 2 [DIED July 31]

Pvt. Isaac W. Mitchell, Company K, 19th Maine, wounded in the hand

Pvt. Jesse Mitchell, Company K, 19th Maine, wounded in the shoulder

Pvt. Simmons A. Mitchell, Company K, 19th Maine, wounded in the back

Pvt. Isaac Moody, Company G, 19th Maine, wounded

***James Moore, Company G, 108th New York, wounded July 2 while supporting Lt. George A. Woodruff's Battery I, 1st U.S. Artillery, transferred to Fort Schuyler, New York

Pvt. James M. Moore, Company G, 11th Virginia, battlefield fracture of thigh on July 3, captured, [DIED July 19, buried behind the Schwartz barn]

Pvt. James S. Moore, Company E, 19th Maine, wounded

Capt. Richard Moroney, 69th New York, wounded July 2

Col. Orlando Harriman Morris, 66th New York, wounded on July 2

Pvt. James K. Morse, Company A, 20th Massachusetts, wounded

First Lt. William S. Mortimer, Company K, 148th Pennsylvania, wounded July 2

Pvt. James W. Morton, Company E, 18th Virginia, wounded in the thigh on July 3, captured, lower third of thigh amputated [DIED July 23, buried in Row 2, Yard B in the cemetery between the Schwartz and Bushman farms under a walnut tree, disinterred to Richmond on June 13, 1872, in Box #18]

Pvt. Ludwell J. Mosher, Company G, 1st Minnesota, wounded in the thigh and wrist on July 2, permanently disabled by his wounds

Pvt. Rascellas Mowry, Company A, 1st Minnesota, wounded in the side on July 2

***Adjt. Joseph W. Muffly, 148th Pennsylvania, wounded July 2

***Pvt. Charles Muller, Company A, 1st Minnesota, wounded in the right thigh on July 2

First Sgt. and Acting Second Lt. Michael Mullin, Company G, 69th Pennsylvania, gunshot fracture of the left hip on July 3 [DIED July 7, buried on the Schwartz Farm back of Rock Creek, reinterred in A-50 in the Pennsylvania Plot]

Pvt. Charles A. Murch, Company D, 19th Maine, wounded in the leg

Pvt. Daniel Murphy, Company A, 20th Massachusetts, wounded

Pvt. Edward Murphy, Company K, 20th Massachusetts, wounded

Pvt. John E. Murphy, Company D, 20th Massachusetts, wounded

Pvt. William B. Murphy, Company A, 19th Maine, wounded in the leg on July 3

Pvt. Winthrop Murray, Company G, 19th Maine, wounded in the head

Pvt. Jacob W. Myers, Company B, 28th Virginia, age 17, blacksmith, shot in the lung on July 3, captured, treated at the First Division Hospital [DIED, date not specified, buried there in Yard B, Row 2,

on the hill between the Schwartz and Bushman farms under a walnut tree; disinterred June 13, 1872, to Richmond with 110 others in ten large boxes marked "S"]

First Lt. Charles E. Nash, Company F, 19th Maine, wounded in the leg on July 3

Cpl. Thomas B. Nason, Company D, 1st Minnesota, wounded in the arm and chest on July 2

Pvt. Lester Nelson, Company K, 126th New York, shot in the abdomen on July 3 [DIED July 5, buried in the back of the Jacob Swisher Farm near the Third Division aid station, age 18]

Cpl. Robert T. Newell, Company D, 19th Maine, mortally wounded [DIED July 9]

Pvt. Joseph Newton, Company D, 81st Pennsylvania, wounded July 2 [DIED July 5 or 6, buried in the Schwartz cornfield near a walnut tree, reinterred in B-31 in the Pennsylvania Plot]

Pvt. Charles H. Nichols, Company D, 27th Connecticut, wounded

Pvt. George H. Nicholson, Company H, 126th New York, shot in the leg on July 3, leg amputated [DIED July 15, buried on the Schwartz Farm near "Red Rock" on the bank of the creek, reinterred in B-73 in the New York Plot, age 40]

Pvt. Henry Nickel, Company A, 1st Minnesota, right thigh fractured on July 2 [DIED August 10]

***Capt. Azor H. Nickerson, 8th Ohio, shot through the lungs and one arm, treated at the Third Division aid station at the Widow Guinn Farm by Surg. Harry McKindree McAbee, the Rock Creek facility, and the Schwartz Farm hospital

***Sgt. Frank B. Nickerson, 4th Ohio, severely wounded on July 2, treated at the Third Division aid station at the Widow Guinn Farm, treated by Surgeon Harry McKindree McAbee

Pvt. Fred A. Nickerson, Company E, 19th Maine, wounded in the hand

Pvt. John E. Nickerson, Company E, 19th Maine, wounded in the leg

Pvt. Ruel Nickerson, Company E, 19th Maine, shot in the right arm on July 3, lower third of arm amputated [DIED July 18, buried in Yard D, in the Schwartz cornfield near Rock Creek, reinterred in B-10 in the Maine Plot, age 26, single]

Pvt. Benjamin F. Noel, Company D, 1st Minnesota, wounded in the leg on July 2, age 21

Cpl. Charles North, Company K, 1st Minnesota, wounded on July 2

Pvt. Joseph H. Norton, Company I, 19th Maine, wounded

Pvt. John B. Nostrand, Company G, 111th New York, mortally wounded and missing July 2 [DIED, buried on the east side of the William

Patterson Farm near the Second Corps Division Hospital near a small house, reinterred in E-56 in the New York Plot, age 23]

Sgt. Henry W. Nye, Company C, 19th Maine, wounded in the head and shoulder

Pvt. Erick Nystedt, Company B, 1st Minnesota, seriously wounded in the thigh on July 2, still hospitalized in Philadelphia as of February 23, 1864

Third Sgt. Thomas C. Oakes, Company B, 38th Virginia, battlefield fracture of the thigh on July 3, captured [DIED August 2, 1863, buried in Yard B, Row 2 on the hill between the Schwartz and Bushman farms; disinterred on June 13, 1872, to Richmond in Box #213]

Pvt. Thomas H. Oakes, Company E, 14th Virginia, shot on July 3, captured, treated at the Third Division Hospital, exchanged August 17, 1863, from Chester Hospital

Cpl. Henry D. O'Brien, Company E, 1st Minnesota, wounded slightly on July 2, and in the head by a spent bullet on July 3 while carrying the colors, awarded Medal of Honor for gallantry in the July 3 action

Pvt. John O'Brien, Company A, 63rd New York, wounded July 2 [DIED July 4, buried on the Schwartz Farm near "Red Rock," reinterred in A-59 in the New York Plot]

Pvt. William O'Brien, Company A, 69th Pennsylvania, shot in the left hip on July 3 [DIED July 19, buried in the Schwartz cornfield near a walnut tree]

Pvt. Daniel O'Harra, Company G, 40th New York [Third Corps], shot in the head July 2 [DIED July 8, buried on the Schwartz Farm opposite White Run, reinterred in A-89 in the New York Plot]

Col. Dennis O'Kane, 69th Pennsylvania, shot in the chest and/or abdomen on July 3 [DIED July 4 at the Second Division Hospital]

Sgt. George Oliver, Company B, 1st Minnesota, wounded in the chest on July 2, celebrated his twenty-eighth birthday on July 1

Pvt. Loring C. Oliver, Company K, 19th Maine, gunshot fracture of the leg on July 2, amputated [DIED July 11 (Busey) or July 20 (regimental history), buried in Yard D, in the Schwartz cornfield near Rock Creek, under a walnut tree, reinterred in B-4 in the Maine Plot, age 34, married]

Pvt. Daniel O'Neal, Company F, 27th Connecticut, wounded

Cpl. John C. Orcutt, Company A, 20th Massachusetts, wounded

Pvt. Rowland L. Ormsby, Company G, 64th New York, gunshot fracture of the right thigh, leg amputated at the upper third of the thigh [DIED July 17, buried in the Schwartz cornfield, reinterred in A-54 in the New York Plot, age 21]

Pvt. Israel Otto, Company A, 148th Pennsylvania, wounded July 2

Musician James A. Overman, 13th Mississippi, left behind to nurse the wounded of his regiment, captured July 5 with the 13th Mississippi wounded, shipped to Baltimore, transferred to Point Lookout Prison, moved to Hammond General Hospital on October 27 due to chronic diarrhea "by order of General Butler," still imprisoned as of February 28, 1865

Pvt. Amos B. Oxton, Company I, 19th Maine, wounded in the hand

Pvt. Ambrose E. Paine, Company F, 42nd New York, gunshot fractures in both legs on July 3, legs amputated [DIED July 23, buried on the Schwartz Farm near "Red Rock," reinterred in B-72 in the New York Plot, age 28]

Second Lt. Sumner Paine, Company A, 20th Massachusetts, wounded in the body by a shell on July 3 [DIED July 3, buried on the Schwartz Farm near Rock Creek, opposite the George Bushman Farm, reinterred in E-1 in the Massachusetts Plot, age 18 (direct descendent of Thomas Paine, Revolutionary War patriot)]

Pvt. Edward Parnell, Company A, 111th New York, shot in the knee on July 2 [DIED July 13, buried on the Michael Trostle Farm on the west side of Rock Creek, age 19]

Pvt. Samuel Parrish, Company E, 28th Virginia, age 19, shot through the lungs on July 3, captured [DIED, date unknown, attended by Jane Boswell Moore]

AND/OR

Pvt. Samuel Parish, 57th Virginia, wounded July 3, captured [DIED, date unknown, attended by Catherine Wert]

First Sgt. Joseph H. Parker, Company K, 20th Massachusetts, wounded

Pvt. William B. Parker, Company I, 20th Massachusetts, wounded

Pvt. Marcus A. Past, Company D, 1st Minnesota, wounded on July 2 [DIED July 5]

Capt. Henry L. Patten, Company D, 20th Massachusetts, wounded

Cpl. Frank A. Patterson, Company E, 19th Maine, wounded in the leg

First Sgt. Robert H. Patterson, Company G, 148th Pennsylvania, wounded July 2

Pvt. Edwin Paul, Company I, 1st Minnesota, battlefield fracture of the left leg on July 2, leg amputated [DIED late July 13 or early July 14]

First Lt. Carl Theodore Pausch, Company C, 39th New York, shot in the abdomen on July 3 [DIED July 9 at the Third Division, reinterred in A-81 in the New York Plot, age 28]

Pvt. Charles Paxden, Company B, 27th Connecticut, wounded

Second Lt. Fielding F. Payne, Company B, 8th Virginia, shot in the head on July 3, captured, treated at the Second Division Hospital [DIED July 13, buried in Yard D in the Jacob Schwartz cornfield by Rock Creek, disinterred to Richmond on June 13, 1872, with 110 others in ten large boxes marked "S"]

Pvt. Joseph T. Payne, Company C, 38th Virginia, wounded and captured on July 3 [DIED July 22 at the Second Corps Hospital, buried there in Yard B, Row 2 on the hill between the Schwartz and Bushman farms; disinterred on June 13, 1872, to Richmond with 110 others in 10 large boxes marked "S"]

Sgt. Benjamin B. Pease, Company I, 20th Massachusetts, wounded

Cpl. William N. Peck, Company I, 1st Minnesota, wounded in the left leg on July 2, leg amputated [DIED July 4 or 21]

First Lt., Adjutant John Peller, Company A, 1st Minnesota, gunshot fracture of the left arm on July 2, transferred to a Baltimore hospital where he had a slow recovery, unfit for duty as of December 1863

Pvt. John Pennington, Company F, 148th Pennsylvania, wounded July 2

Sgt. Ira Penoyar, Company D, 111th New York, shot in the head on July 3 [DIED July 10 at the Third Division Hospital, buried on Michael Trostle's "Walnut Row," reinterred in B-67 in the New York Plot, age 27]

Capt. Joseph Per(r)iam, Company K, 1st Minnesota, shot in the head on July 2, the ball entering at the nose and exiting behind the ear, last day completely delirious [DIED late July 6 or early July 7 at the Second Division Hospital, reinterred in B-9 in the Minnesota Plot, age 30]

Color Sgt. Ellet P. Perkins, Company D, 1st Minnesota, wounded in the knee on July 2

Cpl. George L. Perkins, Company G, 19th Maine, severely wounded on July 2 [DIED July 2, probably in a Second Corps aid station, age 32, married]

Pvt. James V. Perrin, Company A, 14th Virginia, captured while sick, treated at First Division Hospital, exchanged September 23, 1863, from Chester Hospital

Pvt. William Perry, Company F, 148th Pennsylvania, wounded July 2
Adjt. George F. Peterson, 27th Connecticut, wounded
Cpl. Jacob Pfeiffer, Company B, 20th Massachusetts, wounded
Pvt. William B. Philbrook, Company I, 1st Minnesota, wounded in the thigh on July 2
Pvt. John Phillips, Company D, 27th Connecticut, wounded
First Sgt. James H. Pierce, Company E, 19th Maine, wounded in the side
Pvt. Legrand Platt, Company B, 86th New York [Third Corps], wounded July 2 [DIED July 6 at the First Division Hospital, buried in the Schwartz cornfield at the edge of the woods under a walnut tree, reinterred in A-68 in the New York Plot, age 19]
Third Cpl. Cornelius Powell, Company E, 9th Virginia, wounded in the thigh on July 3, captured, leg amputated [DIED July 21, buried there behind the Schwartz barn in Grave #17]
Cpl. John Powers, Company F, 20th Massachusetts, wounded
Second Lt. John R. Presgraves, Company I, 8th Virginia, gunshot fracture of left leg on July 3, captured, treated at the Second Division Hospital, leg amputated July 13 by Surgeon Charles Squire Wood of the 66th New York [DIED on July 15 of tetanus, buried in Yard C west of the Schwartz farm house in the woods on the red hill above the creek; cared for by one of his two brothers in the 8th Virginia (Pvt. George W. Presgraves, released from Fort Delaware on June 20, 1865), who secured a pine coffin for his burial; his remains were removed sometime prior to the general disinterment of Confederate dead in the 1870s]
First Lt. Charles P. Prince, Company F, 27th Connecticut, wounded
Sgt. J. Proctor, Company D, 20th Massachusetts, wounded
Cpl. Warren Proctor, Company K, 19th Maine, wounded in the groin
Pvt. Edgar Proseus, Company E, 111th New York, shot in the left leg on July 3, leg amputated [DIED July 10 at the Third Division Hospital, buried on Michael Trostle's "Walnut Row," age 21]

Pvt. Andrew P. Quist, Company B, 1st Minnesota, wounded in the thigh on July 2

Pvt. Herman Rabaca, Company I, 1st Minnesota, wounded on July 2
First Sgt. James O. B. Racer, Company K, 7th Virginia, age 20, farmer, wounded on July 3, captured [DIED July 15, buried there in Yard D, Row 3, in the Schwartz's cornfield, disinterred to

Richmond on June 13, 1872, with 110 others in 10 large boxes marked "S"]

Pvt. Jacob Raisch, Company I, 125th New York, wounded July 2 [DIED July 5, buried on Michael Trostle's "Walnut Row," reinterred in C-60 in the New York Plot, age 38]

Pvt. Frederick Rambmeier, Company B, 52nd New York, shot in the hip on July 2 [DIED July 18, buried in the Schwartz cornfield near Rock Creek, reinterred in A-57 in the New York Plot, age 22 (*state Adjutant General's Office also shows him as having been killed at the Battle of Cold Harbor, June 1, 1864*)]

Pvt. James Y. Ramsey, Company E, 14th Virginia, age 25, farmer, shot in the left knee on July 3, captured, probably accompanied William B. Ramsey, exchanged November 17, 1863, from West's Buildings Hospital

Pvt. William B. Ramsey, Company E, 14th Virginia, age 23, farmer, battlefield wound fracture of the thigh on July 3, captured [DIED July 25, buried in Grave #3 behind the Schwartz barn]

Pvt. Marshall H. Rand, Company B, 19th Maine, wounded

Pvt. James W. Rawlings, Company B, 8th Virginia, age 27, shot in the thigh and right shoulder on July 3, captured, treated at the Second Division Hospital, paroled on August 22, 1863 from West's Buildings Hospital

Cpl. James Ray, Company C, 148th Pennsylvania, wounded July 2

Pvt. Emanuel Raybuck, Company E, 148th Pennsylvania, wounded July 2

Pvt. Fred W. Raymond, Company H, 1st Minnesota, wounded on July 3, transferred to a general hospital, serious infection developed [DIED October 10, 1863, committed suicide]

Pvt. George O. Raymond, Company C, 15th Massachusetts, wounded July 2 or 3 [DIED July 22, buried on the Schwartz Farm near Rock Creek under a walnut tree, age 32]

Pvt. David Read, Company A, 59th New York, vertebra fractured by a gunshot and/or wounded in the right arm by a grapeshot on July 2, upper third of the humerus resected [DIED July 3 or 5 at the Second Division Hospital, reinterred in B-50 in the New York plot, age 23]

First Sgt. Charles W. Reed, Company G, 8th Virginia, wounded in the arm on July 3, captured, arm amputated [DIED July 17, buried in Grave #14 in back of the Schwartz barn]

Pvt. Reuben Reed, Company G, 148th Pennsylvania, wounded July 3

Pvt. Walter S. Reed, Company G, 1st Minnesota, wounded in the eye on July 2

Col. Paul J. Revere, 20th Massachusetts, severely wounded by shell fragment through the left lung on July 2 [DIED July 4 or 5 at the Second Division Hospital on the Schwartz Farm, age 30, (direct descendant of Revolutionary War patriot Paul Revere)]

Capt. John William Reynolds, 145th Pennsylvania, wounded on July 2

Pvt. Malachia Rhodes, Company E, 148th Pennsylvania, wounded July 2

Pvt. John M. Rhorer, Company G, 1st Minnesota, wounded in the neck on July 2

Second Lt. Edwin H. Rich, Company F, 19th Maine, wounded in the arm on July 3

Pvt. Isaac H. Rich, Company H, 106th Pennsylvania, wounded in the abdomen on July 2 [DIED July 4 or 5, buried in the Schwartz cornfield, reinterred in A-52 in the Pennsylvania Plot]

Sgt. William K. Richards, Company I, 1st Minnesota, wounded in the leg on July 3

Pvt. Luke T. Richardson, Company H, 19th Maine, wounded in the side

First Sgt. Thomas P. (or T.) Rideout, Company F, 19th Maine, shot through the lungs and in the shoulder on July 3 [DIED July 18, buried in Yard D, in the Schwartz cornfield near Rock Creek, reinterred in C-10? in the Maine Plot, age 21, single]

Sgt. Samuel Smith, of Company F, 19th Maine wrote this of First Sergeant Rideout: "No better soldier nor one more highly esteemed by his comrades ever lived in the State of Maine than First Sgt. Thomas T. Rideout, of Company F. While we were making the flank movement to the right at the time of Pickett's charge, he fell by my side. When he fell, I stopped and asked him where he was hit. His reply was 'I am hit in the back.' He was lying in a very exposed position and I laid down my gun and took hold of his shoulders and dragged him about one rod and behind a large boulder, which would shield him somewhat from further danger from bullets which were singing about there pretty lively at the time. I then picked up my own gun and rejoined the Company. Sgt. Rideout was taken later to the field hospital, where I visited him after the battle. There I found him shot through the lungs, the bullet lodging in his shoulder, where he first felt it and thought he was hit in the back. He was cheerful at the time and fully expected to recover and live to go home. When I saw the Surgeon in charge of the hospital, he informed me that Rideout could not live. I afterwards learned that he died about fifteen days after he was wounded." [John Day Smith, *The History of the Nineteenth Maine Regiment of the Maine Volunteer Infantry 1862-1865*, p. 90]

Capt. John S. Rickers, Company C, 5th New Hampshire, wounded

Cpl. Edward J. Riley, Company K, 111th New York, shot in the stomach on July 2 [DIED July 11 at the Third Division Hospital, buried on the Schwartz Farm, age 21]

Pvt. James A. Riley, Company E, 12th New Jersey, shot in the left lung on July 2 [DIED July 4 at the Third Division Hospital, reinterred in B-18 in the New Jersey Plot]

Pvt. Charles H. Rines, Company D, 1st Minnesota, wounded in the side on July 2

Pvt. Arthur M. Rivers, Company I, 20th Massachusetts, wounded

Pvt. James P. Robbins, Company B, 53rd Virginia, age 22, farmer, shot in the leg on July 3, captured, treated at the Third Division Hospital [DIED July 20, buried there in Yard B, Row 2 on the hill between the Schwartz and Bushman farms; disinterred June 13, 1872, to Richmond with 110 others in 10 large boxes marked "S"]

David B. Robertson, Company I, 2nd New York, wounded? [DIED, buried on the Schwartz Farm, *no other record of this man available in any other sources*]

?First Lt. J. N. Robertson, 5th Alabama, wounded and captured

Cpl. Robert A. Robertson, Company C, 18th Virginia, age 23, farmer, wounded in the arm and leg on July 3, captured [DIED July 24, buried in Grave #9 behind the Schwartz barn]

G. H. Roe, Company G, 45th Georgia, wounded and captured

Pvt. Martin V. Roe, Company K, 111th New York, leg fractured by a shell on July 2 [DIED July 11 at the Third Division Hospital, buried on the Jacob Swisher Farm, reinterred in D-109 in the New York Plot, age 22]

Sgt. William J. Roe, Company I, 1st Minnesota, wounded in the leg on July 2 (or 3) [DIED July 2 or 3]

Pvt. Franklin Rollins, Company D, 1st Minnesota, wounded on July 2 [DIED August 3]

Pvt., Pioneer John H. Rue, Company B, 11th New Jersey [Third Corps], shot in both legs on July 2, legs amputated [DIED July 11, buried in the Schwartz cornfield near a walnut tree, reinterred in B-5 in the New Jersey Plot]

Cpl. George M. Rupp, Company A, 148th Pennsylvania, wounded July 2

Pvt. James R. Russell, Company A, 20th Massachusetts, wounded

Pvt. Patrick Ryan, Company A, 5th New Jersey [Third Corps], shot in the face and leg on July 2 [DIED July 26, buried on the Schwartz Farm lane, under a walnut tree near White Run, reinterred in B-1 in the New Jersey Plot]

Pvt. John Salsbury, Company E, 64th New York, wounded July 2 [DIED July 5, buried in the Schwartz cornfield at the edge of the woods under a walnut tree, reinterred in A-67 in the New York Plot, age 21]

Pvt. Benjamin F. Sanders, Company A, 1st Minnesota, wounded on July 2

Cpl. Weld Sargent, Company K, 19th Maine, wounded in the arm

Pvt. John H. Saulpaugh, Company E, 126th New York, wounded July 3 [DIED July 4, buried on Michael Trostle's "Walnut Row," reinterred in B-69 in the New York Plot, age 22]

Pvt. Addison Sawyer, Company K, 19th Maine, wounded in the hand

Pvt. John H. Sc(h)ammel, Company C, 1st Virginia, wounded in the abdominal cavity (and possibly the thigh) on July 3 by shell fragment, captured [DIED July 4 or 5]

Michael Scannel, 19th Massachusetts, wounded on July 2

Pvt. Conrad Schmidt, Company D, 82nd New York, wounded July 3 [DIED July 10, buried in the Schwartz cornfield, age 25]

Pvt. John P. Schoenbeck, Company B, 1st Minnesota, wounded in the thigh on July 2, age 38

Daniel Schout, 108th New York, wounded during the July 3 Confederate attack

Pvt. William K. Schrack, Company I, 72nd Pennsylvania, wounded July 2 [DIED July 5, buried in the Schwartz cornfield]

Cpl. William Schultz, Company I, 71st Pennsylvania, wounded in both thighs on July 2, transferred to Letterman General Hospital, [DIED September 29, 1863, buried temporarily at Camp Letterman, reinterred in the National Cemetery at Gettysburg]

Pvt. George Schumacher, Company B, 39th New York, gunshot fracture of the leg on July 2, leg amputated [DIED July 25, buried on the Schwartz Farm, reinterred in D-40 in the New York Plot, age 21]

Second Lt. Leroy S. Scott, Company B, 19th Maine, wounded by a shell in both legs and thighs on July 2 or 3, right leg amputated [DIED July 13 at Second Division Hospital, age 25, married]

Pvt. Thomas E. Scott, Company K, 19th Maine, wounded in the leg, leg amputated

***John M. Scoville, Battery B, 1st New York Light Artillery, shot through the shoulder blades and upper arm on July 2, begged not to have arm amputated, saved arm, recovered from his injuries

Lt. James M. Seals, 42nd Mississippi, wounded in five places, captured, at least one amputation performed [DIED July 19, buried in Yard B, Row 2 between the Jacob Schwartz and George Bushman farms, grave's identity lost, disinterred south with the other Confederate dead from the Schwartz Farm]

Cpl. Edwin Searson, Company B, 148th Pennsylvania, wounded twice on July 3

Pvt. Albert Sebers, Company B, 1st Minnesota, wounded in the head and leg on July 2, still recovering at the convalescent camp in Alexandria, Virginia, as of February 23, 1864

Pvt. Thomas Sebring, Company I, 126th New York, wounded July 2 [DIED July 8, buried on Michael Trostle's "Walnut Row," reinterred in A-80 in the New York Plot, age 24]

Second Lt. Henry Sewall, Company G, 19th Maine, wounded in the face

Pvt. Henry C. Shark, Company I, 4th Ohio, wounded by a shell in the ankle on July 2 [DIED July 11 at the Third Division Hospital, buried on the Michael Trostle's "Walnut Row," reinterred in B-17 in the Ohio Plot, age 21]

Pvt. Johnson Shaw, Company C, 19th Maine, wounded in the foot, foot amputated

Pvt. Samuel B. Shea, Company K, 19th Maine, wounded in the chest on July 2 [DIED July 9 (Busey) or July 20 (regimental history), buried in the Schwartz cornfield near a walnut tree, reinterred in B-5 in the Maine Plot, age 30, single]

Lt. Albert S. Sheldon, Battery B, 1st New York Light Artillery, shot on July 3 during the Confederate assault

Pvt. Edward B. Sheldon, Company F, 19th Maine, wounded in the arm, arm amputated

Col. Eliakim Sherrill, 126th New York, mortally wounded on July 3 [DIED July 4]

Duncan Sherwood, Company A, 19th Massachusetts, wounded on July 2

Cpl. Rufus Shibbles, Jr., Company I, 19th Maine, wounded in the hand

Third Sgt. Octavius M. Shifflett, Company H, 57th Virginia, shot in the arm on July 3, captured [DIED July 13, buried in Yard D, Row

1 in the Schwartz cornfield; disinterred on June 13, 1872, to Richmond with 110 others in 10 large boxes marked "S"]

Pvt. Samuel Shilling, Company E, 148th Pennsylvania, wounded July 2

Pvt. William H. Shorey, Company F, 19th Maine, mortally wounded July 2 [DIED July 4]

Pvt. William H. Shultz, Company H, 148th Pennsylvania, wounded July 2

Pvt. Joseph Simmons, Company C, 13th Vermont [First Corps], wounded July 3 [DIED July 14, buried on the Schwartz Farm opposite the George Bushman Farm in back of Rock Creek, reinterred in Vermont A-22 in the Vermont Plot]

Pvt. Hans M. Simonson, Company A, 1st Minnesota, gunshot fracture of the thigh on July 2 [DIED August 3]

Pvt. William Simpson, Company D, 145th Pennsylvania, gunshot fracture of the thigh on July 2 [DIED July 16, buried in the Schwartz cornfield, reinterred in D-15 in the Pennsylvania Plot]

Capt. Thomas Sinclair, Company B, 1st Minnesota, wounded in the arm on July 2

Pvt. Alexander Skelton, Company A, 53rd Virginia, shot in the left hip on July 3, captured, treated at the First Division Hospital [DIED December 4, 1863, of complications from the wound and chronic diarrhea at Fort Wood, Bedloe's Island, New York Harbor, buried in Grave #953 of the Cypress Hill Cemetery, Long Island, New York]

Darwin Skinner, 108th New York, wounded during the July 3 Confederate attack

Pvt. William B. Small, Company G, 19th Maine, wounded in the shoulder

Pvt. William S. Small, Company F, 19th Maine, wounded in the arm

Pvt. Orrin P. Smart, Company G, 19th Maine, wounded in the chest

Pvt. Audubon C. Smith, Company C, 56th Virginia, shot through both shoulders on July 3, captured, given a drink and carried out of the line of fire by Albert N. Hamilton of the 72nd Pennsylvania (Second Brigade, Second Division, Second Corps)—the two men recognized each other at the 50th anniversary of the battle in July 1913, exchanged September 23, 1863, from Chester Hospital

Pvt. Benjamin J. Smith, Company H, 1st Minnesota, wounded on July 3

Pvt. David Smith, Company E, 148th Pennsylvania, wounded July 2

Capt. George D. Smith, Company I, 19th Maine, mortally wounded in the left lung on July 2 [DIED at 1:00 a.m. on July 3, in transport to the First Division Hospital, buried in L. Bushman's field west of the barn, reinterred in F-1 in the Maine Plot, age 27, single]

Cpl. George S. Smith, Company I, 64th New York, gunshot fracture of the hip on July 2 [DIED July 26, buried on the Schwartz Farm, reinterred in A-71 in the New York plot, age 18]

First Sgt. Henry E. Smith, Company F, 14th Virginia, age 25, planter, shot in the arm and spine on July 3, captured, treated at the Second Division Hospital, exchanged August 17, 1863, from Chester Hospital

Pvt. Matthew Smith, Company G, 71st Pennsylvania, shot in the right portion of the chest on July 3 [DIED July 5 at the Second Division Hospital, reinterred in A-49 in the Pennsylvania Plot]

Pvt. William C. Smith, Company D, 1st Minnesota, wounded in the shoulder on July 2

Pvt. Joseph Smithyman, Company D, 1st Minnesota, wounded in the side on July 2

Col. Thomas A. Smyth, 1st Delaware, wounded by flying debris during the cannonade on July 3

Pvt. William J. Snow, Company B, 14th Virginia, age 28, farmer, shot in the shoulder, hand and leg on July 3, captured, treated at the Second Division Hospital, exchanged September 23, 1863, from Chester Hospital

Sgt. Tyler J. Snyder, Company G, 126th New York, shot in the right groin on July 3 [DIED July 3 at the Third Division Hospital, reinterred in E-58 in the New York Plot, age 21]

Pvt. Sidney Southard, 5th Massachusetts Battery [Artillery Reserve] (unit noted as "I," 5th Battery, First Corps), shot in the abdomen July 1 or 2 [DIED at the Third Division Hospital, *not in state Adjutant General Office records*]

Pvt. William Spaulding, Company C, 19th Maine, wounded in the arm

Pvt. Henry Sprouse, Company F, 19th Virginia, shot in the leg on July 3, captured, treated at the First Division Hospital, exchanged September 27, 1863, from DeCamp Hospital

Cpl. Leonard J. Squire, Company F, 1st Minnesota, shot in the hip on July 2 [DIED July 7]

Cpl. Gideon L. Squires, Company C, 1st Minnesota, wounded in the arm on July 3

Cpl. William H. Stannis, Company G, 27th Connecticut, wounded

Cpl. Benjamin F. Staples, Company E, 1st Minnesota, wounded on July 2

Capt. Isaac W. Starbirg, Company F, 19th Maine, wounded July 3

Sgt. George L. Starkey, Company D, 19th Maine, wounded in the leg July 2, leg amputated

Pvt. Anthony Starr, Company G, 106th Pennsylvania, shot in the thigh on July 2, leg amputated [DIED July 15, buried in the Schwartz cornfield, reinterred in D-16 in the Pennsylvania Plot]

First Sgt. Charles Steen, Company A, 1st Minnesota, wounded in the leg on July 2, leg amputated

Cpl. John B. Stephens, Company B, 1st Minnesota, wounded in the chest on July 2

Pvt. Albert W. Stetson, Company D, 20th Massachusetts, wounded

Pvt. James W. Stevens, Company F, 38th Virginia, battlefield fracture of the thigh on July 3, captured [DIED July 29, buried in Yard B, Row 2 on the hill between the Schwartz and Bushman farms; disinterred June 13, 1872, to Richmond in Box #200]

Second Lt. Robert Stewart, Company D, 72nd Pennsylvania, wounded in the ankle, thigh, and testicles on July 3

Pvt. John W. Stewart, Company G, 19th Virginia, age 18, clerk, shot in the thigh on July 3, captured, treated at the First Division Hospital, exchanged September 8, 1863, from DeCamp Hospital

Pvt. Stephen B. Stewart, Company A, 20th Massachusetts, wounded

Pvt. Adams C. Stites, Company E, 1st Minnesota, wounded in the head on July 2

Sgt. Samuel B. Stites, Company E, 1st Minnesota, wounded in the arm on July 2

Pvt. John R. Stockton, Company I, 71st Pennsylvania, shot in the left leg, leg amputated [DIED July 12, buried in the Schwartz cornfield, reinterred in A-45 in the Pennsylvania Plot]

Pvt. Henry S. Stockwell, Company K, 12th New Jersey, shot in the back on July 3 [DIED July 4 at the Third Division Hospital]

Cpl. John F. Stone, Company F, 4th Maine [Third Corps], mortally wounded in the groin on July 2 [DIED July 2, buried beside the Schwartz farm lane, near the creek, under a walnut tree]

Cpl. David Stoup, Company E, 63rd Pennsylvania [Third Corps] [DIED July 24 of rheumatism, buried on the Jacob Schwartz farm lane, reinterred in A-72 in the Pennsylvania Plot]

Frank Stoughton, Company D, 14th Connecticut, wounded on July 3, shot just below the neck

Pvt. William M. Stuart, Company C, 82nd New York, shot in the side on July 2 or 3 [DIED July 8, buried in the Schwartz cornfield at the edge of the woods near a walnut tree, reinterred in B-44 in the New York Plot, age 28]

Pvt. Daniel Sullivan, Company D, 1st Minnesota, wounded in the foot on July 2

Cpl. James Sullivan, Company A, 20th Massachusetts, wounded

Pvt. Isaac Summerfield, Company I, 7th West Virginia, right thigh terribly lacerated by a shell on July 2 or 3 [DIED July 4 at the Third Division Hospital]

Pvt. John Sutter, Company H, 7th West Virginia, wounded by a shell in both thighs, compound fracturing of one femur [DIED July 4 at the Third Division Hospital]

Capt. John F. Sutton, Company E, 148th Pennsylvania, wounded July 2

John Swager, 108th New York, wounded July 3

First Sgt. George T. Swank, Company D, 27th Connecticut, wounded

Pvt. Isaac Sweetwood, Company H, 148th Pennsylvania, wounded July 2

Pvt. Joseph A. Tanner, Company B, 1st Minnesota, severely wounded in the shoulder on July 3, still recovering in a New York hospital as of February 23, 1864, age 34

Capt. Bennett Taylor, Company F, 19th Virginia, age 24, teacher, shot in the side on July 3, captured, treated at the Second Division Hospital, exchanged March 22, 1865, from Johnson's Island, Ohio

Pvt. George Taylor, Company G, 111th New York, shot in the leg on July 2 or 3 [DIED July 20, buried on Michael Trostle's "Walnut Row," body removed prior to reinterment in the National Cemetery, age 23]

First Lt. John S. Taylor, Company D, 14th Virginia, farmer, shot in the thigh on July 3, captured, treated at the Second Division Hospital, released June 12, 1865 from Fort Delaware

Cpl. Mathew F. Taylor, Company E, 1st Minnesota, wounded in the chest on July 2

Pvt. Roland Taylor, Company G, 5th New Hampshire, gunshot fracture of the leg on July 2, leg amputated [DIED July 11, buried on the J. Bair Farm, reinterred in A-6 in the New Hampshire Plot, age 33]

Sgt. William P. Temple, Company C, 18th Virginia, age 29, blacksmith, shot in the thigh and captured July 3, treated at Second Division Hospital, exchanged from West's Buildings Hospital September 8, 1863

Pvt. Richard A. Tenner, Company D, 27th Connecticut, wounded

Pvt. Samuel S. Tenney, Company K, 1st Minnesota, wounded in the leg on July 2

Pvt. John Tennison, Company K, 82nd New York, gunshot fracture of the leg on July 3 [DIED July 19, buried in the Schwartz cornfield near Rock Creek, reinterred in B-40 in the New York Plot, age 34]

Lt. Col. Max A. "Jack of Diamonds" Thoman, 59th New York, right shoulder fractured by a shell on July 2 [DIED July 11, buried on the Schwartz Farm back of Rock Creek opposite the George Bushman Farm, reinterred in A-70 in the New York plot, age 31]

Pvt. Abraham J. Thomas, Company D, 38th Virginia, wounded and captured on July 3 [DIED July 9, buried in Yard D in Jacob Schwartz's cornfield by Rock Creek; disinterred on June 13, 1872, to Richmond with 110 others in 10 large boxes marked "S"]

Pvt. Hushai C. Thomas, Company D, 19th Maine, mortally wounded [DIED July 2]

***Capt. Benjamin W. Thompson, 111th New York, wounded in the head by a flying board and rock chips on July 3

Pvt. Elbridge E. Thompson, Company G, 86th New York [Third Corps], wounded in the side on July 2 [DIED July 3, buried on the Schwartz Farm opposite White Run, reinterred in A-88 in the New York plot, age 21]

Pvt. James A. Thompson, Company G, 148th Pennsylvania, wounded July 3

Cpl. John A. Thompson, 4th New York Light Battery [Third Corps], mortally wounded July 2 [DIED July 2, buried on the Schwartz Farm opposite White Run, reinterred in C-58 in the New York Plot, age 27]

Pvt. Ole Thompson, Company B, 1st Minnesota, wounded on July 2, left arm amputated [DIED August 8]

Pvt. Thomas C. Tiernan, Company A, 20th Massachusetts, wounded

Pvt. Lyman F. Tilton, Company A, 20th Massachusetts, wounded

Lt. Francis A. Timberlake, Company B, 7th Tennessee, wounded through the body (just to the right of the stomach, deflected internally and emerging near the backbone), captured, transferred to Johnson's Island, Ohio

Pvt. Joseph A. Tobey, Company F, 19th Maine, wounded in the face

Sgt. John A. Toothaker, Company K, 4th Maine [Third Corps], wounded in the neck on July 2 [DIED July 20, buried beside the

Schwartz farm lane, near the creek, under a walnut tree, age 18, single]

Pvt. Josiah Tosh, Company B, 53rd Virginia, age 24, wounded in the right hip on July 3, captured, treated at the First Division Hospital, exchanged September 27, 1863, from DeCamp Hospital

Sgt. Philip Tracy, Company G, 8th Ohio, shot in the shoulder on July 3 [DIED July 5 at the Third Division Hospital, buried on Michael Trostle's "Walnut Row," reinterred in B-22 in the Ohio Plot, age 24]

Cpl. Stephen P. Trafton, Company K, 19th Maine, wounded in the leg

Pvt. Charles Triscut, Company E, 145th Pennsylvania, gunshot fracture of the hip on July 2 [DIED July 15, buried in the Schwartz cornfield, reinterred in D-17 in the Pennsylvania Plot]

Pvt. Samuel Try, Company I, 148th Pennsylvania, wounded July 2

Pvt. George F. Tufts, Company D, 19th Maine, wounded in the arm and leg

Cpl. Abial Turner, Company B, 19th Maine, wounded in the side on July 2

Pvt. George S. Turner, Company I, 19th Maine, mortally wounded [DIED July 19]

Pvt. Elias Tyler, Company G, 19th Maine, shot in the left portion of the chest on July 2 [DIED July 14 or 15 at the Second Division Hospital, age 21, single]

Pvt. A. B. Usher, Company D, 125th New York, wounded July 3 [DIED July 9, buried on the Michael Trostle Farm under a sycamore tree, reinterred in A-91 in the New York Plot, age 21]

Cpl. Oliver Valentine, Company C, 74th New York [Third Corps], shot in the left lung on July 2 [DIED July 3, buried on the Schwartz Farm opposite White Run, age 20]

Sgt. Francis Vanderveher, Company H, 71st Pennsylvania, wounded in the chest and/or the right side of the neck on July 3 [DIED July 5 at the Second Division Hospital, reinterred in A-80 in the Pennsylvania Plot]

Cpl. Oliver W. Vanvalin, Company B, 148th Pennsylvania, wounded July 2

Pvt. Myron H. Van Winkle, Company E, 111th New York, gunshot fracture of the leg on July 3, leg amputated [DIED July 27, buried on the Schwartz Farm, reinterred in A-72 in the New York Plot, age 26]

Pvt. Gilman N. Varell, Company K, 19th Maine, wounded in the legs

Pvt. Louis Vigne, Company A, 19th Maine, wounded July 3

Cpl. John Vinal, Company I, 19th Maine, wounded in the hand

?Pvt. Eli Vincent, Company G, 1st United States Sharpshooters, shot in the right shoulder and lung on July 2 [DIED July 16, reinterred in B-36 in the United States Plot, from Milton, Wisconsin]

? Sgt. William Henry Voss, Company D, 21st North Carolina, wounded and captured

Pvt. Peter Vosz, Company K, 1st Minnesota, wounded in the bowels on July 3 [DIED July 3]

Pvt. Robert M. Wadding, Company I, 148th Pennsylvania, wounded July 2

Sgt. Maj. George A. Wadsworth, 19th Maine, wounded in the head

Pvt. Christian Wagner, Company B, 20th Massachusetts, wounded

Pvt. Warren Wagner, Company A, 1st Minnesota, wounded in the back on July 2 or 3 [DIED July 6]

Pvt. Daniel H. Waite, Company E, 1st Minnesota, wounded in the leg on July 2

Sgt. James T. Waldron, Company H, 19th Maine, wounded in the thigh

First Lt. Charles F. Walker, Company B, 7th New Jersey [Third Corps], shot in the hip on July 2 [DIED July 3, buried on the Schwartz Farm opposite White Run]

Adjt. William H. Walker, 20th Massachusetts, wounded

Pvt. Francis M. Wallace, Company C, 14th Indiana, shot in the back on July 2 [DIED July 4 at the Third Division Hospital, reinterred in F-3 in the Indiana Plot]

Pvt. James W. Walsh, Company D, 1st Minnesota, wounded in the shoulder on July 2

Col. George Hull Ward, 15th Massachusetts, wounded July 2, left leg amputated [DIED July 3]

Sgt. Thomas Ward, Company F, 27th Connecticut, wounded

Third Sgt. Edwin S. Ware, Company I, 19th Virginia, shot in the right leg on July 3, captured, treated at the First Division Hospital, leg amputated by Surgeon Charles Squire Wood of the 66th New York on July 6, exchanged November 17, 1863, from West's Buildings Hospital

Pvt. James G. Warren, Company D, 20th Massachusetts, wounded

First Lt. John C. Warren, 52nd North Carolina, wounded and captured—Warren was attended by his brother, Dr. L. P.

Warren, left behind to care for the Confederate wounded (per Page)

Pvt. Augustus Washburn, Company H, 19th Maine, wounded in the right arm, arm amputated

Pvt. Melcher Wasser, Company K, 148th Pennsylvania, wounded on either July 2 or 3, transferred to the Veteran Reserve Corps

Pvt. Fred L. Waterhouse, Company E, 19th Maine, wounded in the leg

Cpl. Alfred P. Waterman, Company D, 19th Maine, wounded July 2 [DIED July 4]

Pvt. Peter Wean, Company H, 6th New Jersey [Third Corps], shot in the back on July 2 [DIED July 11, buried in the Schwartz cornfield near a walnut tree, reinterred in D-13 in the New Jersey Plot]

Pvt. Daniel S. Weaver, Company I, 1st Minnesota, wounded in the leg on July 2

Pvt. Elijah Weaver, Company E, 1st Minnesota, wounded in the neck on July 2

Brig. Gen. Alexander S. Webb, Second Corps, Second Division, Second Brigade commander, wounded in the groin

Pvt. Reuben Webb, Company C, 19th Maine, wounded in the thigh

Sgt. George E. Webber, Company H, 19th Maine, mortally wounded [DIED July 7]

Pvt. Lorenzo Webster, Company K, 19th Maine, wounded

Pvt. Henry Wedges, Company I, 1st Minnesota, wounded on July 2

Pvt. John Weight, Company A, 148th Pennsylvania, wounded July 2 [DIED July 24, buried in Rebersburg, Pennsylvania]

Cpl. Siegmund Weil, Company B (of Company F, 7th New York detachment), 52nd New York, wounded July 2 [DIED July at the First Division Hospital, buried on the Schwartz Farm at the edge of the woods near a walnut tree, reinterred in B-52 in the New York Plot, age 22]

Pvt. Charles W. Weiser, Company A, 148th Pennsylvania, wounded July 2

Maj. James W. Welch, 19th Maine, wounded in the scalp

Color Cpl. William Welch, Company I, 8th Ohio, shot in the head on July 3 [DIED July 10 at the Third Division Hospital, buried on Michael Trostle's "Walnut Row," reinterred in B-23 in the Ohio Plot, age 18]

Pvt. Peter Welin, Company E, 1st Minnesota, shot in the thigh on July 2, leg amputated [DIED July 29]

Cpl. William Fix Wellman, Company I, 1st Minnesota, wounded in the leg on July 2, leg amputated [DIED August 2, age 20]

Cpl. Edwin Wells, Company B, 1st Minnesota, wounded in the leg on July 2, still recuperating at a Providence, Rhode Island, hospital as of February 23, 1864

Pvt. James K. Wells, Company E, 148th Pennsylvania, wounded July 2

Pvt. Jeremiah Y. Wells, Company H, 19th Massachusetts, shot in the foot and leg on July 2 or 3, leg amputated [DIED July 14, buried on the Schwartz Farm near Rock Creek, opposite the George Bushman Farm, reinterred in C-32 in the Massachusetts Plot, age 34]

Cpl. James C. Welsh, Company H, 8th Ohio, wounded July 3 [DIED July 5 at the Third Division Hospital, buried on Michael Trostle's "Walnut Row," age 18]

First Sgt. Edward Welton, Company H, 20th Massachusetts, wounded

Pvt. Peter West, Company K, 42nd New York, shot in the right leg on July 3, leg amputated [DIED July 23, buried on the Schwartz Farm, reinterred in C-43 in the New York Plot, age 22]

Pvt. George E. Wheeler, Company H, 19th Maine, wounded in the legs

Pvt. Wessel T. Whitbeck, Company E, 111th New York, gunshot fracture of the thigh on July 2, leg amputated [DIED July 14, buried in the Schwartz cornfield, reinterred in D-31 in the New York Plot, age 18]

Pvt. George O. White, Company F, 19th Maine, wounded in the shoulder

Pvt. Henry P. White, Company G, 57th Virginia, shot in the leg and arm on July 3, captured, arm amputated [DIED July 27, buried there in Yard B, Row 2 on the hill between the Bushman and Schwartz farms; disinterred on June 13, 1872, to Richmond in Box #3]

Pvt. John E. White, Company D, 53rd Pennsylvania, wounded in the hand and in the side of the abdomen on July 2 [DIED July 11, buried in the Schwartz cornfield, reinterred in A-48 in the Pennsylvania Plot]

Cpl. Lishur G. White, Company K, 20th Massachusetts, wounded

Pvt. Luther White, Company K, 20th Massachusetts, hit in the head, tearing off a portion of his ear, shattered his jaw, laid open his throat, revived at graveside by a violent drop of his stretcher, transferred to Chestnut Hill Hospital, Philadelphia, where he was expected to live

Pvt. Emmet M. Whitmore, Company E, 111th New York, shot in the intestines on July 3 [DIED July 11 at the Third Division Hospital, buried on Michael Trostle's "Walnut Row," reinterred in D-58 in the New York Plot, age 21]

Pvt. Mark L. Whitney, Company B, 19th Maine, wounded in the leg on July 2

James Whitson, Virginia, mortally wounded in the leg, leg amputated [probably DIED]

Cpl. Lindley H. Whittaker, Company C, 19th Maine, wounded

Pvt. Henry Widger, Company I, 1st Minnesota, wounded in the hip on July 2

Capt. Ephraim Wood, 125th New York, shot through the bowels on July 3

Pvt. James W. Wickham, Company E, 122nd New York [Sixth Corps], mortally wounded July 3 [DIED July 3, buried on the Schwartz Farm opposite White Run, reinterred in E-31 in the New York Plot, age 37]

Pvt. Timothy Wiley, Company H, 20th Massachusetts, wounded

Junior Second Lt. Henry S. Wilkinson, Company B, 9th Virginia, age 27, clerk, shot in the head on July 3, captured, treated at the Second Division Hospital [DIED on April 21, 1864, at Johnson's Island, Ohio, of chronic diarrhea, buried there in Block 23, Grave #4]

Cpl. George H. Willey, Company H, 19th Maine, wounded in the abdomen [DIED July 24, reinterred in D-7 in the Maine Plot, age 20, single]

Sgt. Albert N. Williams, Company G, 19th Maine, mortally wounded [DIED July 3]

Pvt. Henry N. Williams, Company K, 19th Maine, mortally wounded [DIED July 18]

Pvt. James A. Williams, Company E, 56th Virginia, gunshot fracture of the hip on July 3, captured [DIED July 19, buried in Row 1, Yard D in the Jacob Schwartz cornfield by Rock Creek; disinterred on June 13, 1872, to Richmond with 110 others in ten large boxes labeled "S"]

Pvt. Peter Williams, Company I, 20th Massachusetts, wounded

Pvt. John E. Williamson, Company D, 27th Connecticut, wounded

Pvt. J. Wilson, Company G, 19th Massachusetts, wounded July 2 [DIED July 2 at the Second Division Hospital of his wounds, *not listed in the unit casualty report or in the state Adjutant General Office reports—this could be Cpl. S. A. Wilson, Company D, 19th Maine (see below), who died the same day in the same hospital*]

Cpl. Jesse A. Wilson, Company D, 19th Maine, mortally wounded on July 3 [DIED July 3 at the Second Division Hospital, age 19, single]
Cpl. S. A. Wilson, Company D, 19th Maine, wounded July 2 [DIED July 2 at the Second Division Hospital]
Cpl. Nehemiah W. Winship, Company K, 86th New York [Third Corps], wounded July 2 [DIED, buried on the Schwartz Farm opposite White Run, reinterred in D-53 in the New York Plot, age 23]
Capt. Ephraim Wood, Company H, 125th New York, shot in the abdomen on July 3 [DIED July 4 at the Third Division Hospital, age 44]
Cpl. Francis C. Wood, Company D, 19th Maine, wounded in the arm
Pvt. George E. Wood, Company A, 20th Massachusetts, wounded
Pvt. James J. Wood, Company I, 114th Pennsylvania [Third Corps], wounded July 2 [DIED July 3, buried on the Schwartz Farm opposite White Run, reinterred in A-79 in the Pennsylvania Plot]
Pvt. William F. Wood, Company H, 19th Maine, wounded in the leg
Pvt. Thomas Woodman, Company F, 20th Massachusetts, wounded
Lt. George Augustus Woodruff, Battery I, 1st U.S. Artillery, "Rickett's Battery," wounded July 3, treated at the Granite School House aid station [DIED July 4]
Pvt. Daniel G. Wright, Company A, 20th Indiana [Third Corps], shot in the left hip on July 2 [DIED July 21 at the Third Division Hospital, reinterred in D-2 in the Indiana Plot]
Sgt. Henry C. Wright, Company A, 1st Minnesota, wounded in the head on July 2 [DIED July 6]
Sgt. James A. Wright, Company F, 1st Minnesota, wounded in the face and neck by splinters and lead fragments when a bullet shattered the stock of his gun on July 3
Pvt. John S. Wynkoop, Company E, 148th Pennsylvania, wounded July 2

Pvt. Thomas G. Yale, Company D, 27th Connecticut [DIED August 26 in a Philadelphia hospital]
Pvt. William P. Yearger, 22nd Georgia, wounded in left leg, leg amputated [DIED between July 11 and 14, burial site not identified at the Schwartz Farm, possibly reinterred south before the general reinterment of 1872]
Pvt. Benjamin Young, Company H, 19th Maine, wounded in the neck

Brig. Gen. Samuel K. Zook, Second Corps, First Division, Third Brigade, wounded in the abdomen on July 2, examined at the First

Division Hospital late July 2 [DIED July 3, in a private home just off the Baltimore Pike]

SOURCES

Federal Civil War Records

Records of the Adjutant General's Office

National Archives and Records Administration Record Group 94

Entry 89, Registers of Regular Army Enlistments 1798-1914

Entry 119, Registers of Deceased Soldiers, Volunteers, 1861-64

Entry 520, General Index to the Carded Records, Volunteer Organizations, Civil War

Entry 544, Field Records of Hospitals, 1821-1912

Entry 621, "File A" and "Bound Manuscripts," 1861-65

Entry 624, "File F," 1861-89

Entry 643, Register of Deaths, Regular Army, 1860-89

Entry 650, Registers of Deaths, Volunteers, 1861-65

Entry 652, Regimental Casualty Lists, Civil War, 1861-65

Entry 653, Army Corps, Army and Departmental Casualty Lists, Civil War, 1861-65

Entry 699, Index to Army Corps Organization-Hospital-Civil War Period

Entry 700, Index to Civil War Hospitals

Books and Articles

Andrews, C. C., *Minnesota in the Civil and Indian Wars 1861*. 2 volumes. (St. Paul, Minnesota: Pioneer Press Company, 1891).

Busey, John, *These Honored Dead: The Union Casualties at Gettysburg*. (Hightstown, New Jersey: Longstreet House, 1988).

Busey, John and David G, Martin, *Regimental Strengths and Losses at Gettysburg*. (Hightstown, New Jersey: Longstreet House, 1986).

Frey, J. G., "J. G. Frey's Book" (of Union interment sites by state). Original at Lee's Headquarter Museum, Gettysburg, Pennsylvania; copy in the Gettysburg National Military Park files.

Harrison, Kathleen Georg and John W. Busey, *Nothing But Glory: Pickett's Division at Gettysburg*. (Hightstown, New Jersey: Longstreet House, 1987).

Krick, Robert K., *The Gettysburg Death Roster*. (Dayton, Ohio: Press of the Morningside Bookshop, 1981).

Raus, Edward, "Union Civil War Veterans Buried at Gettysburg." Manuscript in the Gettysburg National Military Park files. (Gettysburg, Pennsylvania, 1977).

Regimental histories of individual regiments in the Second Corps.

Stryker, William S., editor, *Record of Officers and Men of New Jersey in the Civil War 1861-65.* 2 volumes. (Trenton, New Jersey: John L. Murphy, Publisher, 1876).

Wills, David, "The Soldiers' National Cemetery, Gettysburg, Pennsylvania." (Gettysburg, Pennsylvania: 1864; 1978 University Microfilm International, Ann Arbor, Michigan, reprint of the 1864 cemetery listing compiled by Wills).

Governmental Publications

Annual Report of the Adjutant Gen. of the State of Maine for the Year Ending December 31, 1863. (Augusta, Maine: Stevens & Sayward, Printers to the State, 1863).

Gettysburg National Military Park. Tablets on the Pennsylvania Memorial listing the names of Pennsylvania troops present at the battle. Alphabetical listing of names compiled by Gettysburg Park staff in the Gettysburg National Military Park files.

History and Roster of Maryland Volunteers, War of 1861-5. Volume 1. Prepared under authority of the General Assembly of Maryland by L. Allison Wilmer, J. H. Jarrett and George W. F. Vernon. (Baltimore: Press of Guggenheimer & Company, n. d.).

History of Pennsylvania Volunteers 1861-5. Volume 1. Prepared in compliance with acts of the legislature by Samuel P. Bates. (Harrisburg, Pennsylvania: B. Singerly, State Printer, 1869).

Massachusetts Soldiers, Sailors and Marines in the Civil War. 8 volumes and index. Compiled under the direction of Jesse F. Stevens, Adjutant General. (Norwood, Massachusetts: Norwood Press, 1931).

New York Monuments Commission for the Battlefields of Gettysburg and Chattanooga. *Final Report on the Battlefield of Gettysburg.* Volume 1. Edited by William F. Fox. (Albany, New York: J. B. Lyon Company, Printers, 1900).

Official Roster of the Soldiers of the State of Ohio in the War of the Rebellion 1861-1866. Compiled under direction of the Roster Commission. Published by authority of the General Assembly. (Cincinnati: The Ohio Valley Press, 1888).

Record of Service of Connecticut Men in the Army & Navy of the U. S. During the War of the Rebellion. Compiled by authority of the General Assembly under direction of the Connecticut Adjutant General's Office. (Hartford, Connecticut: Press of the Case, Lockwood & Brainard Company, 1899).

Record of Service of Michigan Volunteers in the Civil War 1861-1865. Published by authority of the Senate and House of Representatives of the Michigan Legislature, under the direction of Brig. Gen. George H. Brown, Adjutant General, Kalamazoo, Michigan: Ihling Brothers & Everard Stationers, Printers and Publishers.

Report of the Adjutant General of the State of Illinois. Volume 5 and 8, containing reports for the years 1861-66. (Springfield, Illinois: Journal Company, Printers and Binders, 1901).

Report of the Adjutant Gen. of the State of Indiana. Volume 4 and 8, containing reports for the year 1861-65. (Indianapolis: Alexander H. Conner, State Printer, 1868).

Revised Register of the Soldiers and Sailors of New Hampshire in the War of the Rebellion 1861-1866. Prepared and published by authority of the legislature by Augustus D. Ayling, Adjutant General. (n. p.: Ira C. Evans, Public Printer, 1895).

Revised Roster of Vermont Volunteers and Lists of Vermonters who Served in the Army and Navy of the United States During the War of the Rebellion 1861-66. Compiled by authority of the General Assembly under direction of Theodore S. Peck, Adjutant General. (n. p.: Press of the Watchman Publishing Company, Publishers and Printers, 1892).

Rhode Island Adjutant General Office. *Annual Report 1861-70.*

Roster of Wisconsin Volunteers War of the Rebellion, 1861-1865. Compiled by authority of the legislature, under the direction of Jeremiah M. Rusk, Governor, and Chandler P. Chapman, Adjutant Gen. (Madison, Wisconsin: Democrat Printing Company, State Printers, 1886).

United States War Department. *The War of the Rebellion: A Compilation of the Official Records of the Union and Confederate Armies.* Series 1, Volume 27, Part 1. (Washington, D. C.: Government Printing Office, 1889).

Appendix 6

SUPPLYING THE SECOND CORPS HOSPITAL

The work of supplying the field hospitals at Gettysburg was a task of monumental proportions. Each field hospital had a hospital fund from which to buy the barest of necessary supplies for hospital maintenance and patient care. The following document details the July 1863 purchases from the Second Corps Hospital fund.

> Abstract of provision issued from the 1st day of July 1863 to the 31st day of July 1863 to sick in field hospital of 2d Army Corps near Gettysburg Pa—under charge of Justin Dwinelle Surgeon U.S.A. by Capt. Thos England U. S. Vols.

A monthly statement of the Hospital fund— Dolls. Cts.

Dr—

To balance due[,] hospital cash [/] month[,] 12800 rations[,] being whole amount due ~~this month~~ at 20 c[en]ts per ration—$2560.00

Cr[edit] — Issued

By the following provisions at contract prices

400	lbs	Pork	@	8c/ per lb.	$32.00
13015	"	Hardbread	"	5 1/2 c/" "	$715.82 1/2

3600	"	Fresh Beef	"	9 1/2 " " $342.00
1.58 1/2	bbls	Flour	"	6.75c/ per bbl $8.76 196
2 bushels of beans			"	3.60c/ " bushel $7.20
1485	lbs	coffee	"	39c/ " lb. $579.15
62 3/16	"	tea	"	95c/ " " $59.08
2703	"	sugar	"	13c/ " " $351.39
264 7/16	"	candles	"	25 1/2 c/ " " $67.43 1/2
249	"	Soap	"	8 " " " $19.92
9 16/50	bushels	Salt	"	64 " " bush. $5.96 1/2
Total issued and expended				$2188.72 1/2
Balance due this month				371.27 1/2[1]

Obviously, the hospital fund was not going to be able to meet the extreme emergency in the aftermath of Gettysburg. For that, the services of the United States Sanitary Commission, the United States Christian Commission, the Adams Express Company, and countless smaller relief agencies and volunteer aid societies were needed. While most of these groups left few if any records, the Sanitary Commission kept scrupulous and detailed accounts of its activities.

The efforts of the Sanitary Commission at Gettysburg stagger the mind, even by twenty-first century standards. In a town overwhelmed by invasion, devastated by three days of intense battle, cut off from the outside world, and stripped of virtually all useful supplies by both

1. Union Field Hospitals Vertical File, Gettysburg National Military Park Library.

friend and foe alike, the accomplishments are truly Herculean. Dietary specialties such as lemons and oranges, chocolate, pickles, oysters, catsup, dried fruit and all types of jellies demonstrated the first stirrings of the fledgling science of nutrition and specialized dietary supplements. The amount and variety of supplies brought by wagon and railroad into town after the battle are best illustrated by the following statement:

TABULATED STATEMENT OF ISSUES

The following is a statement of the quantities of the principle articles distributed by the Commission to the wounded upon the field at Gettysburg, subsequent to the battle. The perishable articles (amounting to over 60 tons) were taken to the ground in refrigerated cars:

Of Articles of Clothing, etc., viz.:

Of Drawers, (woolen)	5,310 pairs
" (cotton)	1,833 "
Shirts, (woolen)	7,158 "
" (cotton)	3,266 "
Pillows	2,114 "
Pillow Cases	264
Bed Sacks	1,630
Blankets	1,007
Sheets	274
Wrappers	508
Handkerchiefs	2,659
Stockings, (woolen)	3,560 pairs
" (cotton)	2,258 "
Bed Utensils	728
Towels and Napkins	10,000
Sponges	2,300
Combs	1,500
Buckets	200
Soap, castile	250 pounds
Oil Silk	300 yards
Tin Basins, Cups, etc	7,000
Old Linen, Bandages, etc	110 barrels
Water Tanks	7
Water Coolers	46

Bay Rum and Cologne Water	225 bottles
Fans	3,500
Chloride of Lime	11 barrels
Shoes and Slippers	4,000 pairs
Crutches	1,200
Lanterns	180
Candles	350 pounds
Canvas	300 sq yds
Mosquito Netting	648 pieces
Paper	237 quires
Pants, Coats, Hats	189 pieces
Plaster	16 rolls

Of Articles of Sustenance, viz.:

Of Fresh Poultry and Mutton	11,000 pounds
" Butter	6,430 "
" Eggs, (chiefly collected for the occasion at farm-houses in Pennsylvania and New Jersey)	8,500 dozen
" Garden Vegetables	675 bushels
" Berries	48 bushels
" Bread	12,900 loaves
Ice	20,000 pounds
Concentrated Beef Soup	3,800 "
" Milk	12,500 "
Prepared Farinaceous Food	7,000 "
Dried Fruit	3,500 "
Jellies and Conserves	2,000 jars
Tamarinds	750 gallons
Lemons	116 boxes
Oranges	46 "
Coffee	850 pounds
Chocolate	831 "
Tea	426 "
White Sugar	6,000 "
Syrups, (Lemon, etc.)	785 bottles
Brandy	1,250 "
Whiskey	1,168 "
Wine	1,148 "
Ale	600 gallons
Biscuit, Crackers, and Rusk	134 barrels
Preserved Meats	500 pounds

Preserved Fish	3,600 "
Pickles	400 gallons
Tobacco	100 pounds
Tobacco Pipes	1,000
Indian Meal	1,621 pounds
Starch	1,074 "
Codfish	3,848 "
Canned Fruit	582 cans
Canned Oysters	72 "
Brandy Peaches	303 jars
Catsup	43 "
Vinegar	24 bottles
Jamaica Ginger	43 jars [2]

2. *Report on the Operations of the Sanitary Commission During and After the Battle of Gettysburg*, pp. 21-22.

Appendix 7
WHO DROWNED IN ROCK CREEK, AND WHEN?

One of the great challenges in telling the story of the Second Corps Hospital is determining exactly when Rock Creek catastrophically flooded its banks, and who (if anyone) was drowned. That the creek did indeed flood is clear from the number and variety of accounts of the event. However, the issue is clouded by several difficulties.

For one thing, Rock Creek has altered significantly since 1863. While the creek bed follows the Warren map very closely, the dam at McAllister's Mill is no longer there. This means that the water impoundment behind it is gone, leaving the level of the stream somewhat lower than it was in 1863.

Second, people were so busy trying to save the wounded in the harried days following the battle that they simply did not take the time to note down the exact date. Pastors worked straight through Sunday without ever once realizing it was the Lord's Day. People often described the same event, but placed it on different dates.

Contemporary accounts and weather records indicate that the heaviest rains fell between July 4 and 6. The actual date for the flooding along Rock Creek, however, is notoriously hard to pin down. The following considerations help narrow down the window of possibility:

1) The only volunteer nurse to mention the flooding (other than Mary Cadwell Fisher, whose July 9 date corresponds only with that of 4th Ohio Hospital Steward Charles H. Merrick) is Ellen Orbison Harris. She arrived at the Second Corps hospitals on Sunday, July 5.

2) Cornelia Hancock, a careful observer and meticulous recorder of camp minutiae, does not mention the flooding. She arrived at the

Second Corps hospitals early in the morning on Tuesday, July 7.

3) Capt. Benjamin F. Thompson, 111th New York, marched away from Gettysburg with his regiment to Quakertown in the late afternoon of Sunday, July 5. After staying the night, he returned to Gettysburg on doctor's orders, arriving on Monday morning, July 6, where he finds the Third Division hospital "on the bank of a stream and led up into a clover field," not in the bottomlands of Rock Creek. He also makes no mention of flooding.

4) When Cornelia Hancock and her party, as well as George Anna Woolsey and her mother, finally reached Gettysburg, their train was forced to halt at Rock Creek. The original bridge, destroyed by the Confederates, had been rebuilt, but the replacement span had been swept away by high water before their arrival on the evening of Monday, July 6.

This seems to indicate early morning, July 6 as the time of the flooding. However, the difficulty is further compounded by trying to correlate all the divergent contemporary accounts:

Samuel Toombs
New Jersey Historian—flooding on July 4
"wounded men . . . some were drowned"

> During the morning of July 4th a heavy rain fell—an occurrence which seemed to succeed every great battle, and hundreds of disabled soldiers were without shelter, and unable to reach any. The water in Rock Creek rose to a considerable height and in immense volume rushed southward with great force, in several instances carrying down with it the wounded men along its banks who were unable to move to higher ground, and some were drowned.[1]

Francis A. Walker
Historian of the Second Corps—flooding on July 4
"helpless prisoners" were in "danger of drowning"

> Towards morning came on a terrible storm, one of those instances which seem to establish a connection between battles and rainfall. In this instance, at any rate, the downpour was in proportion to the violence of the cannonade. The soldiers were drenched in an instant; and

1. Toombs, *New Jersey Troops in the Gettysburg Campaign*, p. 327.

sudden torrents swept over the hills, as if to wash out the stains of the great battle. One of the Second Corps hospitals, around which had been collected hundreds of the Confederate wounded, was flooded; and some of the helpless prisoners were actually in danger of drowning where they lay, but were with great haste dragged or carried to higher ground.[2]

Lt. Charles Fuller
61st New York—flooding on July 4—secondhand
"some men . . . it was said, drowned"

The day of July 4 we had a drenching rain. Some men out lying in the low places and who could not move were, it was said, drowned. On the whole, I presume the rain was a benefit to the wounded.[3]

Pvt. Elbert Corbin
1st New York Light Artillery, Battery B, detailed to care for twelve men from the First New York Light Artillery at the Second Corps Hospital—heavy rain on July 4
"thousands of the wounded were exposed"

SUNDAY, July 5—9 P.M. I was kept very busy in the rain all day yesterday, taking care of the wounded. It was a hard storm, and thousands of the wounded were exposed, without cover.[4]

Sgt. T. P. Meyer
148th Pennsylvania Pioneers—flooding on or after July 4
"a number of wounded" drowned

In the field hospital a mile to our rear on the low banks of Rock Creek, many desperately wounded were lying upon the ground. Consequent on the heavy rains of the 4th, the stream rose suddenly, and overflowed the ground, so that a number of the wounded were drowned before they could be moved to higher ground.[5]

---

2. Walker, *History of the Second Army Corps*, pp. 306-7.
3. Fuller, *Personal Recollections*, p. 102.
4. Letter of Pvt. Elbert Corbin, July 5, 1863, courtesy of Mr. Stephen J. Dreher.
5. Muffly, *The Story of Our Regiment*, p. 467.

Philadelphia Public Ledger
flooding on July 5—no one drowned

An account in the *Philadelphia Public Ledger* states that a violent thunder storm yesterday (Sunday, July 5th) would have drowned some of the wounded "had not the most extraordinary efforts been put forward to prevent it."[6]

Dr. Theodore Dimon
General Agent of the State of New York for the Relief of Sick, Wounded, and Discharged Soldiers—flooding on July 5
"the wounded did not suffer appreciably"

Doctor Dimon does not mention drownings, but he does mention flooding and a date.

> While the surgeons were toiling night and day for this vast number of wounded (about 4,000), the freshet occurred which followed the battle on Sunday July 5th. The creeks at this point commenced overflowing their banks, and in the midst of the storm new ground had to be selected, cleared up, and the wounded conveyed to it. . . . So carefully and systematically was this sudden removal affected, that the wounded did not suffer appreciably thereby.[7]

As General Agent of the State of New York for the Relief of Sick, Wounded, and Discharged Soldiers, had any New York troops been washed downstream, Dimon would certainly have discovered it and reported it to his superior, John F. Seymour, General Agent of the State of New York. With sixteen regiments and two battalions of New Yorkers in the Second Corps, it is highly unlikely that there would be no New York casualties involved in a wholesale drowning of both Union and Confederate wounded.

Capt. Louis C. Duncan
Medical Corps, U. S. Army—flooding after July 5
some patients "were in danger of drowning, scrambling out as best they could"

> The division hospitals were now located together among the trees in a bend on the west side of Rock Creek, as shown

---

6. *Philadelphia Public Ledger*, July 6, 1863.
7. Dimon, *Report of the General Agent of the State of New York*, p. 53.

in a number of maps. The location was safe and convenient, but the site was on very low ground. There was rain on the fourth and still more on the fifth, overflowing the low ground, and a part of the hospital. Some patients were in danger of drowning, scrambling out as best they could. Many were left lying in the mud.[8]

John B. Linn
battlefield visitor from Philadelphia—flooding on July 8
"six rebels" drowned

The diary of battlefield visitor John B. Linn seems to indicate that only Confederates perished in the flash flood. Lodging with Gettysburg Pastor Bucher, discussion over dinner turned to events out at the Second Corps hospitals. "He told us of six rebels drowning today [July 8] from the rising of the streams in which they were lying wounded. The suffering in the 2nd Corps [is] pitiful, men particularly rebels still lying there unattended." Sadly, neither Linn nor any of his companions made any efforts to go to the Schwartz Farm and see if there was any way that they could be of assistance to the "pitiful" sufferers; instead, they sat and swapped stories of the battle with various visitors that dropped by the house until it was time for bed.[9]

Hospital Steward Charles H. Merrick
4th Ohio Volunteer Infantry—flooding on July 9
needed to "wade in water" to remove "several hundred wounded and dying men"
no mention of drowning

The mean little creek got mad and rose over seven feet. It flooded our Camp so quick we had to wade in the water to remove the wounded. It was an awful thing to hurry out several hundred wounded and dying men, the rain falling in torrents all the time. How I did work, and how the poor fellows did suffer.[10]

---

8. Duncan, *The Medical Department of the United States Army*, p. 241.
9. Linn, "Journal of my trip to the battlefield at Gettysburg," p. 10.
10. Charles H. Merrick, letter to his sister Min, July 10, 1863, William P. Palmer Collection, Container 1, Folder 3, MSS 3088, Western Reserve Historical Society, Cleveland, Ohio [underlining is by Merrick]. Merrick dated the flooding as taking place July 9; however, by July 9, all the Second Corps hospitals were high and dry on the farmland of Jacob Schwartz.

Mary Cadwell Fisher
volunteer relief worker from York, Pennsylvania—flooding on July 9 three men from Massachusetts, two Georgians, a "raw Irish boy," and a man from Maine drowned

The account of Mary Cadwell Fisher, who, along with her son and two other ladies, had personally delivered a load of relief supplies to Gettysburg, writes of a mixed group of Confederates and Union men who were drowned. On Monday, July 6, Mary was "by request, assigned to the Second Army Corps' Hospital, temporarily located on the ground along Rock creek, about two and a half miles south of Gettysburg." Although she did not officially start work there until Tuesday, she visited the Second Corps Hospital on Monday evening.

> One of the saddest of all the saddest incidents crowded into this week of suffering was the fate of some boys whom I found on Wednesday [July 8] evening as I was about to leave the ground. When I had reached the ravine which lay below the sloping hills [a tributary of the Rock Creek floodplain], I found a little group of young men who had not been badly wounded, but were temporarily unfit for duty. They had kindled a fire and drawn around it some logs, upon which they had stretched themselves to dry their soaked uniforms. Three of them were from the old "Bay State." There were also two Georgians, prisoners; one raw Irish boy, who was the life of the party, and a down Easter from the forests of Maine. In spite of their discomforts they were a jolly set, the oldest not more than eighteen years. As usual they begged me for a "chaw of tobaker." Unfortunately, I had exhausted my supply, but found in the depths of my pocket some calamus root and some cinnamon bark which they willingly took as a substitute. "Oh," said one, "this makes me think of home and the pies my mother made! When I had to grind the cinnamon for her she always gave me a piece." They all began to talk about their homes, telling me their simple stories. Even the Irish boy fondly recalled the memory of the little cabin in the Green Island where he was born, and longed to see his sisters and brothers with whom he shared his scanty meal.
>
> They begged me to stay with them, but it was late, and my faithful escort was impatiently waiting to take me to my night quarters in town, and I reluctantly left them with the promise

to go at noon the next day and take the tobacco and some pies if I could procure them. *A sharp, sudden shower came up in the night and converted the little stream into a roaring torrent. The little band of light-hearted merry boys, who had borne hunger, thirst and fatigues of many a weary day's march, had escaped the deadly battle and fatal shell only to die in the midst of safety. They were all swept away without a moment's warning and drowned in the flood.*"[11]

Capt. Thomas Livermore
Second Corps Ambulance Chief—flooding on an uncertain date
"drove some of the wounded from the right bank"
no drownings

Second Corps medical director Alexander N. Dougherty had charged Livermore to select a new site for the corps hospitals, one that was "removed from the range of projectiles for a general field hospital, where all the wounded could be carried and provided with shelter and treatment until the battle was over."

After riding the countryside seeking a good location, Livermore found what appeared to be an ideal spot.

> I selected a spot on Rock Creek about a mile and a half down the stream from the crossing of the Baltimore road, I should think. At this point it was of sufficient volume to afford water for all necessary purposes. The left bank was a hillside, and the right bank was level and low and perfectly accessible from the road leading from the field of battle, and both hillside and level were clothed with trees nearly free from undergrowth. The hillside afforded a fine place for the wounded, being sheltered by the trees and having perfect drainage, and the level was needed for hospital wagons. My selection met with the approval of the medical director. I believe that the creek was raised by a rain which followed the battle, and drove some of the wounded from the right bank, but they ought not to have been there.[12]

---

11. Fisher, "A Week on Gettysburg Field." Emphasis added.
12. Livermore, *Days and Events*, pp. 258-59.

Rev. Andrew Boyd Cross
Christian Commission—flooding on an uncertain date at the Second Corps, Third Division Hospital site
"some of the wounded were drowned"

The rain not only made the ground at this [Third] division hospital muddy, but at times so overflowed, that some of the wounded were drowned for want of help to move them from the low and flat places; at times it was with difficulty we could walk through the hospital.[13]

Reverand Williams
Sanitary Commission—flooding on an uncertain date at the Second Corps, Third Division Hospital site
"the sudden rise of the little stream" caused flooding

There were nearly or quite a thousand Rebels, most of them severely wounded, lying on the outskirts of the hospital, shrieking and continually crying for assistance. The appearance of those connected with the Third Division of this corps beggars description. Destitute of clothing, many of them nearly naked, lying in the mud—for the sudden rise of the little stream by which they had been placed rendered it impossible to avoid this—cursing, praying, begging their visitors to put an end to their sufferings; here one and there another laid out by himself to die, these wretched men made the strongest appeal to Christian sympathy and benevolence.[14]

Capt. Azor Nickerson
8th Ohio Volunteer Infantry—flooding on an uncertain date
"quite a number of the more helpless ones" drowned

Of course no one foresaw that the little stream which ran around us would soon overflow its banks, or doubtless more men would have been left, at least for this emergency. As it was, the stream, swollen to an unusual height, did soon overflow its banks, and sweeping through our dismal ranks, drowned many helpless fellows before the few attendants there could get them out of the way. . . . The overflow was

---

13. Cross, *Battle of Gettysburg and the Christian Commission*, p. 14.
14. *United States Sanitary Commission Report*. Quote of either Rev. E. F. Williams or Rev. J. W. M. Williams—no first name is given.

probably not over two feet in depth, but to men who could not raise their heads, this, like Mercutio's wound, was enough—it sufficed. The few attendants there worked like Trojans, but it was impossible to save all, and quite a number of the more helpless ones were drowned within the range of my limited vision.[15]

Robert Laird Stewart
Historian of the 140th Pennsylvania—flooding on an uncertain date
"helpless patients" were saved from drowning

The field hospital, which had been so directly in range of the enemy's guns in the afternoon was now threatened with a new peril. In the lower levels of the valley the ground quickly flooded and it required prompt action to save some of the helpless patients from drowning.[16]

John M. Scoville
1st New York Light Artillery, Battery B—flooding on uncertain date
"men who were lying on the banks of the stream . . . drowned"

It was terrible! Men who were lying on the banks of the stream and were unable to move, remained in their helplessness and drowned. We who were equally helpless were lying where we could see the waters cover them, extinguishing the little spark of life left from the wounds.[17]

Charles Minard
1st New York Light Artillery, Battery B—flooding on uncertain date
rescued two men from going "under the water"

Minard had stayed behind to help his wounded comrade, John M. Scoville. After making sure that his friend was out of danger, Minard rushed back to the water's edge to assist in getting the helpless away from the danger.

I pulled two of the wounded up the hill at one time; I had one by the arm and the other by the hair; I had no time to get

---

15. Nickerson, "Personal Recollections of of Two Visits to Gettysburg," pp. 22-23.
16. Stewart, *History of the One Hundred and Fortieth Regiment*, p. 127.
17. "Wounded at Gettysburgh. The War Experiences of Commander Scoville, of Moses Summers Post," *The Syracuse Sunday Herald*, March 8, 1885, p. 5.

a better hold, for if I had let go of either he would have gone under the water.[18]

Unknown Newspaper Writer
The Syracuse Sunday Herald—flooding on an uncertain date
"the creek had risen very rapidly, flooding the whole space...."

A heavy rain had been falling and the creek had risen very rapidly, flooding the whole space where Scoville and his comrades were.[19]

J. Howard Wert
local resident and historian—flooding on an uncertain date
"twenty are supposed to have been lost," and "a considerable number" drowned

After Gettysburg, as after every great battle, there were copious rains. The men who brought the wounded back from the front to the field hospitals were unaware of the treacherous character of the little streams along which these were pitched. Not much more than rivulets in dry weather, they became wide and swollen onrushing torrents after heavy showers. Many wounded were placed in rows in the meadows and flats along the streams, wherever trees afforded shade to wait the erection of tents. With the sudden rising of the streams numbers of these helpless men were washed away. On White Run some twenty are supposed to have been lost from the meadows of Moses Schwartz and Aaron Sheely in front of the Second Corps Hospital. A considerable number met the same fate along the flats of Rock Creek. Some of the corpses were subsequently discovered lodged on bushes along the Monocacy river in Maryland.[20]

Rev. Mr. Parvin
Christian Commission—flooding on an uncertain date
many "in danger of drowning"

After the battle in the heavy showers, many of the wounded on the bank of a brook were in danger of drowning

---

18. *Ibid.*
19. *Ibid.*
20. Wert, "In the Hospitals of Gettysburg, July, 1863."

from the rapid rise of the water. There were no stretchers, and some of the badly wounded could not be carried in the arms of the men without great pain. "Lay them on my back," said a Delegate, going into the water on his hands and knees, and thus, bent with his face to the ground, he conveyed them tenderly out of the reach of danger.[21]

Ellen Orbison Harris
Secretary of the Ladies' Aid Society of Philadelphia—flooding on an uncertain date
"our wounded in numbers have been drowned"

Ellen Orbison Harris, who had been at the Second Corps hospitals since July 4, penned a weary letter on July 9:

> My Dear Dr.: . . . Am full of work and sorrow. The condition of things here beggars all description. Our dead lie unburied, and our wounded neglected. . . . Our wounded in numbers have been drowned by the sudden rising of the waters around, and thousands of them are still naked and starving. God pity us! pity us![22]

Surgeon-in-Charge Justin Dwinelle
Second Corps Hospital—flooding on an uncertain date
several of "our men" were rumored to have been "swept down the creek and drowned," but were not

One of the more mystifying aspects of this entire incident is the response of Surgeon Justin Dwinelle, head of the combined Second Corps hospitals, in his official report to Doctor Dougherty.

> We have not escaped the usual silly storys [*sic*] put in motion by foolish, mischievous, and excitable characters of both sexes who always congregate where there are scenes of horror and blood to gratify a disgusting morbid curiosity. It has been reported that the number of deaths in our hospital amounted to one hundred & twenty five a day. Not one sixth of that number died in any one twenty four hours. *It has also extensively circulated that several of our men*

21. Rev. Edward P. Smith, *Incidents of the United States Christian Commission.* (Philadelphia: J. B. Lippincott & Co., 1869), p. 173.
22. *Fifth Semi-Annual Report of the Ladies' Aid Society*, p. 13.

were swept down the creek and drowned. I am happy to state that no such occurance [*sic*] *took place.* One would suppose that the realities were bad enough to satisfy even a sensationalist without adding to their horrors by falsehood.[23]

Doctor Dwinelle consistently shows himself to be a man of accuracy, precision, and honor in his medical report, his other wartime correspondence, and in the comments of those that came in contact with him. Can there be a discrepancy here, or could the drownings have been of Confederates only—note carefully his phrase "several of *our men* were swept down the creek and drowned?"[24]

Mr. R. L. Jones
Historical Technician of the National Park Service, October 25, 1933—flooding on an uncertain date
"a group of Confederate wounded" drowned

That this is the case seems to be borne out in a letter from Mr. R. L. Jones, Historical Technician of the National Park Service, to Mr. Ambrose Cort, Sr., on October 25, 1933, in which he says: "We have found reference to a group of Confederate wounded left on the bank of a creek, a sudden rise of which drowned and carried some of them away."[25] As to what that "reference" was, Jones does not say, nor could Mr. Cort shed any additional light on the issue.

Jane Boswell Moore
Independent Maryland Nurse and Newspaper Columnist—flooding on an uncertain date
Confederate wounded near the banks of Rock Creek, no mention of drowning

Jane Boswell Moore also seems to bear out the fact that it was Confederates who perished, although not directly mentioning drownings.

---

23. Justin Dwinelle, Final Report of Wounded in Second Corps Hospital, August 10, 1863 [Manuscript report of the Second Corps hospital operations during the Battle of Gettysburg, MSC 129, National Library of Medicine, Bethesda, Maryland; copy in the Union Field Hospital Vertical File, Gettysburg National Military Park Library]. Emphasis added.
24. Emphasis added.
25. R. L. Jones, letter to Ambrose Cort, Sr., October 25, 1933, photocopy in the Hospitalization after Gettysburg: Personal Accounts Vertical File, Gettysburg National Military Park Library

> For more than four weeks (beginning the first few days after the fight) we were engaged in the field hospitals of the Second Army Corps. . . . Words utterly fall short in describing the appearance of those woods in the morning we reached the hospital, after riding through swollen streams, amid the still unburied bodies of men and horses that lay putrefying on the field.
>
> The site of the hospital, which had been hurriedly chosen, was in a grove of trees on a piece of rising ground. Surrounded nearly on all sides by a ravine, along which ran a creek near whose banks lay hundreds of wounded and dying Rebels, most of whom were exposed to the pitiless pelting of the storm. . . . Miserable little shelter-tents alone protected them from the rain, whilst numbers of the poor wretched Rebels had not even these, but were exposed through all the heavy rain of Tuesday night, with scarcely covering enough to keep warm in dry weather.[26]

The United States Christian Commission for the Army and Navy. For the Year 1863. Second Annual Report
flooding on an uncertain date
Confederates "lying in the mud" due to "the sudden rise of the little stream"

The second annual report of the Christian Commission also seems to bear out the fact that Confederates were caught in the flash flood along Rock Creek; however, there is no mention of drownings.

> In addition to the twenty-five hundred [Union wounded] previously mentioned, there were nearly or quite a thousand rebels, most of them severely wounded, lying on the outskirts of this hospital, shrieking and crying for assistance continually. The appearance of those connected with the hospital of the Third Division of this corps beggars description. Destitute of clothing, many of them nearly naked and covered with filth, without tents, lying in the mud—for the sudden rise of the little stream by which they had been placed rendered it impossible to avoid this.[27]

---

26. Moore, "An Incident in Gettysburg," pp. 104-5.
27. *The United States Christian Commission for the Army and Navy. For the Year 1863. Second Annual Report*, p. 71.

There is another account that gives a concrete date and time for the flooding:

First Sgt. Levi W. Baker
9th Massachusetts Battery—flooding on July 7

Baker was wounded in the "hip and shoulder, twice, severe" during the frantic July 2 action at the Trostle Farm. "I found myself completely disabled, and was ordered to the rear. . . . I was directed to the 3d Corps hospital on the Taneytown road, the east side of Little Round Top." There the ball was cut from his thigh by a hospital steward.[28]

> At daylight, every man that could walk was ordered to start for the new hospital on Rock Creek. As the present place was unsafe, it was vacated, and one or two miles southeast, in a piece of woods on either side of the creek, I found a large number of tents pitched, and under a gun tarpaulin, in the artillery hospital of the 3d Corps, I made my home from Saturday to Wednesday morning, July 7. Four yards from our shelter ran Rock Creek, three yards wide, with three to six inches of water running over a stony channel, two feet below the bank we were on. Of my companions not one had I ever seen before, and like myself they could care for themselves. The most severely wounded—a ball through both thighs–was the most cheerful. Considerable rain fell, but Rock Creek was not full.
>
> Wednesday morning at daylight, orders were, "All that can walk start for Gettysburg town." *It had rained all night; Rock Creek was a torrent, impassable, and we were obliged to start, as the ground where we were would soon be flooded.* We toiled on, scattering more and more, according to our ability to walk. *One of the causeways on the Baltimore pike was covered with eight or ten inches of water.*[29]

Sergeant Baker's account is significant for several important reasons:

1) He was in an ideal position to record the date and time—not well enough to be rushing about helping the more grievously wounded, but

---

28. Baker, *History of the Ninth Massachusetts Battery*, pp. 64, 86.
29. *Ibid.*, pp. 86-87. Emphasis added.

not so gravely injured as to be overwhelmed by concern for his life. Isolated as he was in an artillery invalid camp, he was free to observe and record what went on around him.

2) He was totally separate from the Second Corps hospital complex—Baker would have no reason to downplay or exaggerate the effects of the flooding in the Second Corps hospitals, as he might have had he actually been at those hospitals.

3) At the Third Corps Artillery Hospital, south of the reverse "S" of the Second Corps position, Rock Creek had cut a nine foot wide, two foot deep channel into the embankment. The effects of the flooding experienced at the flat floodplain position of the Second Corps Hospital on July 6 might very well not have overflowed the banks at Baker's higher location until the next day. Note his comment that "the ground where we were *would soon be flooded*." But would not Baker and his comrades have noticed any bodies floating downstream from the Second Corps Hospital if it had happened a day earlier?

4) The amount of water flowing over portions of the Baltimore Pike—"eight or ten inches"—indicates that considerable flooding was already well under way by the time Sergeant Baker and the other wounded from the invalid hospital were on the road to "Gettysburg town." If there was nearly a foot of standing water in parts of the Baltimore Pike, how much more would have already been raging through the low-lying ground of Captain Livermore's ill-chosen hospital position?

In the light of extensive research on this hospital, very early morning of July 6 still seems to be the date with the least contradictions, especially against the accounts of those who were present on the other dates and fail to mention such major occurrences as torrential rain, flooding, and drownings.

It appears certain that an indefinite number of Confederates were carried away by the rapid rise of the water, and drowned. That it was Confederates who perished, and not Northerners, is all the more likely in light of standard Civil War medical care. As Assistant Surgeon Francis M. Wafer of the 108th New York Volunteers points out: "I can confidently and earnestly assert that I have never seen any distinction in their [the Confederates'] treatment—more than attending to our own first, which is our duty."[30] Doctors, attendants, and volunteers

30. Wafer diary.

apparently rescued "our own" first, and some Southerners were consequently lost to the waters before they could be saved.

Until such a time as Historical Technician Jones' illusive "reference," or further documentation, is found concerning the date and time of the flooding, we may never know the full extent of the losses sustained by the Confederates in this tragic event.

Appendix 8
MEDICAL DEPARTMENT ORGANIZATIONAL POLICIES BEFORE AND AFTER THE BATTLE OF GETTYSBURG

In spite of the medical chaos created by the influx of so many wounded following the Battle of Gettysburg, the corps hospital system was a highly organized and well-thought-out system, as this 1862 Field Hospital Order from Jonathan Letterman shows. The order was drawn up based on the experiences of the Medical Department of the Army of the Potomac at Antietam, and reflects the valuable lessons learned there:

> Headquarters Army of the Potomac,
> Medical Director's Office, October 30, 1862
>
> Sir: In order that the wounded may receive the most prompt and efficient attentions during and after an engagement, and that the necessary operations may be performed by the most skillful and responsible surgeons at the earliest moment, the following instructions are issued for the guidance of the medical staff of this army, and medical directors of corps will see that they are promptly carried into effect:
>
> Previous to an engagement, there will be established in each corps a hospital for each division, the position of which will be selected by the medical director of the corps.
>
> The organization of the hospital will be as follows:

1st. A surgeon in charge; one assistant surgeon to provide food and shelter, &c.; one assistant surgeon to keep records.

2d. Three medical officers to perform operations; three medical officers as assistants to each of these officers.

3d. Additional medical officers, hospital stewards, and nurses of the division.

The surgeon in charge will have general superintendence, and be responsible to the surgeon-in-chief of the division for the proper administration of the hospital. The surgeon-in-chief of a division will detail one assistant surgeon, who will report to and be under the immediate orders of the surgeon in charge, whose duties shall be to pitch the hospital tents and provide straw, fuel, water, blankets, &c.; and, when houses are used, put them in proper order for the reception of wounded. This assistant surgeon will, when the foregoing shall have been accomplished, at once organize a kitchen, using for this purpose the hospital mess chests and the kettles, tins, &c. in the ambulances. The supplies of beef stock and bread in the ambulances, and of arrowroot, tea, &c., in the hospital wagon, will enable him to prepare quickly a sufficient quantity of palatable and nourishing food. All the cooks, and such of the hospital stewards and nurses as may be necessary, will be placed under his orders for these purposes.

He will detail another assistant surgeon, whose duty it shall be to keep a complete record of every case brought to the hospital, giving the name, rank, company, and regiment; the seat and character of injury; the treatment; the operation, if any be performed; and the result; which will be transmitted to the medical director of the corps and by him sent to this office.

This officer will also see to the proper interment of those who die, and that the grave is marked with a head-board, with the name, rank, company, and regiment legibly inscribed upon it.

He will make out two tabular statements of wounded, which the surgeon-in-chief of division will transmit within thirty-six hours after the battle, one to this office (by a special messenger, if necessary) and the other to the medical director of the corps to which the hospital belongs.

There will be selected from the division, by the surgeon-in-chief, under the direction of the medical director of the corps, three medical officers, who will be the operating staff of the hospital, upon whom will rest the immediate responsibility of the performance of all important operations. In all doubtful cases they will consult together, and a majority of them shall decide upon the expediency and character of the operation. These officers will be selected from the division without regard to rank, but solely on account of their known prudence, judgment, and skill. The surgeon-in-chief of the division is enjoined to be especially careful in the selection of these officers, choosing only those who have distinguished themselves for surgical skill, sound judgment, and conscientious regard for the highest interests of the wounded.

There will be detailed three medical officers to act as assistants to each one of these officers, who will report to him and act entirely under his direction. It is suggested that one of these assistants be selected to administer the anaesthetic. Each operating surgeon will be provided with an excellent table from the hospital wagon, and, with the present organization for field hospitals, it is hoped that the confusion and the delay in performing the necessary operations so often existing after a battle will be avoided, and all operations hereafter be primary.

The remaining medical officers of the division, except one to each regiment, will be ordered to the hospital to act as dressers and assistants generally. Those who follow the regiments to the field will establish themselves, each one at a temporary depot, at such a distance or situation in the rear of his regiment as will insure safety to the wounded, where they will give such aid as is immediately required; and they are here reminded that, whilst no personal consideration should interfere with their duty to the wounded, the grave responsibilities resting upon them render any unnecessary exposure improper.

The surgeon-in-chief of the division will exercise general supervision, under the medical director of the corps, over the medical affairs in his division. He will see that the officers are faithful in the performance of their duties in the hospital and upon the field, and that by the ambulance corps, which has heretofore been so efficient, the wounded are removed from the field carefully and with dispatch.

Whenever his duties permit, he will give his professional services at the hospital, will order to the hospital as soon as located all the hospital wagons of the brigades, the hospital tents and furniture, and all the hospital stewards and nurses. He will notify the captain commanding the ambulance corps, or, if this be impracticable, the first lieutenant commanding the division ambulances, of the location of the hospital.

No medical officer will leave the position to which he shall have been assigned without permission, and any officer so doing will be reported to the medical director of the corps, who will report the facts to this office.

The medical directors of corps will apply to their commanders on the eve of a battle for the necessary guard and men for fatigue duty. This guard will be particularly careful that no stragglers be allowed about the hospital, using the food and comforts prepared for the wounded.

No wounded will be sent away from any of these hospitals without authority from this office.

Previous to an engagement, a detail will be made by medical directors of corps of a proper number of medical officers, who will, should a retreat be found necessary, remain and take care of the wounded. This detail medical directors will request the corps commanders to announce in orders.

The skillful attention shown by the medical officers of this army to the wounded upon the battle-fields of South Mountain, Crampton's Gap, and the Antietam, under trying circumstances, gives the assurance that, with this organization, the medical staff of the Army of the Potomac can with confidence be relied upon under all emergencies to take charge of the wounded intrusted to its care.

Very respectfully, your obedient servant,

JONA. LETTERMAN,
Medical Director.[1]

Letterman had also taken some time to rethink the supply system of the military hospitals. The problem had been an ongoing one ever since the beginning of the war. "Hitherto large amounts of medical supplies had been lost and in various ways wasted," wrote the Army of the Potomac Medical Director, "and not unfrequently all the supplies for a regiment had been thrown away for want of transportation, and, of course were not on hand when wanted. It was necessary that this should be remedied, and in order to do so it was necessary to diminish the amount that was furnished a regiment at one time, which would affect the whole existing system and make the change a radical one. The objects which it was considered as desirable to attain were to reduce the waste which took place when large supplies were at one time issued to regiments, to have a supply given them, small, but sufficient for all immediate wants, and to have these supplies easily obtainable and replenished without difficulty when required, and without a multiplicity of papers and accounts. It was necessary also that they should be transported with facility, and that no trouble should be experienced in having them in abundance at the field hospitals in time of action and yet at the same time to preserve a proper degree of accountability."[2]

In a circular issued from his office to the Medical Department of the Army of the Potomac on October 4, 1862, Letterman outlined his new supply strategy:

Hereafter in the Army of the Potomac the following supplies will be allowed to a brigade for one month for

1. *OR*, vol. 19, pt. 1, pp. 114-16.
2. *Ibid.*, pp. 113-14.

active field service, viz: One hospital wagon, filled; one medicine chest for each regiment, filled; one hospital knapsack for each regimental medical officer, filled. The supplies in the list marked A to be transported in a four-horse wagon.

The surgeon in charge of each brigade will require and receipt for all these supplies, including those in the hospital wagons, and will issue to the senior surgeons of each regiment the medicine chests and knapsacks, taking receipts therefor. The hospital wagon, with its horses, harness, &c., will be receipted for by the ambulance quartermaster.

The surgeon in charge of the brigade will issue to the medical officers of the regiments such of these supplies as may be required for their commands informally, taking no receipts, demanding no requisitions, but accounting for the issues as expended.

The surgeons in charge of brigades will at once make out requisitions in accordance with these instructions, and transmit them, approved by the medical director of the corps, to the medical purveyor of this army. These supplies being deemed sufficient for one month only, or for an emergency, medical directors of corps will see that they are always on hand, timely requisitions being made for that purpose.[3]

After the disastrous affair of the stranded medical wagon trains, left far to the rear during the Gettysburg Campaign, Medical Director Letterman revamped and updated his orders of October 4, 1862, significantly tightening up the regulation of medical supplies in the Army of the Potomac:

SUPPLY TABLE FOR THE MEDICAL
DEPARTMENT OF THE ARMY OF THE POTOMAC.
HEADQUARTERS ARMY OF THE POTOMAC,

Medical Director's Office
September 3, 1863

3. *Ibid.*, p. 114.

[Circular.]

The following table of supplies for the Medical Department of this Army is published, instead of the one contained in the Circular from this office of October 4, 1862.

Experience has more fully shown the expediency of the manner of supplying the Department, as ordered by the Circular referred to, and it will be kept up.

There will be allowed, in the Army of the Potomac, the following supplies to a Brigade for one month, for active field service, viz.:

One Medicine Wagon, filled.

One Medicine Chest for each Regiment, filled.

One Hospital Knapsack for each Regimental Medical Officer, filled.

Supplies in the list marked 'A,' which will be carried in an ordinary Army wagon.

The Surgeon-in-Chief of each Brigade will require and receipt to the Medical Purveyor for all these supplies, and will issue to the senior Medical Officer of each Regiment in his Brigade the Medicine Chest and Knapsacks, taking the receipt therefor. The Wagons, both Medicine and Army, will be receipted for by the Ambulance Quartermaster.

The Surgeon-in-Chief of Brigade will issue to the Regimental Medical Officers such of the supplies from the Medicine and Army Wagon as may from time to time be required. These issues will be informal, the Surgeons-in-Chief giving no invoices, demanding no receipts, but accounting for them as expended. At the same time they will be particular that no improper expenditure or wastage is permitted. These officers are especially directed, when they shall have drawn the monthly supply, not to divide it out among the Regiments, but only to issue the articles at such times and in such quantities as they are needed for use, or to keep the Medicine Chests and Knapsacks supplied.

Requisitions will be made in duplicate, and in strict conformity with this table; and in all cases the articles will be enumerated in the order in which they occur in it. Supplies will only be issued by the Medical Purveyor upon requisitions approved by Medical Directors of Corps, and these officers are particularly enjoined to revise all requisitions with care, that sufficient supplies may be on hand, and yet that no unnecessary expenditure be permitted. As far as possible, requisitions will be made but once a month, and special requisitions avoided as far as possible.

The supply allowed will be kept up, and Medical Directors will see, especially before a march or battle, that timely requisitions are made, and the supplies obtained.

In all ordinary cases, the amount on hand at the time the requisition is made, will be given, as well as the amount required, and requisitions will be made only for such articles, and in such amounts, as may be necessary to fill the Brigade Supply to the amount ordered to be kept on hand.

Should the welfare of the sick demand a greater amount than is given by this table, or for articles which are not allowed by it, the reasons therefor must be fully and clearly stated, and the requisitions approved by this office. The Medical Purveyor will keep on hand only such articles as are contained in this table.

Instruments, except such as are enumerated in this table, will be issued only upon requisitions approved at this office.

When articles, such as Instruments, Medicine Chests, are from any cause unserviceable, they will not be turned in to the Medical Purveyor, unless inspected and ordered to be disposed of in accordance with the instructions contained in General Order No. 37, Headquarters of Army of the Potomac, April 2, 1863. Whenever it becomes necessary for any other cause to turn in supplies to the Medical Purveyor, applications, with reasons therefore will be made to this office. The knapsacks will be carried in each regiment, when on the march, by a hospital steward.[4]

---

4. Duncan, *The Medical Department of the United States Army*,pp. 122-23. The medical purveyor was in charge of all reserve supplies of the entire army.

The hard lessons learned at Gettysburg were also reflected in the further clarifying of the duties and organizational status of the Ambulance Corps during late August. While Captain Livermore had handled his Second Corps ambulances remarkably well, especially considering how rapidly he had gone into a combat situation after assuming command, the Army of the Potomac's Ambulance Corps was barely a year old, and still going through its initial shake-down period, and there were still some areas that needed better supervision. In the grueling marches to Gettysburg, weary men had fallen out without passes, or packed the ambulances with unsanctioned passengers, often leaving no room for those with serious cases of sunstroke or heat exhaustion. During the battle, generals still exercised their perogative of requitioning ambulances to use as personal sleeping quarters, making removal of the wounded on the field all that much harder.

Doctor Letterman was determined to put an end to all such unauthorized use of his ambulances. General Orders No. 85 served to carefully define the role of officers, medical passes, the interaction of the Ambulance Corps and the Medical Corps, corps insignia, the specific use of ambulance vehicles, march regulations, and camp regulations—a move that successfully completed the transition of the ambulance corps from an innovative experiment in patient care into a vital and normative part of army life.

AMBULANCE CORPS ORDERS.

Headquarters, Army of the Potomac
August 24, 1863

[General Orders, No. 85]

The following revised regulations for the organization of the Ambulance Corps, and the management of the Ambulance Trains, are published for the government of all concerned, and will be strictly observed:

1. The Army Corps is the unit of organization for the ambulance corps, and the latter will be organized upon the basis of the Captain as the commandant of

the corps, one 1st Lieutenant for each division, one 2d Lieutenant for each brigade, one Sergeant for each regiment.

2. The Privates of the corps will consist of two men and one driver for each ambulance, and one driver to each medicine wagon.

3. The two-horse ambulances only will be used, and the allowance, until further orders, to each corps, will be upon the basis of three to each regiment of infantry, two to each regiment of cavalry, one to each battery of artillery, to which it will be permanently attached, and two to the headquarters of each army corps, and two army wagons to each division. Each ambulance will be provided with two stretchers.

4. The captain is the commander of all the ambulances, medicine and other wagons in the corps, under the immediate direction of the Medical Director of the Army Corps to which the ambulance corps belongs. He will pay special attention to the condition of the ambulances, wagons, horses, harness, etc., and see that they are at all times in readiness for service; that the officers and men are properly instructed in their duties, and that these duties are performed, and that the regulations for the corps are strictly adhered to by those under his command. He will institute a drill in his corps, instructing his men in the most easy and expeditious method of putting men in and taking them out of the ambulances, lifting them from the ground and placing and carrying them on stretchers, in the latter case observing that the front man steps off with the left foot and the rear man with the right, etc.; that in all cases his men treat the sick and wounded with gentleness and care; that the ambulances and wagons are at all time provided with attendants, drivers, horses, etc.; that the vessel for carrying water are constantly kept clean and filled with fresh water; that the ambulances are not used for any other purpose than that for which they are designed and ordered. Previous to a march he will receive from the Medical Director of the Army Corps his orders for the distribution of the ambulances for gathering up the sick and

wounded previous to, and in time of, action; he will receive orders from the same officer where to send his ambulances, and to what point the wounded are to be carried. He will give his personal attention to the removal of the sick and wounded from the field in time of action, going from place to place to ascertain what may be wanted; to see that his subordinates (for whose conduct he will be responsible) attend faithfully to their duties in taking care of the wounded, and removing them as quickly as may be found consistent with their safety to the field hospital, and see that the ambulances reach their destination. After every battle he will make a report, in detail, of the operations of his corps to the Medical Director of the Army Corps to which he belongs, who will transmit a copy, with such remarks as he may deem proper, to the Medical Director of this Army. He will give his personal attention to the removal of sick when they are required to be sent to general hospitals, or to such other points as may be ordered. He will make a personal inspection, at least once a month, of everything pertaining to the ambulance corps, a report of which will be made to the Medical Director of the Corps, who will transmit a copy of the report to the Medical Director of this Army. This inspection will be minute and made with care, and will not supersede the constant supervision which he must at all times exercise over his corps. He will also make a weekly report, according to the prescribed form, to the same officer, who will forward a copy to the Medical Director of this Army.

5. The 1st Lieutenant assigned to the ambulance corps for a division, will have complete control, under the captain of his corps and the Medical Director of the Army Corps, of all ambulances, medicine and other wagons, horses, etc., and men in that portion of the ambulance corps. He will be the Acting assistant Quartermaster for that portion of the corps, and will receipt and be responsible for all the property belonging to it, and be held responsible for any deficiency in anything appertaining thereto. He will have a traveling cavalry force, a blacksmith and a saddler, who will be under

his orders to enable him to keep his train in order. His supplies will be drawn from the depot Quartermaster, upon requisitions approved by the captain of his corps, and the Commander of the Army Corps to which he is attached. He will exercise a constant supervision over his train in every particular, and keep it at all times ready for service. Especially before a battle will he be careful that everything be in order. The responsible duties devolving upon him in time of action, render it necessary that he be active and vigilant and spare no labor in their execution. He will make reports to the captain of the corps, upon the forms prescribed, every Saturday morning.

6. The 2d Lieutenant will have command of the portion of the ambulance corps for a brigade, and will be under the immediate orders of the commander of the ambulances for a division, and the injunctions in regard to care and attention and supervision prescribed for the commander of the division he will exercise in that portion under his command.

7. The Sergeant will conduct the drills, inspections, etc., under the orders and supervision of the commander of the ambulances for a brigade, be particular in enforcing all orders he may receive from his superior officer, and that the men are attentive to their duties.

The officers and non-commissioned officers will be mounted. The non-commissioned officers will be armed with revolvers.

8. Two Medical Officers, and two Hospital Stewards will be detailed, daily, by roster, by the Surgeon-in-Chief of Division, to accompany the ambulances for the Division, when on the march, whose duties will be to attend to the sick and wounded with the ambulances, and see that they are properly cared for. No man will be permitted, by any line officer, to fall to the rear to ride in the ambulances, unless he has written permission, from the senior Medical Officer of his regiment, to do so. These passes will be carefully preserved, and at the close of the march be transmitted, by the senior Medical Officer with the train, with such

remarks as he may deem proper, to the Surgeon-in-Chief of his Division. A man who is sick or wounded, who requires to be carried in an ambulance, will not be rejected, should he not have the permission required; the surgeon of the regiment who has neglected to give it, will be reported at the close of the march, by the senior surgeon with the train, to the Surgeon-in-Chief of his Division. When on the march, one-half of the privates of the ambulance corps, will accompany, on foot, the ambulances to which they belong, to render such assistance as may be required. The remainder will march in the rear of their respective commands, to conduct, under the order of the Medical Officer, such men as may be unable to proceed to the ambulances, or who may be incapable of taking proper care of themselves until the ambulances come up. When the case is of so serious a nature as to require it, the surgeon of the regiment, or his assistant, will remain and deliver the man to one of the Medical Officers with the ambulance. At all other times the privates will be with their respective trains. The medicine wagons will, on the march, be in their proper places, in the rear of the ambulances for each brigade. Upon ordinary marches, the ambulances and wagons belonging to the train will follow immediately in the rear of the division to which it is attached. Officers connected with the corps must be with the train when on the march, observing that no one rides in any of the ambulances except by the authority of the Medical Officers. Every necessary facility for taking care of the sick and wounded upon the march will be afforded the Medical Officers by the officers of the ambulance corps.

9. When in camp, the ambulances will be parked by divisions. The regular roll-calls, reveille, retreat, and tattoo, will be held, at which at least one commissioned officer will be present and receive the reports. Stable duty will be at hours fixed by the captain of the corps, and at this time, while the drivers are in attendance upon their animals, the privates will be employed in keeping the ambulances to which they belong in order, keeping the vessels for carrying water filled with

fresh water, and in general police duties. Should it become necessary for a regimental Medical Officer to use one or more ambulances for transporting sick and wounded, he will make a requisition upon the commander of the ambulances for a division who will comply with the requisition. In all cases when the ambulances are used, the officers, non-commissioned officers, and men belonging to them, will accompany them; should one ambulance only be required, a non-commissioned officer as well as the men belonging to it shall accompany it. The officers of the ambulance corps will see that ambulances are not used for any other purposes than that for which they are designed, viz.: the transportation of sick and wounded, and in urgent cases only, for medical supplies. All officers are expressly forbidden to use them, or require them to be used, for any other purpose. When ambulances are required for the transportation of sick or wounded at Division or Brigade Headquarters, they will be obtained, as they are needed for this purpose, from the Division train, but no ambulances belonging to that corps will be retained at such Headquarters.

10. Good, serviceable horses will be used for the ambulances and medicine wagons, and will not be taken for any other purpose except by orders from these Headquarters.

11. This corps will be designated by Sergeants, by a green band one and one-quarter inches broad around the cap, and chevrons of the same material, with the point toward the shoulder, on each arm above the elbow. For Privates, by a band the same as for Sergeants around the cap, and a half chevron of the same material on each arm above the elbow.

12. No person except the proper Medical Officers, or the officers, non-commissioned officers, and privates of this corps, will be permitted to take or accompany sick or wounded to the rear, either on the march or upon the field of battle.

13. No officer or man will be selected for this service except those who are active and efficient, and

they will be detailed and relieved by Corps Commanders only.

14. Corps Commanders will see that the foregoing regulations are carried into effect.

By Command of Major General Meade:

S. Williams
Assistant Adjutant General[5]

While much has been written about how the battle of Gettysburg affected the ultimate outcome of the war, there is little doubt that it led directly to the streamlining of the medical and ambulance corps, transforming them into a highly skilled team of medical professionals that would set the standard for military medical care in the years to follow.

5. *Ibid.*

Bibliography

MANUSCRIPTS

Ames, Albert. Letter to Father, June 30, 1963. Transcribed copy in the 1st New York Light Artillery Vertical File, Gettysburg National Military Park (GNMP) Library.

Ames, Lyman D. Unpublished diary in possession of Edwin L. Ames, San Francisco, California.

Bachelder, John. "Notes Relating to the Services of the Troops at Gettysburg, 1863." Manuscript in the Nicholson Collection, Huntington Library.

-----. Papers. New Hampshire Historical Society, Concord, New Hampshire.

Belknap, Charles W. Copy of diary in files at GNMP Library. Camp Letterman Papers, GNMP Library.

Biddle, James C. Letter to General Alexander S. Webb. November 31, 1886. Alexander S, Webb Collection, Yale University Library.

Bingham, Henry H. Letter to Winfield Scott Hancock. January 5, 1869, GNMP Library.

Breck, George. Letter to Ellen. July 2, 1863. Transcribed copy in the 1st New York Light Artillery Vertical File, GNMP Library.

-----. Letter to Ellen. July 8, 1863. Transcribed copy in the 1st New York Light Artillery Vertical File, GNMP Library.

Burns, William J. Diary. Philadelphia Brigade Vertical File, GNMP Library.

Carpenter, Alfred P. Letter. July 30, 1863. Minnesota Historical Society.

Cassidy, Robert A. Letter to Mrs. William Barksdale. n. d. *Mississippi Index*, June 13, 1866, Ethelbert Barksdale Papers, Mississippi Department of Archives and History.

Cavada, Adolfo F. Diary. Transcribed copy in the Lt. Col. Adolfo F. Cavada Vertical File, GNMP Library.

Colvill, William. Letter to John B. Bachelder. June 9, 1886. John B. Bachelder Papers, New Hampshire Historical Society, Concord, New Hampshire.

Corbin, Pvt. Elbert. Letter. July 5, 1863. Courtesy of Mr. Stephen J. Dreher.

Cort, Sr., Ambrose. Letter to R. L. Jones. October 25, 1933. Photocopy in Hospitalization after Gettysburg: Personal Accounts Vertical File, GNMP Library.

Cowan, Andrew. Letters of July 2, December 5, and December 10, 1913. Copies in the GNMP Library.

Cuyler, John. Letter to Justin Dwinelle. July 24, 1863. Copy in the Union Field Hospital Vertical File, GNMP Library.

Dougherty, Alexander N. Order for establishment of Corps hospital at Gettysburg. July 5, 1863. Courtesy of Scott Michael Dwinelle.

Dwinelle, Justin. Letter to brother. June 20, 1863. Courtesy of Scott Michael Dwinelle.

-----. Manuscript report of the Second Corps hospital operations during the Battle of Gettysburg, MSC 129, National Library of Medicine, Bethesda, Maryland.

England, Thomas. Abstract of provisions issued in the Second Corps field hospital, July 1 to July 31, 1863. Copy in the Union Field Hospital Vertical File, GNMP Library.

Gibson, Col. William. Letter to Capt. R. H. Ford. July 30, 1863. Courtesy of Scott Michael Dwinelle.

Hale, Charles A. "With Colonel Cross at the Wheatfield." John Rutter Brooke Papers, Historical Society of Pennsylvania, Philadelphia, Pennsylvania. Reprinted in *Civil War Times Illustrated.* Vol. 13, No. 5, August 1974, pp. 30-38.

Hammond, Surgeon General William A. Letter to Pennsylvania Governor Andrew G. Curtin. July 5, 1863. Office of the Surgeon General, Letters and Endorsements Sent 1818-1889, General Correspondence, volume 35, Record Group 112, National Archives and Records Administration.

Hancock, Winfield Scott. Papers and Scrapbook. Pennsylvania State Library.

-----. Letter to Maj. William G. Mitchell. August 24, 1863. Hartzell Collection.

-----. Letter to Peter F. Rothermel. December 31, 1868. Civil War Library and Museum, Philadelphia, Pennsylvania.

-----. Letter to Peter F. Rothermel. January 9, 1869. Rothermel Papers, Pennsylvania Historical and Museum Commission, Division of Archives and Manuscripts.

-----. Letter to Francis A. Walker. November 5, 1885. Sessler Collection, Civil War Library and Museum, Philadelphia, Pennsylvania.

-----. Letter to ? November 16, 1885. Sessler Collection, Civil War Library and Museum, Philadelphia, Pennsylvania.

-----. Letter to Francis A. Walker. December 12, 1885. Sessler Collection, Civil War Library and Museum, Philadelphia, Pennsylvania.

Harvey, Edward B. and Betty A. Typed transcipt of their fragmentary diaries. Courtesy of the Appomattox Court House National History Park.

Hilton, John C. Letter to Mrs. J. H. W. Stuckenberg. June 7, 1906. Stuckenberg Collection, Musselman Library, Gettysburg College.

Jacobs, Rev. Dr. Michael. Detailed Gettysburg weather reports, July 1863. Copy in the Professor Jacobs Vertical File, GNMP Library.

Janes, Henry. Letter to Justin Dwinelle. July 7, 1863. Copy in the Union Field Hospital Vertical File, GNMP Library.

-----. Medical Officers Files, Record Group 94, National Achives, Washington, D.C.

Jones, R. L. Letter to Ambrose Cort, Sr. October 25, 1933. Copy in the Hospitalization after Gettysburg: Personal Accounts Vertical File, GNMP Library.

Keaton, Frank M. Letter to O. P. Morton. July 10, 1863. Correspondence of the Indiana Military Agencies, Archives Division, Indiana State Library, Indianapolis.

Lambert, George Washington. Journal. Indiana Historical Society Library.

Lee, Robert E. Letter to George G. Meade. July 4, 1863. Formerly in the collection of Ted and Mary Sutphen, Gettysburg, Pennsylvania.

Leister, Lydia. Account of damages to her property during the Battle of Gettysburg, 1865. Transcribed copy in the Leister Farm Vertical File, GNMP Library.

Letterman, Jonathan. Order to Medical Director's Office. July 5, 1863. Copy in the Union Field Hospital Vertical File, GNMP Library.

-----. Letter to Alexander N. Dougherty. July 5, 1863. Copy in Union Field Hospital Vertical File, GNMP Library.

Linn, John B. "Journal of my trip to the battlefield at Gettysburg." Diary of John B. Linn, Centre County Library and Historical Museum, Bellefonte, Pennsylvania. Typescript copy in the Hospitalization after Gettysburg Vertical File, GNMP Library.

Marian, Mathew. Diary. Mathew Marian Papers, 1861-1863, Minnesota Historical Society, St. Paul, Minnesota.

Meade, Maj. Gen. George. Orders to the Union Corps hospitals. Copy in Union Field Hospitals Vertical File, GNMP Library.

Merrick, Charles H. Letters to his wife, Dr. Myra H. Merrick, and sister, Min Merrick. June 27, July 6, July 7, July 10, July 12, July 13, July 15, July 23, and July 24, 1863. Charles H. Merrick Papers, 1861-1866. William P. Palmer Collection, Container 1, Folder 3, Manuscript Collection Number 3088. Gift of Dr. Eliza J. Merrick, 1947. Western Reserve Historical Society, Cleveland, Ohio.

"Minnesota at Gettysburg." Winfield Scott Hancock Papers. Scrapbook of his death and obituaries, United States Army Military History Institute (USAMHI), Carlisle Barracks, Pennsylvania.

Mitchell, William. G. Letter to Dr. L. W. Read. September 20, 1880. Transcribed copy in the General Winfield Scott Hancock Vertical File, GNMP Library.

Moore, James. Letter. July 3, 1863. Copy in the 108th New York Vertical File, GNMP Library. Copied by permission of the USAMHI, Carlisle, Pennsylvania. Original at the University of Rochester.

-----. Letter to "My Dear Friend." July 15, 1863. Copy in 108th New York Vertical File, GNMP Library. Original at University of Rochester.

Mott, Marianna. Letter to Agnes Hopper. July 10, 1863. Garrison Family Papers.

-----. Letter to Martha Wright. July 12, 1863. Garrison Family Papers.

Mulholland, St. Clair A. Statement to John B. Bachelder. John B. Bachelder Papers, New Hampshire Historical Society.

Muller, Charles. Papers. Minnesota Historical Society, St. Paul, Minnesota.

Richardson, C. A. Letter to John B. Bachelder. May 8, 1868. John B. Bachelder Papers, New Hampshire Historical Society.

Shearer, F. E. Letter to Justin Dwinelle. July 22, 1863. Copy in the Union Field Hospital Vertical File, GNMP Library.

Shields, David. Letter to John B. Bachelder. August 27, 1884. John B. Bachelder Papers, New Hampshire Historical Society.

Silliman, Justus M. Letters of Justus M. Silliman. New Canaan Historical Society, New Canaan, Connecticut.

Slade, Richard. Letter to his sister. June 28, 1864. Dallas, Texas Historical Society.

Smith, Acting Surgeon General J. R. Letter to John M. Cuyler. July 6, 1863. Office of the Surgeon General, Letters and Endorsements Sent 1818-1889, General Correspondence, volume 35, Record Group 112, National Archives and Records Administration.

Stannard, George G. Diary. Typescript in the John B. Bachelder Papers, New Hampshire Historical Society.

-----. Letter to Abner Doubleday. September 3, 1865. Abner Doubleday Papers, Baseball Hall of Fame, Cooperstown, New York.

Stewart, George R. Letter to Glenn Tucker. July 3, 1959. In the possession of Glenn Tucker.

Stiles, R. C. Manuscript report of the First Division, Second Corps hospital operations during the Battle of Gettysburg, MSC 129, National Library of Medicine, Bethesda, Maryland (page 5 only extant).

Stuckenberg, J. H. W. Report of part taken by 145th Pennsylvania Regiment in the Battle of Gettysburg. RG 94, War Records Office, Union Battle Reports, volume 27, boxes 48-52, National Archives and Records Administration. Copy in 145th Pennsylvania Vertical File, GNMP Library.

Thompson, Benjamin W. "Personal Narrative of Experiences in the Civil War." Manuscript owned by John A. Thompson, Minneapolis, Minnesota. Copy of original typescript edition in 111th New York Vertical File, GNMP Library.

Tucker, Glenn. "Hancock at Gettysburg." Manuscript courtesy of GNMP Library.

Vander Veer, Albert. Vander Veer Papers, DB 560, Albany Institute of History and Art, Albany, New York. Transcribed copy in the 66th New York Infantry Vertical File, GNMP Library.

Wafer, Francis Moses. 108th New York, 41, Archives. Original diary. Douglas Library, Queen's University at Kingston, Kingston, Ontario, Canada K7L 5C4. Transcript copy in the 108th New York Vertical File, GNMP Library.

Wagner, Dr. Clinton. Letter to George Torney. August 7, 1911. GNMP Library.

Webb, Alexander S. Letter to H. M. Haskell. Haskell Papers, Pennsylvania Historical and Museum Commission.

Wills, John C. Wills Papers, Adams County Historical Society, Gettysburg, Pennsylvania.

Wright, James A. "Story of Company F." Unpublished manuscript, Minnesota Historical Society.

Yost, Lt. George. Letter to his father. July 4, 1863. Copy in the 126th Vertical File, GNMP Library.

NEWSPAPERS

Adams Sentinel & General Advertiser. July 21, 1863; August 18, 1863; March 22, 1864.

Buffalo Enquirer. March 14, 1911.

Buffalo Evening News. May 29, 1894.

Concord [North Carolina] *Tribune*. May 11, 1986.

Coos Democrat. [Lancaster, New Hampshire]. Undated.

Coos Republican. [Lancaster, New Hampshire]. July 14, 1863.

Democratic Watchman. [Bellefonte, Pennsylvania]. December 12, 1902.

Detroit Advertiser and Tribune. August 7, 1863.

Erie Observer. July 11, 16, 18, 23, 1863.

Erie Weekly Gazette. July 16, 1863.

Fredonia Censor. July 11, 1900.

Gettysburg Compiler. March 15, 1887; June 7, 1887; February 3, 1891.

Harrisburg Telegraph. July 2, 25, 27; August 6, 8, 16, 28, 30; September 9, 16, 20; October 7, 1907; July 1, 3, 5, 11, 1913.

Indianapolis Daily Journal. July 23, 1863.

Minneapolis Atlas. August 26, 1863.

Minneapolis Journal. June 30, 1897.

Montgomery [Pennsylvania] *Ledger*. August 4, 1863.
National Tribune. May 31, 1864; November 28, 1886; September 1, 1887.
New York Times. July 16, 1863.
New York World. July 7, 1863.
Norristown [Pennsylvania] *Republican*. August 28, 1863.
Norristown [Pennsylvania] *Times Herald*. July 31, 1863; February 11, 1924.
Philadelphia Inquirer. July 23, 1863; August 1, 1863.
Philadelphia North American. Sunday, June 29, 1913.
Philadelphia Public Ledger. July 6, 15, 1863.
Philadelphia Press. Undated July, 1863 clipping.
Philadelphia Times. January 6, 1864; December 23, 1882; June 28, 1---, undated clipping.
Philadelphia Weekly Times. May 31, 1879; March 26, 1881.
Pittsburgh Gazette. July 8, 1863.
St. *Louis Globe Democrat*. March 9, 1913.
Territorial Enterprise. March 2, 1868.
Syracuse Sunday Herald. March 8, 1885.
Washington D.C. Sunday Herald. July 4, 1880.

OTHER PERIODICALS

Blue and Grey. July, 1988; October, 1993.
Buffalo Medical and Surgical Journal. October and November, 1889.
The Bulletin of the Historical Society of Montgomery County, Pennsylvania. Vol. 18, No. 2, Spring, 1972; Vol. 23, Spring 1982, No. 2.
California Freemason. June, 1992.
Civil War. Vol. 17, April 1989.
Civil War Times Illustrated. May, 1963; May, 1967; October, 1967; June, 1978; January, 1981; May, 1986.
C*onfederate Veteran*. Vol. 8, 1900.
The General Magazine and Historical Chronicle. 1942-43, Vol. 45.
Gettysburg Magazine. No. 3, 6, 7, 8, 9. (Dayton, Ohio: Morningside House, Inc.).
Harper's New Monthly Magazine. Vol. 38, February, 1864.
Journal of Military Service Institution of the United States. Vol. 41, November-December, 1907.

Lutheran Observer. August 21, 1863.
Magazine of American History. July 1887.
Papers of the Military Historical Society of Massachusetts. (Boston, Massachusetts: 1905), 5.
Pennsylvania Magazine. Vol. 72, October, 1951.
Resident & Staff Physician. Vol. 27, No. 11, November 1991.
The Rochester Historical Society. Vol. 22, 1944.
Scribner's Magazine. Vol. 14, 1893.
Southern Historical Society Papers. Vols. 7, 8, 31, 34.

UNIT HISTORIES

Adams, John G. B. *Reminiscences of the Nineteenth Massachusetts Regiment*. Boston: Wright and Potter Printing Company, 1899.
Aldrich, T. A. *History of Battery A, First Regiment, Rhode Island Light Artillery*. Providence, Rhode Island: Snow and Farnham, 1904.
Levi W. Baker. *History of the Ninth Massachusetts Battery*. Lancaster, Ohio: Vanberg Publishing, 1996.
Banes, Charles H. *History of the Philadelphia Brigade*. Philadelphia: J. B. Lippincott & Co., 1876.
Bates, Samuel P. *History of the Pennsylvania Volunteers 1861-5*. 5 vols. Harrisburg, Pennsylvania: B. Singerly, 1869-71.
Baxter, Nancy Niblack. *Gallant Fourteenth: The Story of an Indiana Civil War Regiment*. Indianapolis: Guild Press, 1980. Reprint. Indianapolis: Guild Press, 1986.
Benedict, George G. *Vermont at Gettysburg*. Burlington, Vermont: The Free Press Association, 1870.
-----. *Vermont in the Civil War: A History of the Part Taken by the Vermont Soldiers and Sailors in the War for the Union, 1861-5*. 2 vols. Burlington, Vermont: Free Press Association, 1886-1888.
Bruce, George A. *The Twentieth Regiment of Massachusetts Volunteer Infantry 1861-1865*. Boston: Houghton, Mifflin and Company, 1906.
Child, Surgeon William A. *A History of the Fifth Regiment, New Hampshire Volunteers in the American Civil War*. Bristol, New Hampshire: R. W. Musgrove, 1893.
Coffin, Howard. *Full Duty: Vermonters in the Civil War*. Woodstock, Vermont: The Countryman Press, Inc., 1995.

Conyngham, D. P. *The Irish Brigade and Its Campaigns: With Some Account of The Corcoran Legion, and Sketches of the Principal Officers*. New York: William McSorley and Company, 1867.

Gates, Theodore B. *The "Ulster Guard" [20th N. Y. State Militia] and the War of the Rebellion.* New York: Benj. H. Tyrrel, 1879.

Haibler, Robert and William. *The First Minnesota Regiment at Gettysburg*. LaGrangeville, New York: The Info Devels Press, 1992.

Haskin, William L. *The History of the First Regiment of Artillery.* Portland, Maine: B. Thurston and Company, 1879.

Holcombe, Return I. (Completed by Jasper N. Searles and Matthew W. Taylor). *History of the First Regiment, Minnesota Volunteer Infantry.* Stillwater, Minnesota: Easton & Masterson, 1916.

Imholte, John Quinn. *The First Volunteers: History of the First Minnesota Volunteers Regiment 1861-1865.* Minneapolis: Ross & Haines, Inc., 1963.

Kepler, William. *History of the Three Months' and Three Years' from April 16th, 1861, to June 22d, 1864, of the Fourth Regiment Ohio Volunteer Infantry in the War for the Union.* Cleveland: Leader Printing Company, 1886. Reprint. Huntington, West Virginia: Blue Acorn Press, 1992.

Moe, Richard. *The Last Full Measure: The Life and Death of the First Minnesota Volunteers*. New York: Henry Holt and Company, 1993.

Muffly, Joseph W., ed., *The Story of our Regiment, a History of the 148th Volunteers.* Des Moines, Iowa: Kenyon Print and Manufacturing Co., 1904.

Mulholland, St. Clair A. *The Story of the 116th Regiment Pennsylvania Infantry.* Philadelphia: F. McManus Jr. & Company Printers, 1889.

Murphey, Chaplain Thomas G. *Four Years in the War. The History of the First Regiment of Delaware Veteran Volunteers, (Infantry.) Containing an Account of Marches, Battles, Incidents, Promotions, The Names of All the Officers and Men who have Been Connected with the Regiment from its Organization in 1861, to the Close of the War, in 1865.* Philadelphia: James S. Claxton, 1866.

Murray, R. L. *The Redemption of the "Harper's Ferry Cowards": The Story of the 111th and 126th New York State Volunteer Regiments at Gettysburg.* Edited by David Hickey. Wolcott: Published by the author, 1994.

Page, Charles Davis. *History of the Fourteenth Regiment, Connecticut Volunteer Infantry.* Meriden, Connecticut: The Horton Printing Co., 1906.

Rhodes, John H. *The History of Battery B, First Regiment Rhode Island Light Artillery, in the War to Preserve the Union, 1861-1865.* Providence, Rhode Island: Snow & Farnham, 1894.

Sheldon, Winthrop Dudley. *The "Twenty-Seventh." A Regimental History.* New Haven, Connecticut: Morris & Benham, 1866.

Simon, Ezra D. *A Regimental History, the One Hundred and Twenty-fifth New York State Volunteers.* New York,: Ezra D. Simons, 1888.

Smith, John Day. *The History of the Nineteenth Regiment of the Maine Volunteer Infantry 1862-1865.* Minneapolis: The Great Western Printing Company, 1909.

Stewart, Robert Laird. *History of the One Hundred and Fortieth Regiment, Pennsylvania Volunteers.* Philadelphia: Regimental Association, 1912.

Sturdivant, Ralph Orson, and Carmi Lathrop Marsh. *History of the 13th Regiment, Vermont Volunteers.* Burlington, Vermont: Regimental Association, 1910.

----- and Eli N. Peck. *Pictorial History of the Thirteenth Vermont Volunteers, War of 1861-1865.* Burlington, Vermont: Regimental Association, 1910.

Toombs, Samuel. *New Jersey Troops in the Gettysburg Campaign from June 5 to July 31, 1863.* Orange, New Jersey: The Evening Mail Publishing House, 1888.

Ward, Joseph R. C. *History of the One Hundred and Sixth Regiment Pennsylvania Volunteers, 2d Brigade, 2d Division, 2d Corps. 1861-1865.* Philadelphia: Grant, Faires & Rodgers, 1883.

Willson, Arabella M. *Disaster, Struggle, Triumph: The Adventures of 1000 "Boys in Blue," August, 1862, to June, 1865.* Albany, New York: The Argus Company, 1870.

PERSONAL LETTERS, MEMOIRS, AND RECOLLECTIONS

Abbott, Henry Livermore. *Fallen Leaves: The Civil War Letters of Major Henry Livermore Abbott.* Edited by Robert Garth Scott. Kent, Ohio: The Kent State University Press, 1991.

Austin, Anne L. *The Woolsey Sisters of New York: A Family's Involvement in the Civil War and a New Profession (1860-1900).* Philadelphia: Memoirs of the American Philosophical Society, Vol. 85, American Philosophical Society, 1971.

Bacon, George Anna Woolsey, and Eliza Newton Woolsey Howland. *Letters of a Family During the War for the Union, 1861-1865.* Printed for Private Distribution: 1899.

Barziza, Decimus et Ultimus. *The Adventures of a Prisoner of War, 1863-1864.* Edited by R. Henderson Shuffler. Austin: University of Texas Press, 1964.

Bassett, M. H. *From Bull Run to Bristow Station.* St. Paul: North Central Publishing Company, 1962.

Bee, Robert L. "Fredericksburg on the Other Leg: Sergeant Ben Hirst's Narrative of Important Events, Gettysburg, July 3, 1863," in Gary Gallagher, ed. *The Third Day at Gettysburg & Beyond.* Chapel Hill: University of North Carolina Press, 1994.

Beidelman, George Washington. *The Civil War Letters of George Washington Beidelman.* Edited by Catherine H. Vanderslice. New York: Vantage Press, 1978.

Benedict, George G. *Army Life in Virginia: Letters from the Twelfth Vermont Regiment and Personal Experiences of Volunteer Service in the War for the Union.* Burlington, Vermont: Free Press Association, 1895.

Beyer, W. F., and O. F. Keydel, eds. *Deeds of Valor: How America's Civil War Heroes Won the Congressional Medal of Honor.* Detroit: Perrien-Keydel, 1901. Reprint. Stamford, Connecticut: Longmeadow Press, 1991.

Biddle, Gertrude Bosler, and Sarah Dick[in]son Lowrie. *Notable Women of Pennsylvania.* Philadelphia: University of Pennsylvania Press, 1942.

Brinton, John H. *Personal Memoirs of John H. Brinton, Major and Surgeon U. S. V., 1861-1865.* New York: Neale Publishing Co., 1914. Reprinted as *Personal Memoirs of John H. Brinton, Civil War Surgeon, 1861-1865.* Carbondale: Southern Illinois University Press, 1996.

Brockett, L. P., and Mary C. Vaughn. *Woman's Work in the Civil War: A Record of Heroism, Patriotism and Patience.* Philadelphia: Zeigler, McCurdy & Co., 1867.

Bucklin, Sophronia E. *In Hospital and Camp: A Woman's Record of Thrilling Incidents among the Wounded in the Late War.* Philadelphia: John E. Potter and Company, 1869.

Buehler, Fannie J. *Recollections of the Rebel Invasion and One Woman's Experience During the Battle of Gettysburg.* Gettysburg, Pennsylvania: 1896.

Byrne, Frank L., and Andrew T. Weaver, eds. *Haskell of Gettysburg: His Life and Civil War Papers.* Kent, Ohio: The Kent State University Press, 1989.

Carr, Austin A. *A Casualty at Gettysburg and Andersonville: Selections from the Civil War Diary of Private Austin A. Carr of the 82nd N. Y. Infantry.* Edited by David G. Martin. Hightstown, New Jersey: Longstreet House, 1990.

Cleaves, Freeman. *Meade of Gettysburg.* Norman: University of Oklahoma Press, 1960. Reprint. Dayton, Ohio: Morningside Press, 1980.

Cole, Jacob H. *Under Five Commanders, or, A Boy's Experience with the Army of the Potomac.* Patterson, New Jersey: News Printing Company, 1906.

Cook, J. D. S. "Personal Reminiscences of Gettysburg." MOLLUS, *War Talks in Kansas.* Kansas City, 1906.

Denison, Rev. C. W. *Winfield, the Lawyer's Son and How He Became a Major General.* Philadelphia: 1865.

Dennison, Chaplain C. W., and Capt. G. B. Herbert. *Hancock "the Superb," The Early Life and Public Career of Winfield Scott Hancock.* Detroit: 1880.

Dimon, Theodore. *From Auburn to Antietam: The Civil War Journal of a Battlefield Surgeon who served with the Army of the Potomac 1861-1863.* Transcribed copy in the Hospitalization after Gettysburg: Personal Accounts Vertical File, GNMP Library.

Dooley, John. *John Dooley, Confederate Soldier, His War Journal.* Edited by Joseph T. Durkin. South Bend, Indiana: University of Notre Dame Press, 1963.

Dwinelle, Justin. *Healer and Comforter: The Civil War Surgeon. A Collection of Orders and Letters belonging to Surgeon J. Dwinelle, 106th Penn. Inf.* Edited by Scott

Michael Dwinelle. n.p., 1989. Copy in the Civil War Hospitals and Medicine Vertical File, GNMP Library.

Favill, Josiah M. *Diary of a Young Officer.* Chicago: R. R. Donnelly & Sons, Company, 1909.

Fuller, Charles A. *Personal Recollections of the War of 1861 as a Private, Sergeant and Lieutenant in the Sixty-First Regiment, New York Volunteer Infantry.* Sherburne, New York: News Job Printing House, 1906. Reprint. Hamilton, New York: Edmonston Publishing, Inc., 1990.

Galwey, Thomas Francis. *The Valiant Hours: The Narrative of "Captain Brevet," an Irish-American in the Army of the Potomac.* Edited by W. S. Nye. Harrisburg, Pennsylvania: Stackpole Books, 1961.

Gibbon, John. *Personal Recollections of the Civil War.* New York: 1903. Reprint. Dayton, Ohio: Press of Morningside Bookshop, 1978.

Glazier, Willard. *Heroes of Three Wars.* Philadelphia: 1879.

Graham, Ziba B. *On to Gettysburg. Ten Days from My Diary of 1863.* Detroit: Winn and Hammond, 1893.

Haight, Theron Wilber. *Three Wisconsin Cushings.* Madison, Wisconsin: 1910.

Haley, John W. *The Rebel Yell & The Yankee Hurrah: The Civil War Journal of a Maine Volunteer.* Edited by Ruth L. Silliker. Camden, Maine: Down East Books, 1985.

Hancock, Almira. *Reminiscences of Winfield Scott Hancock by his Wife.* New York: Charles L. Webster & Co., 1887.

Hancock, Cornelia. *South After Gettysburg.* Edited by Henrietta Stratton Jaquette. Philadelphia: University of Pennsylvania Press, 1937.

Haskell, Frank Aretas. *The Battle of Gettysburg.* Edited by Bruce Catton. Cambridge: Houghton Mifflin Company, 1958.

Haupt, Herman. *Reminiscences of General Herman Haupt.* Milwaukee: Wright and Joys Co., 1901.

Hays, Alexander. *Life and Letters of Alexander Hays.* Edited and arranged with notes and contemporary history compiled by George T. Fleming from data compiled by Gilbert A. Hays. Pittsburgh: 1919.

Hoke, Jacob. *The Great Invasion of 1863, or General Lee in Pennsylvania.* Dayton, Ohio: W. J. Shuey, 1887.

-----. *Historical Reminiscences of The War; or Incidents which Transpired In and About Chambersburg, during the War of the Rebellion.* Chambersburg, Pennsylvania: M. A. Foltz, 1884.

Holland, Mary A. Gardner. *Our Army Nurses. Interesting Sketches, Addresses, and Photographs of nearly One Hundred of the Noble Women who Served in Hospitals and on Battlefields during Our Civil War.* Boston: B. Wilkins & Co., 1895.

H[olstein], Mrs. [William H. (Anna Morris Ellis)], *Three Years in Field Hospitals of the Army of the Potomac.* Philadelphia: J. B. Lippincott & Co., 1867.

Jacobs, Michael. *Notes on the Rebel Invasion of Maryland and Pennsylvania, and the Battle of Gettysburg, July 1st, 2d and 3d, 1863.* Philadelphia: J. B. Lippincott & Company, 1864.

James, Bushrod W. *Echoes of Battle.* Philadelphia: Henry T. Coates and Company, 1895.

Letterman, Jonathan. *Medical Recollections of the Army of the Potomac.* New York: D. Appleton and Co., 1866.

Livermore, Thomas. *Days and Events, 1860-1866.* Boston: H. Mifflin Company, 1920.

Longacre, Edward G. *To Gettysburg and Beyond.* Hightstown, New Jersey: Longstreet House, 1988.

McCrea, Tully. *Dear Belle: Letters from a Cadet & Officer to his Sweetheart, 1858-1865.* Edited by Catherine S. Crary. Middletown, Connecticut: Wesleyan University Press, 1965.

McCreary, Albertus. *Gettysburg: A Boy's Experience of the Battle.* Gettysburg, Pennsylvania: Albertus McCreary, 1909.

McKay, C. E. *Stories of Hospital and Camp.* Philadelphia: Claxton, Remsen & Haffelfinger, 1876.

Meade, George. *The Life and Letters of George Gordon Meade, Major General United States Army.* Edited by George Gordon Meade. 2 vols. New York: Charles Scribner's Sons, 1913.

Meade, Jr., George G. *With Meade at Gettysburg.* Philadelphia: John C. Winston Co., 1930.

Morgan, William Henry. *Personal Reminiscences of the War of 1861-5.* Lynchburg, Virginia: J. P. Bell Company, 1911.

Morton, Jr., Joseph W., ed. *Sparks from the Camp Fire. Or Tales of the Old Veterans. Thrilling Stories of Heroic Deeds, Brave Encounters, Desperate Battles, Bold Achievements, Reckless Daring, Lofty Patriotism, Terrible Suffering and Wondrous Fortitude. As Retold To-day Around the Modern Camp Fire. New and Revised Edition with Contributions from One Hundred and Fifty Comrades.* Philadelphia: Keystone Publishing Co., 1893.

Munson, Edward L. "The Army Surgeon and His Work." In William T. Miller, ed. *The Photographic History of the Civil War.* 10 vols. New York: The Review of Reviews Co., 1911. Reprint. New York: Castle Books. Vol. 7.

Azor H. Nickerson. "Personal Recollections of Two Visits to Gettysburg." *Scribner's Magazine.* Vol. 14, 1893.

Patrick, Marsena R. *Inside Lincoln's Army: The Diary of Marsena Rudolph Patrick, Provost Marshal General, Army of the Potomac.* Edited by David S. Sparks. New York: Thomas Yoseloff, 1924.

Pierce, Matilda J. *At Gettysburg, Or, What a Girl Saw and Heard of the Battle. A True Narrative.* New York: W. Lake Borland, 1889.

Potter, William Warren. *Three Years with the Army of the Potomac: A Personal Military History.* Buffalo, New York: n.p., 1888.

Powell, Robert M. *Recollections of a Texas Colonel at Gettysburg.* Edited by Gregory Coco. Gettysburg, Pennsylvania: Thomas Publications, 1990.

Reichardt, Theodore. *Diary of Battery A, First Regiment Rhode Island Light Artillery.* Providence, Rhode Island: N. Bangs Williams, 1865.

Rhodes, Elisha Hunt. *All for the Union: The Civil War Diary and Letters of Elisha Hunt Rhodes.* Edited by Robert Hunt Rhodes. New York: Random House, Vintage Civil War Library Edition, 1992.

Rollins, Richard, ed. *Pickett's Charge!: Eyewitness Accounts.* Redondo Beach, California: Rank and File Publications, 1994.

Ropes, Hannah. *Civil War Nurse, The Diary and Letters of Hannah Ropes.* Edited by John R. Brumgardt. Knoxville: The University of Tennessee Press, 1980.

Sawyer, Franklin. *A Military History of the 8th Regiment, Ohio Volunteer Inf'y*. Cleveland: Fairbanks and Company, 1881.

Skelly, Daniel A. *A Boy's Experience During the Battles of Gettysburg*. Gettysburg, Pennsylvania: Daniel A. Skelly, 1932.

Small, Abner. *The Road to Richmond: The Civil War Memoirs of Major Abner Small of the 16th Maine Vols.; With His Diary as a Prisoner of War*. Edited by Harold Adams Small. Berkeley: University of California Press, 1959.

Souder, Edmund A. *Leaves from the Battle-field of Gettysburg. A Series of Letters from a Field Hospital and National Poems*. Philadelphia: Caxton Press of C. Sherman, Son & Co., 1864.

Stevens, Henry S. *Souvenir of Excursion to Battlefields by the Society of the Fourteenth Connecticut Regiment and Reunion at Antietam, September 1891; with History and Reminiscences of Battles and Campaigns of the Regiment on the Fields Revisited*. Washington, D.C.: Gibson Bros., 1893.

Straubing, Harold Elk, ed. and comp. *In Hospital and Camp: The Civil War through the Eyes of Its' Doctors and Nurses*. Harrisburg, Pennsylvania: Stackpole Books, 1993.

Strong, George Templeton. *Diary of the Civil War*. New York: 1982.

Stuckenberg, J. H. W. *I'm Surrounded by Methodists: The Civil War Diary of a Lutheran Chaplain*. Edited by David T. Hedrick and Gordon Barry Davis, Jr. Gettysburg, Pennsylvania: Thomas Publications, 1994.

Trobriand, P. Regis de. *Four Years with the Army of the Potomac*. Trans. George K. Dauchy. Boston: Ticknor and Company, 1889.

Walker, Francis A. *General Hancock*. New York: D. Appleton and Company, 1894.

-----. *History of the Second Army Corps in the Army of the Potomac*. New York: Charles Scribner's Sons, 1886.

Watson, William. *Letters of a Civil War Surgeon*. Edited by Paul Fatout. West Lafayette, Indiana: Purdue University Press, 1961.

Weld, Stephen Minot. *War Diary and Letters*. Boston: Privately Published, 1912.

Welsh, Peter. *Irish Green and Union Blue: The Civil War Letters of Peter Welsh, Color Sergeant, 28th Regiment Massachusetts Volunteers*. Edited by Lawrence Frederick Kohl and Margaret Cosse Richard. New York: Fordham University Press, 1986.

Young, Jesse Bowman. *The Battle of Gettysburg: A Comprehensive Narrative.* New York: Harper & Brothers, 1913.

GENERAL STUDIES

Adams, George Worthington. *Doctors in Blue*. New York: Henry Schuman, Inc., 1952. Reprint. Dayton, Ohio: Press of Morningside, 1985.

Max Allen. *Medicine Under Canvas: A War Journal of the 77th Evacuation Hospital*. Kansas City: The Sosland Press, 1949.

Ambrose, Stephen E. *Citizen Soldiers: The U. S. Army from the Normandy Beaches to the Bulge to the Surrender of Germany, June 7, 1944 to May 7, 1945*. New York: Simon and Schuster, 1997.

Andrews, J. Cutler. *The North Reports the Civil War.* Pittsburgh: University of Pittsburgh, 1955.

The Annals of the Civil War: Written By Leading Participants North and South. Originally published in the *Philadelphia Weekly Times*. Philadelphia: The Times Publishing Company, 1879. Reprint. New York: Da Capo Press, 1994.

Anonymous. *In Memoriam Alexander Stuart Webb.* Albany, New York: n.p., 1916.

Anonymous "The Great Battlefield Forty-Five Years Ago." *Gettysburg Scrapbook*, GNMP Library.

Brooks, Stewart. *Civil War Medicine.* Springfield, Illinois: Charles C. Thomas, 1966.

Brown, Kent Masterson. *Cushing of Gettysburg: The Story of a Union Artillery Commander.* Lexington: The University Press of Kentucky, 1993.

Busey, John W. *The Last Full Measure: Burials in the Soldiers' National Cemetery at Gettysburg*. Hightstown, New Jersey: Longstreet House, 1988.

-----. *These Honored Dead.* Hightstown, New Jersey: Longstreet House, 1988.

----- and David G. Martin. *Regimental Strengths at Gettysburg.* Baltimore: Gateway Press, Inc., 1982.

Catton, Bruce. *The Army of the Potomac: Glory Road.* Garden City, New York: Doubleday and Company, 1952.

Clark, Champ. *Gettysburg: The Confederate High Tide.* Alexandria, Virginia: Time-Life Books, 1985.

Coco, Gregory A. *A Strange and Blighted Land—Gettysburg: The Aftermath of a Battle.* Gettysburg, Pennsylvania: Thomas Publications, 1995.

-----. *A Vast Sea of Misery: A History and Guide to the Union and Confederate Field Hospitals at Gettysburg, July 1-November 20, 1863.* Gettysburg, Pennsylvania: Thomas Publications, 1988.

-----. *Killed in Action: Eyewitness Accounts of the Last Moments of 100 Union Soldiers who Died at Gettysburg.* Gettysburg, Pennsylvania: Thomas Publications, 1992.

-----. *On the Bloodstained Field.* Gettysburg, Pennsylvania: Thomas Publications, 1987.

-----. *On the Bloodstained Field II.* Gettysburg, Pennsylvania: Thomas Publications, 1989.

-----. *War Stories: A Collection of 150 Little Known Human Interest Accounts of the Campaign and Battle of Gettysburg.* Gettysburg, Pennsylvania: Thomas Publications, 1992.

-----. *Wasted Valor: The Confederate Dead at Gettysburg.* Gettysburg Pennsylvania: Thomas Publications, 1990.

Coddington, Edwin B. *The Gettysburg Campaign: A Study in Command.* New York: Charles Scribner's Sons, 1968.

Colver, Michael. Article. Pennsylvania College yearbook, *The Spectrum.* 1902.

Conklin, E. F. *Women at Gettysburg 1863.* Gettysburg, Pennsylvania: Thomas Publications, 1993.

Cunningham, Horace H. *Doctors in Gray: The Confederate Medical Service.* Baton Rouge: Louisiana State University Press, 1958.

-----. *Field Medical Services at the Battles of Manassas (Bull Run).* University of Georgia Monographs, No. 16. University of Georgia Press, 1968.

Dammann, Gordon. *Pictorial Encyclopedia of Civil War Medical Instruments and Equipment, Volume I.* Missoula, Montana: Pictorial Histories Publishing Company, 1983.

-----. *Pictorial Encyclopedia of Civil War Medical Instruments and Equipment, Volume II.* Missoula, Montana: Pictorial Histories Publishing Company, 1988.

-----. *Pictorial Encyclopedia of Civil War Medical Instruments and Equipment, Volume III.* Missoula, Montana: Pictorial Histories Publishing Company, 1997.

Dannett, Sylvia G. L., comp. and ed. *Noble Women of the North.* New York: Thomas Yoseloff, 1959.

Eide, Brad and Lawrence, Robert, "Samuel Zook," *The Gettysburg Discussion Group Web Site.* February 28, 1999. www.gdg.org/szook.html.

Forty, George. *At War in Korea.* London: Ian Allen Ltd., 1982. Reprint. The Cassell Group, 1997.

Fox, William F. *Regimental Losses in the American Civil War, 1861-1865.* Albany, New York: Brandon Printing Company, 1898.

Frassanito, William A. *Early Photography At Gettysburg.* Gettysburg, Pennsylvania: Thomas Publications, 1995.

-----. *Gettysburg: A Journey in Time.* New York: Charles Scribner's Sons, 1975.

-----. *Gettysburg: Then and Now.* Gettysburg, Pennsylvania: Thomas Publications, 1996.

-----. *The Gettysburg Then and Now Companion.* Gettysburg, Pennsylvania: Thomas Publications, 1997.

Freed, A. T. *The Life and Public Services of Winfield Scott Hancock.* Chicago: 1880.

Gambone, A. M. *Hancock At Gettysburg . . . and Beyond.* Baltimore: Butternut and Blue, 1997.

Greenbie, Marjorie Barstow. *Lincoln's Daughters of Mercy.* New York: G. P. Putnam's Sons, 1944.

Grimm, Herbert L., and Paul L. Roy. *Human Interest Stories of the Three Days' Battles at Gettysburg.* Gettysburg, Pennsylvania: Times and News Publishing Co., 1927.

Hall, W. W. "Take Care of Your Health: Advice to Soldiers." GNMP Library Specimen Collection, Hospitalization after Gettysburg—General Information Vertical File.

Hansen, Arlen J. *Gentlemen Volunteers: The Story of the American Ambulance Drivers in the Great War, August, 1914—September, 1918.* New York: Arcade Publishing, 1996.

Harrison, Kathleen Georg, comp. Detailed roster of known Confederate dead, compiled from the handbook and burial lists of Dr. John W. C. O'Neal, J. G. Frey, the Weaver family and others, GNMP Library.

----- and John W. Buse. *Nothing But Glory*. Hightstown, New Jersey: Longstreet House, 1987. Reprint. Gettysburg, Pennsylvania, Thomas Publications, 1993.

Hospital Markers [at Gettysburg of the] Army of the Potomac Department. n.p., n.d. USAMHI, Carlisle, Pennsylvania.

Hunter, Alexander. *Johnny Reb and Billy Yank*. New York: Neale Publishing Co., 1905.

Johnson, Robert U., and Clarence C. Buel, eds. *Battles and Leaders of the Civil War*. 4 vols. New York: The Century Company, 1884-1887. Reprint. Secaucus, New Jersey: Castle, 1995.

Jordan, David M. *Winfield Scott Hancock: A Soldier's Life*. Bloomington: Indiana University Press, 1988.

Kamm, Samuel Richey. *The Civil War Career of Thomas A. Scott*. Philadelphia: 1940.

Krick, Robert K. *Lee's Colonel's: A Biographical Register of the Field Officers of the Army of Northern Virginia*. Dayton, Ohio: Morningside Bookshop, 1979.

Leech, Margaret. *Reveille In Washington, 1860-1865*. New York: Harper and Brothers, 1941.

Leisch, Juanita. *An Introduction to Civil War Civilians* Gettysburg, Pennsylvania: Thomas Publications, 1994.

Livermore, Thomas L. *Numbers and Losses in the Civil War in America 1861-1865*. Bloomington, Indiana: Periodicals Service Company, 1957.

Lochren, William. "Narrative of the First Regiment." *Minnesota in the Civil and Indian Wars, 1861-1865*. vol. 1. St Paul: Pioneer Press Company, 1891.

McLaughlin, Jack. *Gettysburg: The Long Encampment*. New York: Bonanza Books, 1963.

Magner, Blake A. *Traveller and Company: The Horses of Gettysburg*. Gettysburg, Pennsylvania: Farnsworth House Military Impressions, 1995.

Maher, Sister Mary Denis. *To Bind Up the Wounds: Catholic Sister Nurses in the U.S. Civil War*. New York: Greenwood Press, 1989.

Minnich, Luther W. *Gettysburg: "What They Did Here." Profusely Illustrated Historical Guide Book.* Chicago: Tipton & Blocher, 1892. Reprint. 14th edition, 1922).

Mitchell, Ralph M. "Appendix 1. Medical Practices and the Handling of Wounded in the Civil War: Theory and Application." *Guide to the Battle of Chickamauga.* Edited by Matt Spruill. Lawrence: University Press of Kansas, 1993.

Moore, Frank, ed. *The Rebellion Record: A Diary of American Events.* New York: D. Van Nostrand, 1864. Vol. 7.

-----. *Women of the War: Their Heroism and Self-Sacrifice.* Hartford, Connecticut: Scranton, 1866.

Motts, Wayne E. *Trust in God and Fear Nothing: General Lewis A. Armistead, C.S.A.* Gettysburg, Pennsylvania: Farnsworth House Military Impressions, 1994.

Patterson, Gerald A. *Debris of Battle: The Wounded of Gettysburg.* Mechanicsburg, Pennsylvania: Stackpole Books, 1997.

Pennypacker, Isaac R. *General Meade.* New York: D. Appleton and Company, 1901.

Pfanz, Harry W. *Gettysburg: The Second Day.* Chapel Hill: University of North Carolina Press, 1987.

Raus, Jr., Edmund J. *A Generation on the March: The Union Army at Gettysburg.* Lynchburg, Virginia: H. E. Howard, 1987.

Robertson, Jr., James I. *Soldiers Blue and Gray.* New York: Warner Books, 1988.

Smith, Nina Bennett. *The Women Who Went to War: The Union Army Nurse in the Civil War.* Ann Arbor, Michigan: Northwest University Microfilm International, 1981.

Stewart, George R. *Pickett's Charge: A Microhistory of the Final Attack at Gettysburg, July 3, 1863.* Cambridge, Massachusetts: The Riverside Press, 1959.

Storrick, W. C. *The Battle of Gettysburg: The Country, The Contestants, The Results.* Harrisburg, Pennsylvania: J. Horace McFarland Company, Mount Pleasant Press, 1931. Reprint. Sixth Edition, 1946.

Tucker, Glenn. *Hancock the Superb.* Indianapolis: The Bobbs-Merrill Company, Inc., 1960.

"VMI Civil War Generals, Biographical sketches of VMI alumni who became general officers, 1861-1865." http://www.vmi.edu/~archtml/cwgen.html.

Warner, Ezra. *Generals in Blue: Lives of the Union Commanders.* Baton Rouge: Louisiana State University Press, 1964.

Weber, Thomas. *The Northern Railroads in the Civil War, 1861-1865.* Columbia University: King's Crown Press, 1952.

Wert, J. Howard. *A Complete Hand-Book of the Monuments and Indications and Guide to the Positions on the Gettysburg Battlefield.* Harrisburg, Pennsylvania: R. M. Sturgeon & Co., 1886. Tipped-in map in the flyleaf.

Wiley, Bell Irvin. *The Life of Billy Yank: The Common Soldier of the Union.* Indianapois: The Bobbs-Merrill Company, Inc., 1952. Reprint. Garden City, New York: Doubleday & Company, 1971.

Young, Agatha. *The Women and the Crisis.* New York: McDowell and Obolensky, 1959.

PAPERS, LECTURES, THESES, AND DISSERTATIONS

Litoff, Judy and David Smith. "Today We Have Lived History: The D-Day Letters of U. S. Women." Paper given at the Eisenhower Center, May 16, 1994.

Lochren, William. "The First Minnesota at Gettysburg." *Glimpses of the Nation's Struggle.* Papers read before the Minnesota Commandery, MOLLUS (Series 3), New York, St. Paul, Minneapolis, 1892, No. 42.

Lyman, Colonel Theodore. Paper. January 9, 1882. *Papers of the Military Historical Society of Massachusetts.* Boston: 1905. Vol. 5.

Pierce, John Edward. "The Civil War Career of Richard Brooke Garnett: A Quest for Vindication." Master of Arts dissertation, Virginia Polytechnic Institute, 1969.

Scott, W. "Pickett's Charge as Seen from the Front Line." MOLLUS Collection, California, *War Papers #1.*

Stuckenberg, J. H. W. Lecture delivered in Warren, Pennsylvania, on January 6, 1864. The Stuckenberg Collection, Gettysburg College.

Vickery, Richard Swanton. "On the Duties of the Surgeon in Action." Thesis at the Bentley Historical Library, Michigan Historical Collections, University of Michigan at Ann Arbor, Michigan. Reprinted as Richard Swanton Vickery, "On the Duties of the Surgeon in Action," Edited by Albert Castel. *Civil War Times Illustrated.* Vol. 17, No. 3. June 1978, pp. 13-23.

Walker, Francis A. Paper. MOLLUS Massachusetts Papers, Vol. 10, p. 49.

COMMISSIONS, GOVERNMENT, STATE, COMMUNITY, AND LOCAL INTEREST PUBLICATIONS

Brown, Francis H. *Harvard University in the War in 1861-1865: A Record of Services Rendered in the Army and Navy of the United States by the Graduates and Students of Harvard College and the Professional Schools.* Boston: Cupples, Upham, and Company, 1886.

Candler, Allen D. and Clement A. Evans, eds. *Cyclopedia of Georgia.* Vol. 2. Atlanta: State Historical Society, 1906.

Confederate Military History, Extended Edition. Wilmington, North Carolina: Broadfoot Publishing Company, 1987.

Cross, Andrew B. *Battle of Gettysburg and the Christian Commission.* Baltimore: n.p., 1865.

-----. *The War and the Christian Commission.* Baltimore: n.p., 1865.

Deaderick, Robert D. *Field Medical Support of the Army of the Potomac at Gettysburg.* Carlisle Barracks, Pennsylvania: U. S. Army War College, 1989.

Dimon, Theodore. *Report of the General Agent of the State of New York for the Relief of Sick, Wounded, and Discharged Soldiers.* New York: Comstock and Cassidy, 1864.

Douglas, J. H. *Report on the Operations of the Sanitary Commission During and After the Battles at Gettysburg, July 1st, 2d, and 3d, 1863. Sanitary Commission No. 71.* Washington, D.C.: Privately Published, 1863.

Duncan, Louis C. *The Medical Department of the United States Army in the Civil War.* Washington, D.C.: U. S. Government Printing Office, 1910. Reprint. Gaithersburg, Maryland: Olde Soldier Books, Inc., 1987.

Fifth Semi-Annual Report of the Ladies Aid Society of Philadelphia with Letters and Extracts from Letters from the Secretary of the Society Written from Various Places While Attending to the Sick and Wounded of the Union Army. Philadelphia: C. Sherman & Son, 1863.

Fourth Semi-Annual Report of the Ladies Aid Society of Philadelphia with Letters and Copious Extracts of Letters from the Secretary of the Society. Philadelphia: C. Sherman & Son, 1863.

Fox, William F., comp. and ed. *Final Report on the Battlefield of Gettysburg: New York Monuments Commission for the Battlefields of Gettysburg and Chattanooga*. 2 vols. New York: J. B. Lyon Company, 1900.

Fuger, Frederick. *Family History*. Detroit: Privately Published, 1904.

The History of Waterford, Oxford County, Maine. A Compilation of Addresses, Records and Proceedings, published at the direction of the Town. Portland, Maine: Hoyt, Fogg, and Donham, 1879.

Lochren, William. "Narrative of the First Regiment." *Minnesota in the Civil and Indian Wars, 1861-1865*. Vol. 1. St Paul: Pioneer Press Company, 1891.

Maxwell, William Quentin. *Lincoln's Fifth Wheel: The Political History of the United States Sanitary Commission*. New York: Longmans, Green, 1956.

Meroni, William. *Harris (or Herris), Miller, and Dunlop*. Privately Published, 1920.

Military Service Institute. *Letters and Addresses Contributed at a General Meeting of the Military Service institute at Governor's Island, New York Harbor, February 26, 1886, in Memory of Winfield Scott Hancock, etc.* New York: Military Service Institute, 1886.

Moss, Rev. Lemuel. *Annals of the United States Christian Commission*. Philadelphia: J. B. Lippincott & Co., 1868.

New York Monuments Commission for the Battlefields of Gettysburg and Chattanooga. *Final Report on the Battlefield of Gettysburg*. 3 vols. Albany New York: J. B. Lyon Company, Printers, 1900.

Nicholson, John P., ed. *Pennsylvania at Gettysburg: Ceremonies at the Dedication of the Monuments Erected by the*

Commonwealth of Pennsylvania. 2 vols. Harrisburg Pennsylvania: William Stanley Ray, 1904.

Official Roster of the Soldiers of the State of Ohio in the War of the Rebellion, 1860-1866. Vol. 2, 1st - 20th Infantry Regiments. Cincinnati: Wilstach, Baldwin & Co., 1886.

Olmstead, Frederick Law. *Hospital Transports: A Memoir of the Embarkation of the Sick and Wounded from the Peninsula of Virginia in the Summer of 1862.* Boston: Ticknor and Fields, 1863.

-----. *The Papers of Frederick Law Olmstead;* vol. 4: *Defending the Union: The Civil War and the U. S. Sanitary Commission, 1861-1863.* Edited by Jane Turner Censer. Baltimore: The Johns Hopkins University Press, 1986.

Philadelphia Brigade Association. *Reply of the Philadelphia Brigade Association to the Foolish and Absurd Narrative of Lieutenant Frank A. Haskell which Appears to be Endorsed by the Military Order of the Loyal Legion Commandry of Massachusetts and the Wisconsin History Commission.* Philadelphia: Bowers Printing Company, 1910.

Report of the Joint Committee on the Conduct of the War, 2nd Session, 38th Congress. 2 vols. Washington, D.C.: Government Printing Office, 1863, 1865. Reprint. New York: Kraus Reprint Company, 1977.

Report on the Operations of the Sanitary Commission During and after the Battle of Gettysburg. New York: 1863.

Roster of Regimental Surgeons and Assistant Surgeons in the U.S. Army Medical Department During the Civil War. n.p.: 1882; Reprint. Gaithersburg, Maryland: Olde Soldier Books, Inc., 1989.

The Sanitary Commission of the United States Army; A Succinct Narrative of Its Works and Purposes. New York: Published for the Benefit of the United States Sanitary Commission, 1864.

Smith, Rev. Edward P. *Incidents of the United States Christian Commission.* Philadelphia, Pennsylvania: J. B. Lippincott & Co., 1869.

Supreme Court of Pennsylvania. May Term, 1891. #20, 30. Middle District. *Appeal of the Gettysburg Battlefield Memorial Association from the Decree of the Court of Common Pleas of Adams County. Paper Book of Appelants.*

Third Semi-Annual Report of the Ladies Aid Society of Philadelphia with Letters and Copious Extracts of Letters from the Secretary of the Society. Philadelphia: C. Sherman & Son, 1863.

Tilberg, F. *Museum Prospectus.* GNMP, January 23, 1947. Confederate and Union Field Hospital Vertical File, GNMP Library.

Turner, Rev. D. K. *History of Neshaminy Presbyterian Church of Warwick.* Philadelphia, Pennsylvania: Culbertson & Bache, 1876.

The United States Christian Commission for the Army and Navy. Work and Incidents. First Annual Report. Philadelphia: United States Christian Commission, 1863.

The United States Christian Commission for the Army and Navy. For the Year 1863. Second Annual Report. Philadelphia: April, 1864.

The United States Christian Commission. Second Report of the Committee of Maryland, September 1, 1863. Baltimore: Sherwood & Co., 1863.

The United States Medical Field Service School. *The Battle of Gettysburg.* Carlisle Barracks, Pennsylvania, 1929.

The United States Sanitary Commission Report for the Army and Navy—[Its] Work and Incidents, First Annual Report. Philadelphia, Pennsylvania: 1863.

The United States War Department. *War of the Rebellion: A Compilation of the Official Records of the Union and Confederate Armies*. 70 volumes in 128 parts. Washington, D.C.: Government Printing Office, 1880-1901. Series 1, Vol. 27, Pts. 1, 3.

Wilson, James. Appendix containing testimony from the Court of Common Pleas of Adams County, In Equity. No. 1, January Term, 1889. *Survivors of the Seventy-second Regiment of Pennsylvania Volunteers, Plaintiffs vs. Gettysburg Battlefield Memorial Association, Commissioners appointed by the Governor of the State of Pennsylvania, Defendants.*

Wormeley, Katherine Prescott. *The United States Sanitary Commission. A Sketch of Its Purposes and Its Work. Compiled from Documents and Private Papers.* Boston: Little, Brown and Company, 1863.

Index

T

Y

Z